AMBULANCE CARE Practice

SECOND EDITION

Disclaimer
Class Professional Publishing have made every effort to ensure that the information, tables, drawings and diagrams contained in this book are accurate at the time of publication. The book cannot always contain all the information necessary for determining appropriate care and cannot address all individual situations; therefore, individuals using the book must ensure they have the appropriate knowledge and skills to enable suitable interpretation. Class Professional Publishing does not guarantee, and accepts no legal liability of whatever nature arising from or connected to, the accuracy, reliability, currency or completeness of the content of Ambulance Care Practice. Users must always be aware that such innovations or alterations after the date of publication may not be incorporated in the content. Please note, however, that Class Professional Publishing assumes no responsibility whatsoever for the content of external resources in the text or accompanying online materials.

Text © Kris Lethbridge and Richard Pilbery 2019
Chapter 19 © Aimee Yarrington

All rights reserved. Without limiting the rights under copyright reserved above, no part of this publication may be reproduced, stored in or introduced into a retrieval system, or transmitted, in any form or by any means (electronic, mechanical, photocopying, recording or otherwise) without the prior written permission of the publisher of this book.

The information presented in this book is accurate and current to the best of the authors' knowledge.

The authors and publisher, however, make no guarantee as to, and assume no responsibility for, the correctness, sufficiency or completeness of such information or recommendation.

Printing history
First edition published 2016. Reprinted 2017, 2018.
This second edition first published 2019. **Reprinted in 2020 (twice), 2021, 2023 (with corrections), 2025.**

The authors and publisher welcome feedback from the users of this book. Please contact the publisher:

Class Professional Publishing,
The Exchange, Express Park, Bristol Road, Bridgwater TA6 4RR
Telephone: 01278 427 826
Email: info@class.co.uk
www.classprofessional.co.uk

Class Professional Publishing is an imprint of Class Publishing Ltd

A CIP catalogue record for this book is available from the British Library

Paperback ISBN: 9781859598542
Ebook ISBN: 9781859598559

Line illustrations by David Woodroffe and S4Carlisle
Cover design by Hybert Design Limited, UK
Designed and typeset by S4Carlisle
Printed in the UK by Hobbs.

This book is printed on paper from responsible sources.

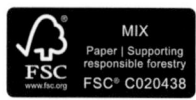
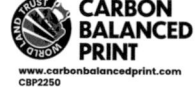

AMBULANCE CARE Practice

SECOND EDITION

Richard Pilbery
and
Kris Lethbridge

Contents

List of Abbreviations — xv

Acknowledgements — xviii

Foreword — xxi

1: Introduction — 1

1. Textbook guide — 1
   - 1.1 Introduction — 1
   - 1.2 Textbook — 1
   - 1.3 Getting started — 1
2. Anatomy of an emergency call — 1
   - 2.1 Introduction — 1
   - 2.2 The emergency operations centre — 1
   - 2.3 Arriving on scene — 2
   - 2.4 Principles of communication — 2
   - 2.5 Patient assessment — 3
   - 2.6 Patient history — 3
   - 2.7 The 12-lead ECG — 3
   - 2.8 Manual handling — 4
   - 2.9 Assist the paramedic — 4
   - 2.10 Hospital arrival — 5
   - 2.11 Clean up and prepare for the next call — 6

2: The Ambulance Service — 7

1. Organisational structure — 7
   - 1.1 Learning objectives — 7
   - 1.2 Introduction — 7
2. Response to a 999 call — 7
   - 2.1 Learning objectives — 7
   - 2.2 Introduction — 8
   - 2.3 Call for help and triage — 8
   - 2.4 Ambulance service response — 8
   - 2.5 Onward care — 9
3. Roles within the ambulance service — 10
   - 3.1 Learning objectives — 10
   - 3.2 Introduction — 10
   - 3.3 Clinical roles — 10
   - 3.4 Clinical leadership roles — 11
   - 3.5 Command and control roles — 12
4. Working relationships — 13

3: Communication — 15

1. Principles of communication — 15
   - 1.1 Learning objectives — 15
   - 1.2 Introduction — 15
   - 1.3 Who will you be communicating with? — 15
   - 1.4 Basics of communication — 15
   - 1.5 Social context — 17
   - 1.6 Barriers to communication — 18
   - 1.7 Summary — 18
2. Practical communication — 19
   - 2.1 Learning objectives — 19
   - 2.2 Record keeping — 19
   - 2.3 Handover — 19
   - 2.4 Pre-alert — 20
   - 2.5 Breaking bad news — 20
3. Electronic communication devices — 21
   - 3.1 Learning objectives — 21
   - 3.2 Introduction — 21
   - 3.3 Radios — 21
   - 3.4 Mobile data terminals — 23
   - 3.5 Electronic patient records — 23

4: Legal, Ethical and Professional Issues — 25

1. Being a healthcare professional — 25
   - 1.1 Learning objectives — 25
   - 1.2 Introduction — 25
   - 1.3 Values-based healthcare — 25
   - 1.4 Duty of care — 27
   - 1.5 Scope of practice and standards — 28
   - 1.6 When things go wrong — 29
   - 1.7 Reflection — 30
2. Provision of healthcare — 32
   - 2.1 Learning objectives — 32
   - 2.2 Introduction — 32

		2.3	Health inequalities	33
		2.4	Person-centred care	33
		2.5	Health promotion	34
	3	Consent and capacity		34
		3.1	Learning objectives	34
		3.2	Introduction	34
		3.3	Consent	34
		3.4	Mental capacity	35
		3.5	Summary	40
	4	Confidentiality and information governance		41
		4.1	Learning objectives	41
		4.2	Introduction	41
		4.3	Maintaining confidentiality	42
		4.4	Key points	44
	5	Equality and diversity		44
		5.1	Learning objectives	44
		5.2	Introduction	45
		5.3	Equality in healthcare	45
		5.4	Discrimination	45
		5.5	Identity, self-image and self-esteem	47
	6	Clinical governance		47
		6.1	Learning objectives	47
		6.2	Introduction to clinical governance	47
		6.3	Purpose of clinical governance	48
		6.4	How to contribute to clinical governance	48

5: Safeguarding 49

	1	Safeguarding adults and children		49
		1.1	Learning objectives	49
		1.2	Introduction	49
		1.3	Learning from previous cases	49
		1.4	Vulnerability	50
		1.5	Forms of abuse	51
		1.6	Domestic violence and abuse	53
		1.7	Managing abuse or disclosures of abuse	53
		1.8	Safeguarding referrals	54
		1.9	Summary	55
	2	Counter-terrorism and anti-radicalisation		55
		2.1	Learning objectives	55
		2.2	Introduction	55
		2.3	PREVENT	56
		2.4	Your role	56

6: Health and Safety 57

	1	Health and safety policies and legislation		57
		1.1	Learning objectives	57
		1.2	Introduction	57
		1.3	Health and Safety at Work, etc. Act	57
		1.4	Management of Health and Safety at Work Regulations	58
		1.5	Manual Handling Operations Regulations	58
		1.6	Provision and Use of Work Equipment Regulations	59
		1.7	Lifting Operations and Lifting Equipment Regulations	59
		1.8	Personal Protective Equipment at Work Regulations	59
		1.9	Control of Substances Hazardous to Health Regulations	60
		1.10	Regulatory bodies	60
		1.11	Why health and safety matters	60
		1.12	Communicating health and safety	61
	2	Risk assessment		61
		2.1	Learning objectives	61
		2.2	Introduction	61
		2.3	Risk assessment	61
	3	Infection prevention and control		64
		3.1	Learning objectives	64

	3.2	Introduction	64
	3.3	Regulations and legislation	65
	3.4	Microorganisms	66
	3.5	Infection and precautions	67
	3.6	Personal hygiene	68
	3.7	Hand hygiene	68
	3.8	Personal protective equipment	72
	3.9	Managing healthcare waste	75
	3.10	Decontamination process	76
	3.11	Handling linen and laundry	80
	3.12	Sharps injury	80
	3.13	Splash contamination	81
	3.14	Legionella awareness	81
	3.15	Occupational health	81
	3.16	Reporting incidents	81
4	Fire safety		81
	4.1	Learning objectives	81
	4.2	Introduction	82
	4.3	Fire prevention	82
	4.4	What to do in case of fire	82
5	Stress		83
	5.1	Learning objectives	83
	5.2	Introduction	83
	5.3	Signs of stress	83
	5.4	Managing stress	84

7: Manual Handling — 85

1	Principles of manual handling		85
	1.1	Learning objectives	85
	1.2	Introduction	85
	1.3	Consequences of poor manual handling	85
	1.4	Risk assessment	87
	1.5	Biomechanics	88
	1.6	General principles	88
	1.7	Handling aids	89
	1.8	Procedure	90
	1.9	Team handling	91
	1.10	Bariatric patients	91
	1.11	Further help and support	92
2	Moving and handling equipment and techniques		92
	2.1	Learning objectives	92
	2.2	Introduction	92
	2.3	Patients on the floor	92
	2.4	Seated patients	102
	2.5	Patients in bed	104
	2.6	Carry chair	106
	2.7	Ambulance trolley	110

8: Drug Administration — 113

1	Drug legislation and guidelines		113
	1.1	Learning objectives	113
	1.2	Introduction	113
	1.3	Legislation and guidelines	113
	1.4	Routes of administration	114
	1.5	Drug administration	114
2	Administering medication to patients		114
	2.1	Learning objectives	114
	2.2	Drawing medication from an ampoule	114
	2.3	Administering oral medication	117
	2.4	Administering nebulised drugs	117
	2.5	Administering intramuscular drugs	118
	2.6	Administering intranasal drugs	120

9: Scene Assessment — 123

1	Scene assessment and safety		123
	1.1	Learning objectives	123
	1.2	Introduction	123
	1.3	Safety	123
	1.4	Cause	123
	1.5	Environment	124

	1.6	Number of patients	124
	1.7	Extra resources	125
2	Major incidents	125
	2.1	Learning objectives	125
	2.2	Introduction	125
	2.3	Interoperability and JESIP	127
	2.4	Classification of incidents	128
	2.5	Role of the ambulance service	128
	2.6	Incident command and control	129
	2.7	First crew on scene	131
	2.8	Subsequent crews on scene	133
	2.9	Triage	133
3	Hazardous materials	135
	3.1	Learning objectives	135
	3.2	Introduction	135
	3.3	Labelling hazardous substances	135
	3.4	Transporting hazardous substances	136
	3.5	Danger labels	136
	3.6	Ambulance crew actions at scene	136

10: Patient Assessment — 141

1	Patient assessment process		141
	1.1	Learning objectives	141
	1.2	Introduction	141
	1.3	Primary survey	141
	1.4	History-taking	143
	1.5	Secondary survey	145
	1.6	Reassessment	147

11: Airway — 149

1	Airway anatomy		149
	1.1	Learning objective	149
	1.2	Introduction	149
	1.3	Nose	149
	1.4	Mouth	149
	1.5	Pharynx	150
	1.6	Lower airway	151
	1.7	Trachea	152
	1.8	Bronchi	152
	1.9	Lungs	152
2	Assessing and managing the airway		152
	2.1	Learning objectives	152
	2.2	Introduction	152
	2.3	Assessing the airway	153
	2.4	Step-wise approach to the airway	154
	2.5	Manual airway manoeuvres	154
	2.6	Suction	158
	2.7	Airway adjuncts	160
	2.8	Supraglottic airway device (SAD)	162
	2.9	Removal of foreign bodies with laryngoscopy in adults	164
3	Tracheostomies		167
	3.1	Learning objectives	167
	3.2	Introduction	167
	3.3	Tracheostomy tubes	168
	3.4	Management of the tracheostomy patient	169
	3.5	Management of the laryngectomy patient	170
4	Choking in adults		171
	4.1	Learning objectives	171
	4.2	Introduction	172
	4.3	Recognition	172
	4.4	Management	172
5	Choking in the paediatric patient		173
	5.1	Learning objective	173
	5.2	Introduction	173
	5.3	The paediatric airway	173
	5.4	Recognition	174
	5.5	Management	175

12: Breathing — 177

1	Respiratory system physiology		177
	1.1	Learning objective	177
	1.2	Introduction	177

	1.3	Respiration	177
	1.4	The lungs	177
	1.5	Mechanics of breathing	178
	1.6	Gas exchange	179
	1.7	Control of breathing	180
	1.8	Oxygen physiology	180
2	Using medical gases safely		181
	2.1	Learning objectives	181
	2.2	Introduction	182
	2.3	Medical gas cylinder storage	182
	2.4	Anatomy of a medical gas cylinder	183
	2.5	Safety first	184
	2.6	Preparing a new cylinder for use	184
	2.7	Oxygen delivery devices	185
	2.8	Assisted ventilation	187
	2.9	Mechanical ventilation	190
	2.10	Oxygen administration	192
	2.11	After use	195
	2.12	Entonox	196
3	Assessment of breathing		200
	3.1	Learning objectives	200
	3.2	Respiratory rate	200
	3.3	Oxygen saturations	200
	3.4	Peak flow	202
	3.5	Capnography	203
	3.6	Auscultation	204
4	Common respiratory conditions		208
	4.1	Learning objectives	208
	4.2	Asthma	208
	4.3	Chronic obstructive pulmonary disease	212
	4.4	Pneumonia	214
	4.5	Pulmonary embolism	215

13: Circulation   217

1	Cardiovascular system anatomy and physiology		217
	1.1	Learning objectives	217
	1.2	Introduction	217
	1.3	Heart	217
	1.4	Blood	220
	1.5	Blood vessels	220
	1.6	Cardiac cycle	221
	1.7	Electrocardiograms	222
2	Lymphatic system and immunity		223
	2.1	Learning objectives	223
	2.2	Introduction	223
	2.3	Anatomy and physiology	223
	2.4	Immunity	224
	2.5	Autoimmune disease	225
3	Assessment of circulation		225
	3.1	Learning objectives	225
	3.2	Introduction	225
	3.3	Pulse	225
	3.4	Capillary refill time	227
	3.5	Blood pressure	228
	3.6	Recording an ECG	231
4	Cardiovascular system disorders		239
	4.1	Learning objectives	239
	4.2	Introduction	239
	4.3	Coronary artery disease	239
	4.4	Stable angina	239
	4.5	Acute coronary syndromes	240
	4.6	Heart failure	242
	4.7	Aortic dissection	244
	4.8	Shock	246
	4.9	Sickle cell disease	247

14: Disability   251

1	Nervous system anatomy and physiology		251
	1.1	Learning objectives	251
	1.2	Introduction	251
	1.3	Anatomy and physiology	251
	1.4	Brain	253
	1.5	Spinal cord	255
	1.6	Somatic nervous system	256

	1.7	Autonomic nervous system	256
	1.8	The eye	257
2	Assessment of disability		259
	2.1	Learning objectives	259
	2.2	Introduction	259
	2.3	Glasgow Coma Scale	259
	2.4	Pupillary response	262
	2.5	Face, arm, speech test	262
3	Disorders of the nervous system		263
	3.1	Learning objectives	263
	3.2	Introduction	263
	3.3	Convulsions	263
	3.4	Stroke	265
	3.5	Meningococcal disease	266
	3.6	Cauda equina syndrome	268
	3.7	Paralysis	269
	3.8	Coma	269

15: Exposure 271

1	Extremes of temperature		271
	1.1	Learning objectives	271
	1.2	Introduction	271
	1.3	Hypothermia	271
	1.4	Heat-related illness	272
	1.5	Assessment of temperature	273
2	Drowning		275
	2.1	Learning objective	275
	2.2	Introduction	275
	2.3	Pathophysiology	275
	2.4	Management	276

16: Medical and Surgical Emergencies 279

1	Anaphylaxis		279
	1.1	Learning objectives	279
	1.2	Introduction	279
	1.3	Signs and symptoms	280
	1.4	Management	281
2	Sepsis		282
	2.1	Learning objectives	282
	2.2	Introduction	282
	2.3	Risk factors for sepsis	282
	2.4	Recognition	284
	2.5	Management	284
3	Endocrine system disorders		284
	3.1	Learning objectives	284
	3.2	Introduction	284
	3.3	Anatomy and physiology of the pancreas	285
	3.4	Anatomy and physiology of the adrenal glands	286
	3.5	Diabetes	288
	3.6	Diabetic emergencies	288
	3.7	Hypoglycaemia	288
	3.8	Severe hyperglycaemia	290
	3.9	Blood sugar measurement	292
	3.10	Addison's disease	294
4	Poisoning		295
	4.1	Toxidromes	295
	4.2	Assessment and management	295
5	The acute abdomen		300
	5.1	Learning objectives	300
	5.2	Introduction	300
	5.3	The abdominal cavity	300
	5.4	Locating abdominal organs	302
	5.5	The digestive system	302
	5.6	Abdominal pain	302
	5.7	Management of abdominal pain	303
6	Urinary system disorders		304
	6.1	Learning objectives	304
	6.2	Introduction	305
	6.3	Anatomy and physiology	305
	6.4	Urinary tract infections	307
	6.5	Renal dialysis	308

17: Trauma 311

1	Major trauma services		311
	1.1	Learning objectives	311
	1.2	Introduction	311

	1.3	Inclusive trauma systems	311		6.3	First-aid techniques	347
	1.4	Major trauma triage tool	313		6.4	Spinal immobilisation	350
2	Mechanism of injury		313		6.5	Splints	357
	2.1	Learning objectives	313	7	Burns		366
	2.2	Introduction	313		7.1	Learning objectives	366
	2.3	Kinetics	313		7.2	Introduction	366
	2.4	Energy	314		7.3	Assessment of burns	366
	2.5	Mechanisms that cause injury	315		7.4	Thermal burns	368
3	Integumentary system anatomy and physiology		319		7.5	Chemical burns including acid attacks	370
	3.1	Learning objective	319		7.6	Radiation burns	370
	3.2	Introduction	319		7.7	Electrical injuries	371
	3.3	Epidermis	319		7.8	The impact of burns	371

18: Assisting the Paramedic — 373

	3.4	Dermis	320
	3.5	Hypodermis	320
	3.6	Physiology	320
4	Wounds and bleeding		320
	4.1	Learning objectives	320
	4.2	Introduction	320
	4.3	Bleeding	320
	4.4	Wounds	325
5	Assessment and management of the trauma patient		326
	5.1	Learning objectives	326
	5.2	Introduction	327
	5.3	Scene assessment	327
	5.4	Primary survey	327
	5.5	Secondary survey	329
	5.6	Head injuries	330
	5.7	Maxillofacial injuries	331
	5.8	Spinal injuries	336
	5.9	Thoracic injuries	337
	5.10	Abdominal injuries	340
	5.11	Pelvic injuries	342
	5.12	Suspension trauma	342
	5.13	Musculoskeletal injuries	342
6	Skeletal immobilisation		347
	6.1	Learning objective	347
	6.2	Introduction	347

1	Tracheal intubation		373
	1.1	Learning objectives	373
	1.2	Introduction	373
	1.3	Tracheal intubation	373
	1.4	DOPES	378
2	Intravenous drug administration		378
	2.1	Learning objectives	378
	2.2	Introduction	378
	2.3	Intravenous cannulation	378
	2.4	Preparing an intravenous infusion	382
	2.5	Intraosseous cannulation	384

19: Obstetrics and Gynaecology — 393

1	Reproduction		393
	1.1	Learning objectives	393
	1.2	Introduction	393
	1.3	Anatomy and physiology	393
	1.4	Normal pregnancy	399
	1.5	Terminology and abbreviations	399
	1.6	Assessing the pregnant woman	400
2	Complications in pregnancy		402
	2.1	Learning objectives	402
	2.2	Ectopic pregnancy	402
	2.3	Antepartum haemorrhage	402

	2.4	Miscarriage	405
	2.5	Pre-eclampsia	405
	2.6	Trauma in pregnancy	406
3	Normal childbirth		407
	3.1	Learning objectives	407
	3.2	Stages of labour	407
	3.3	Equipment for childbirth	408
	3.4	Management of the first stage of labour	409
	3.5	Management of the second stage of labour	409
	3.6	Management of the third stage of labour	413
4	Childbirth complications		413
	4.1	Learning objectives	413
	4.2	Cord prolapse	413
	4.3	Shoulder dystocia	414
	4.4	Breech presentation	415
	4.5	Post-partum haemorrhage	417
	4.6	Multiple births	418
	4.7	Preterm labour	418
5	Newborn life support		419
	5.1	Learning objectives	419
	5.2	Introduction	419
	5.3	Management	419
	5.4	The preterm infant	421
6	Gynaecological emergencies		421
	6.1	Learning objectives	421
	6.2	Introduction	422
	6.3	Vaginal tissue damage	422
	6.4	Heavy menstrual bleeding (menorrhagia)	422
	6.5	Termination of pregnancy	422
	6.6	Uterine prolapse	423
	6.7	Gynaecological cancers	424

20: Children and Infants — 425

1	Why paediatric patients are different		425
	1.1	Learning objective	425
	1.2	Introduction	425
	1.3	Anatomy and physiology	425
	1.4	Cognitive development	427
2	Initial assessment and management of the paediatric patient		428
	2.1	Learning objectives	428
	2.2	Introduction	428
	2.3	Developmental approach to the paediatric patient	428
	2.4	Recognising the sick infant and child	429
	2.5	Primary survey	430

21: Mental Health — 437

1	Mental health legislation and codes of practice		437
	1.1	Learning objectives	437
	1.2	Introduction	437
	1.3	The Mental Health Act 1983 (as amended 2007, MHA)	437
	1.4	Transporting patients	439
2	Mental disorders		439
	2.1	Learning objectives	439
	2.2	Introduction	439
	2.3	Organic disorders	440
	2.4	Schizophrenia and delusional disorders	440
	2.5	Mood (affective) disorders	440
	2.6	Neurotic, stress-related and somatoform disorders	441
	2.7	Personality disorders	441
	2.8	Suicide and deliberate self-harm (DSH)	441
	2.9	Assessment of patient with mental health problems	442
	2.10	Management of patients with mental disorders	442
3	Caring for yourself and colleagues		445
	3.1	Learning objectives	445
	3.2	Introduction	445
	3.3	Mental well-being	445
	3.4	Building resilience	445

		3.5	Seeking help	445
		3.6	Supporting a colleague	446

22: Learning Disabilities — 447

	1	Supporting the care of people with learning disabilities		447
		1.1	Learning objectives	447
		1.2	Introduction	447
		1.3	Learning disabilities legislation and rights	447
		1.4	Causes of learning disabilities	448
		1.5	Categories of learning disabilities	448
	2	Disabilities, healthcare and discrimination		448
		2.1	Learning objectives	448
		2.2	Inequality in healthcare	449
		2.3	Tackling inequality	449
		2.4	Communication	449
		2.5	Learning difficulties and vulnerability	450
		2.6	Further support	450

23: Older People — 451

	1	Ageing		451
		1.1	Learning objective	451
		1.2	Introduction	451
		1.3	Anatomy and physiology of ageing	451
	2	Caring for older patients		455
		2.1	Learning objectives	455
		2.2	Age-related conditions	455
		2.3	Patients with co-morbidities	457
		2.4	Attitudes to ageing	457
	3	Dementia		457
		3.1	Learning objectives	457
		3.2	Introduction	457
		3.3	Dementia	458
		3.4	Communication	463
		3.5	Challenging behaviour	463
	4	Frailty		464
		4.1	Learning objectives	464
		4.2	Introduction	464
		4.3	Recognising frailty	464
		4.4	Living with frailty	464
		4.5	Supporting patients with frailty	465
	5	Falls		465
		5.1	Learning objectives	465
		5.2	Introduction	465
		5.3	Assessing people who fall	465

24: Cardiac Arrest — 467

	1	Adult basic life support		467
		1.1	Learning objectives	467
		1.2	Introduction	467
		1.3	Chain of survival	467
	2	Paediatric basic life support		470
		2.1	Learning objectives	470
		2.2	Introduction	470
		2.3	Infant BLS	470
		2.4	Child BLS	472
	3	Defibrillation		474
		3.1	Learning objectives	474
		3.2	Introduction	474
		3.3	Shockable rhythms	475
		3.4	Non-shockable rhythms	475
		3.5	Defibrillators	476
	4	Cardiac arrest in special circumstances		482
		4.1	Learning objectives	482
		4.2	Introduction	482
		4.3	Cardiac arrest in pregnancy	482
		4.4	Cardiac arrest in hypothermic patients	482
		4.5	Cardiac arrest in drowned patients	483
		4.6	Traumatic cardiac arrest	483
	5	Post-resuscitation care		484
		5.1	Learning objectives	484

	5.2	Introduction	484
	5.3	Management	484
6		Cardiac arrest decisions	485
	6.1	Learning objectives	485
	6.2	When to start and stop resuscitation	485
	6.3	End of life decisions	485
	6.4	Recognition of life extinct (ROLE)	486
	6.5	Sudden unexpected death in infants, children and adolescents	488

25: End of Life Care — 489

1		End of life care	489
	1.1	Learning objectives	489
	1.2	Introduction	489
	1.3	Palliative care and end of life care	489
	1.4	Care of dying adults in the last days of life	489
	1.5	Religious and spiritual influences on end of life care	491
	1.6	Advance care planning	491
	1.7	Disclosures of patient wishes	492
	1.8	Hospices	492
	1.9	End of life care in the community	492
	1.10	Resuscitation in end of life care	493
	1.11	Supporting carers and relatives	493
2		Bereavement	493
	2.1	Learning objectives	493
	2.2	Introduction	493
	2.3	Bereavement and grieving process	494
	2.4	Referring for additional help	494
	2.5	Sources of help	494
	2.6	Support for health professionals	495

References — 497

Glossary — 536

Index — 542

List of Abbreviations

AAA	abdominal aortic aneurysm
AACE	Association of Ambulance Chief Executives
AAP	ambulance associate practitioner
ABC	airway, breathing, circulation
ABCDE	airway, breathing, circulation, disability, exposure/environment
ACP	advance care plan
ACS	acute coronary syndrome
ADRT	advance decision to refuse treatment ('living will')
AED	automated external defibrillator
AHF	acute heart failure
AIC	ambulance incident commander
AMHP	approved mental health professional
ANS	autonomic nervous system
APH	antepartum haemorrhage
ATMIST	age, time of incident, mechanism of injury, injuries, signs and symptoms, treatment given/immediate needs
ATP	adenosine triphosphate
AV	atrioventricular
AVPU	alert, voice, pain, unresponsive
BASICS	British Association for Immediate Care
BLS	basic life support
BP	blood pressure
BURP	backwards-upwards-rightwards pressure
BVM	bag-valve-mask
CABCDE	catastrophic haemorrhage, airway, breathing, circulation, disability, exposure/environment
CAD	coronary artery disease
CBRNE	chemical, biological, radiological, nuclear, explosive
CCO	casualty clearing officer
CCP	critical care paramedic
CCS	casualty clearing station
CES	cauda equina syndrome
CNS	central nervous system
CO	Carbon monoxide
CoP	College of Paramedics
COPD	chronic obstructive pulmonary disease
COSHH	Control of Substances Hazardous to Health
CPP	cerebral perfusion pressure
CPR	cardiopulmonary resuscitation
CQC	Care Quality Commission
CRT	capillary refill time
CSF	cerebrospinal fluid
CVP	central venous pressure
DKA	diabetic ketoacidosis
DoH	Department of Health
DoLS	Deprivation of Liberty Safeguards
DNA	deoxyribonucleic acid
DNACPR	do not attempt cardiopulmonary resuscitation
DRA	dynamic risk assessment
DSH	deliberate self harm
DVT	deep vein thrombosis
ECA	emergency care assistant
ECG	electrocardiogram
ED	emergency department
EDS	Equality Delivery System
EEG	electroencephalogram
EMR	emergency medical responder
EMT	emergency medical technician
EOC	emergency operations centre
EoLC	end of life care
EPCR	electronic patient clinical record
EPRR	emergency preparedness, resilience and response
ET	endotracheal
ETA	estimated time of arrival
EtCO$_2$	end-tidal carbon dioxide

FGM	female genital mutilation	**MAP**	mean arterial pressure
FRS	fire and rescue service	**MCA**	Mental Capacity Act 2005
FTSU	Freedom to Speak Up	**MDT**	mobile data terminal
GCS	Glasgow Coma Scale	**MTC**	major trauma centre
GDPR	General Data Protection Regulations	**METHANE**	major incident, exact location, type of incident, hazards, access, number of casualties, emergency services
GFR	glomerular filtration rate		
GI	gastrointestinal		
GSL	general sales list	**MHA**	Mental Health Act
GTN	glyceryl trinitrate	**MHFA**	mental health first aid
HART	hazardous area response team	**MHOR**	Manual Handling Operations Regulations 1999
HCAI	healthcare-associated infection		
HCPC	Health and Care Professions Council	**MHSWR**	Management of Health and Safety at Work Regulations 1992
HHS	hyperosmolar hyperglycaemic state		
HIN	Hazard Identification Number	**MILS**	manual in-line stabilisation
HIV	human immunodeficiency virus	**MIU**	minor injuries unit
HSCIC	Health and Social Care Information Centre	**MOI**	mechanism of injury
		MRI	magnetic resonance imaging
HSE	Health and Safety Executive	**MRSA**	methicillin-resistant Staphylococcus aureus
HSWA	Health and Safety at Work Act 1974		
ICP	intracranial pressure	**MSC**	motor, sensory, circulation [function]
IHD	ischaemic heart disease		
IM	intramuscular	**MTA**	marauding terrorist attack
IMCA	independent mental capacity advocate	**NAI**	non-accidental injury
		NARU	National Ambulance Resilience Unit
IPAP	Intent, plans, action, protection	**NEAD**	non-epileptic attack disorder
ISS	injury severity score	**NEWS**	National Early Warning Score
IV	intravenous	**NHS**	National Health Service
JESIP	Joint Emergency Services Interoperability Programme	**NIBP**	non-invasive blood pressure measurement
kPa	kilopascal	**NICE**	National Institute for Health and Care Excellence
KTD	Kendrick Traction Device		
LAD	left anterior descending artery	**NIHR**	National Institute for Health Research
LCA	left coronary artery		
LOC	level of consciousness	**NILO**	national inter-agency liaison officer
LOLER	Lifting Operations and Lifting Equipment Regulations 1998	**NNBC**	National Network for Burn Care
		NOF	neck of femur
LPA	lasting power of attorney	**NOI**	nature of illness
LVH	left ventricular hypertrophy	**NPA**	nasopharyngeal airway
MAD	mucosal atomiser device	**NPIS**	National Poisons Information Service

NSTEMI	non-ST segment elevation myocardial infarction	**SBAR**	situation, background, assessment, recommendation
OCD	obsessive compulsive disorder	**SCD**	sickle cell disease
OPA	oropharyngeal airway	**SCENE**	safety, cause including NOI/MOI, environment, number of patients, extra resources needed
PAT	paediatric assessment triangle		
PDA	posterior descending artery		
PE	pulmonary embolism	**SCI**	spinal cord injury
PEA	pulseless electrical activity	**SOBOE**	shortness of breath on exertion
PEF/PEFR	peak expiratory flow/peak expiratory flow rate	SpO_2	blood oxygen saturation
		SPCC	specialist paramedic (critical care)
pPCI	primary percutaneous coronary intervention	**SPUC**	specialist paramedic (urgent care)
		STEMI	ST-segment elevation myocardial infarction
PNS	peripheral nervous system		
POM	prescription only medicines	**STI**	sexually transmitted infection
PPE	personal protective equipment	**SUDICA**	sudden unexpected death in infancy, children and adolescents
PPV	positive pressure ventilation		
PUWER	Provision and Use of Work Equipment Regulations 1998	**SVC**	superior vena cava
		SW	support worker
RBC	red blood cell	**T1DM**	type 1 diabetes mellitus
RCA	right coronary artery	**TARN**	Trauma Audit Research Network
RCGP	Royal College of General Practitioners	**T2DM**	type 2 diabetes mellitus
		TBI	traumatic brain injury
RCN	Royal College of Nursing	**TBSA**	total body surface area
REAP	Resourcing Escalatory Action Plan	**TCA**	traumatic cardiac arrest
ReSPECT	Recommended Summary Plan for Emergency Care and Treatment	**TEP**	tracheo-oesophageal puncture
		TETRA	terrestrial trunk radio
RNA	ribonucleic acid	**TIA**	transient ischaemic attack
ROLE	recognition of life extinct	**TILEE**	task, individual, load, environment, equipment
ROSC	return of spontaneous circulation		
RSV	respiratory syncytial virus	**TRiM**	Trauma Risk Management
RTC	road traffic collision	**UA**	unstable angina
SA	sinoatrial	**UTI**	urinary tract infection
SAD	supraglottic airway device	**VF**	ventricular fibrillation
SAMPLE	signs and symptoms of presenting complaint, allergies, medications, past medical history, last oral intake, events leading to current illness/injury	**VT**	ventricular tachycardia
		VTE	venous thromboembolism
		VZV	varicella-zoster virus
		WHO	World Health Organization
SARS	severe acute respiratory syndrome		

Acknowledgements

Class Professional Publishing would like to thank the following for their co-operation in the production of the Ambulance Care series:

- Iris Murch, Mervyn Murch, Sarah Petter, Steven Petter, Karina Pilbery, Megan Pilbery, Vicky Pilbery, Peter Williams, the students at Coventry University and the teams at SWAST, WMS and YAS for modelling
- Charles L. Till and colleagues at Coventry University for the use of their facilities and equipment
- Daniels for the loan of patslide equipment
- Mike Page for consulting
- Ken Wenman and Claire Warner at SWAST and James Short at WMS for the loan of the ambulances
- Tasnim Ali at YAS for sourcing volunteers for the photoshoot
- Mangar for the loan of the Mangar ELK
- Nigel Wilson for photography work
- SP Services for the loan of first aid and medical devices
- Ferno for the loan of the stretcher.

We would like to thank the following for their invaluable feedback on earlier drafts of this book:

- The National Education Network of Ambulance Services (NENAS) for their contribution to the development of the text throughout
- Sinead Blanchette, West Midlands Ambulance Service
- John Ellison, West Midlands Ambulance Service
- Claire Gedge, South Central Ambulance Service
- Gary Heaps, North West Ambulance Service
- Clive James, St John Ambulance
- Stephen Jeffries, West Midlands Ambulance Service
- Jim Lewis, St John Ambulance
- Sid Marshall, South Central Ambulance Service
- Clare McGonigle, South Central Ambulance Service

- Ken Morgan, North West Ambulance Service
- Carol Offer, North West Ambulance Service
- Julian Rhodes, West Midlands Ambulance Service
- Lizzie Ryan, South West Ambulance Service Trust
- Rob Slee, University of Greenwich
- Allan Sunderland, East of England Ambulance Service
- Sam Taylor, University of Hertfordshire
- Ken Wheeler
- Steve Knowles, South West Ambulance Service
- Trevor West, East Midlands Ambulance Service.

The following images are © Richard Pilbery:

- Figure 1.6 An example of a 12-lead ECG
- Figure 6.2 Non-latex disposable gloves
- Figure 6.3 Face masks
- Figure 9.8 A hazard warning panel from a diesel tanker
- Figure 9.9 Annotated hazard warning panel
- Figure 12.6 Oxyhaemoglobin dissociation curve
- Figure 12.8 An ambulance station medical gas cylinder store
- Figure 13.7 An example of a 12-lead ECG
- Figure 13.8 Basic components of an ECG complex
- Figure 13.17 An ECG showing artefact
- Figure 13.19 A normal 12-lead ECG
- Figure 13.20 Contiguous leads on a 12-lead ECG
- Figure 13.21 An inferior MI
- Figure 13.22 An anterolateral STEMI
- Figure 13.23 An anterolateral STEMI
- Figure 13.24 LBBB on a 12-lead ECG Child BLS procedure
- Chapter 16 Procedure – Accu-Chek® Aviva blood glucose meter images
- Figure 19.18 Resuscitation of the newborn
- Figure 20.1 Infant positive-pressure ventilation
- Figure 20.2 An infant with their airway in neutral alignment

- Chapter 24 Procedure – To perform basic life support on an infant images
- Chapter 24 Procedure – To perform basic life support on a child images
- Figure 24.2 Ventricular fibrillation
- Figure 24.3 Ventricular tachycardia following a 200J shock
- Figure 24.4 Asystole
- Figure 24.5 An example of an ECG showing an pulseless electrical activity
- Figure 24.6 A Corpuls3 monitor/defibrillator commonly used by ambulance services.

We would like to thank the following for their kind permission to publish material:

- Chapter 6 Alcohol handrub procedure. Based on the 'How to Handrub' poster © World Health Organization 2009. All rights reserved
- Chapter 6 Handwashing procedure. Based on the 'How to Handwash' poster © World Health Organization 2009. All rights reserved
- Figure 6.5 Clinell® wipes. Republished with permission of GAMA Healthcare Ltd. Best practice guidance for infection control wet wipes developed by Clinell and GAMA Healthcare Ltd © 2016
- Figure 7.3 A Ferno mechanically powered ambulance stretcher. Republished with kind permission of Ferno.
- Figure 9.1 Dynamic Risk Assessment Model. Reproduced by the kind permission of the National Ambulance Resilience Unit (NARU).
- Figure 9.2 CBRN(e) first responder flowchart. Reproduced by the kind permission of JESIP.
- Figure 9.3 JESIP joint decision-making model taken from 'Joint Doctrine – The Interoperability Framework Edition Two'. Reproduced by the kind permission of JESIP.
- Figure 9.4 An incident command structure showing examples of the additional support roles that may be required. Reproduced by the kind permission of the National Ambulance Resilience Unit (NARU)
- Figure 9.5 The triage sieve. Reproduced by kind permission of the National Ambulance Resilience Unit (NARU)
- Figure 10.6 Royal College of Physicians. *National Early Warning Score (NEWS) 2: Standardising the assessment of acute-illness severity in the NHS.* Updated report of a working party. London: RCP, 2017 © Royal College of Physicians 2017
- Figure 11.10 Mechanical suction device. Image reproduced by the kind permission of Laerdal Medical
- Figures 11.16, 11.17, 11.18 and 11.19 Tracheostomy tubes. Images reproduced by the kind permission of Kapitex Healthcare Ltd
- Figure 11.22 Adult choking algorithm. Reproduced with the kind permission of the Resuscitation Council (UK)
- Figure 11.23 Paediatric choking algorithm. Reproduced with the kind permission of the Resuscitation Council (UK)
- Figure 12.12 A Firesafe. Image reproduced by the kind permission of BPR Medical
- Figure 12.14 Bag-valve-mask with oxygen reservoir bag attached and inflated. Image reproduced by the kind permission of Ambu A/S
- Chapter 12 Instructions for use of oxygen images © BOC Ltd 2014. Image reproduced by the kind permission of BOC healthcare
- Figure 12.17 The Pneupac paraPAC® plus 310. Image property of Smiths Medical and reprinted with permission from Smiths Medical, ASD, Inc
- Figure 12.22 Normal peak flow values. Image reproduced by the kind permission of Clement Clarke International
- Chapter 12 salbutamol, Chapter 13 aspirin and Chapter 13 GTN drugs guidelines are republished with permission of AACE.
- Figure 13.15 An aneroid sphygmomanometer. Image reproduced by the kind permission of Welch Allyn
- Figure 14.13 Petechial non-blanching rash. Courtesy Meningitis Research Foundation www.meningitis.org

- Figure 14.14 Maculopapular rash with scanty petechiae. Courtesy Meningitis Research Foundation www.meningitis.org
- Chapter 16 Procedure – for Jext® auto-injector. Images reproduced with the kind permission of ALK
- Figure 17.23 Orthopaedic stretcher. Image reproduced by the kind permission of Ferno (UK) Ltd
- Chapter 18 EZ-IO® procedure images. Republished with kind permission of Teleflex
- Figure 19.17 Newborn life support algorithm. Reproduced with the kind permission of the Resuscitation Council (UK)
- Figure 23.4 The Abbey pain scale. Reproduced by permission of MA Healthcare Ltd
- Figure 24.1 The chain of survival. Image reproduced by the kind permission of Laerdal Medical

Every effort has been made to secure permission to reproduce copyright images. If any have been inadvertently overlooked, the copyright holders are invited to contact Class Professional Publishing and the omission will be rectified in the next printing as well as all further editions.

Foreword

The Association of Ambulance Chief Executives welcomes the second edition of *Ambulance Care Practice* to its portfolio of endorsed publications. This innovative textbook will continue to assist many in learning essential ambulance skills at the start of their careers and provides a solid foundation for those who later undertake paramedic studies. The progressive manner of introducing new concepts, skills and knowledge gives the reader a complete understanding of what is required of today's multi-skilled ambulance staff. The second edition has been brought up-to-date with current guidance and introduces additional information on key topics such as Care of the Elderly, Safeguarding, and issues regarding Mental Health. We look forward to future editions.

Steve Irving, Executive Officer, the Association of Ambulance Chief Executives

Welcome to this revised edition of *Ambulance Care Practice*, written by Richard Pilbery and Kris Lethbridge. This textbook provides essential underpinning learning for Level 4 emergency ambulance Diploma programmes in place across the UK ambulance services.

The emergency and urgent care systems are undergoing significant and continual change and the development of a suite of qualifications for UK ambulance services will ensure that the ambulance workforce is able to continue working at the heart of these changing systems.

The textbook will assist learners to develop their knowledge and skills as a part of taught programmes and apprenticeships and will provide a strong understanding of what is required of today's ambulance workforce and a solid foundation for continued learning.

Carol Offer, Chair, National Education Network for Ambulance Services (NENAS) and Assistant Director of Workforce and OD, North West Ambulance Service

Chapter

1 Introduction

1 Textbook guide

1.1 Introduction

This textbook is designed to help prepare you to work as an ambulance associate practitioner (AAP, although this role may be named differently in your organisation, for example, emergency medical technician). The content is suitable for any Level 4 diploma course, or similar, that qualifies you to practise as an AAP.

Each chapter comprises a number of topics centred on a theme, such as health and safety, or the airway. The learning objectives for each chapter have been mapped to objectives from a range of courses that are used by ambulance services to prepare their staff for the role of AAP.

1.2 Textbook

This textbook is designed to be read from start to finish on the first reading because concepts introduced later on in the book assume that you already have knowledge of the content that has been covered in earlier chapters. However, this textbook will also be a useful reference to which you can return again and again, reflecting on the learning points that are highlighted.

1.3 Getting started

To help get you orientated to the book and the relevance of the various chapters to clinical practice, the next section, 'Anatomy of an emergency call', will take you step by step through an emergency attended by an ambulance crew. It will highlight the variety of knowledge and skills that you will require in order to be an effective AAP.

Each chapter is split into sections, which are typically laid out in the following way:
- **Learning objectives:** To clearly highlight what you are expected to learn in the chapter.
- **Introduction:** Setting the scene for the theme of the chapter.
- **Content:** The content!

2 Anatomy of an emergency call

2.1 Introduction

This book consists of a number of chapters that are completed in sequence and all play an essential part in your role as an AAP. It can be helpful to find out why you need to learn something. In order to see the themes of this book in context, let's review a typical clinical scenario that you may be faced with when working on an emergency ambulance (Figure 1.1).

2.2 The emergency operations centre

When Mr Brown's daughter makes a 999 call, she speaks to a telephone operator who asks her which service she requires. She asks for the ambulance service and is put through to her local

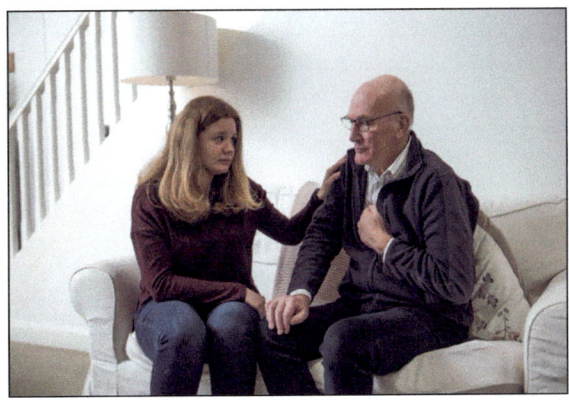

Figure 1.1 Mr James Brown, a 59-year-old man who has chest pain, with his daughter.

Chapter 1 – *Introduction*

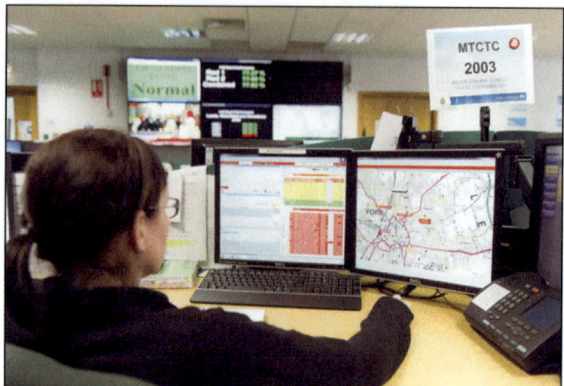

Figure 1.2 A dispatcher in the EOC.

ambulance service's emergency operations centre (EOC; see Figure 1.2).

While she talks to the call handler, the dispatcher allocates the ambulance that you are working on to the emergency call. Since it has been categorised as a high-priority call by the medical priority dispatch system, you need to arrive as soon as possible.

You will learn more about the ambulance service, including the roles and responsibilities of its staff, and ambulance and clinical quality indicators in Chapter 2, 'The Ambulance Service'.

2.3 Arriving on scene

You will have been conducting a scene assessment before arriving at the address. This will include the location, time of day and type of incident, and is a dynamic process, i.e. it should be constantly reviewed as the scene can change rapidly. You will learn about scene assessment and safety later on in the book.

In addition to scene safety, you will consider the need for personal protective equipment. At a residential address, this may be limited to a pair of disposable gloves, but at the scene of a road traffic collision, you will need a helmet and high-visibility jacket as well.

With the help of your paramedic colleague, you carry the immediate aid kit, oxygen, drugs bag and monitor/defibrillator to the front door, where the patient's daughter is anxiously waiting (Figure 1.3).

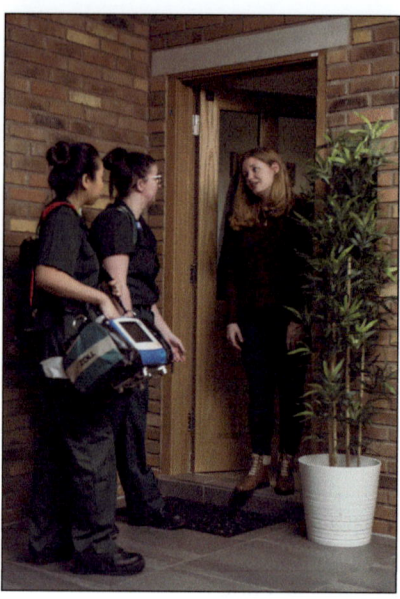

Figure 1.3 The crew arrive at the address.

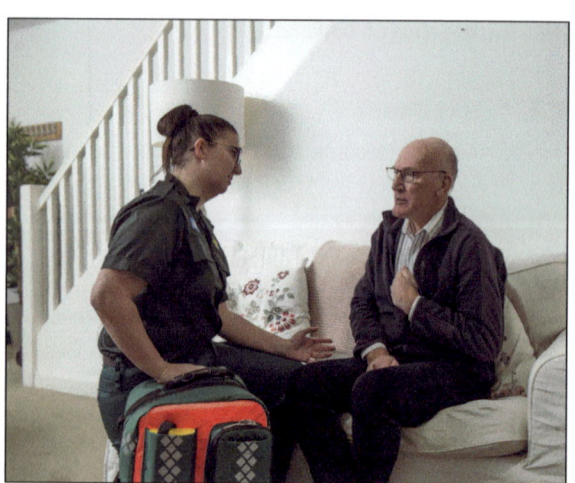

Figure 1.4 The paramedic talking to Jim.

2.4 Principles of communication

You are shown into the living room where Mr Brown is sitting on the sofa, clutching his chest and looking rather grey and sweaty. Your paramedic colleague introduces you both to Mr Brown and his daughter, and clarifies what Mr Brown prefers to be called. He tells you to call him Jim (Figure 1.4).

Communication is a fundamental aspect of all ambulance work and your role as an AAP. It is not always easy as you will have to communicate with patients, friends and family members, as well as other healthcare professionals, and will need to adapt your approach and style appropriately. In addition, you cannot communicate the same way with an elderly person as you would a two-year-old child. Some patients will not, or cannot, communicate with you, because they are depressed or don't speak English, for example. Chapter 3, 'Communication' will cover this in more detail.

2.5 Patient assessment

Your paramedic colleague completes an initial airway, breathing, circulation, disability, exposure (ABCDE) assessment of Jim and asks you to obtain a set of baseline observations to support this. Jim's airway is patent; he is breathing at a rate of 16 breaths per minute, which is in the normal range. After obtaining permission (correctly termed 'consent', an important legal concept, covered in Chapter 4, 'Legal, Ethical and Professional Issues') from Jim, you apply a pulse oximeter to one of his fingers. His oxygen saturations are 93% on air and, having excluded the presence of chronic obstructive pulmonary disease (COPD, which you will learn about in Chapter 12, 'Breathing'), you confirm with the paramedic before administering low-flow oxygen via a simple face mask.

Continuing with the assessment of Jim's circulation, you measure his blood pressure and apply electrodes to each of his limbs in order to record a 3-lead electrocardiogram (ECG), put on your disposable gloves to check his blood sugar (covered in the assessment of disability lesson in Chapter 14, 'Disability') and, finally, check his temperature.

2.6 Patient history

Jim explains that he experienced a sudden onset of central chest pain radiating to his jaw, back and both arms an hour prior to his daughter's 999 call. It feels like a heavy pressure, which he scores as 7 out of 10, and is associated with shortness of breath, nausea and sweating. His daughter states that he has been very pale since the onset of pain.

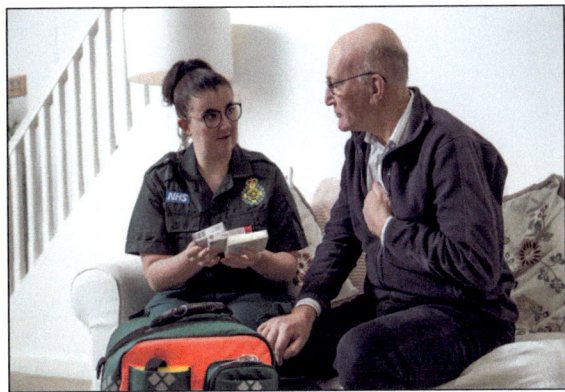

Figure 1.5 Reviewing the patient's medication is an important part of the history.

The paramedic asks about Jim's past medical history and is told that he has high cholesterol and hypertension, for both of which he takes medication (Figure 1.5). He has never suffered from a heart attack (myocardial infarction, MI), but does admit to suffering from occasional chest pain on exertion over the past month or so.

2.7 The 12-lead ECG

The paramedic asks you to record a 12-lead ECG, while she administers aspirin and glyceryl trinitrate (GTN) to Jim, having checked that there are no contra-indications to administration (criteria as to when the drugs should not be given to the patient) (Figure 1.6).

After obtaining consent, you open Jim's shirt and prepare his chest for the electrodes, which is not easy as his skin is greasy with sweat. Having prepared the skin (covered in Chapter 13, 'Circulation'), you identify the anatomical landmarks to ensure you place the electrodes in the correct location. Once completed, you connect up the ECG leads to the monitor/defibrillator, enter the patient's age and gender, and press the 12-lead ECG button.

There is a short pause while the machine acquires the ECG and prints it out. You review the 12-lead ECG with the paramedic and come to the conclusion that it shows signs of a heart attack. Knowing that patients with a heart attack should

Chapter 1 – *Introduction*

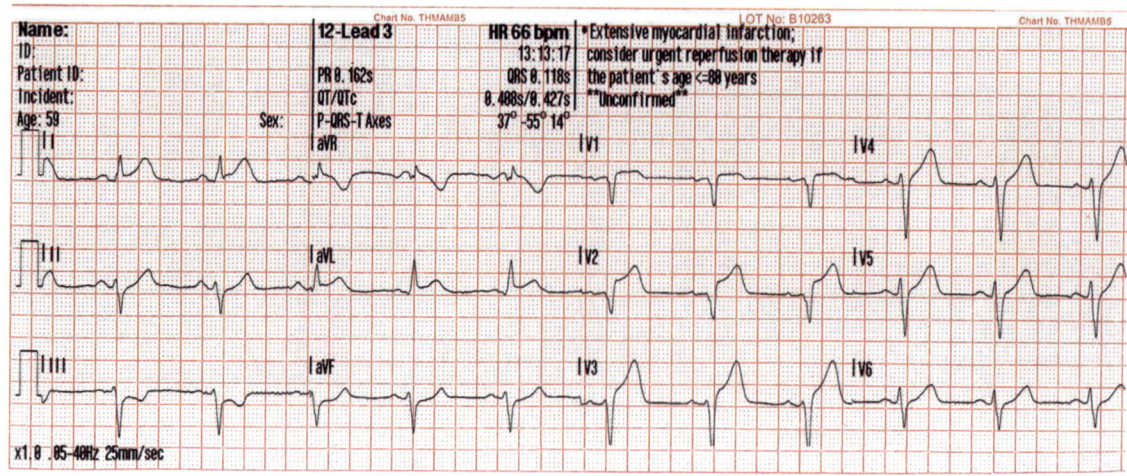

Figure 1.6 A 12-lead ECG showing signs of a heart attack.

not walk, you fetch the carry chair from the ambulance.

2.8 Manual handling

You return with the carry chair, complete a task, individual, load, environment, equipment (TILEE) assessment and explain to Jim how you would like him to transfer to the carry chair. Ensuring that you have a hand on the back of the chair at all times, you assist Jim into the chair and fasten the safety strap across his chest. Before tipping the chair backwards onto the rear wheels, you warn Jim, and then proceed out of the house, stopping to allow your colleague to exit first to lift the chair over the lip of the doorframe and the outside step.

You wheel Jim around to the rear of the ambulance, up the ramp, and alongside the ambulance stretcher so that he can transfer onto it (Figure 1.7).

The TILEE manual handling assessment tool and the equipment used for manual handling are covered in sections 1 and 2 of Chapter 7, 'Manual Handling': 'Principles of manual handling' and 'Moving and handling equipment and techniques'.

2.9 Assist the paramedic

With the patient safely aboard the ambulance, you reconnect the monitor/defibrillator so that the paramedic can observe changes in Jim's condition

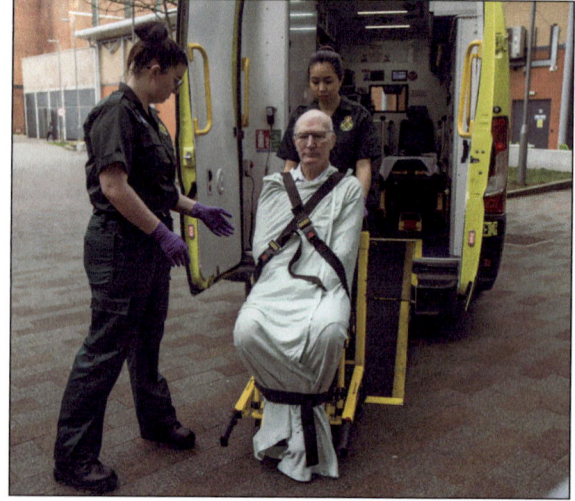

Figure 1.7 The crew loading Jim into the ambulance.

en route to hospital. However, the paramedic would like to cannulate before leaving and asks you to help.

Assisting the paramedic is part of the AAP role, although you will be expected to take the lead when working with junior staff. You quickly gather the equipment required, including a selection of cannulas, a dressing pack, alcohol wipes, syringes and a saline flush (Figure 1.8). Having identified a vein and prepared the site, the paramedic

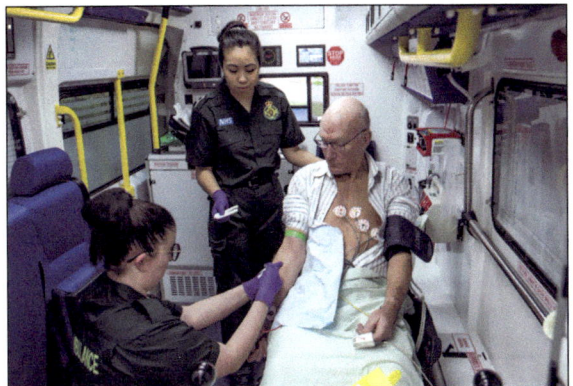

Figure 1.8 Assisting the paramedic with cannulation.

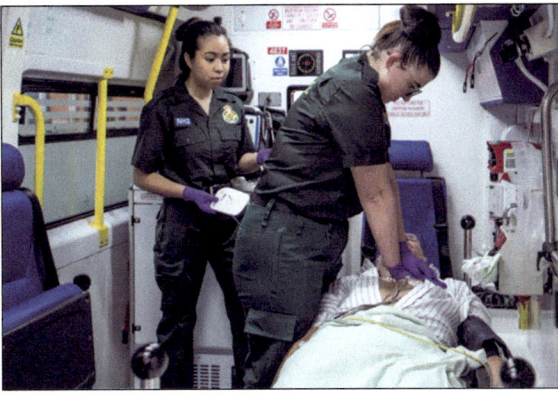

Figure 1.9 Jim suffers a cardiac arrest in the back of the ambulance.

inserts the cannula and advances it, releasing the tourniquet and removing the needle, which is safely deposited in a sharps bin that you have already placed close to her.

With this completed, and due to the fact that Jim is having a heart attack, the paramedic requests that you drive on blue lights and sirens to the local heart attack centre and not the local emergency department (ED). Thanks to your knowledge of the ambulance service, you are aware of this pathway and know which hospital is the regional centre capable of performing primary percutaneous coronary intervention (pPCI). You pass the paramedic the mobile phone to alert the hospital and head for the driver's seat.

2.10 Hospital arrival

Traffic is light and you make good progress, arriving at the heart attack centre within 30 minutes. Just as you are pulling up outside the doors to the hospital, the paramedic shouts through that Jim has suffered a cardiac arrest.

You park up and leap into the back of the ambulance to assist. The paramedic is already performing chest compressions and asks you to connect the defibrillator pads (Figure 1.9).

You apply the pads as you have been taught, removing the ECG chest leads that are obstructing the placement of one of the pads. The paramedic pauses chest compressions so that you can check the rhythm and you recognise it at once as ventricular fibrillation (VF), one of the shockable rhythms. You resume chest compressions as the paramedic charges the defibrillator (covered in Chapter 24, 'Cardiac Arrest').

The tone of the defibrillator tells you it is ready to deliver the shock and, after checking that the paramedic is not touching the patient, you press the shock button. Jim jolts upwards slightly as his chest muscles contract and you take over chest compressions while the paramedic inserts an oropharyngeal airway (OPA) and connects the bag-valve-mask (BVM) to high-flow oxygen.

After two minutes of cardiopulmonary resuscitation (CPR), you briefly pause chest compressions to assess the rhythm. The ECG shows an organised rhythm and a pulse check reveals that Jim's heart is beating again. His breathing is not adequate, however, and the paramedic ventilates Jim with the BVM en route to the cardiac catheter lab. By the time you arrive at the catheter lab, Jim is making some respiratory effort.

The paramedic provides a handover to the waiting staff, explaining Jim's history, findings on examination, treatment administered and the cardiac arrest, for which Jim has just been successfully resuscitated.

Chapter 1 – *Introduction*

2.11 Clean up and prepare for the next call

With Jim safely in the hands of the cardiac catheter lab staff, you return with the paramedic to the ambulance to clean up, restock and get ready for the next emergency call.

You find out later that Jim had an occluded left anterior descending coronary artery, which was cleared and reopened by the cardiac catheter lab staff. He is recovering well and due to be discharged from hospital soon.

Working as an AAP in the ambulance service will frequently involve meeting patients like Jim, but often it is the non-life-threatening calls that are the most challenging. This book, together with clinical practice and hands-on training, will provide you with the knowledge and skills you require to become a competent AAP and a valued member of the ambulance service.

Chapter 2 The Ambulance Service

1 Organisational structure

1.1 Learning objectives
By the end of this section, you will be able to:
- identify which NHS organisations influence ambulance services
- list the regulators relevant to providing ambulance services in the UK.

1.2 Introduction
Ambulance services are primary care organisations that form part of the NHS; some are NHS trusts, others are NHS foundation trusts. NHS foundation trusts have more control over their own functioning and budgets than standard trusts [UK Government, 2018].

Individual paramedics are regulated by the Health and Care Professions Council (HCPC). The HCPC sets out standards of proficiency which paramedics must meet in order to remain registered. It oversees continuing professional development for paramedics, which is a requirement of the job role.

All ambulance services, be they part of the NHS, private or voluntary, are monitored by the Care Quality Commission (CQC). The CQC is tasked with ensuring that health and social care delivered across the UK is safe, effective and compassionate. It carries out inspections of ambulance services led by the Chief Inspector of Hospitals. It provides a rating for the service, ranging from outstanding and good to requires improvement or inadequate.

The National Institute for Health and Care Excellence (NICE), established in 1999, exists to promote best practice in clinical settings across the NHS. It issues guidance, procedures and standards on areas of practice ranging from handwashing to the appropriate drugs used to treat cancer. NICE works to the principle of evidence-based practice.

Other organisations you should be aware of include the following:
- NHS Improvement is responsible for overseeing foundation trusts. It offers support to providers in delivering services and holds trusts to account, helping the NHS to meet its overall aims.
- NHS Digital is the national information and technology partner to the NHS, helping to transform services with the aid of technology.
- The Association of Ambulance Chief Executives (AACE) is an organisation that provides a structure to co-ordinate, manage and implement key national work programmes and policies that are fundamental to the ongoing improvement of English ambulance services and their delivery of care.
- The College of Paramedics is the professional body for paramedics and ambulance professionals throughout the UK. It represents the profession at a national level and undertakes activity to drive the profession forwards.
- The Faculty of Pre-Hospital Care is a part of the Royal College of Surgeons of Edinburgh. Its purpose is to promote the highest standards of clinical care throughout the speciality of pre-hospital emergency medicine from first aiders to multi-disciplinary critical care teams.

2 Response to a 999 call

2.1 Learning objectives
By the end of this section you will be able to:
- explain how the ambulance service manages an emergency call
- state some of the alternative services that callers may be directed to when an emergency ambulance is not required.

2.2 Introduction

The response to a 999 call can be complex and varies between each incident depending on the degree of need. The three main stages of a response are:
- call for help and triage
- ambulance service response
- onward care of patient.

2.3 Call for help and triage

When someone calls 999 (or 112) in the UK, they are connected to an operator from the national telephone network. Once the nature of the emergency has been established, the call will be forwarded to the police, fire service, ambulance service or coastguard, depending on the most appropriate response(s) required.

Once the call is connected to the ambulance service emergency operations centre (EOC), a qualified call handler will ask a series of questions. These pre-set questions are designed to triage calls and identify those that need an ambulance most urgently. They can also identify those callers who do not need an ambulance and for whom an alternative care pathway, such as visiting a GP or self-presenting at a minor injuries unit (MIU), would be more appropriate.

As the call handler works through the questioning, the triage system will identify how urgently an ambulance is required and arrive at a triage code and a response category. Two systems are used for triage: NHS Pathways and the Advanced Medical Priority Dispatch System. Although there are significant differences between the two systems, they both ultimately generate a diagnostic code, which is then allocated to one of four priorities for response.

These systems can be helpful in identifying to the dispatcher which callers need an ambulance most urgently. They can be subject to error, however, especially if the person calling is scared, confused or struggling to answer the questions asked.

Following a large review of ambulance services responses in 2015/16 called the Ambulance Response Programme, the old categories of response were dropped and new response standards were introduced (Table 2.1) [NHS England, 2018a].

During the triage process, a clinician is often available to assist in 'enhanced triage'. This is particularly useful when dealing with patients who have complex needs that the standard pathways system may not be set up to deal with.

Also during triage, the call handler will identify if there is a need for other emergency services, or whether there may be any dangers to the responding ambulance clinicians present (such as an assailant still at a scene). Where required, other services will be contacted and ambulance crews can be advised of the risks.

2.4 Ambulance service response

Based on the information gathered during the triage process, the most appropriate response can be determined. There are two main types of response, which are:
- hear and treat
- physical response.

2.4.1 Hear and treat

Hear and treat is where the patient is advised how to look after themselves, or recommended to self-present to a more appropriate care provider, such as a GP or MIU. In late 2018 the number of patients being managed in England through this route was around 5% of all 999 calls [NHS England, 2018b].

2.4.2 Physical response

For the majority of 999 calls, the ambulance service will send a physical response. Depending on the need of the patient and the scale of the incident, this may include:
- air ambulance (including critical care teams)
- community responder
- rapid response car
- response motorbike/pedal bike
- emergency ambulance
- specialist practitioner in urgent care
- hazardous area response team (HART)

Table 2.1 Ambulance Response Programme call categories.

Category	Description	Details	Average response target	90th percentile response target
1	Life-threatening	A time-critical life-threatening event requiring immediate intervention or resuscitation	7 minutes	15 minutes
2	Emergency	Potentially serious conditions that may require rapid assessment and urgent on-scene intervention and/or urgent transport	18 minutes	40 minutes
3	Urgent	An urgent problem (not immediately life-threatening) that needs treatment to relieve suffering and transport or assessment and management at the scene with referral where needed within a clinically appropriate timeframe	None (mean indicator of 60 minutes)	2 hours
4	Less urgent	Problems that are less urgent, but require assessment and possibly transport within a clinically appropriate timeframe	None	3 hours

- ambulance service officer/commander
- specialist operations response team
- medical support such as the British Association for Immediate Care (BASICS).

2.5 Onward care

Where necessary, patients will be transported to hospital for emergency care and treatment. This is frequently to emergency departments (EDs) but now also includes an increasing number of specialist emergency care departments, such as stroke units or cardiac centres.

In addition to this, ambulance clinicians now have a range of alternative care pathways available to them in order to avoid hospital admission where appropriate. During late 2018 in England, in 29% of incidents where patients had a response from the ambulance service, they were not transported to an ED, but were either managed at the scene ('see and treat') or taken to an alternative care provider [NHS England, 2018b].

Alternative care providers may include:
- specialist paramedics in urgent care: paramedics with additional training who can manage a range primary and urgent care presentations within the community
- GP surgeries
- GP drop-in centres
- out-of-hours services

- mental health teams
- minor injury units
- pharmacies
- 111
- social services
- 'Hospital at Home' teams
- emergency residential care
- community hospitals.

The exact nature of alternative care providers available in your local area will depend on how local services are arranged and commissioned, but it is likely you or your patients will be able to access a number of those listed above.

3 Roles within the ambulance service

3.1 Learning objectives

By the end of this section you will be able to:
- identify a number of clinical and leadership roles within the ambulance service and briefly explain what the role entails
- describe the importance of good working relationships.

3.2 Introduction

There are ten NHS ambulance trusts in England, as well as NHS ambulance services in Scotland, Wales, Northern Ireland and the Channel Islands, which are statutory providers of ambulance services for the government within the UK [AACE, 2019]. There are also a range of voluntary services, including St John Ambulance and the British Red Cross, and a variety of independent sector services, ranging from the very small to national scale organisations.

Each service is structured differently, so it is not possible to give a definitive list of the different roles. However, over the following pages, descriptions are given of some of the roles you may find, which could be broadly divided into:
- clinical
- clinical leadership
- command and control.

3.3 Clinical roles

3.3.1 Community responder

Community responders come from a variety of backgrounds and volunteer their time for the ambulance service. They respond to incidents close to where they live or work, often in remote settings, which can take longer for an ambulance to reach. Responders carry basic life-saving equipment including an automated external defibrillator (AED) and devices for managing a patient's airway [SCAS, 2019]. In some places the fire service and other similar agencies may also act as first responders for the ambulance service.

3.3.2 Support worker (SW)

SWs (sometimes referred to as emergency care assistants, ECAs) work alongside paramedics on front-line ambulances. They are trained in providing emergency care, basic emergency interventions and life support, and are qualified emergency drivers. SWs normally work under the supervision of a qualified clinical colleague. They may also work on support vehicles that are used to transport patients to hospital when they have been assessed by another healthcare professional and are viewed as needing a less urgent admission to hospital. SWs have different names in different places, though common names are emergency care assistants or emergency care support workers.

3.3.3 Associate ambulance practitioner

AAPs (sometimes referred to as emergency medical technicians, EMTs), are non-registered clinicians who normally work alongside a paramedic, but sometimes may also work on their own. They have a range of skills relevant to emergency and urgent care and can undertake a number of pre-hospital procedures and administer a limited range of medications. There is national variation in the skill sets of AAPs and the way in which they are deployed by different services.

AAPs are similar to, but not the same as, the previous role of IHCD technician, which may also still be found in some ambulance trusts. They are also unregistered clinicians who may work independently to a limited scope of practice or under supervision.

3.3.4 Paramedic

Paramedics are qualified and registered clinicians who specialise in working in the urgent and emergency care setting. They are trained in the examination and treatment of emergency conditions, have a wide range of skills and treatment options, and are considered specialists in emergency care. Registered with the Health and Care Professions Council (HCPC), paramedics have a degree of autonomy in their practice and can be held accountable to the HCPC for actions and omissions that arise from providing clinical care to patients.

To become a new paramedic, students must complete a course equivalent to a certificate of higher education. From September 2021, only education programmes at degree level or above will lead to paramedic registration [HCPC, 2018].

3.3.5 Specialist paramedic – urgent care (SPUC)

Specialist paramedics have been known by a range of titles including emergency care practitioner and paramedic practitioner. They have undertaken an enhanced course of learning, usually at postgraduate level, along with a range of placements that equip them with the skills and knowledge to treat urgent care patients. These patients include those with acute illnesses such as respiratory tract and urinary tract infections or minor injuries and wounds. Specialist paramedics have a broad range of skills in the management of urgent patients and can administer a greater variety of medications [CoP, 2015].

3.3.6 Specialist paramedic – critical care (SPCC)

Also known as critical care paramedics (CCPs), these clinicians have also undertaken enhanced study, but with a focus on dealing with the most critically ill or injured. Specialist paramedics in critical care will often work as part of a multi-disciplinary team alongside a doctor who specialises in emergency pre-hospital care. Like their SPUC colleagues, they will have completed additional study, normally at postgraduate level [CoP, 2015].

3.3.7 Advanced paramedic

Advanced paramedics are experienced paramedics who have completed master's level study relevant to their practice. They will be very experienced, most likely having worked in a number of different settings and will be able to demonstrate an expert knowledge base, complex decision-making, and clinical leadership in their area of practice. Advanced paramedics may have roles that mix clinical practice and clinical leadership or development [CoP, 2015].

3.3.8 Hazardous area response team (HART)

HART are groups of paramedics who have been specially trained to work in difficult situations and alongside the police and fire services at large and dangerous incidents. They have a special set of skills and equipment, which can include water rescues, working at heights and the use of breathing apparatus. This allows them to safely access patients in remote and difficult settings. There is a network of HART bases around the country and their help can normally be requested through the emergency operations centre (EOC).

3.4 Clinical leadership roles

Running any ambulance service requires a large range of clinical leaders. Some of the common roles include:
- consultant paramedic
- clinical development manager
- pharmaceutical adviser
- medical director.

3.4.1 Consultant paramedic

The consultant paramedic is a relatively new role in some ambulance trusts throughout the UK. The role of the consultant is to act as a senior clinical leader involved in service development; clinical leadership; research and evaluation; and education and professional development. Consultants will normally work in a mixed role providing advanced clinical support to operational staff while also undertaking their other responsibilities. After the medical director, a consultant paramedic is normally the most senior clinical leader in an ambulance trust.

3.4.2 Clinical development manager (CDM)
The CDM is responsible for ensuring that clinical policies and procedures are up to date. They also consider what new procedures and medication may be beneficial for patients.

3.4.3 Pharmaceutical adviser
Most organisations will have a pharmacist working for them at least part-time. This is to ensure that the use of medications by the service is safe and appropriate and that the relevant laws are being followed.

3.4.4 Medical director
The medical director, normally a doctor with a background in emergency and/or critical care, is the ultimate person responsible for the clinical care inside an organisation. They are a very senior clinical leader and are answerable for clinical errors and omissions within an organisation.

3.5 Command and control roles
Inside every large organisation is a command and control structure. This structure is required to co-ordinate and effectively deliver the functions of the organisation, but it becomes particularly relevant in emergency services at times of complex or major incidents. All commanders receive specific training relevant to their role. Different command roles do not necessarily indicate rank or seniority within an organisation, but are instead allocated so that those involved understand their role in managing an incident. Following criticism of emergency services not communicating effectively at previous major incidents, the national Joint Emergency Services Interoperability Programme (JESIP) has been launched in the UK so that commanders from all the emergency services know better how to work together and communicate at complex and multi-agency incidents [JESIP, 2019].

3.5.1 Operational commanders
Operational commanders, broadly equivalent to what were formerly known as 'bronze' commanders, are present at the scene of an incident and are responsible for organising the delivery of care and the safety of those working at a scene. They have to assess what resources are available to them or have been made available to them by tactical and strategic commanders, and utilise those resources in the most effective way possible.

Depending on the size of the incident, operational commanders work alongside a number of officers from both the ambulance and other emergency services to ensure services are being provided in an effective and co-ordinated manner.

Operational commanders receive direction from tactical commanders, with whom they have to liaise closely to ensure they have the resources they require to manage an incident.

3.5.2 Tactical commanders
Formerly known as 'silver' commanders, the tactical commander is responsible for ensuring that all the tactical resources an operational commander requires for the management of the incident are in place. They will communicate closely with other emergency services and agencies, and may or may not be present at the actual incident, depending on the scale and nature of the incident, as well as the length of time it goes on for. At some incidents, there may be multiple operational commanders, each dealing with different sections of the incident, in which case the tactical commander will be responsible for co-ordinating their actions.

The tactical commander achieves a level of oversight for an incident that cannot normally be achieved by an operational commander on the ground. From this position, the tactical commander can ensure there is effective joint working of agencies and that the deployment of resources and the tactics being used to manage an incident are appropriate.

3.5.3 Strategic commanders

Formerly known as 'gold' commanders, strategic commanders are responsible for devising strategic plans and making available the resources to implement a strategy for managing an incident. The strategic commander usually has control over all of the organisation's resources and is responsible for making these resources available to the tactical and operational commanders.

Strategic commanders, like tactical commanders, get an oversight of the management of an incident and are responsible for ensuring the tactics being used are appropriate, that all services are working effectively together and that clear lines of communication are in place. Where necessary, strategic commanders are responsible for national level communication to make available further resources if they are required.

3.5.4 National inter-agency liaison officer (NILO)

The NILO is a nominated person who has had specific training and experience to ensure that agencies such as fire, police and ambulance services can communicate effectively during a major or serious incident [NARU, 2019].

4 Working relationships

As you can see, there are a wide range of roles in the ambulance service and it is likely that you will need to work collaboratively with all of them at some time or another. Key to successful collaborative working will be building successful working relationships.

A good relationship with your manager is particularly important. Key principles of good working relationships are:
- knowledge of the responsibilities and limits of your own role
- regular, face-to-face meetings
- performance feedback sessions
- opportunities to ask questions so you can develop your skills.

Should you have a problem with or encounter bullying from your manager, escalate this to your employer. The NHS Constitution details that all staff have a right to 'a good working environment with flexible working opportunities, consistent with the needs of patients' [DoH, 2015a]. NHS employers must strive to provide 'a positive working environment for staff and to promote supportive, open cultures that help staff do their job to the best of their ability' [NHS Employers, 2017].

Chapter

3 Communication

1 Principles of communication

1.1 Learning objectives

By the end of this section you will be able to:
- identify the different reasons why people communicate
- explain how communication affects relationships in the work setting
- describe the factors to consider when promoting effective communication
- explain how people from different backgrounds may use and/or interpret communication methods in different ways
- identify barriers to effective communication
- explain how to access extra support or services to enable individuals to communicate effectively.

1.2 Introduction

Communication will be at the core of your role in your day-to-day management of patients and when attending incidents. As inter-personal communication forms such a fundamental aspect of our daily lives we rarely stop to think about how we do it. But, as will be discussed throughout this chapter, effective communication, especially in a high-stress environment, is a skill that requires development and practice.

Poor communication is the leading cause of complaints for healthcare organisations, including the NHS [NHS Digital, 2017]. The World Health Organization (WHO) recognises that communication is a key aspect of improving medical safety; poor communication has previously been responsible for disastrous medical and surgical errors, including the removal of incorrect organs and limbs [WHO, 2009b].

As a health professional, effective communication will be a key standard against which your employer will expect you to perform. For registered professionals, including paramedics, being able to communicate effectively is one of the fundamental standards of registration [HCPC, 2014].

1.3 Who will you be communicating with?

Over the course of one day at work, you are likely to communicate with many different people, who may include:
- service users
- other health and care professionals
- colleagues
- members of the public
- staff in the EOC
- other professional services (police, fire, etc.).

This communication is likely to take place through a variety of methods including:
- verbal
- body language
- written
- electronic written (e-mail or electronic patient record)
- radio
- telephone.

This will often be under pressure or personal stress, where poor communication or misinformation can have a detrimental effect on patient outcomes. Therefore, mastering communication in the emergency environment is a core skill of any ambulance practitioner.

1.4 Basics of communication

Traditionally, communication has been regarded as the sending of a message from one person to another (Figure 3.1) [Corcoran, 2013]. The sender (person A) has a message they wish to pass to the receiver (person B). The message exists within the consciousness of the sender initially; they then

Chapter 3 – Communication

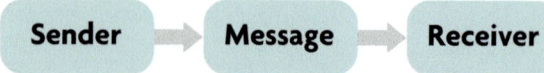

Figure 3.1 Basic model of communication.

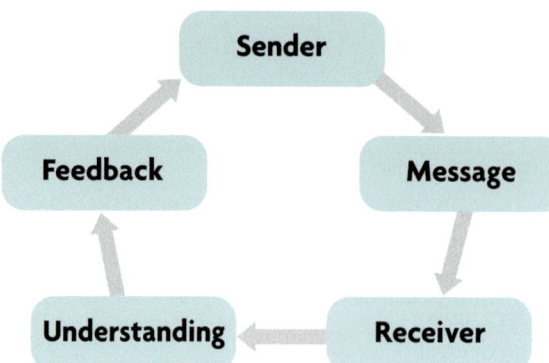

Figure 3.2 Modified model of communication.

decide how to pass on that message. Before it can be passed it must be 'encoded'. This encoding may be the selecting of certain words, certain emphasis during part of the sentence or other verbal or non-verbal features. The receiver must then 'decode' the message as they receive it and try to interpret the original message from all the verbal and non-verbal information they have received. Clearly, this model is not sufficient in healthcare, as it implies a one-way communication, not the two-way communication that is essential for providing best care to patients.

A revised model which would be more appropriate includes the variables of understanding and feedback, which forms a cyclic process (Figure 3.2). This inclusion of checking the understanding of the message given, and receiving feedback, is fundamental to ensure that messages have been understood in the way in which they were intended [Corcoran, 2013].

This is particularly important in high-stress situations or when communicating information which may not be easily understood (such as a medical history) to ensure that the correct message has been received and understood. In these situations, it is very easy for a message to be misinterpreted, with potentially disastrous consequences.

1.4.1 Verbal skills

Verbal communication can be divided into two broad areas [Blaber, 2008]:
- language and vocabulary
- paralinguistic features of communication.

Language and vocabulary

Working in healthcare, you must be able to adjust your language and vocabulary so that it is suited to the person you are communicating with. When communicating with colleagues and other health professionals, you will need to use more complex and professional language. However, there will be times when you need to adjust to communicate with those who have a narrower range of language skills, which may include children or those with cognitive impairment, such as dementia patients or those with learning difficulties.

Guidance for ensuring clear verbal communication includes the following:
- Do not try to say too much at one time; people can only process a certain amount of new information at once.
- Avoid using jargon.
- Speak in a clear manner and be as concise as possible.
- Frequently check that what you are trying to communicate is being understood.
- Think about what you want to say and then consider the easiest way to communicate that to someone else.
- Do not use overly complex language to try and appear knowledgeable; lots of medical language can be complicated and similar-sounding words have different meanings, which if used incorrectly can cause confusion, e.g. dysphasia (difficulty with language) and dysphagia (problems with swallowing).

Paralinguistic features of communication

Paralinguistics refers to the modification of the way in which we speak and place emphasis in communication. This includes:
- volume
- rhythm

Principles of communication

- pitch
- pace
- tone.

1.4.2 Non-verbal communication

Non-verbal communication can have a dramatic impact on the message you are sending and the way that it is then interpreted. It can be possible to communicate entirely by non-verbal means, especially if you know the person well [Blaber, 2008].

Examples of non-verbal communication include:
- eye contact
- facial expression
- gesture and posture
- personal space and touch.

All of these should be used in a manner that is appropriate to the situation. For example, when gathering a history from a patient, if your head is down and you are writing as they speak, the patient may get the impression you are not paying attention to them and might leave out key details. In contrast, if you are making eye contact, nodding your head and acknowledging their communication with small verbal cues, such as 'OK' and 'yes' as they are speaking, known as active listening, they are more likely to continue communicating and reveal all the information you need in order to assess them properly.

Equally, you should observe the body language of those you are communicating with. If the person you are talking to looks as though they are becoming increasingly agitated and frustrated, you should respond to this visual reaction and change the conversation or method of communication.

1.4.3 Written communication

It is likely that every patient contact you have will involve some form of communication, most commonly as part of the patient record, but may include writing to other healthcare professionals.

It is important that all written communication is neat, legible, concise and follows a logical structure. Completing patient clinical records will become a routine part of your role and something you will need to master based on your local record-keeping procedures, but some general guidelines include the following:
- Avoid unnecessary abbreviations.
- Ensure that your writing is legible and has transferred through to the copy if carbon paper is being used.
- Diagrams can be beneficial, but these need to be clear and labelled appropriately.
- Ensure you follow a structure; most organisations use some form of standardised 'medical model' to aid this.

1.5 *Social context*

Communication relies heavily on the social context in which it takes place. Consider the following two scenarios and how the changing social context may influence how you communicate:
- **Scenario A:** You attend a small child who has fallen and injured their wrist. As part of your assessment you need to look at the wrist, but the child is wary of letting you get close, due to fear that you will cause more pain.
- **Scenario B:** You are called to give evidence in court at the case of a serious assault you attended. You are placed in the witness box and asked a series of questions by the prosecution, prior to cross-examination by the defence.

In both these scenarios, effective communication is critical to ensure that others receive the message you intended to send. However, the way in which you communicate these messages will be very different. Your role is to ensure you encode the message, using both verbal and non-verbal features of communication, in such a way that it is likely it will be decoded in the manner you intended.

This concept extends well beyond the extreme examples cited above and into your daily role as a healthcare provider. Every day, you will meet people from a wide range of social and cultural backgrounds. Every one of these people will have a different social context in which they exist, and you will need to be mindful of modifying your communication, based on the needs of the individual, to ensure that accurate messages are passed on and misunderstanding does not occur.

1.6 Barriers to communication

Barriers to communication are anything that influences your ability to effectively pass on and receive back the message you need. You will frequently encounter difficult-to-manage barriers to communication and will need to think of ways of dealing with them. Here are some examples of barriers to communication and how they can be overcome [RCN, 2018].

- **Sensory problems:** Many patients will have sensory impairments to their hearing, sight or speech, making communication more challenging. Speak slowly; listen carefully. Don't shout at someone who has a hearing impairment – just pronounce your words clearly and make sure the person can see your lips. Use communication aids such as hearing aids and think about alternative methods of communication such as writing things down.
- **Language:** You will inevitably meet people with whom you cannot communicate in their native language. Many simple issues can be communicated through imitating and actions – such as eating and drinking. For more complex messages, using a family member as a translator can be helpful. Alternatively, your service may have provided you with other tools such as phrase books or access to Language Line, a telephone service that provides translators for a wide range of languages over the phone.
- **Emotions:** You will frequently encounter patients and situations where those involved are experiencing extreme emotions. At these times people are less able to understand what is being said to them or asked of them. Using your verbal and non-verbal skills of communication will be key here to ensure clarity of message.
- **Age:** Young patients in particular will need to be communicated with in a way that is suitable to them and that they can understand. Using pictures, drawings and other props can be an effective means of overcoming barriers to communication.

This is just a short list of examples of barriers that you may experience in communicating. It is worth noting that whenever you adapt your communication to overcome such difficulties there is an increased risk of your message being misinterpreted, so you should make doubly sure that what you wanted to communicate is the message the person has received.

As with all elements of your practice, you should constantly reflect on your communication skills to learn from both positive and negative experiences in order to continue improving your abilities in this fundamental skill of clinical practice.

1.6.1 Clarify misunderstandings

In the emergency and urgent care setting it is inevitable that, at times, you will be communicating large quantities of information in a short space of time. Due to the emotions that are frequently present in scenarios that accompany emergency situations, it is inevitable that misunderstandings can develop. To combat this, you should:
- observe for non-verbal cues that the person you are talking to has not understood what you are trying to communicate
- confirm the person understands what you are saying to them
- repeat what you are trying to communicate in a different manner if you suspect misunderstanding.

Misunderstandings can be costly and lead to treatment errors, including serious mistakes such as drug errors, which can ultimately harm or even kill a patient. If you are ever not sure, then ask; you may be very relieved that you did!

1.7 Summary

Communication is a natural skill that we all use on a daily basis. However, in your frontline role you will routinely be faced with challenging and demanding communication scenarios. To help overcome these, having an understanding of the theory of communication and a strong working knowledge of what resources are available to you locally will be helpful. You will also need to be adaptive, creative, responsive and innovative in overcoming barriers to communication on a daily basis. Only when you can overcome barriers can you be sure of providing the right care to your patient.

Long after your patients have forgotten what you did for them, they will remember the way in which you went about doing it. Communication may be one of the most frequently received complaints for healthcare services, but being treated with care and compassion, and effectively communicated with, is also one of the most frequently praised attributes of individual health professionals.

2 Practical communication

2.1 Learning objectives

By the end of this section you will be able to:
- explain the importance of clear, concise reporting of findings to the clinician
- explain the importance of recording patient observations
- describe the procedure for clinical handover to medical professionals
- describe a structured approach to breaking bad news.

2.2 Record keeping

In your role, it is likely that you will frequently need to undertake examinations and record observations. Keeping accurate records and gaining accurate observations is critical to safe patient care as it forms a part of the continuity of their care. Changes in observations can indicate a deteriorating or improving patient, so if there are errors in the recorded observations it can create a false perception of the patient's changing state of health.

The following tips will help to ensure patient safety when undertaking this part of your role:
- Pass on, or record, all the information you obtain (even if you are not sure of its relevance) to the clinician responsible for the patient's care.
- If you are asked to undertake procedures, observations or interventions that are outside your skill set, politely inform the responsible clinician that you are not able to do this.
- Make your supervising clinician aware if you are struggling or unsure.
- Never fabricate, estimate or make up observations; doing so not only exposes the patient to risk, but would also be considered unprofessional conduct when discovered.

2.3 Handover

The process of a handover is passing on the care of your patient to another healthcare provider(s). During handover, all information relevant to the care of the patient should be provided in a concise and effective manner.

You may, on occasion, be required to undertake a handover, whether it be to hospital staff, GPs or anyone from the vast range of clinicians or other services involved in the provision of care to your patients. It is well recognised that handovers are a high-risk aspect of a patient's care, where important information can be forgotten or missed out [BMA, 2014a]. This can lead to errors or omissions on the part of the receiving clinician and then harm to the patient as a result.

This risk of error is increased in high-stress situations where patients are critically ill or injured; just the time when that information needs to be passed on accurately.

There are many models to help facilitate clinical handover and thereby reduce the risk of key information being forgotten. It may be necessary to use different models in different circumstances. You should use your organisation's preferred models as they will be familiar to your colleagues and the other health professionals you come into contact with. Two that are particularly common are SBAR and ATMIST.

2.3.1 Medical handover

SBAR is usually the most appropriate tool when conducting a handover of a patient whose primary concern is a medical problem [NHS Institute for Innovation and Improvement, 2010]:

S: Situation
- Identify yourself and your role.
- Identify the patient by name and the reason you have come into contact with them.
- Outline your concerns.

B: Background
- Describe the reason the patient has called for help.
- Describe the history of the presenting condition.
- List any other pertinent information about the patient's background, which may include: medical history, previous illnesses, current medications, allergies, social situation, etc.

A: Assessment
- Relate details of the patient's vital signs.
- Pass on your clinical impressions and concerns.

R: Recommendations
- Explain what you need – be specific about the request and timeframe.
- Make suggestions.
- Clarify expectations.

In some scenarios you may not need to make a recommendation. For example, if you are handing a patient over in an ED resuscitation bay, it is unlikely you will need to make recommendations to the medical team. However, if you are giving a verbal handover to a GP on the phone, you may describe what you think is the most appropriate next step for the patient. If the GP agrees, you will need to clarify what you need to do and what the GP will be doing as part of the ongoing care of the patient.

2.3.2 Trauma handover

The UK Ambulance Services Clinical Practice Guidelines recommend the use of the ATMIST model as a quick and easy way of conducting a handover for trauma patients [JRCALC, 2019]:

A: Age of patient (include a date of birth, if you know it)
T: Time of incident
M: Mechanism of injury
I: Injuries sustained
S: Signs and symptoms
T: Treatment given/immediate needs.

Other principles to consider when conducting a handover include the following:
- Make sure the person to whom you are handing over is the person responsible for the patient's care.
- Have your handover ready: make notes in advance to help if necessary.
- Make it concise: you will have a very limited period of time (often less than 60 seconds) in which to provide a handover, especially for the critically ill and injured patient.
- Make sure you have everyone's attention prior to beginning your handover.
- Provide written copies of all information as well as a verbal account whenever you hand over the care of your patient.

2.4 Pre-alert

When transporting a critically unwell patient to hospital, it is routine practice to call the hospital in advance and provide a pre-alert. Different hospitals will use pre-alert in different ways and you should be familiar with local expectations. Providing a timely pre-alert allows the hospital to prepare for your arrival. For example, if you are bringing in a major trauma patient, it is common for a 'trauma call' to be placed, as this will gather all the correct medical experts in the ED waiting for your arrival.

A pre-alert can be provided via phone or radio. It will follow the same models used for handover, although it should also include an estimated time of arrival (ETA). This ETA should be given in a time format, e.g. 'We will arrive at 13:30' and should include the transport method, e.g. ground ambulance or air ambulance. Wherever possible, it should be the person directly caring for the patient that provides the pre-alert and not passed via a third party such as the EOC.

2.5 Breaking bad news

At some point, you will inevitably have to break bad news to patients, relatives or friends of patients. This may be after an unsuccessful resuscitation attempt, for example.

Breaking bad news can be a difficult and very emotive issue. To help prepare yourself for when you need to break bad news, consider the **SPIKES** mnemonic below [Baile, 2000]:

- **Setting up:** Consider what you can do in preparation so that the situation goes as smoothly as possible. Do not begin the conversation until you have a plan for what you are going to do. Consider what you are going to say. Turn off or silence your radio and consider how the person or people may react to the news; be prepared to manage this.
- **Perception:** When you begin, try to gain an understanding of what the person thinks is going on already. Often patients or relatives will have good insight into a situation and the bad news will not come as a shock. However, sometimes they will not, and these can be particularly challenging scenarios to manage.
- **Invitation:** As the conversation is progressing, find out how much the person wants to know. Most people want to know a lot of detail, but this is not always the case.
- **Knowledge:** Remember you may be speaking to someone who does not fully understand the situation. Avoid using complex medical language. Try to speak in a way that matches their communication. Most importantly, be sensitive, honest and informative.
- **Emotions and empathy:** Use empathetic statements to respond to emotions. Do not rush to provide reassurance that you cannot be sure will happen. Statements such as 'It will all be OK' are not necessarily helpful and can give false hope.
- **Strategy and summarise:** Summarise the situation and come up with concrete next steps for what the person needs to do so that they are not in doubt or confused. Continue to clarify using statements such as 'Does this make sense to you?' or 'Are you clear about what to do next?' until you are satisfied that they understand.

Breaking bad news can also be difficult on you, so remember to talk to colleagues afterwards or seek help managing your own emotions.

3 Electronic communication devices

3.1 *Learning objectives*

By the end of this section you will be able to:
- describe the different forms of electronic communication that may be used by ambulance services
- explain the procedure for communicating via radio.

3.2 *Introduction*

Effective communication is essential to being able to deliver patient care. In order to do this, you are likely to come into contact with a range of electronic communication technology, including:
- radios
- mobile data terminals (MDTs)
- electronic patient clinical records.

Your employing organisation should train you how to use the specific equipment that they have, but below you will find some general information on these systems.

3.3 *Radios*

Most ambulance services use radios in one form or another as a key means of communication and it is likely you will use the device frequently (Figure 3.3).

All NHS ambulance services and some private providers use radios on the Airwave network. This network is a digital, encrypted system allowing for secure communication between ambulance staff, control rooms and other emergency services [Airwave, 2019]. The project to move to Airwave radios was a response to criticism following the 7/7 bombings, during which old analogue radio systems severely hampered effective communications.

As well as providing enhanced communications, these radios form a part of your personal protective equipment (PPE) as they have an emergency button on them that you can depress when in danger. This

Chapter 3 – Communication

button will alert the EOC that you are in difficulty and will allow them to listen in on your situation to decide how best to help.

The Airwave network has extensive coverage across the whole of the UK, but, as with all mobile networks, there are areas where the radios will not work. You may become aware of areas that are 'black spots' and should have a plan of how to communicate with the EOC in the event of losing signal. Various options for doing this may be available. On some vehicles, it is possible to set the vehicle-mounted radio as a 'booster' for the hand portables; this can often boost signal strength significantly.

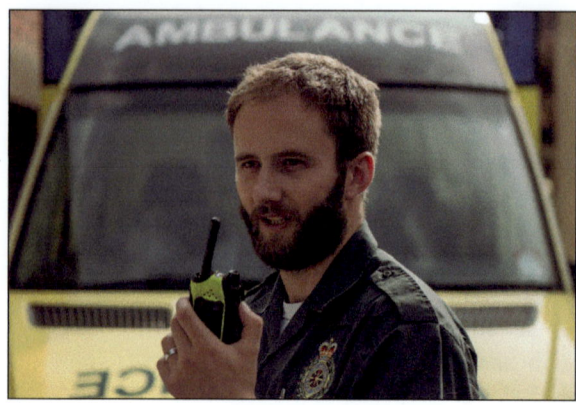

Figure 3.3 Communicating by radio.

3.3.1 Radio security

The new generation of radios use encrypted technology, meaning that no one can 'eavesdrop' as used to be possible with old radio scanners. This significantly increases the security of communications. However, it means that each radio becomes a potential security threat.

Although radios can be remotely disabled, if they fell into the wrong hands it would be possible to monitor the response of the emergency services to incidents; this would be particularly dangerous in the case of a major incident following a terrorist attack. To avoid radios falling into the wrong hands, their use and security should be closely guarded. When not in use, radios should be securely stowed in vehicles or on stations, in line with your employer's guidelines. If you lose a radio as part of your duties, you should immediately report this, either to your line manager or your communications hub, so it can be remotely disabled.

3.3.2 Use of radios

Your employer will train you in the use of the radios they use, but below are some general good practice guidelines for the use of radios for communication:
- **One person speaks:** Unlike on a mobile phone, only one person at a time can talk on a radio, so check frequently with the person you are talking to that they are receiving your message.
- **Be concise:** Often several people will share the same radio channel or be trying to talk to the same person (the EOC, for example) so keep your messages as concise as possible so as not to jam up the line.
- **Be clear:** Radios often distort sounds, especially if the receiving party has a poor signal; speak slightly slower than usual, in a normal tone of voice.
- **Consider security:** Think about who could be listening to your broadcast; do not pass sensitive or confidential information over the radio unless you are authorised to do so.
- **Know your call sign and the call sign of the person you are speaking to:** When making a call, you should use the call sign of the person you are calling, followed by your call sign. For example: *'Control, this is Alpha two six, come in, over.'*

Certain phrases that have specific meanings may be used when talking via the radio (Table 3.1).

When spelling out words, use the phonetic alphabet to avoid confusion of letter sounds:
- **A:** Alpha
- **B:** Bravo
- **C:** Charlie
- **D:** Delta
- **E:** Echo
- **F:** Foxtrot
- **G:** Golf
- **H:** Hotel

Electronic communication devices

- **I:** India
- **J:** Juliet
- **K:** Kilo
- **L:** Lima
- **M:** Mike
- **N:** November
- **O:** Oscar
- **P:** Papa
- **Q:** Quebec
- **R:** Romeo
- **S:** Sierra
- **T:** Tango
- **U:** Uniform
- **V:** Victor
- **W:** Whiskey
- **X:** X-Ray
- **Y:** Yankee
- **Z:** Zulu

3.4 Mobile data terminals

Mobile data terminals are vehicle-mounted systems that act as a text communication system between an ambulance and the EOC. There are many different types available, but generally they:
- display address and clinical details of incidents you have been dispatched to
- act as a way of sending text messages/status updates back to control
- communicate with the on-board satellite navigation system so that it is automatically set to navigate to the address of an incident.

3.5 Electronic patient records

It is increasingly common for ambulance services to move away from paper records in preference of electronic patient clinical records (EPCRs). The advantages of these systems are:
- data is far more secure on the electronic patient records than on paper copies, which can be misplaced or lost
- it is easier to perform audits on records completed electronically
- it should be possible to securely send information about your patient either to hospital or to other healthcare services
- it is possible to access historic records or summary care records for any patient you are attending, giving you far more information about their medical history.

Table 3.1 Phrases to use when communicating by radio.

Phrase	Meaning
Go ahead	Indicates you are ready to receive a message
Wait one	I need to pause for a few seconds
Stand by	Acknowledge the other party, but you are not able to reply immediately
Negative	No
Affirmative	Yes
Say again	Repeat last message
Over	You have finished your message and are ready for the other party to reply
Out	The conversation between you and the other party has finished and others can now use the same channel
Copy	You have understood the message
Wilco	You 'will comply' with the broadcast message
Come in	You are requesting priority over other radio traffic as you have an urgent message
Priority	Indicates your message is urgent and you should be allowed to broadcast before other routine messages
So far?	When broadcasting a longer message, you should stop periodically and check if the person is receiving the message clearly

Chapter 4 Legal, Ethical and Professional Issues

1 Being a healthcare professional

1.1 Learning objectives
By the end of this section you will be able to:
- explain what it means to have a duty of care
- explain how duty of care contributes to the safeguarding or protection of individuals
- describe potential conflicts or dilemmas that may arise between the duty of care and an individual's rights
- describe how to manage risks associated with conflicts or dilemmas between an individual's rights and the duty of care
- explain where to get additional support and advice about conflicts and dilemmas
- explain how to respond to complaints
- explain the main points of agreed procedures for handling complaints
- define duty of candour
- explain expectations about your work role as expressed in relevant standards
- explain the importance of reflective practice in continuously improving the quality of service provided
- describe how your values, belief systems and experiences may affect working practice
- explain how a working relationship is different from a personal relationship
- describe different working relationships in health and social care settings
- describe why it is important to adhere to the agreed scope of the job role
- explain how and why person-centred values must influence all aspects of health and social care work
- explain why it is important to work in partnership with others.

1.2 Introduction
This section will describe what it means to be a healthcare professional, with a focus on:
- values-based healthcare
- duty of care
- scope of practice
- standards
- complaints
- reflection.

1.3 Values-based healthcare
Working as a healthcare professional is an extraordinarily privileged role. As an ambulance clinician, you will often be caring for people when they are at their most vulnerable. The majority of people have less than a handful of contacts with the ambulance service throughout their lifetime so, when they do call during extreme life events, patients will look to you for help, guidance and support in whatever situation they find themselves. Being in this privileged role, it is important to recognise that you should be patient-focused and the attitudes and beliefs that you hold can influence the care you provide to your patient.

1.3.1 County Hospital, Stafford
County Hospital in Stafford is an acute hospital that became the focus of a national outcry about standards of care. Following concerns raised by the families of patients around poor standards of care and further concerns around unusually high mortality rates, especially for emergency admission patients [Cure the NHS, 2014], the Healthcare Commission (HC) conducted an investigation in 2008 looking into care at the hospital. This uncovered deficiencies

at virtually every stage of the pathway of emergency care [HC, 2009].

The resulting public inquiry and report, widely known as the Francis report, painted a damning picture of a place where there were fundamental failures of care. These included [Francis, 2013]:
- Patients were left in excrement-soiled bedclothes for lengthy periods.
- Patients who could not eat without help were not provided with assistance.
- Water was left out of reach of patients.
- Staff treated patients and those close to them with what appeared to be callous indifference.

Although a definitive number has never been published, it is suspected that hundreds of patients died unnecessarily and thousands more suffered as a result of poor care.

The final report made 290 recommendations in total, many of which have been adopted nationally. A number of other reports have since been published looking at improving care within the NHS, but perhaps the most influential is that conducted by the National Advisory Group on the Safety of Patients in England [NAGSPE, 2013]. This review made a number of key recommendations including:
- The NHS should continually and forever reduce patient harm by embracing wholeheartedly an ethic of learning.
- Patients and their carers should be present, powerful and involved at all levels of healthcare organisations from 'wards to the boards'.

Not only does this philosophy make the NHS an organisation that learns from and builds on its errors, but it puts the patient at the core of all activities. Health professionals must always apply a culture of compassionate care when looking after patients, a culture that is best summarised by the 6 Cs (Figure 4.1) [NHS England, 2019a]:
- care
- compassion
- competence
- communication
- courage
- commitment.

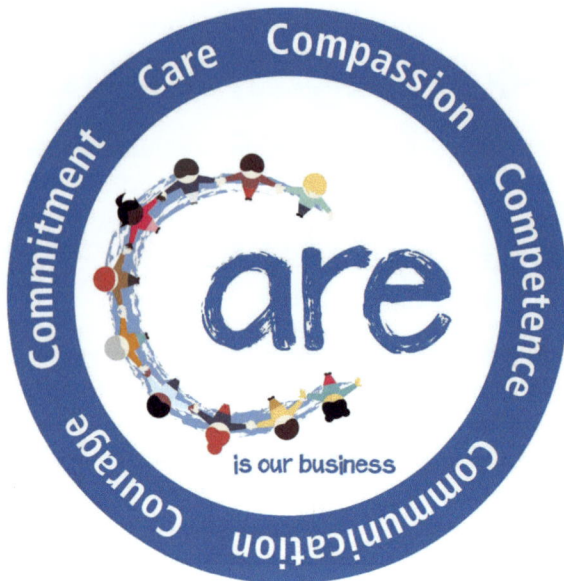

Figure 4.1 The 6Cs describe the core values of a caring, safe and effective healthcare culture.
Source: NHS England, 2019: https://www.england.nhs.uk/leadingchange/about/the-6cs/.

1.3.2 What influences your values and attitudes?

There are multiple aspects that influence our own attitudes, but understanding this and understanding how our attitudes have an impact on the management of our patients is an important distinction to make. Everyone harbours pre-judgements about certain people or groups of people. These can be positive or negative and these stereotypes are used as a form of mental shortcut [Paul, 1998]. However, this can also be dangerous, as it can lead to judgements being made about people based on limited information. These judgements can even influence the way in which a patient is treated, which in turn can lead to errors.

Consider the following scenario:

You are working a Friday night shift in a busy urban setting. It's 03:00 and for the last three hours you've attended four different patients, all of whom are worse for wear through the consumption of alcohol. You're overdue your meal break and are beginning to run low on fuel, but the emergency operations centre has just allocated you to attend a 20-year-old male who is lying on the pavement outside a city-centre nightclub. On arrival, you are greeted by a crowd of his friends, who tell you that it is his birthday, he (and they) have been drinking excessively during the evening and he is known for being a 'lightweight'. It appears the alcohol has got the better of him. The senior clinician quickly checks him out; there are no signs of injury, so he advises the man's friends to call a taxi and take him home.

Is there a risk of stereotyping influencing your practice in this scenario? The answer is almost certainly yes, particularly if you approach the incident thinking 'here we go again', wondering how long it will be until you get your meal break, and whether you will make it to the fuel station before running out of diesel. If you think in this way, you are not focused on how best to care for your patient.

Alcohol consumption can mask a range of conditions, which, if not carefully looked for, can easily go unnoticed. If you attend multiple drink-related incidents in the course of one shift, your brain will naturally want to shortcut or apply a stereotype ('they're just drunk'), especially if you are hungry, tired and late for a rest period.

Stereotyping in this manner is natural and to a degree unavoidable, but you should be aware of the impact it has on you and mentally check yourself frequently to make sure that biasing factors are not adversely affecting your decision-making.

1.4 *Duty of care*

Duty of care is a civil law concept within the UK and exists to ensure that one party does not allow unreasonable harm or loss to occur to another [Dimond, 2015]. This concept is mainly established from case law and two key cases you should make yourself familiar with are *Caparo Industries plc v Dickman* and *Donoghue v Stevenson*.

As a healthcare professional, you owe a duty of care to your patient from the point at which they are accepted as a service user [HCPC, 2016]. From that point onwards, you must act in a way to prevent harm where a reasonable person could see that harm might occur. If you breach this duty of care and someone suffers as a result, this can lead to the civil wrong of negligence.

This duty of care and responsibility to act in such a way as to avoid harm occurring to patients forms one of the fundamental principles that guides the NHS and can be found within the NHS Constitution [DoH, 2015a]. Upholding your duty of care is most likely a condition of your contract of employment and a standard of registration for registered clinicians.

1.4.1 Duty of care vs patient rights

There will be situations where you perceive that a person's rights come into conflict with you trying to achieve your duty of care. For example, if you attend an intoxicated patient who has been assaulted you may well want to take them to hospital for further treatment. However, the patient may want to go home rather than attend hospital.

In this scenario, it is important to consider whether the patient has the capacity to make such decisions as ultimately, if they do, they can make what you perceive to be a bad decision – see section 3, 'Consent and capacity' later in this chapter.

In such cases, you should document fully what course of action the patient is declining, their reasons for doing so, a capacity assessment and what follow-up treatment or advice you have given.

1.4.2 Negligence

Negligence occurs when duty of care is breached and reasonably foreseeable harm occurs as a result. If a party is guilty of negligence, they can be pursued through the civil courts for damages. There are three stages for negligence to be proven [Tovey, 2008]:
- establish a duty of care
- breach of duty
- the claimant's damage has been caused by the defendant's breach of duty.

Establishing a duty of care is usually straightforward, since as a healthcare professional you owe a duty to any patient you encounter.

Breach of duty occurs when a reasonably foreseeable consequence of a person's action leads to harm. The difficult part to measure in this section is what counts as 'reasonably foreseeable' and this is a point that the courts may have to decide upon. Special legal tests based on the *Bolam* and *Bolitho* cases can be used to determine what is or is not reasonable. In these tests, a body of professional opinion will be consulted to determine whether the actions of a practitioner were reasonable, but they must also stand up to logical analysis [Dimond, 2015].

A claimant must be harmed or suffer a loss in order for a claim to be successful. Normally this will be physical harm, but may also include:
- emotional distress
- loss of income, future earnings or enjoyment of life.

For each harm the claimant alleges they suffered, they must be able to prove it was due to the actions or omissions of the practitioner.

Causation is the final step in proving negligence. It is not enough for a duty of care to exist and for that duty to be breached. That breach of duty has to go on to cause harm and it should be evident that this breach was the cause. Also sometimes referred to as the 'but for' principle, it is applied by asking 'But for the (action or omission) would harm have occurred?' If the answer to this is 'Yes', then negligence is not proven; if the answer is 'No', then it is likely that negligence exists.

There are a number of previous cases that illustrate this principle, including the sad case of *Bolitho v City and Hackney HA*, which can help you to understand this better.

As a health professional, you need to bear in mind the principle of duty of care and always consider whether you are providing care in the best interests of your patient.

1.5 Scope of practice and standards

Your scope of practice will most likely be established by your employer through a series of standards. Such standards are treated as the benchmark for determining whether or not a person is working within their scope of practice and also whether or not they are fit to be a health professional for other reasons.

Standards can cover a wide range of topics, not just clinical skills. It is not possible to list the standards for associate practitioners here, as they will vary from organisation to organisation, but standards for paramedic colleagues are set nationally by the Health and Care Professions Council (HCPC) [HCPC, 2016]. These standards include:
- **Standards of proficiency:** The skills required to do the job.
- **Standards of conduct, performance and ethics:** Ensuring that registered health professionals conduct themselves and their business in an ethical and moral fashion.
- **Standards of education and training:** To ensure that each registrant receives, and the educational institution provides, a satisfactory level of education and training.

You should be aware of the standards expected of you from your organisation and make sure you practise within them. You should not attempt to undertake any activity outside your scope of practice as you are not likely to have the knowledge, skill or experience to do so safely and would therefore be putting the patient and yourself at risk.

What constitutes negligence was outlined earlier. It should be noted that any activity undertaken outside of your scope of practice, and which leads to harm, is likely to be grounds for a claim of negligence.

If at any point it becomes unavoidable for you to step outside your scope of practice, you should report this through the usual reporting mechanisms within your organisation. This is not just to protect yourself, but so that the organisation as a whole can learn from the experience.

1.6 When things go wrong

All ambulance services strive to be a 'no harm' organisation, but it is probably an unavoidable fact that systems as large and complex as modern ambulance services will always have adverse incidents. However, these errors should not lead to patient harm, and lessons should be learnt from mistakes when they occur.

The National Advisory Group on the Safety of Patients in England made recommendations in the light of the Francis report discussed above, advising that the NHS needs to become a learning organisation and that a blame culture should be abandoned in preference for a just and reporting culture, which in turn leads to a learning culture. It is also noted that many failings in the NHS are not down to staff; instead they are caused by poor processes and systems, which in turn lead to errors [NAGSPE, 2013].

All health organisations should learn from mistakes. They should also be promoting a learning culture where staff are not unnecessarily blamed for mistakes and where people feel safe in reporting incidents, even small ones, so that the larger organisation can learn from those incidents. Only when organisations can learn from their mistakes will they be able to prevent events from being repeated, meaning that a well-functioning complaints system plays a major role in service improvement and preventing patient harm.

1.6.1 Failure to achieve standards

This concept of reporting extends to yourself and your own practice as well. You should make it known if you recognise that in the course of your duty you have failed to achieve the expected standards for someone in your role. Different organisations will have different methods of reporting, but most now have a central system for reporting incidents and a dedicated team that deals with those reports.

1.6.2 Complaints

During the course of your duty, it may be the case that someone wishes to make a complaint about you, your colleagues, your organisation or another organisation. This can be challenging, as the natural response is to be defensive, but remember that the principles of a learning organisation, together with opportunities to reflect, should be seen as a way of improving services and should be welcomed as such.

It is likely that your service will have specific guidelines or a policy on handling complaints, which you should be familiar with, but good general guidelines for the actions you should undertake include the following:

- Record facts and pass them on to appropriate people; do not undertake the investigation yourself.
- If someone wishes to make a complaint, take the details and pass them on to relevant parties, or give the person the contact details of the relevant people inside your organisation.
- Do not challenge facts about a complaint; if necessary, this can be done later on, once all the facts have been established.
- Provide contact details so that patients know how to get in touch should they wish to.

If you become involved in an investigation or complaint, you should do all you can to support the investigation. Withholding key information may be seen as a misconduct offence, which is likely to be handled very differently from learning from a genuine error.

1.6.3 Whistleblowing

Improving patient safety relies on staff identifying when things are not right, or when mistakes have been made, so that organisations can learn and prevent similar circumstances from arising again in the future. Whistleblowing is the act of reporting suspected wrongdoing at work. Whistleblowers should be supported and congratulated for speaking up and thereby providing an opportunity to remedy the problem. However, whistleblowers are not always treated fairly by their employers, with instances of bullying and dismissal occurring [Francis, 2015].

Changing an organisation's culture takes time, but all organisations should be committed to embracing a learning culture and taking staff concerns seriously, while treating the staff involved fairly.

1.6.4 Freedom to speak up

Following the findings by the Francis review, NHS trusts were required to implement a Freedom to Speak Up (FTSU) policy [NHS Improvement, 2018]. The purpose of the policy is to outline how concerns should be raised and handled inside NHS trusts. It includes safeguards for staff to protect them from bullying and harassment if they should raise a concern.

Several channels are normally available to raise a concern, including your manager or a formal written reporting process, but each trust should also have a FTSU Guardian. This is a senior person who can be confidentially contacted with concerns you do not feel you can raise with other managers.

You could also raise a serious concern directly with the regulator, most often the Care Quality Commission (CQC), but this should be an option of last resort in most situations. If it was necessary, it would be a sign of a major failure of leadership and the FTSU principle within an NHS organisation.

Ultimately, a culture that supports raising concerns should result in improving patient care and the safety of both patients and staff. Most managers and leaders want to hear concerns so that they can work to improve standards.

1.6.5 Duty of candour

Duty of candour is a direct result of the Francis report and places a legal obligation on healthcare providers to inform a patient if they have been harmed by the provision of healthcare and offered an appropriate remedy, regardless of whether a complaint has been made or a question asked. For healthcare organisations, this is a standard of their regulation by the Care Quality Commission [CQC, 2015].

This extends to you as a healthcare professional. If you believe that the actions you have undertaken have caused patient harm, or may cause harm at some future point, you should report this immediately (through the normal reporting channels) in an open and honest manner. If possible, you should also apologise to the patient at the time. For example, if you were to cause a minor injury to a patient's arm whilst wheeling them out of the house in a chair, then once the injury has been treated, apologise for the mistake.

Do not wait for a complaint to be received or for a question to be asked before highlighting the issue. Ultimately, the longer a lot of mistakes are left, the worse the outcome may be for the patient. It is also likely that any wilful failure to observe your duty of candour would be a breach of your duty of care, contract of employment and conditions of registration, for registered clinicians.

1.6.6 Additional sources of support

Dealing with situations where things have gone wrong can be a challenging time and you may well need further advice and support. In those circumstances, you may find that some of the options below are able to assist you:
- organisational policy
- your line manager
- a Making Experiences Count (or similar) investigation team within your organisation
- Freedom to Speak Up Guardian.

1.7 Reflection

Everyone reflects on a near-constant basis throughout their life, but lending structure to reflection can make it a powerful tool for learning and developing. The ability to reflect critically on one's own performance should be seen as a key skill for any health professional and for many, including paramedics, it is a standard of their ongoing registration that they undertake regular reflection [HCPC, 2016].

There are several models for reflection you can use to help focus your reflective practice. Popular models include Gibbs [1988], Johns [1994] and Rolfe et al. [2001]. Below we will discuss Gibbs, which is a frequently used model within the ambulance service.

1.7.1 Gibbs' reflective cycle

Gibbs' reflective cycle is probably one of the most commonly used models in healthcare reflection (Figure 4.2). This is a simple-to-follow model that invites you to look back on an experience and then consider the different elements in specific stages [Gibbs, 1988]. If applied correctly, you should analyse your actions, in detail, before deciding on what could have been done differently and planning how to implement those changes in your practice.

When undertaking reflection, it is tempting to focus on mistakes exclusively. Although reflecting on errors is a helpful process and provides insight into how to avoid similar mistakes in the future, you should do this not only when things have not gone as you would have liked, but also when things have gone well. It is just as important to identify the good things, so that they can become a part of ongoing practice, as well as those things you may wish to change.

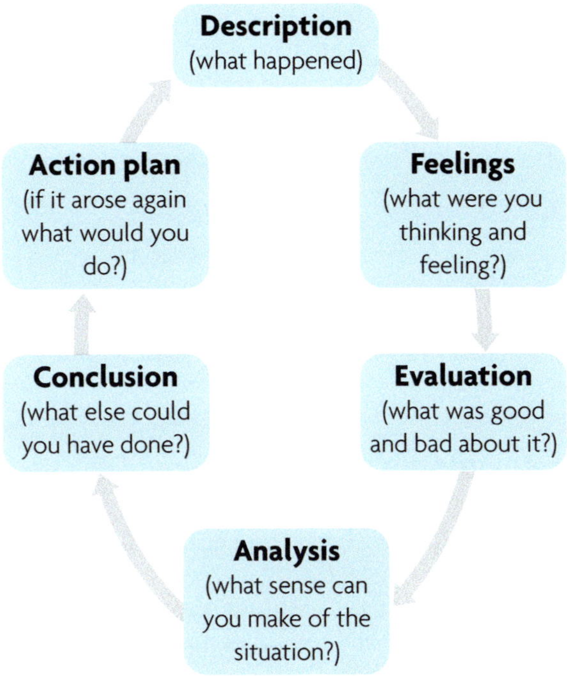

Reflective models such as Gibbs' reflective cycle are primarily intended for formal, written reflections, but this is not always required. A brief chat with your colleagues following a challenging incident may be all that is necessary [Jasper, 2003], though, even in this informal setting, having an idea of the things to discuss can be helped by following the Gibbs process. Gibbs' reflective cycle has six separate stages. Each stage is described below in detail.

1.7.2 Description

This should provide a brief overview of what happened. It needs to be an objective account, i.e. just the facts. Although you need to cover the incident from start to finish, you do not need to elaborate on aspects that you will not discuss further in your reflection. For example, if the journey to hospital was uneventful, then that is all you need to say about it. On the other hand, if the journey to the emergency department was the most important part of the incident, then you will need to say more. If this reflection is going to be read by someone else, you need to alert your reader to the aspects of the incident you intend to discuss (i.e. flag important points). It may help to use some of the following questions [Jasper, 2003]:

- Where were you?
- Who else was there?
- Why were you there?
- What were you doing?
- What were other people doing?
- What was the context of the event?
- What happened?
- What was your part in this?
- What parts did other people play?
- What was the result?

1.7.3 Feelings

Recall and explore the things that were going through your mind:

- How were you feeling when the event started?
- What were you thinking about at the time?
- How did it make you feel?

Figure 4.2 Gibbs' reflective cycle.
Source: Gibbs G (1988). *Learning by Doing: A guide to teaching and learning methods.* Further Education Unit, Oxford Polytechnic: Oxford. Available at: https://shop.brookes.ac.uk/product-catalogue/oxford-centre-for-staff-learning-development/books-publications/ebooks/learning-by-doing-a-guide-to-teaching-and-learning-methods-by-graham-gibbs-ebook.

Cycle stages:
- **Description** (what happened)
- **Feelings** (what were you thinking and feeling?)
- **Evaluation** (what was good and bad about it?)
- **Analysis** (what sense can you make of the situation?)
- **Conclusion** (what else could you have done?)
- **Action plan** (if it arose again what would you do?)

- What did other people's actions/words make you think?
- How did you feel about the outcome?
- What do you think about it now?

1.7.4 Evaluation

Evaluation gives you the opportunity to consider what went well and what did not go so well in any experience. This may be based on your own actions or the actions of other individuals or groups. Your reflections here should try to balance positives and negatives. You should be searching for experiences you would repeat in the future and also experiences where, given the opportunity again, you would do things differently. Where possible you should base your evaluations against a standard. For example, you may reflect positively that you treated the patient with chest pain in accordance with the pharmacological section of the JRCALC guidelines.

Relevant questions may include:
- What was good about the experience?
- What would I like to change about the experience?

Be careful when evaluating that you only talk about the events that have occurred. Do not try to explain them or analyse them in detail, or say what you would do differently in the future as that is what analysis and conclusion, discussed below, are for.

1.7.5 Analysis

Analysis should be the largest part of any reflection. In this part of the cycle you get to explore all of the issues that you have highlighted as part of your description, feelings and evaluation. You should now consider these points one at a time and review what made them particularly positive or an area for development. As part of this you should refer back to established academic literature and professional opinion on the relevant topics. You may also want to compare the experience to previous similar situations and consider what was unique about that particular experience that had an impact on your performance.

Questions you should be asking yourself are:
- Why did I take that decision?
- What was influencing my thinking or decision-making at the time?

- How would I do it differently in the future?
- What choices did I make and what impact did they have?

1.7.6 Conclusion

Now you have successfully taken the incident apart, you need to make sense of what you have found out in order to prepare for the next section – the action plan. In addition, you will need to show that you have developed some insight into your own and other people's behaviour in terms of how they contributed to the event.

1.7.7 Action plan

Now you have reassembled the incident, you are in a position to plan for next time. Factors you might like to consider are:
- What do you want to achieve as a result of your action?
- How will you do it?
- When will you do it?
- Where will you do it?
- Who will be part of the action?

2 Provision of healthcare

2.1 Learning objectives

By the end of this section, you will be able to:
- define the right to healthcare
- discuss some common inequalities in healthcare
- describe the concept of person-centred care
- define health promotion.

2.2 Introduction

The World Health Organization (WHO) determines that health is a fundamental right, a principle that is enshrined in law in the UK within the Human Rights Act. The NHS Constitution sets out the rights of patients and the public. Key rights relevant to urgent care outlined in this constitution are [DoH, 2015a]:
- 'To be treated with a professional standard of care, by appropriately qualified and experienced staff, in a properly approved or registered organisation that meets required levels of safety and quality.'

- 'To be treated with dignity and respect, in accordance with your human rights.'
- 'To accept or refuse treatment that is offered to you, and not to be given any physical examination or treatment unless you have given valid consent.'

Everyone in the UK, regardless of age, gender or disability, has the same right to access healthcare. It should therefore follow that life expectancy and health expectancy is uniform. However, that is far from the case.

2.3 Health inequalities

2.3.1 Social factors

Although it may not appear obvious initially, social factors such as class, gender, age, ethnicity, location and education have an impact on a person's health. On average, adults living in the least-deprived areas of the UK can expect to live over 16 years longer in good health than those living in the most-deprived areas [UK Government, 2015].

The Marmot report, published in 2010, covered poverty and inequality in the UK. The report found that not only are people in the most-disadvantaged groups more likely to die earlier, they are also more likely to be living with a long-term condition. Marmot summarises that this is a major challenge for the contemporary welfare system, stating: 'People with higher socioeconomic position in society have a greater array of life chances and more opportunities to lead a flourishing life. They also have better health. The two are linked: the more favoured people are, socially and economically, the better their health. This link between social conditions and health is not a footnote to the "real" concerns with health – health care and unhealthy behaviours – it should become the main focus' [UCL Institute of Health Equity, 2010].

The reasons behind this inequality are complex, but include access to healthcare (more-deprived areas often have a shortage of local services such as GPs), lower education (which can impact on individuals' ability to care for themselves) and more behavioural risk factors such as smoking, inactivity and poor diet [UK Government, 2017a].

2.3.2 Psychology

In addition to social factors, psychology has an impact on a person's health. The cognitive approach outlined by Beck (1961) explains that a person's negative thoughts can prevent them from making positive change in their lives. This explains repeated negative behaviour by patients, e.g. a lung cancer patient who continues to smoke.

2.4 Person-centred care

The concept of person-centred care is a simple one: the patient should be at the core of their healthcare. This means that care should be provided 'with' people rather than 'to' or 'for' them. 'Person-centred care' as a term describes the ethos and approach that enables this to happen. It requires a whole system and team approach [RCGP, 2018a].

'Person' in this context refers to individual patients, but includes their carers and significant support networks if appropriate.

Key aspects of person-centred care include:
- respect for the person's values, preferences and expressed needs
- personalised, co-ordinated and integrated health and social care and support
- equal partnership in the relationship between healthcare professionals and patients
- involvement of family, friends and carers
- continuity of care
- high-quality education and information

2.4.1 Example of patient-centred care

Consider this scenario:

A young woman presents to her GP having heavy periods. She wants some help in managing these, but is also trying to get pregnant. A routine treatment for the management of heavy periods is the prescribing of oral contraceptives, but clearly this would not be appropriate if the patient is trying to get pregnant at the same time. Instead, a different medication, such as tranexamic acid, could be prescribed, which will help with the heavy periods, but does not reduce the chances of pregnancy.

Chapter 4 – Legal, Ethical and Professional Issues

This is a very simple example of patient-centred care, but it is obvious that if the patient was not considered in the whole, the wrong treatment could have been prescribed which would have had a negative impact on the patient's well-being.

2.4.2 Patient-centred care in the ambulance service

Much of the work in the ambulance service is of an urgent or emergency nature, but this does not mean that patients should not be in control of their own care. You should discuss all treatment plans with your patient and work with them to come up with the most appropriate management option for them.

Do not see your patients as just a disease process, or an injury that needs fixing; consider them in the whole. How might your actions have an impact on other parts of their lives? Include the patient in decision-making and not only will they feel more involved, but treatment is also more likely to be successful as the patient will own their treatment and be more likely to ensure it succeeds.

2.5 Health promotion

Health promotion is a strand of the public health discipline and can be defined as 'any activity that improves health status' (Green and Tones, 2015).

A key model of health promotion was published by Tannahill in 2008. The author, working for the public health department of NHS Scotland, categorises health promotion activities into three areas:
- **Health education:** e.g. a poster encouraging people to wash their hands to prevent the spread of flu.
- **Health protection:** e.g. breast cancer screening, cervical cancer smear testing.
- **Illness prevention:** e.g. a campaign to encourage people to wear seat belts.

As an ambulance clinician, you have a responsibility to engage in health promotion where possible. This might be fairly simple activities, such as:
- promoting smoking cessation services
- providing education on appropriate recommended daily allowance of alcohol
- encouraging people to wear helmets when riding a pushbike.

3 Consent and capacity

3.1 Learning objectives

By the end of this section you will be able to:
- assess capacity
- gain consent
- maintain consent
- analyse factors that influence the capacity of an individual to express consent
- describe different ways of applying active participation to meet individual needs
- describe how to support an individual to question or challenge decisions concerning them that are made by others.

3.2 Introduction

In your frontline role, you will regularly have to apply the concepts of consent and mental capacity to your work, often in challenging and confusing situations where a rapid assessment and fast action may be required to determine a defendable and lawful decision.

Having a good understanding of the basic principles will make this easier and help to remove doubt when tackling challenging and potentially confusing scenarios.

3.3 Consent

In the UK, case law has determined that adult patients with mental capacity must give consent before they are touched or treated. Failure to do this leaves the ambulance crew open to civil claims for trespass against the person, which includes assault and battery [BMA, 2018]. Therefore, you must seek valid consent to treat your patient.

3.3.1 Valid consent

In order for consent to be valid, there are three criteria that must be met [BMA, 2018]. These stipulate that:
- **Consent must be given voluntarily:** i.e. Consent must be given free from pressure exerted by relatives, partners, ambulance staff or police officers, etc.

- **Consent must be informed:** The patient must understand what course of action is being proposed, what the benefits and significant risks are, what alternatives are available, and what the consequences are of doing nothing.
- **The person consenting needs to have the mental capacity to do so:** This is usually the patient, but includes someone with parental responsibility for patients less than 18 years of age, or a person who has been given a lasting power of attorney (LPA) or authority by a court to make treatment decisions [DoH, 2009b].

3.3.2 Communicating consent

Communicating consent may take many forms. For elective procedures in hospital, it will often be written. For the majority of time working on an ambulance it will be verbal, but it may take another form, particularly if the patient has a disability that would make written or verbal communication impossible. Other forms that you may encounter include, but are not limited to:
- sign language
- use of props
- blinking
- movement of limbs
- use of technology, such as speech generators.

3.3.3 Best-interest decisions

As a rule, if your patient is over 18 years of age, only they can consent to any intervention. Lying unconscious in the street covered in vomit after consuming a litre of vodka and Red Bull® does not imply consent. Prior to the Mental Capacity Act 2005 (MCA), you would have cared for this individual in the absence of consent as part of your duty of care for the patient and out of necessity in an emergency. Now, this is covered by the Mental Capacity Act whereby you act in the patient's best interests.

3.4 *Mental capacity*

Imagine the following scenario:

It's 02:00 on a Friday morning and you are called to a pub for two males that have been fighting. On arrival, you find a male in his mid-thirties. He has a nasty head wound that will need treating in hospital and is, by his own admission, 'quite drunk' after consuming multiple pints of larger. After examining the wound, he declines to come to hospital with you, suggesting instead he will go home to sleep it off. To you this appears to be an unwise decision but, if he has capacity, he is within his rights to make it. If he does not have capacity, what are you going to do?

Case law has clearly laid out the right of a mentally competent adult to refuse any treatment, including life-saving interventions, regardless of the reason, or for no reason at all. This has now been incorporated into several statutory frameworks. In England and Wales, this framework is the Mental Capacity Act 2005, and in Scotland, the Adults with Incapacity (Scotland) Act 2000. The purpose of this legislation is to protect the rights of individuals from having treatment forced upon them in all but rare circumstances, normally related to the treatment of a mental health condition, but also to protect them in situations when they are unfit to make decisions for themselves.

Central to capacity and consent is the concept of personal autonomy, that is, the right of an individual to 'govern themselves' according to their own set of personal values, preferences, commitments and character traits [Freyenhagen, 2009]. This can come into conflict with an ambulance crew's tendency towards beneficence (i.e. serving the best interests of patients [Moye, 2007]) and wanting to safeguard their job.

Mental capacity is the ability to make a decision and covers everything from when to get up to how much alcohol to drink and whether to go to hospital as advised by the ambulance crew. A lack of capacity is defined as an inability of your patient to make a specific decision at the time they are required to make it, due to an impairment of or disturbance in the functioning of the mind or brain. It does not matter if this impairment or disturbance is temporary or permanent. Examples of a potential impairment include:
- Temporary:
  - post-ictal following a convulsion
  - a diabetic suffering a hypoglycaemic event
  - ingestion of alcohol or drugs.

Chapter 4 – Legal, Ethical and Professional Issues

- Permanent:
  - dementia
  - significant learning disabilities
  - long-term effects of brain damage.

3.4.1 MCA code of practice

All patients have the right of autonomy over decisions relating to their healthcare (in all but a few specific circumstances) if they have the 'capacity' to make those decisions and these decisions are made voluntarily.

The MCA code of practice explains the five statutory principles that need to be foremost in your mind when making capacity decisions [DCA, 2014]:

- A person must be assumed to have capacity unless it is established that they lack capacity.
- A person is not to be treated as unable to make a decision unless all practicable steps to help them to do so have been taken without success.
- A person is not to be treated as unable to make a decision merely because they make an unwise decision.
- An act done, or decision made, under this Act for, or on behalf of, a person who lacks capacity must be done, or made, in that person's best interests.
- Before the act is done, or the decision is made, regard must be had to whether the purpose for which it is needed can be as effectively achieved in a way that is less restrictive to the person's rights and freedom of action.

It is important to note that a person cannot be said to generally have capacity or to lack capacity; instead, capacity relates to a specific decision needing to be made at a specific point in time. For example: a patient with mild dementia may have capacity to make simple decisions such as day-to-day control of their finances for purchasing essential items, but may lack the capacity to make more complex long-term investment decisions. On certain days, when their dementia is particularly bad, they may not have the capacity to make even simple decisions. Capacity varies, especially for those who have an underlying pathology, and you are responsible for making a capacity assessment on your patient at the time you are with them, in relation to the decision they are being asked to make.

Another important consideration is whether a decision can be delayed. If a person is experiencing a temporary disturbance or impairment, it may be reasonably foreseeable that they will regain capacity and can then make the decision for themselves in the future. There are several situations in the emergency setting where this will not be the case, for example patients suffering from stroke or severe breathing difficulties. However, if the decision is not urgent, and the patient is not likely to come to harm as a result of not making the decision immediately, then it should be delayed where possible, pending the return of normal capacity [DCA, 2014].

3.4.2 Assessing capacity

The MCA describes a two-stage test to determine whether your patient has mental capacity. Stage 1 requires you to identify whether the patient has an impairment of, or a disturbance in the functioning of, their mind or brain. If they do not, then you cannot say that the patient lacks capacity under the Act. Stage 2 requires you to determine whether this impairment or disturbance means that the person cannot make the specific decision currently required of them.

Stage 1

Evidence of impairment is required for stage 1 to be positive. Impairments may be temporary or permanent, as discussed above, but impairment must be present before moving on to the next stage. If no such impairment is present, the person will not lack capacity under the Act. If the patient does have such impairment, this does not in itself mean that they lack capacity, but instead the healthcare person undertaking the assessment should progress to stage 2 of the test. Otherwise, you should assume that the patient does have capacity and it is not necessary to undertake stage 2 of the test.

Stage 2

To help define whether a person is unable to make a specific decision there are four aspects to test during stage 2:

Consent and capacity

- **Is the person able to understand relevant information about the decision to be made?**
  Relevant information includes:
  - the nature of the decision to be made
  - the reason why the decision is needed
  - the likely effects of deciding one way or another, or of making no decision at all.

All the information required to cover these three points should be conveyed, in a suitable manner, for the person receiving the information to understand. The healthcare person undertaking the capacity assessment should then check, by whatever means is most suitable, that the patient understands the relevant information:

- **Is the person able to retain the information in their mind for the period of time required to make the decision?** The patient must be able to hold the information in their mind long enough to make an effective decision. The Act makes it clear that being able to retain information for only a short period does not in itself mean that a person lacks capacity; it depends on the complexity of the decision needing to be made.
- **Is the person able to use or weigh information as part of the decision-making process?** To have capacity, a person must have the ability to weigh up information and use it to arrive at a decision. That decision does not have to be the right one in the view of the person undertaking the assessment, but instead the person being assessed must show they have used the information to arrive at their decision. Some patients with brain damage may understand the information, but not be able to use it to arrive at a decision and may make impulsive decisions regardless of the information they have been given.
- **Is the person able to communicate their decision?** A person must be able to communicate their decision, although this does not have to be in verbal or written form.

If the answer to any of these questions in stage 2 is 'No', it is likely the person lacks capacity. If the answer to all is 'Yes', then it is presumed the patient has mental capacity.

3.4.3 Supporting patients with capacity assessments

A person can only be said to lack capacity if all reasonable steps to help them to reach the decision themselves have been made. These may include:
- presenting information in a way that is easy for them to understand
- using illustrations to help describe certain procedures
- exploring alternative methods of communication where possible
- taking time to give the patient the best opportunity to make a decision for themselves
- utilising a relative or carer who understands a particular barrier and how to overcome it.

Capacity in emergency situations

In certain time-critical situations, such as a stroke affecting a patient's speech or understanding, it may not be possible to take the additional time to help the person to make their own decisions, as to do so may lead to the patient suffering harm due to delaying treatment.

In these circumstances, healthcare staff should work on the basis of a patient lacking capacity and should act in their best interests. However, you should still communicate with the patient and keep them informed of what is happening. Work on the principle that only those actions that must be immediately taken are taken, and that other decisions, which can be safely delayed, should be.

3.4.4 Refusal of treatment

For many different reasons, patients will sometimes refuse certain treatments or examinations. As with consent, a patient must have the relevant capacity to refuse a certain treatment or examination. If they lack this capacity, you should continue to treat them under the 'best interests' principle.

It is likely that your employer will have specific guidelines on how to manage patient treatment refusals. However, you should ensure the following as general principles:
- Firstly, confirm the patient has had all the necessary facts required to make a decision. If

Chapter 4 – Legal, Ethical and Professional Issues

they are unaware of any key facts, make these known to them.
- Document all refusals, including why they are making the refusal, if the patient discloses this. Note: patients are not required to disclose why they refuse treatment.
- Explain the potential consequences of a refusal and record this.
- Get the patient to sign a refusal of treatment form, which should be independently witnessed to demonstrate they have not been coerced into their decision.
- Give any alternative treatment options or advice. Refusal of one specific medical examination or intervention is not necessarily the same as refusing all treatments and you may need to explore potential alternatives, even if these are less preferable to your first plan.

Although it can be uncomfortable for healthcare professionals, you should respect a patient's decision and not put pressure on them to accept your advice, even if you think their decision is unwise (GMC, 2018a).

3.4.5 Patients who lack capacity

When a patient lacks capacity, it will become necessary for you to undertake decisions for them in their best interests. This is a significant responsibility and you should always consider that, while trying to safeguard your patient, you limit their rights and freedoms as little as possible for the given situation.

Making 'best interests' decisions

All acts undertaken and decisions made on behalf of a person who lacks capacity should be done in the 'best interests' of that person. Establishing what is in a person's best interests for the management of emergency conditions is usually simple, but there may be occasions where more complex decisions are required. We all have our own attitudes and beliefs, and therefore what we believe to be in someone's best interests may differ from someone else's idea.

When considering what is in the best interests of a person lacking capacity, you should try to make it person-centred, i.e. keep the patient, their wishes, desires and welfare at the core of all decisions, rather than concerns you may have around your own liability. You should particularly attempt to keep the following in mind:
- **Encourage participation:** Do whatever is possible to encourage the person to take part in the decision-making process.
- **Identify all relevant circumstances:** Try to identify all the things that the person who lacks capacity would take into account if they were making the decision or acting for themselves.
- **Consider safeguarding:** Consider what options would be suitable to safeguard a patient, but are least restrictive to their rights and freedoms.
- **Find out the person's views:** Find out as much as you can about the patient's views, such as:
  - past and present wishes and feelings
  - beliefs and values that would be likely to influence the decision in question
  - any other factors the person themselves would be likely to consider if they were making the decision.
- **Avoid discrimination:** Do not make any decisions based purely on discriminating factors such as age, gender, appearance or behaviour.
- **If the decision concerns life-sustaining treatment:** Do not be motivated in any way by a desire to bring about the person's death. You should not make assumptions about the person's quality of life.

In making these decisions, you should specifically consider whether any of the following are present or relevant:
- lasting power of attorney (LPA)
- deprivation of Liberty Safeguards (DoLS)
- independent mental capacity advocate (IMCA)
- advance decision to refuse treatment (ADRT).

Lasting power of attorney (LPA)

Any adult with capacity can register a lasting power of attorney (LPA). This is another person who they appoint to make decisions on their behalf, including healthcare decisions, should they no longer be able to. An LPA must be registered with the Office of the Public Guardian and has wide-ranging powers to make decisions in the event of the patient being incapacitated. You should know there are two forms of LPA: one for health and welfare and one for property and financial affairs. Only an LPA for health and welfare can make treatment decisions.

Deprivation of Liberty Safeguards (DoLS)
DoLS are a way of protecting patients who are necessarily having their liberty deprived to keep them safe and apply to patients that lack capacity and are resident in either hospital or care homes [Alzheimer's Society, 2016]. Liberty they are deprived of may include not allowing them to leave when they wish to do so, medication being administered against a person's will and staff restricting a person's access to family and friends.

In these circumstances, the hospital or care home will apply for a DoLS, stating what liberty they intend to deprive and why it needs to be done to keep the patient safe. If a DoLS is in place, you should be aware of the content and reason for it being instigated.

Independent mental capacity advocate (IMCA)
The IMCA service is designed to support those particularly vulnerable patients who lack capacity and have no friends or family who could be consulted about important decisions the patient is no longer able to make. In these circumstances, an independent person will be appointed and should be consulted on decisions where possible. However, in an emergency, you should continue to work in a patient's best interests if you are unable to contact the relevant dedicated IMCA.

Advance decision to refuse treatment (ADRT)
An ADRT is an order made by a person over the age of 18 years when they still have capacity to refuse specified medical treatment at a future point in time when they may lack the capacity to consent to or refuse treatment.

If faced with an ADRT, you should be confident that it is valid before working to it. For it to be valid, you should, where possible, confirm whether the patient:
- has done anything that clearly goes against their advance decision
- has withdrawn their decision
- would have changed their decision if they had known more about the current circumstances
- has subsequently conferred the power to make that decision to an LPA.

Generally, an ADRT does not have to be written, but if it refers to life-saving treatment then it must fulfil three criteria. It must:
- be in writing
- be witnessed and signed
- state clearly that the decision applies even if life is at risk.

If you believe an ADRT exists, is valid and applicable, then you should follow the instructions contained within it.

3.4.6 Use of restraint

In some rare circumstances, it may be necessary to utilise restraint in order to keep a patient safe when they lack capacity, although this should be a last resort [Mental Health Network, 2014]. The MCA code of practice defines 'restraint' as either of the following:
- use of force, or threatened use of force, to make someone do something they are resisting
- restricting a person's freedom of movement whether they are resisting or not.

Clearly from this description, there is more to restraint than physically holding someone. Shutting and locking the ambulance doors or physically placing yourself in a position so that the patient cannot get out of the ambulance are both forms of restraint, as is verbally threatening to physically restrain a patient if they do not comply. Remember, to do any of this, you must have first demonstrated the patient lacks capacity and is at risk of further harm if you were not to restrain them.

Chapter 4 – Legal, Ethical and Professional Issues

It is only permissible to restrain someone if both of the following conditions are met:
- you reasonably believe that restraint is necessary to prevent harm to the person who lacks capacity
- the amount or type of restraint used and the amount of time it lasts must be a proportionate response to the likelihood and seriousness of the harm the patient faces.

If you restrain someone outside of these conditions, or otherwise deprive them of their liberty, you may face litigation for doing so and you will not be protected by the MCA. This is particularly true if the level of force used is disproportionate. For example, if an elderly patient falls causing a potential, but minor, fracture of their wrist, it would be grossly disproportionate to physically restrain and remove the patient from the property to the ambulance.

Increasingly, ambulance staff are being trained in some forms of restraint. There remains significant variation in this across the country, so you should follow your own local service protocols and training when considering the use of restraint.

Caring for a restrained patient
It is essential that you closely monitor any patient who is being restrained. Be aware of restraint asphyxia and know how to recognise it. If your patient is becoming quiet, it may not be a good sign and you should be continually monitoring (while also considering your own safety) for signs of deterioration. Often patients who are physically agitated can have other physiological processes going on that put them at risk of becoming very unwell very quickly. Sadly, there have been a number of cases where patients have died either as a direct result of being restrained, or because serious conditions were missed whilst patients were being restrained [MIND, 2013].

3.4.7 Further support and raising concerns
Decisions relating to mental capacity are complex and often present during out-of-hours when clinical decision-making support is limited. Know your local channels for support in relevant decision making, which may include:
- clinical supervisors
- colleagues with specialist experience in mental health and capacity
- key workers
- mental health team (particularly if the patient is known to them).
- specialist or advanced paramedic colleagues.

You should also know where patients and families can get further help and support. This will most likely come from:
- mental capacity leads in hospitals, care homes or in a local authority
- charities
- publications, both printed and online.

At times, you may be concerned that a person is having their rights and liberties excessively restricted. In that scenario, you should be prepared to raise a concern on a patient's behalf. You should have local reporting channels, but most likely this will be undertaken as a safeguarding referral to your local organisation safeguarding lead.

3.5 Summary
Decisions relating to capacity and consent can be difficult and often present themselves at the least opportune moment, frequently out-of-hours when other advice and support is limited. These decisions can also be emotive and charged with ethical dilemmas.

Having a good understanding of the law and the principles that accompany these laws is vital and will give you a strong base from which to practise. Remember these key concepts:
- The Mental Capacity Act applies to anyone aged 16 years or over.
- All persons are assumed to have capacity unless shown otherwise.
- A person with capacity has the right to make their own decisions, even if unwise.
- When a person lacks capacity, you should act in their best interests and know what other options for decision-making support may be available.
- For a person with capacity, you must seek consent before giving treatment.

4 Confidentiality and information governance

4.1 Learning objectives

By the end of this section, you will be able to:
- explain the meaning of the term 'confidentiality'
- demonstrate ways to maintain confidentiality in day-to-day communication
- describe the potential tension between maintaining an individual's confidentiality and disclosing concerns
- define information governance
- explain your role in information governance.

4.2 Introduction

All health professionals have a duty of confidentiality to their patients, whereby they must protect all patient information and handle it in an approved manner. This is emphasised in the professional standards for all registered professions, including paramedics [HCPC, 2016], but equally applies to other roles within the ambulance service (see Chapter 2, 'The Ambulance Service'). Failure to follow strict organisation policies and, where relevant, codes of conduct in relation to handling information can be a source of distress for patients and embarrassment for organisations. It can also result in legal or disciplinary action for both organisations and individuals [NHS England, 2018c].

Information governance is broadly defined as the frameworks that organisations have in place to bring together all the legal rules, guidance and best practice that apply to the handling of information. These rules and guidelines include, but are not limited to [NHS Digital, 2018b]:
- the General Data Protection Regulations (GDPR)
- the Code of Practice on Confidential Information
- the Records Management Code of Practice for Health and Social Care 2016
- the Information Security Management NHS Code of Practice.

Within your role, you will routinely have access to confidential, patient-identifiable information. This information, or data, should be protected. This means that you should record, handle and store this information in such a way that you are not likely to misplace any information or accidentally breach confidentiality by making an unauthorised or unnecessary disclosure that could lead to civil or criminal legal proceedings being brought against you or the organisation you work for.

4.2.1 What should be considered patient-identifiable information?

Patient-identifiable information is anything that may enable a patient to be identified, either directly or indirectly [JRCALC, 2019]. This includes obvious personal information, such as name, address, date of birth, etc. However, it also includes less commonly considered things, such as:
- clinical record numbers
- images or voice recordings of a patient
- rare disease information.

Consider the following scenario:

You work in a small town with a population of around 25,000 people. In this town lives a patient who suffers with Addison's disease, a rare endocrine disorder. The patient frequently suffers from attacks due to their condition, and when this happens family members call for an ambulance. You attend this patient suffering an attack one day. As this is not a condition you are familiar with, on returning to the ambulance station you decide to ask colleagues for some information about the condition. You are mindful not to disclose the name or location of the patient (to prevent a breach of confidentiality), but instead describe the incident and ask for advice.

Considering that Addison's is a rare disease and this one person, in a small community, frequently requires ambulance assistance, is it reasonable that on the balance of probabilities your colleagues would be able to identify whom you are talking about, just by describing the condition?

Any information that has the potential to identify the patient, however remotely, should be considered potentially identifiable and managed in such a way as to help avoid a breach of confidentiality from occurring [JRCALC, 2019].

Chapter 4 – Legal, Ethical and Professional Issues

4.3 Maintaining confidentiality

Organisations should have policies in place to describe how they handle information and protect confidentiality. As a healthcare worker, you have a legal obligation to maintain confidentiality so you should have a good working knowledge of these policies [NHS Digital 2018c].

During the course of a working day, it may be necessary to discuss or share patient-identifiable information on a number of occasions. Such occasions may include:
- discussing the care of your patient with another health and social care professional
- handing over the care of your patient to another health and care professional
- requesting support in clinical decision-making for your patient
- contacting other organisations or services to help provide care or support.

These communications can take many forms including:
- face to face
- written
- telephone
- mobile data systems
- e-mail.

Different systems will have different strengths and weaknesses in their security of managing data. Most records in the out-of-hospital setting are recorded either on paper or on electronic patient record devices. Below are some of the security features of each type of storage.

4.3.1 Physical records
- Once completed, physical records should be submitted into a secure storage system.
- Copies of the record are only passed to patients or patients' relatives with permission once completed.

4.3.2 Electronic record-keeping
- All data is transferred and stored securely; no data is left 'hanging around' once it is no longer required.
- No physical copies of records means it is less likely records will be 'misplaced'.
- Records are easily accessed again in the future when required.

Regardless of which system you use, you should consider how best to maintain confidentiality. Your employing organisation should make a copy of its policy available, but some good practice guidelines include [NHS England, 2018c]:

- **Seek consent before sharing information:** Before you share patient information, you should seek consent from the patient to do so. However, in a limited range of situations, it may be appropriate to share information without the patient's consent. Examples include:
  - It is not possible to gain consent.
  - There is a legal requirement to make certain disclosures.
  - It is in 'the public interest' to make a disclosure.
- **Share only that information which is necessary:** If you phone a GP to discuss the care of your patient, it may be necessary to discuss all aspects of the patient, their medical history and the current episode in order to reach an appropriate management plan. In contrast, when you initially phone the surgery and speak to a receptionist, it would not normally be necessary to provide more than a name and address of your patient (so that their notes can be identified) and a brief description of the reasons for your call (so that it can be triaged for priority).
- **Maintain security of information:** Patient information is collected and held in a range of physical and electronic devices, including written records, mobile data terminals, mobile phones, e-mail inboxes and a range of clinical monitoring equipment, such as ECG machines. At all times, consider how the security of this equipment and the data it contains is being managed. If clinical records are completed on paper, where are these stored? If you are working in an ambulance setting, these records should be safely stored, out of view from those looking into the vehicle and in such a manner that they

could not accidentally fall out when a door to the ambulance is opened. Other security measures include:
- Keep the environment secure: lock doors and close windows when a building or vehicle is unattended.
- Log off or 'lock' computers when leaving your desk.
- Delete electronic records on insecure monitoring equipment, in line with local policy, once relevant information has been collected and recorded.
- If it is necessary to share identifiable information via e-mail then you should do so via a secure system.
- When speaking on the phone, have you taken all reasonable steps to ensure you are speaking to the correct person?
- When discussing the care of a patient either over the phone or face to face, could you be overheard? If so, move to a private place where this could not happen.
- Never temporarily place paper clinical records on the roof of a car or similar when checking a vehicle. They have a tendency to fly off and scatter all over the road when you drive off after having forgotten to remove them!

- **Access only the information that you need:** During the working day, you may have access to a wide range of information about a large number of individuals. This access should be used only when you have reasonable grounds to do so. You should not access records or information about incidents or individuals that are not of relevance to you. Most electronic systems have means for monitoring those who access personal information and any unauthorised access will not only likely breach local policy but may also constitute an offence under the General Data Protection Regulations (GDPR).

4.3.3 Further sources of information

Issues relating to confidentiality can be complex and you should know where to turn in order to find further information or support if required. Sources of support in different organisations vary, but may include:
- All organisations should have a policy detailing how they handle information and maintain confidentiality.
- The NHS has a published code of conduct in respect to confidentiality [DoH, 2003].
- All organisations should have a lead of confidentiality, normally an 'information governance manager' or 'data protection officer'. They can be approached with any queries in relation to confidentiality and the handling of data.
- All NHS organisations have a Caldicott Guardian who is responsible for ensuring that standards of confidentiality are maintained and that appropriate information-sharing arrangements are in place [HSCIC, 2014a].
- Larger organisations will have entire information governance teams. These teams frequently have on-call advice available for assisting with urgent queries. The roles mentioned above are normally key parts of information governance teams along with other staff responsible for the storing and processing of records and requests for information.

Making a disclosure
In the course of your role, you may be faced with the need to disclose information to other bodies or organisations. The primary principle here is that, wherever possible, consent should be gained prior to sharing information. However, in certain circumstances, it may be necessary to make a disclosure without that consent [NHS England, 2018c].

Below is an outline of some scenarios where it may be necessary to share information without patient consent [JRCALC, 2019; GMC, 2019]:
- **Police:** The police have the right to personal information (name, address, contact details, etc.) in the detection and prevention of a crime. However, this does not extend to personal health information unless it is part of the investigation or prevention of a serious crime (rape, arson, murder, etc.) or related to terrorism offences. On most occasions, this information

- **can be requested by the police** through locally agreed channels, and only information required immediately in the prevention and detection of crime should be shared by ambulance crews.
- **Local authorities:** A local authority officer who believes a person to be at risk is allowed access to health, financial and other records in order to determine whether any action needs to be taken to protect them.
- **Coroner:** An ethical duty of confidentiality continues after a patient has died, but relevant information should be disclosed to a coroner or similar officer in the investigation of an inquest or fatal accident inquiry.
- **Notifiable diseases:** There is a legal requirement to disclose if a patient suffers from a notifiable disease, even without patient consent. However, patients should still be informed that this has happened.
- **Risk of well-being:** In certain situations, there may be a risk to a patient's well-being by not informing other professionals and/or the relevant authorities; for example, safeguarding concerns relating to vulnerable adults and children.
- **Unable to gain consent:** If a person lacks the capacity to consent to their information being shared, it is possible to share that information which is relevant to the situation. However, information should be shared cautiously; a proxy, guardian or parent should be consulted first, if available.
- **Public interest:** It may be permissible to share information if it is in the public interest. This may be to prevent or detect a serious crime or in cases where others are placed at risk. Examples include:
  - The release of information relevant to serious crimes. For example, if you were to attend an incidence of physical violence and the victim does not want the police contacted, but they or others remain at serious risk of further harm or injury, then contacting the police and giving details without their consent would likely be justified.
  - Releasing relevant confidential information to social services where there is a risk of significant harm to children. In all cases, consent should be sought prior to disclosure unless it is not practical to do so, or it would be inappropriate because, for example, they lack capacity to consent, or they are suspects who should not be informed that they are under criminal investigation.

Services should have policies in place that cover the majority of the above circumstances and these policies should be studied and followed when making a disclosure. In the absence of a specific policy, wherever possible, the organisation's data protection officer/information governance manager/Caldicott Guardian should be consulted prior to releasing information, but this should not be at the cost of endangering patient care due to the delay in passing on information.

4.4 Key points

Remember these key points relating to confidentiality:
- Patients are the owners of information or data relating to them.
- Patient-identifiable information comes in many forms and is communicated in a range of ways.
- Patient-identifiable information should not be shared without consent except in specific circumstances.
- Only share information that is necessary.
- Consider how to maintain security of data in order to prevent accidental disclosures.
- In certain circumstances, it may be permissible to share information without patient consent; you should be aware of these.
- Organisations should have policies in place for protecting information and you should be familiar with these.
- If you require further information, speak to your information governance manager, data protection officer or Caldicott Guardian.

5 Equality and diversity

5.1 Learning objectives

By the end of this section you will be able to:
- explain what is meant by diversity, equality, inclusion and discrimination

Equality and diversity

- explain the links between identity, self-image and self-esteem
- explain the purpose and objectives of the Equality Delivery System
- analyse factors that contribute to the well-being of individuals
- describe the potential effects of discrimination
- explain how inclusive practice promotes equality and supports diversity
- explain how legislation and codes of practice relating to equality, diversity and discrimination apply to your own work role
- describe how to challenge discrimination in a way that promotes change.

5.2 Introduction

Promoting equality should be at the heart of a healthcare organisation's values. It ensures that organisations work in a way that is fair, so that no community, group or individual is left behind. The NHS Equality and Diversity Council [2017] identified three key strategic objectives for the NHS in implementing equality and diversity strategy:

- inclusive workplaces – longstanding equality issues across NHS workplace
- workforce equality – continuous equality improvements
- inclusive healthcare – spearheading best practice for disadvantaged groups.

It is helpful to understand what the terms 'diversity', 'equality' and 'inclusion' mean:

- **Diversity:** This involves recognising and valuing the difference between individuals across groups. Such differences should be seen as 'assets to be valued and affirmed, rather than as problems to be solved' [Thompson, 2006].
- **Equality:** In its simplest form, equality is about being treated fairly. Equality recognises that people are different (diversity), but that those differences do not mean that a person should be discriminated against as everyone should be treated fairly and equally. Equality also recognises that inequality exists and needs to be overcome for a truly fair society.
- **Inclusion:** This means positively striving to meet the needs of different people and taking deliberate action to create environments where everyone feels respected and able to achieve their full potential [NIHR, 2012].

5.3 Equality in healthcare

In 2011, the NHS first launched the Equality Delivery System (EDS), a system designed to help NHS organisations improve the services they provide for their local communities and also to provide better working environments, free from discrimination, for all those working in the NHS [NHS England, 2019b].

In 2013, a new, streamlined version of EDS, EDS2, was launched. The purpose remains the same and the four primary goals of EDS2 are:
- better health outcomes
- improved patient access and experience
- a representative and supported workforce
- inclusive leadership.

At first glance, it may not be obvious how equality and diversity can have an influence on healthcare or influence outcomes. However, various health inequalities do exist [NHS England, 2019c]. Despite significant advances in health and social care in England, people living in the least-deprived areas of the country live around 20 years longer in good health than people in the most deprived areas [Public Health England, 2017].

Issues thought to influence health inequality include:
- employment
- education
- availability and accessibility to healthcare
- housing.

Working in healthcare, you should be doing all you can to ensure the equitable provision of healthcare to all of your patients and supporting your patients to overcome health inequalities where they exist. This may be as simple as helping someone to work out what bus they need to take in order to visit their GP, or may be more complex and involve referring patients directly to various forms of help or support they require.

5.4 Discrimination

Discrimination occurs when someone treats one person less favourably than they would another

Chapter 4 – *Legal, Ethical and Professional Issues*

because of a personal characteristic. This is often due to stereotyping.

Under the Equality Act 2010, it is unlawful for a person to discriminate against another with respect to certain protected characteristics. The nine characteristics are:
- age
- disability
- gender
- gender reassignment
- marriage and civil partnership
- pregnancy and maternity
- race
- religion and belief
- sexual orientation.

As well as the Equality Act, the Human Rights Act 1998 also provides for ensuring certain equalities, including:
- the right to life
- the right to a fair trial
- the right to education
- the right to participate in free elections.

5.4.1 Discrimination in your role

In order to make sense of society and those in it, we naturally group individuals together when they share common characteristics. Based on these characteristics, we may expect people within the group to act in similar ways or to have similar responses to the same situations; this is the process of stereotyping [Judd, 1993].

Using these stereotypes is a natural process as it allows us to 'shortcut' our thinking, but often they are not accurate. Making such shortcuts in healthcare can be dangerous as we will make incorrect assumptions about our patients and fail to challenge our own thought processes.

Applying such stereotypes is probably unavoidable, but we must be prepared to challenge our own thinking and the assumptions made on the basis of that thinking. For example, elderly patients have very varied life expectancies. Some patients may suffer a multitude of medical conditions in their early seventies and therefore have a relatively limited life expectancy, whereas many people will live late into their nineties and beyond with very few medical concerns. If all of these patients were treated the same purely on the basis of their age, you would not be treating patients as individuals and would be likely to provide poor care as a result, potentially even leading to the avoidable early death of a patient. Remember that age is a protected characteristic and it is both unethical and unlawful to discriminate against someone on the basis of one of these characteristics.

Applying the same thought process to all patients is clearly inappropriate and could lead to your making unreasonable, unjustifiable and unethical decisions. You must actively practise treating all patients equally and base your care on their specific circumstances, rather than on those of a group they may fit into.

5.4.2 Challenging discrimination

When you observe signs of discrimination in practice it should be challenged, not least because, in healthcare, discrimination based on stereotypes, whether it be on purpose or unthinking, can lead to patient harm. It can also lead to an uncomfortable or hostile work environment, within which staff and patients are likely to feel threatened, uncomfortable and ultimately not perform at their optimum as a result. If discrimination is allowed to continue unchallenged, it is likely to become a normal part of the way in which an organisation works and be embedded as part of the organisational culture. Therefore, it is essential that people speak up and challenge this discrimination.

Challenging discrimination can be difficult and could lead to conflict if not done in an appropriate manner. Each situation will be unique, so there is no single solution that can be described here. However, some general guidance includes:
- promoting discussion, rather than telling someone they have got it wrong; during discussion, most people will realise their mistakes
- encouraging an open environment, where people can feel safe to discuss a wide range of difficult and complex issues
- providing sources of further information
- avoiding appearing judgemental.

5.4.3 Further support

If you observe serious discrimination, or you are not able to challenge it yourself, then you may need further support in understanding how best to resolve the situation. In this instance, further help would normally be available from your:
- line manager
- organisation's equality and diversity lead.

If a patient wishes to make a complaint in relation to being discriminated against, you should support them in doing this. See section 1.6, 'When things go wrong' earlier in this chapter for information on how to support patients in making complaints.

Remember, you are responsible for promoting equality, recognising diversity and challenging discrimination. Only by doing this will you be able to ensure your patients are receiving the best care possible and you are practising in a non-discriminatory manner. Do not assume that others will tackle the issue.

5.5 Identity, self-image and self-esteem

The way in which we see others is, in part, based on the way in which we see ourselves.

5.5.1 Identity

Your identity is 'what makes you the person you are'. It is normally a collection of characteristics that, when brought together, make you a unique individual. It may include things like your:
- beliefs and values
- outstanding personal attributes
- life goals
- political, social and ethical beliefs
- life experiences that have moulded you.

5.5.2 Self-image

Self-image is similar to identity, but rather than consisting of what goes together to make you, it is about how you see yourself. It may include:
- how you think you look
- what your place is in society
- how you believe others see you and think of you
- what job you have.

5.5.3 Self-esteem

Self-esteem is about how you feel about yourself and your self-image. For example, you may not have the physical attributes you would like to, or you may not be in a job you enjoy or that you feel gives you sufficient status. Although we all have times where we lack confidence, prolonged periods of low self-esteem can have harmful effects on our mental health and our lives [MIND, 2016a].

Being aware of what influences our self-esteem means we can, with time, change it and also support those around us who wish to change their own image or identity.

When dealing with patients, you should bear in mind a person's self-image and be careful not to do anything that may offend or cause unnecessary upset to that image, as to do so may have a harmful effect on that person's psychological well-being and also on your relationship with them.

6 Clinical governance

6.1 Learning objectives

By the end of this section you will be able to:
- define the term clinical governance
- describe why clinical governance is relevant to your role
- outline how you should engage in clinical governance procedures.

6.2 Introduction to clinical governance

Public Health England [2018b] describes clinical governance as: 'the system through which NHS organisations are accountable for continuously improving the quality of their services and safeguarding high standards of care by creating an environment in which clinical excellence will flourish'.

Rather than being a single idea or set of actions, clinical governance and the ethos of improving standards of care should be at every level of health service design, commissioning and implementation. This means the principles of good clinical governance affect everyone from the top of government through to the clinicians and support staff working to deliver patient care.

6.3 Purpose of clinical governance

Five major themes are often identified as key parts of clinical governance [RCN, 2017]. They include:
- patient focus – how services are based on patient needs
- information focus – how information is used
- quality improvement – how standards are reviewed and attained
- staff focus – how staff are developed
- leadership – how improvement efforts are planned.

6.4 How to contribute to clinical governance

In your role, you should strive to deliver the highest possible standards of care to your patients. The following are examples of how you can contribute to high standards of clinical governance in your organisation:

- **Report incidents and near misses:** As discussed above in relation to being a healthcare provider, you have a responsibility to report any adverse incidents or near misses. This is not so individuals can be blamed but so that lessons can be learned to improve future care.
- **Propose and support service improvement:** Working on the front line, you may be able to identify ways in which care can be delivered more effectively and safely. These don't have to be big changes and can be as simple as changing the layout of equipment in bags. Working operationally, you are best placed to identify how small changes could improve patient care. You should approach your management or use a staff suggestion scheme to propose improvements.
- **Personal reflection:** Every incident you attend offers the opportunity for reflection and learning. Earlier in this chapter, we looked at how models of reflection can be used to formally reflect, but not all reflection needs to be in this format. Simply taking time to think about what went well and what you would do differently in a similar situation is a good way to slowly learn and improve your practice.
- **Team reflection:** As well as reflecting personally, you should support and encourage reflections as a team. Bringing together lots of individuals' personal reflections can be a powerful tool, as others will have ideas that have not occurred to you. Your organisation may host 'clinical supervision' sessions to help facilitate this.
- **Support the development of others:** As you gain experience, it is likely that you will be asked to work alongside new staff and those with less experience than you. You should support these people to develop their skills and offer them potential development ideas based on your own experience.
- **Training:** One of the best ways to improve your knowledge and skills is to complete training. This can be formal training, such as your initial training, or less formal training, for example, an online CPD course. You should also be sure to regularly complete refresher and mandatory training, which helps to ensure that your skills are always kept up to date.

5 Safeguarding

1 Safeguarding adults and children

1.1 Learning objectives

By the end of this section you will be able to:
- define the various types of abuse
- identify the signs and/or symptoms associated with each type of abuse
- describe factors that may contribute to an individual being more vulnerable to abuse
- explain the actions to take if there are suspicions that an individual is being abused
- explain the actions to take if an individual alleges that they are being abused
- identify ways to ensure that evidence of abuse is preserved
- identify reports into serious failures to protect individuals from abuse
- identify sources of information and advice about your own role in safeguarding and protecting individuals from abuse
- explain how the likelihood of abuse may be reduced
- describe unsafe practices that may affect the well-being of individuals
- explain the actions to take if unsafe practices have been identified
- describe the action to take if suspected abuse or unsafe practices have been reported, but nothing has been done in response.

1.2 Introduction

Abuse or neglect is a commonly encountered scenario for those working in healthcare. You are likely to be in a key position to identify and assist victims of abuse or neglect. In order to do this, you will need to have a good understanding of the forms abuse can take, the signs and symptoms of those suffering, what increases a person's risk of being a victim of abuse, and also how to get help and support for victims.

Before going further, consider some of the key terms associated with safeguarding:
- **Safeguarding:** Safeguarding is the process of promoting the welfare of individuals and groups and protecting them from harm, often putting controls and measures in place to do so.
- **Protection:** To keep safe from harm.
- **Abuse:** Any action that causes significant harm to an individual.
- **Harm:** Physical or psychological damage or injury.
- **Maltreatment:** Includes all forms of physical and emotional ill-treatment or abuse.

1.3 Learning from previous cases

The vast majority of abuse and neglect happens behind closed doors and rarely reaches the attention of the public. However, over recent years there have been a number of notable cases, including these two examples:
- **Winterbourne View:** In 2011, a BBC *Panorama* programme showed staff at Winterbourne View, a private hospital caring for patients with disabilities, abusing their patients in a range of both physical and psychological manners. A national outcry followed. As a result of the subsequent investigation, 11 staff were convicted of criminal offences and the hospital was shut. The investigation also identified that serious warning signs, which had not been properly looked into, had been evident at the hospital for a long time prior to the discovery of abuse [DoH, 2013c]
- **Daniel Pelka:** Daniel died aged 4 years and 8 months following a period of sustained abuse and neglect by his mother and her partner. His death was caused by a serious head injury, but he had been physically beaten and starved for a prolonged period prior to his death. In the serious case review following his death, it was identified that, although the family and Daniel

Chapter 5 – *Safeguarding*

were well known to police, social services, healthcare services and his school, the warning signs had not been correctly picked up on, nor had appropriate action been taken. The report said that Daniel was 'invisible against the backdrop of his mother's controlling behaviour' and that professionals involved in his case had failed to 'think the unthinkable' [CSCB, 2014].

Sadly, this failure to notice warning signs is not unique and other equally tragic cases, such as the murders of Victoria Climbié and Peter Connelly (Baby P), had very similar findings in their investigations.

Abusers can be skilled at explaining away injuries or unusual behaviour and reassuring professionals about the situation they find. In your frontline role, you may be the only person who comes into contact with a vulnerable person over a prolonged period of time, so you must be prepared to identify and raise concerns when necessary in order to help prevent further similar cases. You must be prepared to 'think the unthinkable'.

Local authorities are usually the leads for safeguarding vulnerable people, but any professional who frequently comes into contact with potentially vulnerable people should be trained in understanding the risk factors and types of abuse, as well as have an understanding of how to spot abuse and who it should be reported to. All health and social care professionals have a moral, ethical and even legal duty to understand their role in safeguarding and to report their concerns.

1.4 *Vulnerability*

People are considered to be vulnerable when they are at a greater-than-normal risk of abuse. For vulnerable adults, this can include [NHS Choices, 2015]:
- those with learning difficulties
- older people who are isolated
- those with memory problems
- those who are dependent on others for support
- those whose carer is addicted to alcohol or drugs
- those who live with a carer.

1.4.1 Abusers of vulnerable adults

Vulnerable adults may be abused by a wide range of people, including relatives and family, professional staff, paid care workers, volunteers, other service users, neighbours, friends and those who deliberately target and exploit the vulnerable [DoH, 2000].

1.4.2 Risk factors for child abuse

All children are vulnerable to abuse, but those who may be more so include those in the following situations [NICE, 2017a]:
- parental or carer drug or alcohol misuse
- parental or carer mental health problems
- intrafamilial violence or history of violent offending
- previous child maltreatment in members of the family
- known maltreatment of an animal by the carer or parent
- vulnerable and unsupported parents or carers
- pre-existing disability in the child.

What is common to most of these scenarios for both adults and children is that the abused tend to have reduced support networks or social contacts around them who they can turn to for help and support. The victims tend to have a degree of reliance on the abuser and this gives the abuser a position of power with which to control and manipulate the victim.

1.4.3 Cultural influences

Culture is well-recognised as influencing abuse in vulnerable groups and can have a major impact on a person's ability to seek help. Examples where cultural beliefs or difference can worsen abuse situations include [NSPCC, 2014]:
- **Fear of cultural isolation:** Family members who do not abide by cultural practices may be cast out and isolated, making it very difficult for them to seek help and therefore making them increasingly vulnerable. In the most extreme cases, so-called honour violence may even be inflicted on these family members.
- **Cultural beliefs overriding self-interests:** An abuser may make a vulnerable person believe that abuse is part of a cultural practice,

warning their victims they will be socially isolated if they reveal the abuse.

1.5 Forms of abuse

There are four main types of abuse common to both adults and children [JRCALC, 2019]:
- physical abuse
- psychological/emotional abuse
- sexual abuse
- neglect.

For vulnerable adults there is also financial abuse.

Additionally, you should also be aware of female genital mutilation (FGM), a form of child abuse, and your responsibilities in reporting this.

1.5.1 Physical abuse

Physical abuse, also known as non-accidental injury (NAI), involves contact intended to cause, or resulting in, pain, injury or other physical harm. It may include striking someone (with or without an object), kicking, grabbing, biting or inappropriate restraint. For older patients in particular, it may also include being handled roughly, or moved in a way that causes pain without the appropriate lifting or moving aids [JRCALC, 2019; Age UK, 2019].

Physical harm can also be caused when a carer or parent fabricates illness, or induces symptoms of an illness, in an adult or child (Munchausen's syndrome by proxy).

Signs of physical abuse may include:
- bruising at multiple stages of repair
- bruises on children who are not yet crawling
- injuries inconsistent with the age of the patient
- frequent attendance at hospital
- inappropriate history for injury demonstrated
- specific injuries, such as cigarette burns and 'hand-grip' bruises
- fear of those around them
- fear of making mistakes
- being very withdrawn and quiet
- delays in seeking help for illness or injury.

You should be particularly mindful of injuries to non-mobile babies. Those aged under a year old are the most vulnerable as they cannot speak for themselves and are totally dependent on others for all of their care. Any injury in a non-mobile baby needs to be reviewed by a suitably qualified clinician, normally a paediatrician at the local hospital.

1.5.2 Psychological/emotional abuse

Psychological, also known as emotional, abuse is a form of abuse characterised by damaging a person's psychological well-being. This is often seen in situations of power imbalance, such as abusive relationships. It may include conveying a feeling of unworthiness, unimportance or being unvalued. It may also include making a person feel ashamed or humiliated through the words or actions of another person.

Over a prolonged period, this form of abuse can allow the abuser to mentally control the abused person and can seriously damage emotional and psychological development. All forms of abuse usually contain an element of psychological abuse, as abusers will try to control the actions and behaviour of their victim [JRCALC 2019; Age UK, 2019].

Signs may include:
- lack of social skills
- low self-worth
- depression
- self-harm
- poor relationships with others
- helplessness
- excessive fear or anxiety.

1.5.3 Sexual abuse

Sexual abuse involves forcing or enticing a person to take part in sexual activity against their wishes, or for which they are not able to consent. Activities may involve physical assault, including penetration (for example, rape or oral sex), or they can be non-penetrative, such as kissing, masturbation or touching the outside of clothing. Sexual abuse can also include non-contact activities such as indecent exposure or forcing a person to watch, or to be involved in the production of, explicit sexual material. Grooming a person in preparation for abuse is also a form of sexual abuse [JRCALC, 2019; Age UK, 2019].

Signs may include:
- physical signs such as anal or vaginal soreness
- sexually transmitted infection
- unusual discharge
- inappropriate use of sexual language for age
- a child being sexually active at a young age
- guilt or shame
- appearing frightened by or avoiding being near to certain people.

Sexual abuse does not have to include contact and is increasingly occurring online. Young people in particular are vulnerable to abusers over the internet befriending them and then asking or demanding sexual favours in return [NSPCC, 2018].

Child sexual exploitation is a particular form of sexual abuse where a child receives something (such as food, accommodation, drugs or alcohol) as a result of performing sexual acts on others and/or others performing sexual acts on them.

1.5.4 Neglect

Neglect is the persistent failure to meet a person's physical and/or psychological needs. A carer or parent should take reasonable steps to prevent harm from occurring to a dependant and failure to do so may be neglect. Neglect can be deliberate or accidental, due to not fully understanding the needs of a dependent person.

Neglect may include:
- failure to provide adequate food, warmth or shelter for a dependant
- failure to ensure adequate access to appropriate medical care.

Signs of neglect include:
- poor appearance and hygiene
- untreated injuries or dental issues
- poor physical development for age
- poor language or communication skills for age
- pressure sores
- signs of malnourishment or dehydration
- dirt, urine or faecal smell in a person's environment.

1.5.5 Financial abuse

This is the unlawful use of a person's property, money or other valuables. It may include an individual being pressured into lending or giving money or other belongings to another person. A carer could start to take control of an individual's personal finances and then use that control to gain profitably without consent. It may also include charging excessive amounts of money for simple services or goods. Relatives are often perpetrators of this kind of abuse and may move into a patient's house in order to be able to exert the influence required to take financial control [Age UK, 2019].

Signs of financial abuse can include:
- unexplained loss of money
- unusual bank account activity
- rapid deterioration in a person's standard of living as they can no longer afford essential goods and services
- a relative or carer moving into the home and taking control.

1.5.6 Female Genital Mutilation (FGM)

FGM is the partial, or complete, removal of the female genitalia, also known as female circumcision or cutting. It is a practice most commonly observed in certain African countries and also the Middle East [UNICEF, 2018].

FGM is a deeply rooted tradition that acts as a complex form of control over women's reproductive and sexual rights. Although it can be performed at any age from birth through to marriage or first pregnancy, it most commonly takes place between the ages of five and eight. Being subject to FGM can have long-term physical and mental health impacts on well-being.

FGM is a criminal offence in the UK, and it is also an offence for anyone to take a child abroad for FGM to be performed [NSPCC, 2019]. As a healthcare professional, you are legally required by the 2003 FGM Act to report to the police if you:
- are informed by a girl under the age of 18 years that she has undergone an act of FGM
- observe physical signs that an act of FGM may have been carried out on a girl under the age of 18 years.

1.6 Domestic violence and abuse

Domestic abuse is categorised as any incident or pattern of incidents of controlling, coercive or threatening behaviour, violence, or abuse between those aged 16 or over who are or have been intimate partners or family members, regardless of gender or sexuality [Met Police, 2018]. The majority of cases are perpetrated by males against females, but it can also occur the other way around and in same-sex relationships.

Some facts to consider in relation to domestic abuse include the following [JRCALC, 2019]:
- The average time that a person is in an abusive relationship before leaving is eight years.
- One-third of all domestic abuse starts or escalates during pregnancy.
- In 90% of domestic abuse cases, children are in the same or the next room.

Domestic abuse occurs in different forms, but it is always about having power and control over the other person. Different forms include [NHS, 2017a]:
- emotional abuse
- threats and intimidation
- physical abuse
- sexual abuse.

A particular form of domestic abuse is coercive control. Coercive control is an act or pattern of acts of assault, threats, humiliation and intimidation or other abuse that is used to harm, punish or frighten the victim [Women's Aid, 2019]. Signs of coercive control include a partner:
- being isolated from family and friends
- being deprived of basic needs, such as food
- monitoring what the partner does with their time
- monitoring the partner's communication via internet and phone, etc.
- taking control of aspects of daily life, such as who the partner can speak to and where they can go
- controlling finances
- making threats or being intimidating.

Managing situations of domestic abuse is challenging. Remember that victims will be scared and feel trapped in their situation. They may believe they are to blame for the abuse and that there is nothing they can do to escape the situation. They may also be scared for their own safety or the safety of others, including their children, if they report the abuse or try to leave. In managing suspected cases of domestic abuse, try to follow these principles [JRCALC, 2019]:
- Remain calm.
- Adopt a sensitive and respectful manner.
- Try to get the patient on their own and promote an open and honest conversation.
- Avoid probing for details; once you suspect domestic abuse, that is enough to raise a concern.
- Support and encourage the patient to report the abuse.
- If children are present, a safeguarding referral must be completed.

Many forms of domestic abuse are criminal offences and you should report all serious crimes to the police, especially if [JRCALC, 2019]:
- the patient has suffered from abuse involving a weapon/strangulation/smothering or has sustained a significant injury
- the patient is in fear of the perpetrator
- the abuse is escalating
- the alleged perpetrator is stalking the patient
- there is an immediate risk to the patient or any child in the household.

Cases of suspected domestic abuse can be challenging and it can take a long time to break out of a cycle of abuse. If you need further guidance on how to manage a situation, contact either a clinical supervisor or a member of your safeguarding team.

Victims can also contact support charities, including for women: Women's Aid (helpline: 0808 2000 247) or for men: Men's Advice Line (helpline: 0808 801 0327).

1.7 Managing abuse or disclosures of abuse

The primary goal in the management of a patient who has suffered abuse should be their long-term safety. The situation may be highly emotionally charged, not least for you as a responder, but your actions in the immediate moments on scene may influence the entire course of protecting a vulnerable person.

You should remain calm and professional, and should not judge those around you. Situations are rarely as simple as they may initially appear, and in the amount of time you will be in contact with a person, it is unlikely that you will discover the full truth.

Here are some suggestions for managing an incident where a safeguarding concern is evident [JRCALC, 2019]:

- Consider not just the patient, but also others present; for example, you may be called to manage an adult with chest pain initially, but if you are concerned about the welfare of a child living in the same house, you have the same duty to report and raise concerns as if that child was the original patient.
- Your first priority should be to manage the presenting condition and ensure medical well-being, i.e. provide the usual clinical management for the presenting complaint and transport anyone with significant illness or injury to further care without delay.
- Limit your questioning to that which is relevant; stop questioning if your suspicions are confirmed. It is not your role to investigate; you should raise the initial concern for others to investigate.
- Accept any given explanation; even if you do not believe the answer, do not make suggestions to the patient on how an incident may have occurred.
- Do not directly accuse parents or carers of abuse as to do so may result in refusal of further care or transport, thereby increasing the risk a patient faces.
- Wherever possible, you should work in partnership with the parents or carers, inform them of your concerns and the need to share these concerns with other agencies. The only exemption to this rule is when you believe that doing so may put the patient at greater risk of harm. You will have to exercise professional judgement on this point and should record in detail your justification for not informing, if that is the option you choose.
- Take any and all accusations seriously; it is not your role to decide on their validity or to investigate further, but instead you should refer your concerns to the appropriate authorities.
- If a person makes a disclosure, make sure you treat them with respect and dignity, and act in a manner that suggests you believe them. Your words and your body language can have a massive influence on a patient's behaviour and confidence in you; if they feel you do not believe them, they may not continue to disclose.
- Complete full and accurate records of events; where possible, try to record word-for-word what the patient has disclosed.
- If transporting your patient, make sure you fully hand over to the receiving staff all details, your concerns and reasons for those concerns, and details of any further action you are going to take.

1.7.1 Reporting an urgent concern

An urgent concern exists where you believe a person may be at immediate risk of further harm. In those circumstances, you should work to ensure the immediate safety of the patient. This can often be best achieved by transporting the patient to hospital where they can be monitored and assessed while awaiting the support of other services.

In the most serious circumstances it may be necessary for you to contact the police via the EOC with your concerns to ensure immediate patient safety. Follow local policy on deciding the urgency of the situation, and where necessary seek further advice from your organisation's safeguarding team, named professional for safeguarding, on-call social worker or ambulance service officer.

In all cases, a safeguarding referral should be completed as soon as possible after the incident, in line with appropriate policies and procedures.

1.8 Safeguarding referrals

Whenever you believe a person is being abused or neglected, or is at risk of either, you should raise your concerns through a safeguarding referral. Different organisations will have different policies based on the local arrangement of who is responsible for the delivery of social care. You should be familiar with arrangements and policies in your local area, but here are some common guidelines:

- **Report all concerns for children:** Any concerns you have, however small, should be reported through your safeguarding referral pathways. Experienced and qualified safeguarding professionals can judge for themselves whether further investigation or action is required. They will also know whether the patient, place of care, or family is known for previous safeguarding concerns, as well as other information that may not be available to you. For adults who have capacity, you should seek consent before making a referral. If they do not consent, you should only make a referral if to do so would be in the public interest. Most agencies will not be able to help if an adult has capacity and has not given consent to the referral being made.
- **Additional sources of help:** All services should have safeguarding teams including named professionals responsible for safeguarding. These teams are experienced in the management of safeguarding issues and have established relationships with the multidisciplinary teams that work around those issues.
- **Role of social services:** In most areas, social services are the main organisation around which safeguarding concerns are managed. Social workers are experienced in dealing with vulnerable people and with cases of abuse and neglect, and can be a great source of support and advice. In some circumstances, social services may want to get in touch with you for more information following a safeguarding referral. You should work fully with social workers to provide whatever information you can in order to ensure the best available support and protection for individuals.
- **Escalating concerns:** All care organisations should be well prepared for managing safeguarding concerns, but in the unlikely event you do not believe that your concerns are being managed in an appropriate manner, you have a duty to escalate your concern. To do this you should speak to a senior manager, colleague or a named professional. Ensure you make records of all concerns that you pass on.
- **Preserve evidence:** If you suspect abuse and will be making a referral, you may need to consider how to preserve evidence. This could take many forms depending on the form of abuse and might include not touching items you believe have been used to assault a victim or encouraging a person not to wash or change their clothes if they have been subject to physical or sexual abuse in order to retain evidence [JRCALC, 2019].

1.9 Summary

Safeguarding can be a highly emotive topic for all concerned, and this should be at the front of your mind when managing a situation where safeguarding is a concern. Try to remain calm, impartial and factual, and keep the immediate safety of patients as your primary goal. Remember the cases of Winterbourne View and Daniel Pelka, where key signs were missed and professionals failed to 'think the unthinkable'.

Be aware of the signs of abuse or neglect and immediately raise any concerns you have through local policy for doing so. Also be mindful that dealing with safeguarding incidents can be emotionally traumatic for responders. Following such incidents, you may need to make use of your organisation's counselling or support services.

2 Counter-terrorism and anti-radicalisation

2.1 Learning objectives

By the end of this section you will be able to:
- define the CONTEST and PREVENT strategies
- define radicalisation
- explain your responsibilities under PREVENT.

2.2 Introduction

It is a sad fact that terrorism and radicalisation are common problems for the modern world and that the UK is no exception to this. The UK Government's counter-terrorism strategy is known as CONTEST [HMG, 2018a].

CONTEST deals with all forms of terrorism and is based around four main areas designed to reduce the threat and the country's vulnerabilities to any threat. These four areas are [HMG, 2018a]:
- **Prevent:** Work to stop people becoming terrorists or supporting terrorism and extremism.
- **Pursue:** The investigation and disruption of terrorist attacks.
- **Protect:** Improving our protective security to stop a terror attack.
- **Prepare:** Working to minimise the impact of an attack and to recover from it as quickly as possible.

2.3 PREVENT

Radicalisation is a process somebody goes through in order to become involved in extremist activities or terrorism [DfE, 2017].

As healthcare professionals working in the community, there is a high possibility you will, at some point, come into contact with groups or individuals who have been, or are vulnerable to being, radicalised. As such, you should understand your role and responsibilities under the PREVENT strategy.

The objectives of the PREVENT strategy are to [HMG, 2018a]:
- tackle the causes of radicalisation and respond to the ideological challenge of terrorism
- safeguard and support those most at risk of radicalisation through early intervention, identifying them and offering support
- enable those who have already engaged in terrorism to disengage and rehabilitate.

The strategy covers all forms of terrorism, including far-right extremism and some aspects of non-violent extremism [HMG, 2018a]. There is a legal duty on healthcare organisations to train their staff in PREVENT in order to help identify and refer people at risk of radicalisation.

2.4 Your role

In line with the PREVENT duty, you will receive specific training from your organisation on the recognition and management of those demonstrating extremist views. However, some key principles you should consider include:
- **Recognise extremist views:** Be prepared to recognise extremist views in those you are responding to. This might be evident through an extreme reaction to certain events, or a history from friends or family of a gradual or sudden change in ideological values.
- **Recognise those who are more at risk:** Some individuals, including those with learning difficulties, the socially isolated or prisoners, are at increased risk of becoming radicalised. Recognise that they represent targets for those seeking to radicalise individuals and report any concerns you may have.
- **Do not investigate:** Pass on your concerns to your nominated organisation lead.

If you identify anyone you believe may be in the process of becoming radicalised, or is at risk of being so, then you should report this via the usual safeguarding report mechanism inside your organisation.

6 Health and Safety

1 Health and safety policies and legislation

1.1 Learning objectives

By the end of this section you will be able to:
- identify legislation relating to health and safety in the ambulance service
- explain the main points of health and safety policies and procedures
- analyse the main health and safety responsibilities for:
  - yourself
  - your employer or manager
  - others in the work setting
- describe types of hazardous substances that may be found in the work setting.

1.2 Introduction

A variety of the legislation that relates to the ambulance service has been reviewed in Chapter 4, 'Legal, Ethical and Professional Issues', but it is also important that you are aware of the legislation relating to health and safety and, in particular, that you know your and your employer's legal responsibilities.

This section will provide an overview of the following legislation that directly applies to health and safety, including manual handling:
- Health and Safety at Work, etc. Act 1974 (HSWA)
- Management of Health and Safety at Work Regulations 1999 (MHSWR)
- Manual Handling Operations Regulations 1992 (MHOR) (as amended 2002)
- Provision and Use of Work Equipment Regulations 1998 (PUWER)
- Lifting Operations and Lifting Equipment Regulations 1998 (LOLER)
- Personal Protective Equipment at Work Regulations 1992
- Control of Substances Hazardous to Health Regulations 2002.

1.3 Health and Safety at Work, etc. Act

All workers have a right to work in places where risks to their health and safety are properly controlled. Health and safety is about stopping you from getting hurt at work or ill through work. Your employer is responsible for health and safety, but you must help [HSE, 2009a].

Employers must do the following in order to comply with the Act [HSE, 2009a]:
- Decide what could harm you in your job and what precautions could prevent it; this is part of risk assessment.
- In a way you can understand, explain how risk will be controlled and tell you who is responsible for this.
- Consult and work with staff and the health and safety representatives to protect everyone from harm in the workplace.
- Provide (free of charge) health and safety training and provide equipment and protective clothing that you need to do your job.
- Provide toilets, washing facilities, drinking water and adequate first-aid facilities.
- Notify the Health and Safety Executive (HSE) in the event of any major injuries and fatalities at work.
- Have insurance that covers staff in the event of injury at work.
- Display a physical or electronic copy of the current insurance certificate where you can easily read it.
- Work with other employers or contractors sharing the workplace to ensure that everyone's health and safety is protected.

Chapter 6 – Health and Safety

You have a number of responsibilities as an employee too [HSE, 2009a]:
- Follow the training you have received when using any work item your employer has provided.
- Take reasonable care of your own and other people's health and safety.
- Co-operate with your employer on health and safety.
- Tell someone (for example, your employer, line manager or safety representative) if you think that a method of working or inadequate precautions are putting anyone's health and safety at serious risk.

1.4 Management of Health and Safety at Work Regulations

The Management of Health and Safety at Work Regulations 1999 require employers to put in place arrangements to control health and safety risks. These include [HSE, 2013b]:
- a written health and safety policy
- assessments of the risks to employees, contractors, customers, partners and any other people who could be affected by work-related activities and recording significant findings in writing
- arrangements for the effective planning, organisation, control, monitoring and review of the preventive and protective measures that come from risk assessment
- access to competent health and safety advice
- providing employees with information about the risks in the workplace and how those employees are protected
- instruction and training for employees in how to deal with the risks
- ensuring there is adequate and appropriate supervision in place
- consulting with employees about their risks at work and current preventive and protective measures.

1.5 Manual Handling Operations Regulations

Any transporting or supporting of a load (including the lifting, putting down, pushing, pulling, carrying or moving thereof) by hand or by bodily force is considered to be a manual handling operation by the Manual Handling Operations Regulations 1992.

Employers are required to make a suitable and sufficient assessment of the risks to the health and safety of their employees while at work. Where this assessment indicates the possibility of risks to employees from the manual handling of loads, the Regulations require a hierarchy of measures that must be adhered to. These are [HSE, 2016]:
- Avoid the need for hazardous manual handling, 'so far as reasonably practicable'.
- Assess the risk of injury from any hazardous manual handling that cannot be avoided.
- Reduce the risk of injury from hazardous manual handling 'so far as reasonably practicable'.

No doubt you have noticed the term 'reasonably practicable' appearing a couple of times. This means that the employer's duty to avoid manual handling or to reduce the risk of injury can be limited, if the employer can show that the cost of any further preventive steps would be grossly disproportionate to their perceived benefit. Employees are also expected to play their part by following appropriate systems of work laid down by their employer to promote safety during the handling of loads [HSE, 2016].

1.5.1 Emergency services

Preventing all potentially hazardous emergency service manual handling operations would result in an inability to provide the general public with an adequate rescue service. As an employee of an ambulance service, you may be asked to accept a greater risk of injury than someone employed to move inanimate objects (like boxes). In this case, additional relevant factors may include:
- the seriousness of the need for the lifting operation
- the ambulance service's duty to the public overall and the patient who requires assistance.

Taking these factors into account, the level of risk that an employer may ask an employee to accept may, in appropriate circumstances, be higher when considering the health and safety of those in danger, although this does not mean that employees can be exposed to unacceptable risk of injury [HSE, 2016].

1.6 Provision and Use of Work Equipment Regulations

Work equipment as defined by the Provision and Use of Work Equipment Regulations 1998 is any machinery, appliance, apparatus, tool or installation for use at work. This includes equipment that employees provide for their own use at work. The scope of work equipment is therefore extremely wide. The use of work equipment is also very widely interpreted: it covers any activity involving work equipment and includes starting, stopping, programming, setting, transporting, repairing, modifying, maintaining, servicing and cleaning.

Employers must manage the risks from that equipment, including [HSE, 2014a]:
- ensuring equipment is constructed or adapted to be suitable for the purpose it is used or provided for
- taking account of the working conditions and health and safety risks in the workplace when selecting work equipment
- ensuring work equipment is only used for suitable purposes
- ensuring work equipment is maintained in an efficient state, in efficient working order and in good repair.

1.7 Lifting Operations and Lifting Equipment Regulations

Lifting equipment includes any equipment used at work for lifting or lowering loads, along with attachments used for anchoring, fixing or supporting it, including hoists and ambulance trolleys.

Employers are required to ensure that all lifting equipment is [LOLER, 1998]:
- sufficiently strong, stable and suitable for the proposed use, and that the load and anything attached must be suitable
- positioned or installed to prevent the risk of injury, e.g. from the equipment or the load falling or striking people
- visibly marked with any appropriate information to be taken into account for its safe use, e.g. safe working loads, accessories (slings, clamps, etc) should be similarly marked.

Additionally, employers must ensure that [LOLER, 1998]:
- lifting operations are planned, supervised and carried out in a safe manner by people who are competent
- equipment used for lifting people is marked accordingly and is safe for such a purpose, i.e. all necessary precautions have been taken to eliminate or reduce any risk
- where appropriate, lifting equipment (including accessories) is thoroughly examined before being used for the first time. Lifting equipment may need to be thoroughly examined in use at periods specified in the Regulations (i.e. at least six-monthly for accessories and equipment used for lifting people and, at a minimum, annually for all other equipment) or at intervals laid down in an examination scheme drawn up by and performed by a competent person (someone with the necessary skills, knowledge and experience).

You should not use any equipment that 'lifts' if you are not trained and competent in doing so. One of the most common lifting pieces of equipment you will come across is likely to be a patient hoist. There are a large range of these available on the market, all of which look similar, but actually operate in slightly different ways. For this reason, it is unlikely that you will ever be able to be competent on all the different hoists you come across. Instead of using them yourself, you should seek help from others present who are competent in their use.

1.8 Personal Protective Equipment at Work Regulations

Personal protective equipment (PPE) is equipment that will protect the user against health or safety risks at work. It can include items such as safety helmets and hard hats, gloves, eye protection, high-visibility clothing, safety footwear and safety harnesses [HSE, 2013d].

PPE should be used as a last resort. Wherever there are risks to health and safety that cannot be adequately controlled in other ways, the Personal

Protective Equipment at Work Regulations 1992 require PPE to be supplied. The Regulations also require that PPE is:
- properly assessed before use to make sure it is fit for purpose
- maintained and stored properly
- provided with instructions on how to use it safely
- used correctly by employees.

1.9 Control of Substances Hazardous to Health Regulations

The Control of Substances Hazardous to Health Regulations 2002 cover substances that are hazardous to health. Substances can take many forms and include:
- chemicals
- products containing chemicals
- fumes
- dusts
- vapours
- mists
- gases and asphyxiating gases
- biological agents (germs).

If the packaging has any of the hazard symbols then it is classed as a hazardous substance.

Employers have a responsibility to manage and minimise the risks from work activities. They must develop suitable and sufficient control measures and ways of maintaining them by [HSE, 2013c]:
- identifying hazards and potentially significant risks
- taking action to prevent and control risks
- keeping control measures under regular review.

To be effective in the long term, control measures must be practical, workable and sustainable.

Good practice in the control of substances that are hazardous to health can be encapsulated in the eight generic principles set out in the Control of Substances Hazardous to Health Regulations 2002:
- Design and operate processes and activities to minimise the emission, release and spread of substances hazardous to health.
- Take into account all relevant routes of exposure – inhalation, skin and ingestion – when developing control measures.
- Control exposure by measures that are proportionate to the health risk.
- Choose the most effective and reliable control options that minimise the escape and spread of substances that are hazardous to health.
- Provide, in combination with other control measures, suitable PPE where adequate control of exposure cannot be achieved by other means.
- Check and review regularly all elements of control measures for their continuing effectiveness.
- Inform and train all employees on the hazards and risks from substances with which they work and the use of control measures developed to minimise the risks.
- Ensure that the introduction of measures to control exposure does not increase the overall risk to health and safety.

1.10 Regulatory bodies

The main regulatory body for overseeing health and safety is the Health and Safety Executive (HSE), formed as part of the 1974 Health and Safety at Work, etc. Act. Although sponsored by the Department for Work and Pensions, the HSE is a national independent watchdog responsible for work-related health, safety and illness, working to reduce work-related death and serious injury across Great Britain [HMG, 2018b].

The HSE achieve this by working with employers to ensure that all practicably reasonable steps are taken to ensure health and safety at work. They also undertake research and investigate incidents that result in death or significant injury. If an employer fails to meet their health and safety obligations, the HSE can issue a range of improvement orders or, where necessary, file a prosecution, which can result in large fines and custodial sentences for those responsible for allowing health and safety breaches to occur.

1.11 Why health and safety matters

Health and safety exists to make work a safer and more enjoyable place for all employees. Although sometimes rules and regulations can appear restrictive, they exist to protect you and to ensure that you are able to continue working and reduce, so far as is reasonably practicable, the risk you face on a daily basis at work.

As previously discussed, you have a responsibility to comply with health and safety regulations at work and to contribute to making your workplace a safer place to be. If you fail to abide by the regulations and protocols put in place by your employer, not only are you making work a less safe place for yourself, your colleagues and ultimately your patients, but you may also be committing an offence that you could be prosecuted for.

1.12 Communicating health and safety

Health and safety should be considered a dynamic process as it is constantly being reviewed to ensure it is suitable for new ways of working, or that new technologies are being used to their maximum potential to reduce risk. Because of this, it is likely that there will frequently be updates to your organisation's health and safety procedure. Updates may come in many forms, including: e-mails, standard operating procedures, updates to policy, local posters or as part of statutory and mandatory training. Some updates will be made very evident, while others might be subtler, such as a change in policy.

You should be aware of where you can find all relevant health and safety information and updates and keep yourself aware of any changes.

Remember, you are responsible for keeping yourself up to date. If you become ill or are injured due to a lack of familiarity with updates, it may be viewed that you have contributed to your own illness or injury and therefore have to take a proportionally greater amount of responsibility for what has happened.

2 Risk assessment

2.1 Learning objectives

By the end of this section you will be able to:
- define the term 'risk'
- describe the process of carrying out a risk assessment
- explain the importance of carrying out a risk assessment
- compare different uses of risk assessment in health and social care
- explain why risk assessments need to be regularly reviewed and revised.

2.2 Introduction

All healthcare staff have a duty to protect patients, their colleagues and themselves as far as is 'reasonably practicable' by minimising the chance that they are harmed by something, whether that be a procedure, drug administration or dangerous environment.

It is helpful to understand what is meant by the terms 'hazard' and 'risk' [HSE, 2018a; NPSA, 2007a]:
- **Hazard:** Anything that might cause harm, such as chemicals, electricity, working from ladders, an open drawer, etc.
- **Risk:** The chance, high or low, that somebody could be harmed by these hazards, together with an indication of how serious the harm could be,
- **Clinical risk:** The chance of an adverse outcome resulting from clinical investigation, treatment or patient care; also known as a healthcare risk.

For an organisation like an ambulance service, there are other risks to consider:
- injury and safety (patients, staff and the public)
- legal and financial
- service interruption
- Resourcing Escalatory Action Plan (REAP) level increases
- regulatory requirements
- reputation.

2.3 Risk assessment

Risk assessment does not have to be difficult. It can be distilled into five steps [HSE, 2018a]:
1. Identify the hazards (What can go wrong?).
2. Decide who might be harmed and how (Who is exposed to the hazard?).
3. Evaluate the risk (How bad? How often?) and decide on the precautions (Is there a need for further action?).

4. Record your findings and proposed action.
5. Review your assessment and update, if required.

2.3.1 Identify the hazards

This step consists of working out what is likely to go wrong and why. Many hazards can be anticipated in advance, allowing time for a formal written risk assessment to be completed, which is then kept on an organisation and/or departmental risk register. Items suitable for this include:
- equipment
- manual handling procedures
- cleaning products
- risk of injury from sharps, etc.
- adverse media coverage.

However, some risk assessments will have to be conducted quickly and mentally, as there will be no time to conduct a formal written risk assessment. This dynamic risk assessment is the type you will perform as you arrive on scene at an incident and may well conduct a number of times during a patient episode, depending on the risk of harm and the volatility of the scene and/or patients and bystanders. You will learn more about this in Chapter 9, 'Scene Assessment'.

Risk may also be identified from previous incidents, which is why it is important you report all adverse advents or near-misses through your organisation's reporting procedure.

2.3.2 Decide who might be harmed and how

Consider who might be harmed by the hazard and the circumstances that might lead to harm occurring. This could be you, for example, when assisting a senior clinician with an injection or cannulation attempt. Patients can be harmed in many ways, for example during manual handling or the administration of a drug. Your colleagues are also at risk during certain procedures, such as when you are reversing the ambulance into the garage.

It is not usually necessary to identify the individual, just groups of people who may be at risk of harm from the hazard you are assessing. In addition to the examples listed above, consider other groups such as [HSE, 2018b]:
- pregnant patients
- children
- non-English speakers
- people with a disability.

2.3.3 Evaluate the risk and decide on precautions

Evaluating risk is a skill that becomes easier with practice. To assist with the evaluation, it can be helpful to use a risk matrix (Table 6.1) to quantify the two aspects of risk evaluation. This was a process that was strongly advocated by the National Patient Safety Agency, a group that was

Table 6.1 Risk matrix.

	LIKELIHOOD				
	1	2	3	4	5
CONSEQUENCE	Rare	Unlikely	Possible	Likely	Almost certain
5 Catastrophic	5	10	15	20	25
4 Major	4	8	12	16	20
3 Moderate	3	6	9	12	15
2 Minor	2	4	6	8	10
1 Negligible	1	2	3	4	5

responsible for leading patient safety in the NHS before it was closed in 2016. Despite this, its risk matrix approach remains widely in use around NHS organisations and revolves around two criteria [NPSA, 2008]:
- **Consequence:** How severe is the risk?
- **Likelihood:** How often is the risk likely to arise?

To calculate the risk rating, the consequence score is multiplied by the likelihood score. In the case of a staff injury at work, the consequence would be scored as follows:
1 = Negligible injury requiring no medical intervention and no time off work.
2 = Minor injury requiring some medical intervention and fewer than three days off work.
3 = Moderate injury requiring hospital or other professional intervention and 4–14 days off work.
4 = Major injury leaving the staff member with long-term incapacity and/or disability and more than 14 days off work.
5 = Catastrophic injury resulting in death.

The likelihood scores are allocated as follows:
1 = **Rare:** Not expected to occur for years.
2 = **Unlikely:** Expected to occur at least annually.
3 = **Possible:** Expected to occur at least monthly.
4 = **Likely:** Expected to occur at least weekly.
5 = **Almost certain:** Expected to occur at least daily.

Precautions
Having identified risks and given them a risk rating, it is necessary to determine what precautions (controls) are most appropriate to try to reduce the likelihood of the risk occurring [HSE, 2018c]. It is quite likely that there will already be policies and procedures in place. As an employee, you will be expected to be familiar with these, although you may also need training to ensure you can comply with them. In addition, you are likely to have a responsibility to report any risks and not undertake any action that would knowingly cause harm to you or anyone else, including your employer.

When assessing the risks and deciding which precautions to take, you should always strive to reduce the risk to the lowest reasonably practicable level. The HSE proposes a hierarchy of control measures. You should use the first viable option and should not jump down the list without first fully discarding the higher options [HSE, 2018d]:
- **Elimination:** If possible, remove the hazard entirely. This may be done by changing working methods or by implementing a system redesign.
- **Substitution:** Replace the equipment or process with a less hazardous one, for example, the introduction of lifting cushions to help patients that have fallen to get up off the floor.
- **Engineering controls:** Use work equipment or other methods to reduce the risk of injury where a task cannot be avoided.
- **Administrative controls:** Identifying and implementing procedures required to work safely. This may also include training about how to work in a safe manner.
- **PPE:** PPE should only be considered when all of the above are found to be either ineffective or only partially effective at managing the risk.

Finally, once you have decided on the most appropriate precautions to take, you should re-evaluate the risk on the basis that your precautions are undertaken.

2.3.4 Record your findings and proposed actions

Formal risk assessments should be documented in a manner that is easily accessible to all of those who may need to access it. It should be suitable and sufficient, meaning it should show [HSE, 2018e]:
- a proper check was made and those who may be affected were identified
- all obvious hazards were dealt with
- the precautions are reasonable and the remaining risk is low
- employees or their representative were included.

To make the process of recording a risk assessment simpler and more accessible, your organisation probably uses a standard template.

Dynamic risk assessments may also need to be documented and this should take place as soon as possible after the incident. This will provide justification for actions taken in the event of any adverse outcomes as well as providing a starting point for future formal risk assessments if the situation is likely to recur.

2.3.5 Review and update

Risk assessments need to be reviewed periodically as things change. New best practices emerge from research, equipment is updated or modified, and new hazards may be identified. To help decide whether a review is necessary, ask yourself the following questions [HSE, 2018f]:
- Have there been any significant changes?
- Are there improvements that you still need to make?
- Have you or colleagues spotted a problem?
- Has anything been learned from accidents or near misses?

Health and safety and risk assessment exist to keep everyone safe; having a good understanding of these and your role in developing and implementing health and safety at work will make for a safer, happier and more effective workplace, ultimately resulting in better patient care.

3 Infection prevention and control

3.1 *Learning objectives*

By the end of this section you will be able to:
- explain what is meant by 'infection' and how infections can occur and be transmitted
- identify a number of microorganisms, the illnesses they cause and how they can enter the body
- describe how to manage and dispose of sources of infection safely while avoiding harm to your self or others
- outline the current regulations, legislation and responsibilities relating to infection control
- describe the different types of personal protective equipment (PPE) and how to use them appropriately
- explain the role of regulators and other bodies in infection prevention and control
- describe the key principles of good personal hygiene
- describe the correct sequence for handwashing and when it should be carried out
- describe the services that occupational health provide to employees.

3.2 *Introduction*

Infection prevention and control is a collective term for those activities intended to protect people from infections [Dougherty, 2015].

An infection is the body's adverse response to the presence of a pathogen, or disease-causing microorganism [Betsy, 2012]. Damage to tissues caused by an infection can either be limited to the site of infection (localised) or spread throughout the body, typically via the blood (systemic). Sometimes, however, a pathogen in or on the body may not lead to an infection. This is known as colonisation [Weston, 2014].

A healthcare-associated infection (HCAI) is any infection acquired as a result of a healthcare-related intervention or an infection acquired during the course of healthcare that the patient may reasonably expect to be protected from. HCAI has replaced the term 'hospital-acquired infection', since many healthcare interactions take place outside of hospital (such as in your ambulance) [Dougherty, 2015]. The scale of the problem is staggering, with an estimated 300,000 patients each year in England acquiring an HCAI, with a significant number of deaths and a cost to the NHS of around £1 billion [NICE, 2012].

3.2.1 Your own and the patient's health

As well as passing diseases and illness on to patients, health professionals can also be made unwell by poor infection prevention and control. Some diseases, such as norovirus, a viral infection that causes gastroenteritis [NHS 2018a], is very infectious and spreads easily from person to person. In winter, when it is most prevalent, it is likely you will come into contact with patients suffering from this on a frequent basis. If you do not apply adequate infection prevention and controls, it is likely that you may also become unwell and contract the illness. This could mean that you are off sick for several days or weeks from work, which will have an impact not only on your health, but potentially the health of family and friends as well.

Equally, you can spread illness to your patient. If you are not well, you should not come in to work as you might spread illness to already unwell people. For many patients, including the elderly, those with chronic lung conditions or receiving chemotherapy, even a small infection will place a major strain on their immune system; an illness that may not be a major issue for a healthy person could kill someone who is already unwell.

If you are unsure if you are fit to return to work, you should see your GP or contact your occupational health team.

3.2.2 Impact on organisations

For organisations, an outbreak of an illness such as norovirus can be disastrous. In a healthcare setting, if a large number of staff were all to become ill with gastroenteritis at the same time, there would be a very significant strain put on the remaining workforce to cover the gaps left by sickness.

3.3 Regulations and legislation

At the beginning of this chapter, some of the relevant legislation relating to infection prevention and control was reviewed, in particular the Health and Safety at Work etc. Act 1974. This requires employers to provide training and appropriate personal protective equipment (PPE) to prevent harm. It also requires employees to follow the training that they have received, use PPE provided, and report any situations where they believe that patients' and/or staff's health and safety are at serious risk.

However, the Health and Social Care Act [2008] specifically highlights health professionals' duty of care to implement effective infection prevention and control procedures and also makes the Care Quality Commission (CQC) responsible for ensuring that ambulance (and other care) services meet the requirements of the code of practice that accompanies the legislation. This code specified ten key elements that ambulance services must demonstrate that they comply with:

- Systems to manage and monitor the prevention and control of infection. These systems use risk assessments and consider the susceptibility of service users and any risks that their environment and other users may pose to them.
- Provide and maintain a clean and appropriate environment in managed premises that facilitates the prevention and control of infections.
- Ensure appropriate antimicrobial use to optimise patient outcomes and to reduce the risk of adverse events and antimicrobial resistance.
- Provide suitable accurate information on infections to service users, their visitors and any person concerned with providing further support or nursing/medical care in a timely fashion.
- Ensure prompt identification of people who have or are at risk of developing an infection so that they receive timely and appropriate treatment to reduce the risk of transmitting infection to other people.
- Systems to ensure that all care workers (including contractors and volunteers) are aware of and discharge their responsibilities in the process of preventing and controlling infection.
- Provide or secure adequate isolation facilities.
- Secure adequate access to laboratory support as appropriate.
- Have and adhere to policies designed for the individual's care and provider organisations that will help to prevent and control infections.
- Have a system in place to manage the occupational health needs and obligations of staff in relation to infection.

There is also additional legislation that does not apply exclusively to the healthcare setting, but which is intent on reducing the risk of infection. This includes regulations relating to food hygiene [Food Safety Act 1990], water supply [DWI, 2012] and waste management [Hazardous Waste Regulations 2005; Control of Substances Hazardous to Health Regulations 2002].

3.3.1 Regulators and other bodies

The regulators of healthcare services in the UK, the Care Quality Commission for England, Care Inspectorate Wales and the Care Inspectorate for Scotland, are responsible for ensuring that organisations that provide health-related services meet the required standards in the management of infection prevention and control. If organisations fail to meet required standards, they can be prosecuted and have their licence to provide care services taken away.

Health protection agencies

Public Health England is responsible for monitoring and helping to control outbreaks of, and providing protection against infectious diseases such as:
- hepatitis
- genital herpes
- measles.

When such outbreaks occur, they provide specialist advice, expertise and equipment to combat the illness and prevent it spreading further [HMG, 2018c]. In Scotland this is provided by Health Protection Scotland and in Wales by Public Health Wales.

World Health Organization (WHO)

The WHO provides advice to member states on infection prevention and control based on the best available evidence from international studies [WHO, 2018]. WHO also respond to large-scale disease outbreaks to support the local response and prevent spreading of the disease.

3.4 Microorganisms

Microorganisms are very small organisms that live outside and inside larger organisms such as the human body. The four main types that enter the body and cause infection are:
- bacteria
- viruses
- fungi
- parasites.

3.4.1 Bacteria

These are probably the most important microorganisms in relation to infection control as they are responsible for many opportunistic infections in healthcare. There are around ten times as many bacteria as there are cells in the human body and many have functions that are essential, such as the microorganism *Escherichia coli (E. coli)*, which aids digestion in the gut. However, it can cause a urinary tract infection (UTI) if it gains access to the urinary tract [Dougherty, 2015].

Bacteria are fairly simple, single-celled microorganisms and are often classified by their shape. For example, they may be termed bacillus (rod-like), coccus (spherical or ovoid) or spiral (corkscrew or curved). Examples of common bacteria include Group A streptococcus, which can cause throat and ear infections, and Staphylococcus, which can cause impetigo and pneumonia. You may have heard of a particularly troublesome strain of Staphylococcus that is resistant to many antibiotics and is called methicillin-resistant *Staphylococcus aureus* (MRSA) [Betsy, 2012].

3.4.2 Viruses

Viruses are even smaller than bacteria and have no cellular structure. They typically consist of just a core containing genetic material such as deoxyribonucleic acid (DNA) or ribonucleic acid (RNA) and are sometimes surrounded by a membrane called an envelope. Viruses can reproduce only by using the cellular machinery of other organisms and so are rather like parasites [Tortora, 2017].

Common viruses include the rhinovirus, which is responsible for the common cold, and the varicella-zoster virus (VZV), which causes chickenpox and shingles [Betsy, 2012].

3.4.3 Fungi

You are probably most familiar with fungi as mushrooms or as yeast used in bread-making and brewing. Some fungi are responsible for opportunistic infections, such as dermatophytes, which can cause athlete's foot, and Candida albicans, yeast that can cause vaginal thrush [Dougherty, 2015].

3.4.4 Parasites

Parasites are organisms that live at the expense of another organism or host. Pathogenic parasites include bacteria, viruses, protozoa (animal-like single-celled microorganisms) and animals such as roundworms, flatworms and arthropods. Examples of parasitic infections include malaria and toxoplasmosis [Betsy, 2012].

3.5 *Infection and precautions*

3.5.1 Chain of infection

Transmission of infection is a complex process, involving a number of factors, which must all be present and are collectively known as the chain of infection (Figure 6.1) [Ross, 2014; Dougherty, 2015].

Pathogen
An infectious agent is required, such as a bacterium, virus, fungus or parasite. This link can be broken by cleaning, sterilisation of equipment and the treatment of the patient, using antibiotics for bacterial infections, for example.

Reservoir
A reservoir is a place where the pathogen can live and replicate; it includes the human body, but also animals, water and the soil, for example. This link can be broken by cleaning equipment and the environment (such as the ambulance) and removing stagnant water.

Exit route
The exit route is a method for the pathogen to leave its reservoir. In humans, this usually involves urine, faeces, vomit, sputum and in aerosolised form, such as after sneezing or coughing. Asking a patient with active tuberculosis to wear a mask would help to break this chain.

Route of transmission
The transmission route can be direct, such as through touching, sexual intercourse and faecal–oral via ingestion, or indirectly via contaminated bedding, clothing, blood and bodily fluids and then the hands of healthcare workers. One of the most effective ways of breaking this chain is with good hand hygiene.

Entry route
Entry routes include the respiratory, gastrointestinal and genitourinary tracts, but also mucous membranes and via the skin. Direct access to the blood is also possible if the pathogen is inadvertently injected into a person. Covering an open wound with a waterproof plaster would be a good example of breaking the chain by blocking the route of entry.

Susceptible host
Some people are more vulnerable to infection than others, for example, those with a weak immune system due to old age, medication or pre-existing disease. Others may have their natural defences compromised by wounds, surgery, intravenous cannulas and urinary catheters. This chain can be broken by ensuring that healthcare workers are vaccinated and that adequate nutrition and personal hygiene is provided to vulnerable groups.

3.5.2 Standard principles

Standard principles are a group of actions that should be taken in every patient contact to reduce the risk of infection. They are [NICE, 2017b]:
- hand decontamination
- use of personal protective equipment
- safe use and disposal of sharps
- waste disposal.

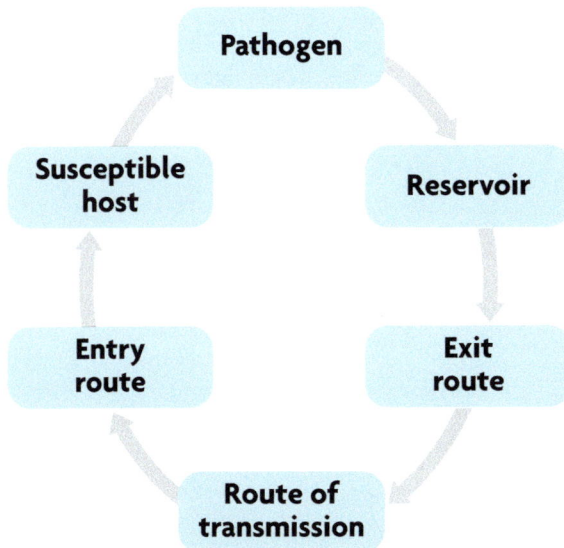

Figure 6.1 Chain of infection.

3.6 Personal hygiene

Personal hygiene is defined as the physical act of cleansing the body to ensure that the hair, nails, ears, eyes, nose and skin are maintained in an optimum condition. It also includes mouth hygiene, which is the effective removal of plaque and debris to ensure that the structures and tissues of the mouth are kept in a healthy condition. In addition, personal hygiene includes ensuring the appropriate length of nails and hair [DoH, 2010a].

Good personal hygiene habits include [DoH, 2010b; Dougherty, 2015]:
- having a shower or bath every day
- brushing your teeth at least once (but preferably twice) a day
- washing your hair with soap or shampoo at least once a week
- washing your hands after going to the toilet
- washing your hands with soap before preparing and/or eating food
- wearing clean clothes.

3.7 Hand hygiene

Good hand hygiene is the primary measure to reduce HCAIs. It is a straightforward method and inexpensive, but poor compliance among healthcare workers is a worldwide problem [WHO, 2009a].

You should clean your hands in the following circumstances [NICE, 2017b]:
- immediately before every episode of direct patient contact or care, including aseptic procedures
- immediately after every episode of direct patient contact or care
- immediately after any exposure to body fluids
- immediately after any other activity or contact with a patient's surroundings that could potentially result in your hands becoming contaminated
- immediately after removal of gloves.

Use a handrub conforming to the latest standards to decontaminate your hands, except when your hands are visibly soiled or potentially contaminated with body fluids, and when it is suspected that alcohol-resistant organisms (such as *Clostridium difficile* or other organisms that cause diarrhoeal illness) are involved, when you should use soap and water instead.

In order to ensure that you can clean your hands while at work, you should [NICE, 2017b]:
- be 'bare below the elbows' when delivering direct patient care
- not wear any wrist or hand jewellery
- ensure that fingernails are short, clean and free of nail polish
- cover cuts and abrasions with waterproof dressings.

3.7.1 Alcohol handrub

Procedure – Hand hygiene with handrub

This is the World Health Organization's (WHO) recommended procedure for hand hygiene with handrub. This procedure should take 20–30 seconds [WHO, 2009a].

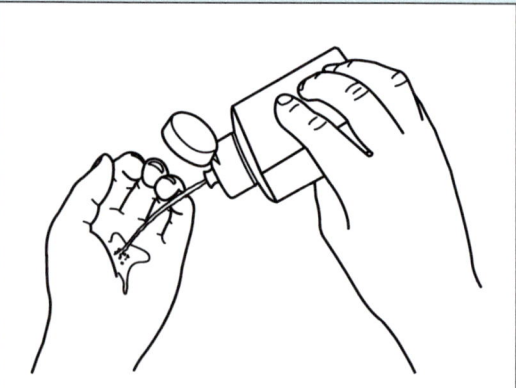

1. Apply a palmful of the handrub in a cupped hand, covering all surfaces.

Infection prevention and control

Procedure – Hand hygiene with handrub – *cont*

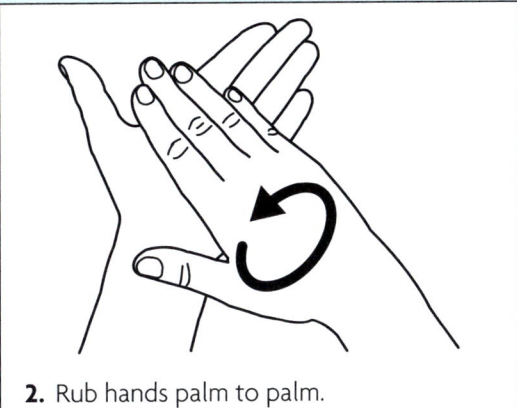

2. Rub hands palm to palm.

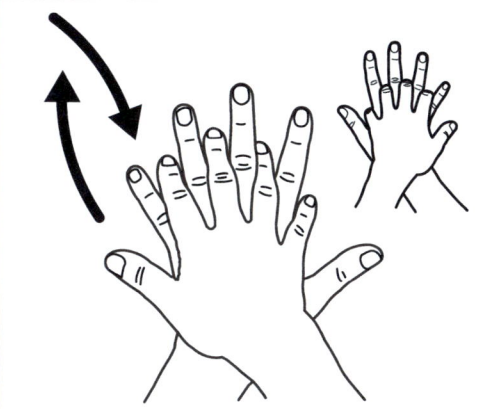

3. Right palm over left dorsum with interlaced fingers and vice versa.

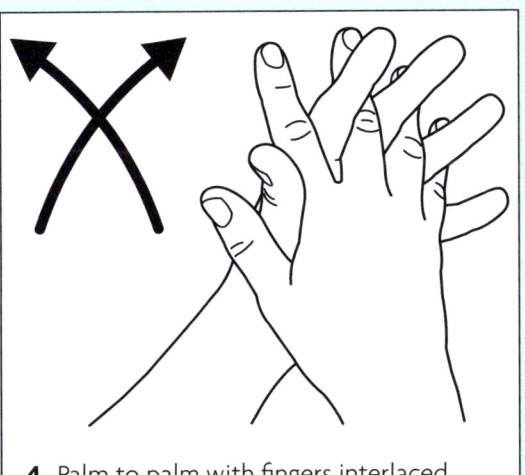

4. Palm to palm with fingers interlaced.

Procedure – Hand hygiene with handrub – *cont*

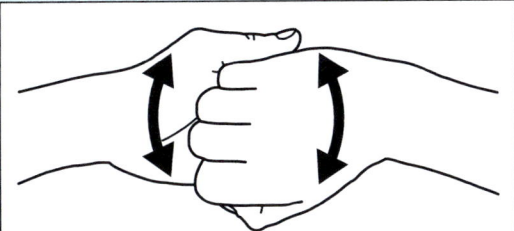

5. Backs of fingers to opposing palms with fingers interlocked.

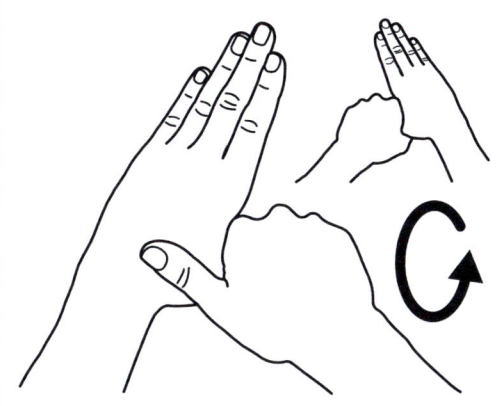

6. Rotational rubbing of left thumb clasped in right palm and vice versa.

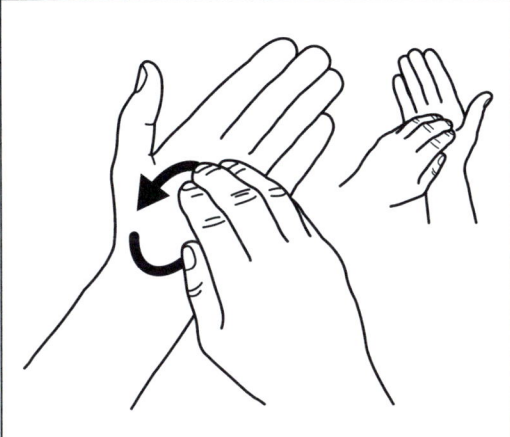

7. Rotational rubbing, backwards and forwards with clasped fingers of right hand in left palm and vice versa.

Chapter 6 – Health and Safety

Procedure – Hand hygiene with handrub – *cont*

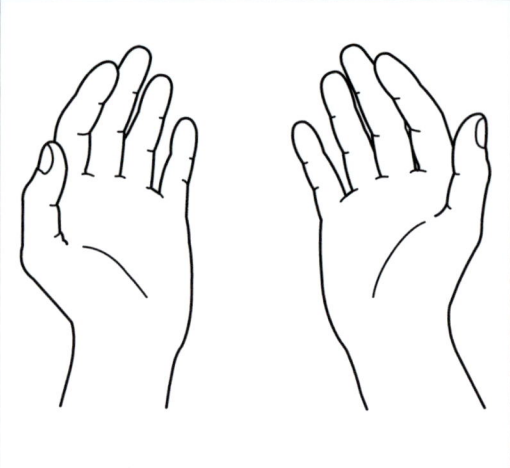

8. Once dry, your hands are safe.

Source: Based on the 'How to Handrub' poster.
© World Health Organization 2009. All rights reserved.

3.7.2 Handwashing

Procedure – Handwashing

This is the WHO recommended procedure for handwashing. This procedure should take 40–60 seconds [WHO, 2009a].

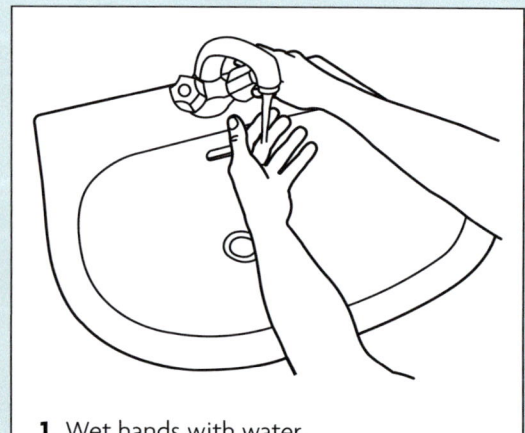

1. Wet hands with water.

Procedure – Handwashing – *cont*

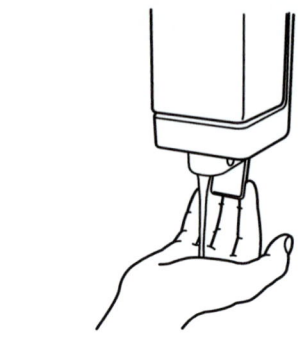

2. Apply enough soap to cover all hand surfaces.

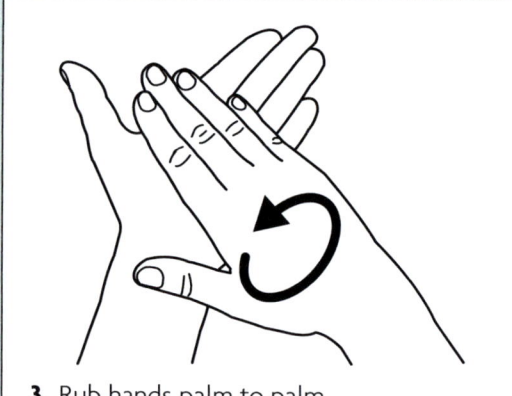

3. Rub hands palm to palm.

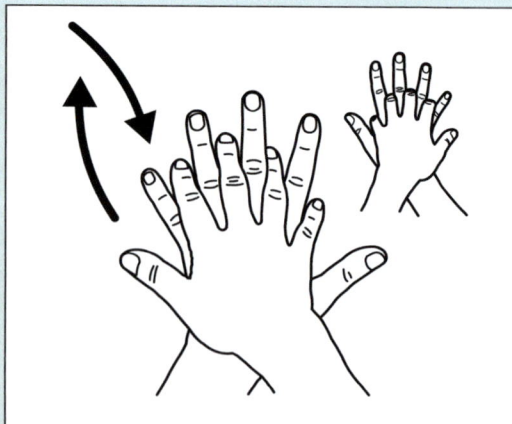

4. Right palm over left dorsum with fingers interlaced and vice versa.

Procedure – Handwashing – *cont*

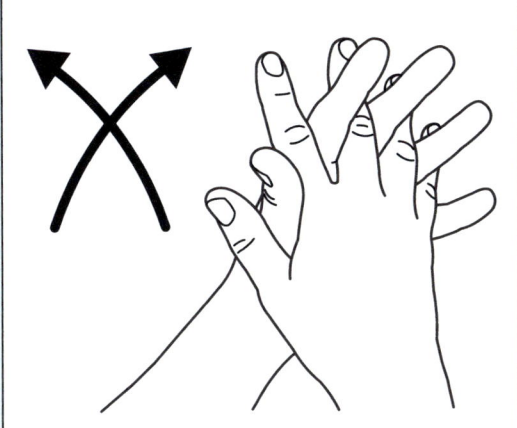

5. Palm to palm with fingers interlaced.

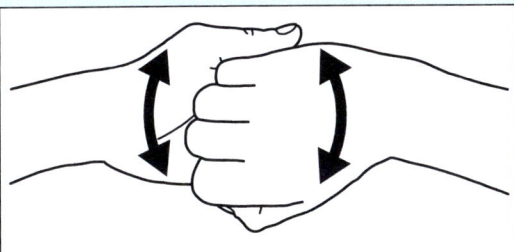

6. Backs of fingers to opposing palms with fingers interlocked.

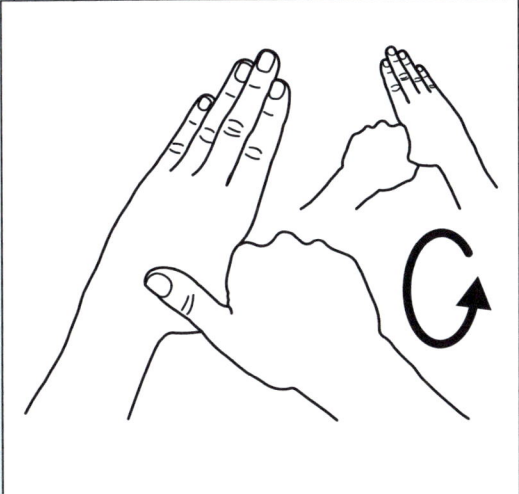

7. Rotational rubbing of left thumb clasped in right palm and vice versa.

Procedure – Handwashing – *cont*

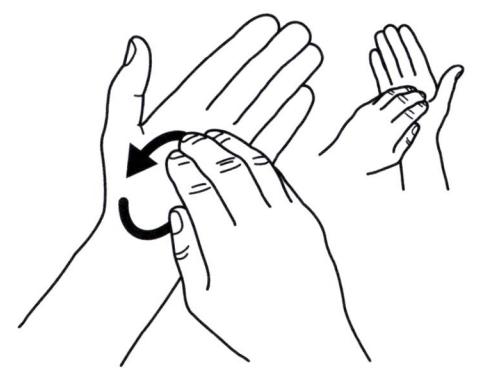

8. Rotational rubbing, backwards and forwards with clasped fingers of right hand in left palm and vice versa.

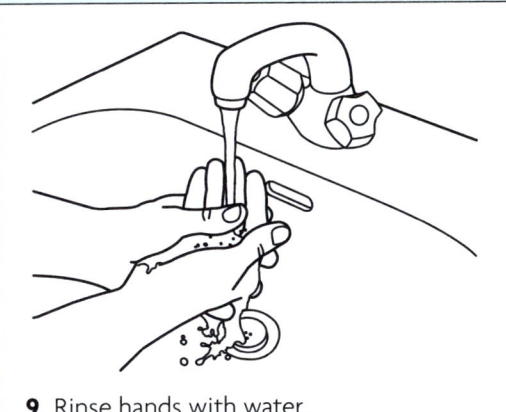

9. Rinse hands with water.

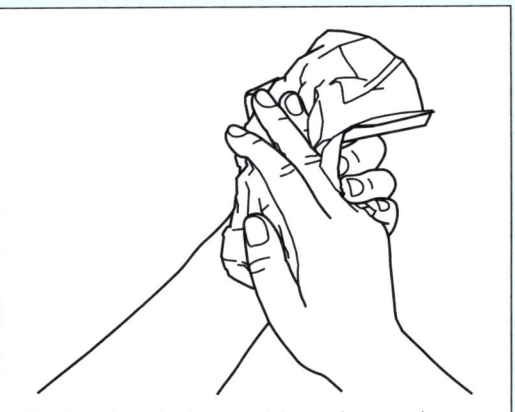

10. Dry hands thoroughly with a single-use towel.

Procedure – Handwashing – *cont*

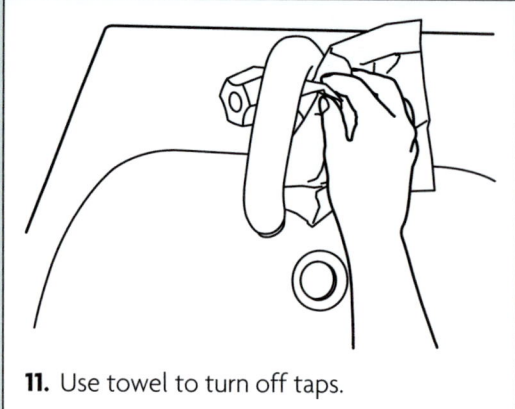

11. Use towel to turn off taps.

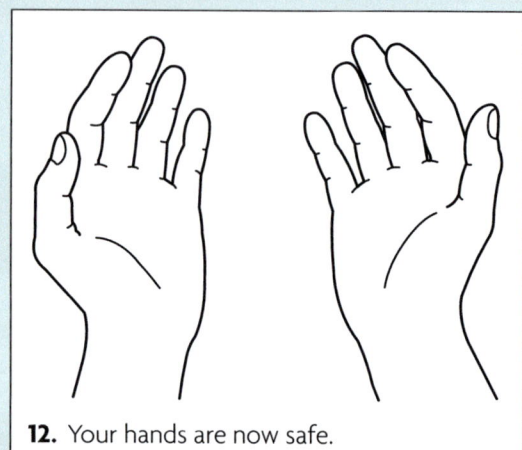

12. Your hands are now safe.

Source: Based on the 'How to Handwash' poster.
© World Health Organization 2009. All rights reserved.

3.7.3 Skincare

Work-related skin problems are very common, with contact dermatitis being the most common form of work-related skin disease. It is more common in healthcare staff due to their need to wash their hands regularly and their skin frequently coming into contact with chemicals or rubber materials as used in personal protective equipment [HSE, 2019b].

When washing your hands frequently, it is important to use hand cream to replace the natural oils that are lost in the washing process [HSE, 2015a]

and to observe for signs of contact dermatitis developing. These signs include:
- dry itchy skin
- reddening
- flaking, cracks or blisters.

If you suffer from contact dermatitis, or any other form of skin disease, you should see your GP or occupational health team to try to find a personal solution for improving your skincare.

3.8 *Personal protective equipment*

Personal protective equipment (PPE) is used to prevent the spread of infection to you, your colleagues, patients and other members of the public. Your choice of PPE (including not wearing any) should be based on an assessment of the risk of transmission of infection [DoH, 2010c].

Typical items of PPE to prevent infection include:
- gloves
- aprons
- face masks
- eye protection
- sleeve protectors
- protective suits (these are generally only for specially trained personnel, such as hazardous area response team (HART) members and are not covered in this text).

3.8.1 Gloves

Gloves should only be worn (Figure 6.2):
- if there is a risk of contact with blood and/or bodily fluids
- when sharp and/or contaminated items are handled
- if there is likely to be contact with non-intact skin or mucous membranes during contact with a patient.

Gloves should not be worn longer than required and never when driving from the scene [SCAS, 2018]. Don't forget that hand hygiene is required before and after wearing gloves. Put gloves on immediately prior to patient contact and change them between each patient task, when caring for different patients, and as soon as they are

Infection prevention and control

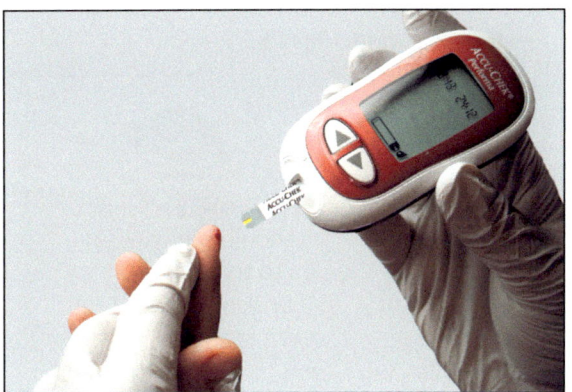

Figure 6.2 Non-latex disposable gloves should be worn when there is a risk of contact with blood, such as when checking a patient's blood sugar.

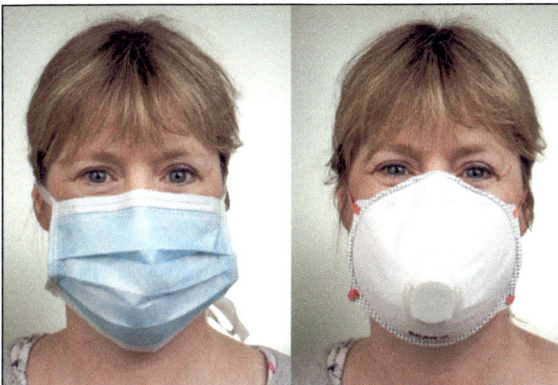

Figure 6.3 Face masks (surgical face mask on left and FFP3 mask on right).

contaminated. Once you have removed your gloves, discard appropriately [DoH, 2010c].

3.8.2 Aprons

Aprons should be worn when:
- your uniform is likely to be contaminated with blood and/or other bodily fluids
- carrying out cleaning that may lead to contamination of your uniform
- transporting infectious patients.

Aprons should be disposed of appropriately following a single use. Unfasten or break the ties and then pull the apron away from your neck and shoulders. Only touch the inside of the apron. Once away from your body, turn it inside out and then fold it into a bundle before discarding appropriately [DoH, 2010c].

3.8.3 Face masks

There are two types of face mask in common use by ambulance services (Figure 6.3):
- surgical face mask
- filtering face piece (FFP3) mask.

Surgical face masks are ineffective against airborne infection, but provide protection against splashes of blood and bodily fluids on to the face and into the mouth and nose. In addition, they are also useful for patients who are prone to bouts of coughing and sneezing. Some surgical face masks come with a clear shield to protect the eyes from splash contamination. These should be used if you believe there may be a risk of you being splashed by bodily fluids from the patient.

FFP3 masks, when fitted correctly, provide protection against airborne infections such as severe acute respiratory syndrome (SARS) [NHS England, 2013a]. To be sure you are correctly protected your organisation will probably test the fit of the mask to your face before you use it for the first time. This is known as a 'fit check'.

3.8.4 Eye protection

Eye protection, such as goggles, should be worn if a procedure is likely to lead to splashing of bodily fluids, including blood, into the eyes, e.g. when assisting the paramedic with intubation. Eye protection used should be single-patient use and disposed of as healthcare waste. Hand hygiene should be completed immediately after the procedure [SCAS, 2018].

3.8.5 Sleeve protectors

Most ambulance services have a 'bare below elbows' policy, making contamination of long-sleeved uniform less likely. However, cross-contamination can occur if you are manually handling multiple patients while wearing long-sleeved clothing such as your high-visibility jacket or fleece. Sleeve protectors can help protect your uniform from wrist to elbow.

Chapter 6 – Health and Safety

They are for single-patient use, can be worn over the top of gloves and should be disposed of as healthcare waste [SCAS, 2018].

3.8.6 Wearing and removing PPE

The amount of PPE required will vary depending on the patient and not all items are always required. In the event that an apron, mask and eye protection are required, adopt the following procedures for putting on and removing PPE [DoH, 2009a].

Procedure – Wearing PPE

Take the following steps when putting on PPE:

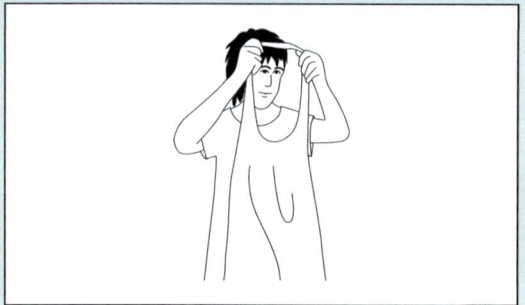

1. Put on apron as shown and fasten at back of waist

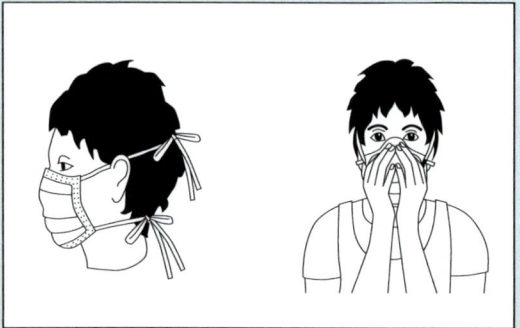

2. Apply face mask:
   - secure ties or elastic bands at middle of head and neck
   - fit flexible band to nose bridge
   - fit snug to face and below chin
   - check fit if using a respirator [NHS England, 2013a].

Procedure – Wearing PPE – cont

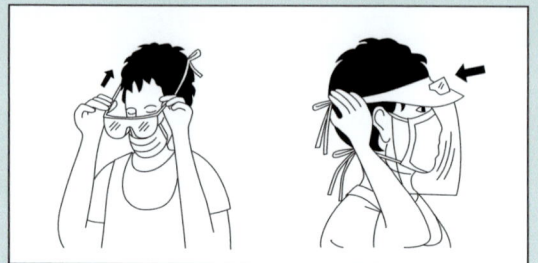

3. Put on eye protection; place over face and eyes and adjust to fit.

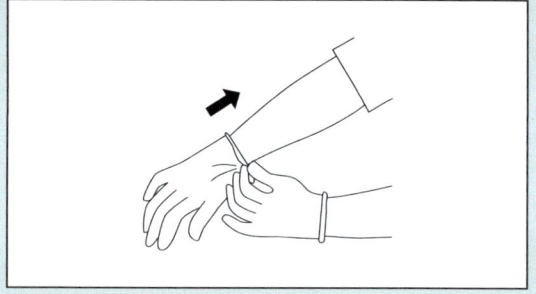

4. Put on disposable gloves; extend to cover wrists.

Procedure – Removing PPE

Take the following steps to remove PPE:

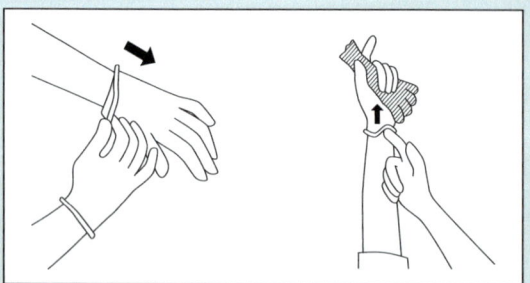

1. Remove gloves:
   - grasp the outside of the glove with the opposite gloved hand; peel off
   - hold the removed glove in the gloved hand
   - slide the fingers of the ungloved hand under the remaining glove at the wrist.

Infection prevention and control

Procedure – Removing PPE – *cont*

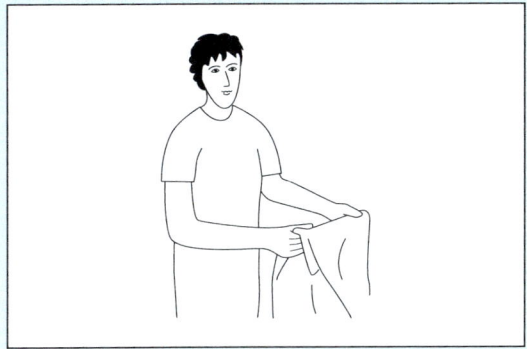

2. Remove apron:
   - unfasten ties
   - pull the apron away from the neck and shoulders, touching the inside of the apron only
   - turn the apron inside out, fold or roll into a bundle and discard.

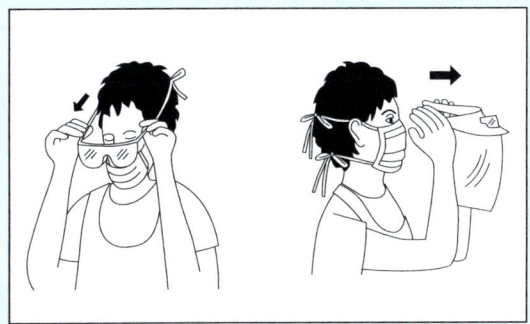

3. Remove eye protection; handle by headband or earpieces and discard appropriately.

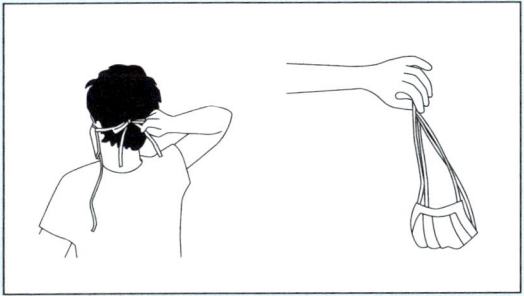

4. Remove face mask. Untie or break bottom ties, followed by top ties or elastic. Remove by handling ties only and discard appropriately.

3.9 *Managing healthcare waste*

Healthcare waste must be segregated immediately by the person generating the waste into appropriate colour-coded waste disposal bags or containers and labelled, stored, transported and disposed of appropriately [NICE, 2017b].

You should be aware of your organisation's policy on managing healthcare waste, but below are a number of basic principles that apply to most healthcare organisations.

3.9.1 Types of healthcare waste

Table 6.2 provides information on the different types of healthcare waste you are likely to encounter within the ambulance service. It's very important that all waste is segregated correctly as the way in which different waste is processed varies greatly based on the risk it presents. There are also significant cost variations, with domestic waste being far cheaper to process than infectious waste. Therefore, if infectious waste was filled with unnecessary packaging, it could lead to substantial unnecessary costs.

There are four main types of waste you will encounter:
- **Mixed sharps:** Sharps are items that could cause cuts or puncture wounds, including: needles, scalpels, knives, broken glass and open drug ampoules.
- **Infectious or potentially infectious waste:** Items where the concentration of harmful microorganisms is likely to be high enough to potentially lead to illness being transmitted. This would include the bodily fluids of a patient known to be suffering from an infectious disease.
- **Offensive/hygiene waste:** Non-infectious waste, from human healthcare. Likely to include items contaminated by bodily fluids, but where the patient is known to not be suffering from an infectious illness.
- **Domestic waste:** This form of waste presents no risk to human health and is similar to the domestic waste you would produce at home. Most of the packaging for products used on an ambulance, gloves without visible signs

Chapter 6 – Health and Safety

Table 6.2 Types of healthcare waste [DoH, 2013b; SWAST, 2016].

Waste type	Example	Disposal method
Mixed sharps	All needles from injections or cannulation, as well as used medicine ampoules	Incineration
Infectious or potentially infectious waste	Items contaminated by body fluids from a patient known, or thought, to be suffering from an infectious disease	Can be disposed of at a licensed alternative plant or through incineration
Offensive/hygiene waste, non-infectious waste	Soiled gloves or dressings, from a non-infectious patient	Landfill
Domestic waste	Uncontaminated packaging and rubbish, including gloves that are not visibly soiled	Landfill

of soiling, and wipes that have been used to clean a patient's finger for a blood glucose reading that is not visibly soiled can all be disposed of this way.

Table 6.3 provides examples of typical waste arising from ambulance service activity.

3.9.2 Storing and handling healthcare waste

All waste should be stored in appropriate receptacles, in line with your organisation's procedures. At times, it may be necessary to transport full bags of waste in the ambulance. If doing this, you should ensure that all bags or containers are sealed and stored safely in the vehicle.

When handling healthcare waste, consider the risks it poses and protect yourself appropriately by using PPE. As a minimum, when handling infectious or offensive waste bags, or containers, wear gloves and also use other appropriate PPE if you anticipate any leakage of waste contained within.

Always label and sign items as appropriate. Note that sharps bins have labels on them that should be completed.

3.10 Decontamination process

Decontamination is a key principle of infection prevention and control. It prevents both healthcare workers and patients from contracting infectious diseases that could be avoided, preventing patient death and patient discomfort as well as reducing costs.

Decontamination is divided into three separate processes:
- Cleaning is defined as the process that removes physical dirt or visible contamination from surfaces, but without necessarily destroying microorganisms [SWAST, 2016].
- Decontamination or disinfection refers to the destruction of microorganisms so that they no longer represent a danger of initiating infection, or other harmful response [HSE, 2015b].
- Sterilisation is the process that removes all viable microorganisms including viruses.

Cleaning, decontamination and sterilisation may not all be required; it depends on the item. Remember back to the chain of infection: decontamination is all about trying to break the transmission of potentially infective processes from reaching a new susceptible host.

Infection prevention and control

Table 6.3 Types of waste arising from ambulance service activity.

Activity	Waste type	Receptacle/bag	Justification	Disposal route
Injections	Contaminated sharps or syringes with medicine residue	Yellow lidded sharps receptacle ('sharps bin'; see Figure 6.4)	Potentially contaminated with medicinal products	Incineration
Items/equipment for treating patients	Contaminated packaging, gloves, aprons, other PPE, dressings, airways, suction liners, laryngoscope blades	Infectious waste in orange waste receptacles	Due to lack of patient records/screening, unlikely to be able to classify as non-infectious	Alternative treatment or incineration
Items/equipment for treating patients	Uncontaminated aprons, other PPE, non-medicated intravenous bags, non-infectious urine, faeces, vomit and their containers	Offensive/unhygienic waste disposed of in yellow and black striped ('tiger') bags	Risk assessment to determine no possible contamination and non-infectious	Non-hazardous municipal incineration/energy from waste or landfill. Note: Liquids (including body fluids) are banned from landfill
Waste packaging as a result of treating patients	Contaminated packaging: plastic and cardboard	Infectious after use, disposed of in orange bag	Due to lack of patient records/screening, unlikely to be able to classify as non-infectious	Alternative treatment or incineration
Refuse/rubbish	Uncontaminated packaging and refuse/rubbish	Non-infectious, black or clear bag	Used packaging, while patient treatment is being carried out in the vehicle, will usually not be infectious/clinical waste	Non-hazardous municipal incineration/energy from waste, materials recycling facilities or landfill

3.10.1 Decontamination process

It is likely that your organisation will have a cleaning schedule, which will cover things like the buildings you work in, the vehicles you work on, and the equipment you use at work. The schedules should detail how often things need to be cleaned, what procedure to use and with what products.

Refer to your organisation's infection prevention and control policy for further details. An example of a cleaning schedule is included in Table 6.4.

Cleaning schedules are designed to protect both healthcare workers and patients. Following the schedules is essential for maintaining a clean environment that reduces the chances of both you and your patients becoming unwell from contact with harmful microorganisms.

3.10.2 National cleaning colour code

The national colour coding of hospital cleaning materials was introduced by the National Patient Safety Agency (NPSA, 2007b) as a unified way of

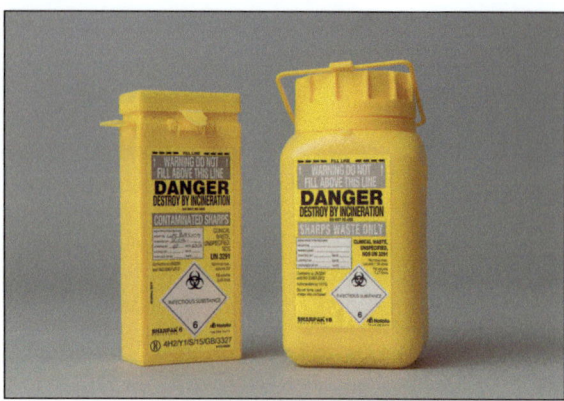

Figure 6.4 Sharps bins.

identifying which cleaning equipment should be used in different settings. The purpose behind this was to reduce the risk of cross-infection from cleaning equipment being used in a variety of different settings throughout hospitals and therefore increasing the likelihood of cross-contamination.

The colours used are:

RED: Bathrooms, washrooms, showers, toilets, basins and bathroom floors

BLUE: General areas, including departments, offices and basins in public areas

GREEN: Kitchen and dining areas

YELLOW: Isolation areas, including inside of ambulances

When cleaning the different areas, you should be sure to use the appropriate equipment for that area. In your place of work, equipment should be clearly segregated and colour-coded to help with this.

3.10.3 Decontamination procedure

Cleaning
Cleaning is the first step of effective decontamination and refers to removing visible dirt, including organic matter, and reducing the presence

Table 6.4 Cleaning schedules.

Item to be cleaned	When it should be cleaned	How to clean
Diagnostic equipment	After each patient contact	Use combined detergent and disinfectant wipes
Ambulance floor	Whenever visibly dirty and at least once per shift	Sweep/mop and bucket using an appropriate detergent or chlorine-based solution as directed locally
Outside of ambulance	Whenever visibly dirty and at least once per shift	Wash with warm water and vehicle detergent as supplied
Internal ambulance surfaces within patient reach	After every patient contact	Clean with disinfectant wipes

of microorganisms. Cleaning should include the use of detergent and hot water to remove all visible contamination and then be allowed to thoroughly dry [SWAST, 2016].

Decontaminating (disinfecting)
This should be carried out after a detergent clean and uses a range of products to reduce the number of viable microorganisms still remaining. A general principle is that disinfection should be minimised and instead single-use equipment used wherever possible [SWAST, 2016].

You may use different products depending on what you are trying to clean, but one product you are likely to have available is some form of sanitising wipes. Clinell® combined detergent and disinfectant wipes are found widely in healthcare settings for decontaminating solid items and

Infection prevention and control

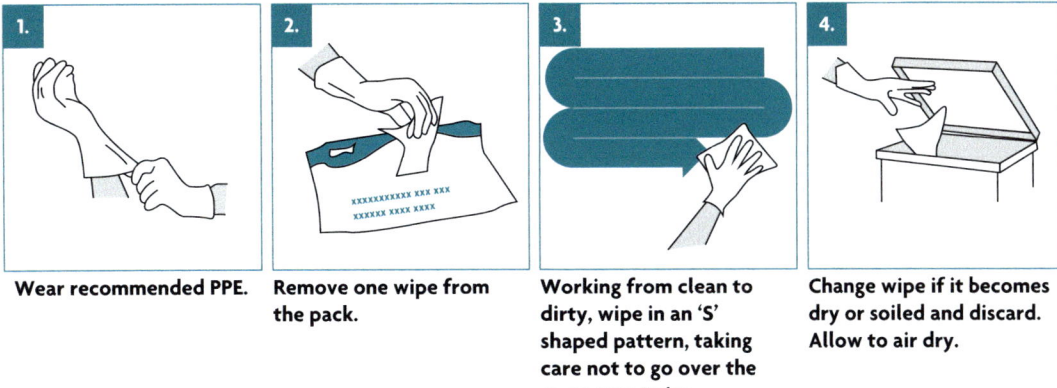

Figure 6.5 Clinell® wipes.
Source: Republished with permission of GAMA Healthcare Ltd. Best practice guidance for infection control wet wipes developed by Clinell and GAMA Healthcare Ltd. © 2016.

surfaces; instructions for their use are shown in Figure 6.5.

3.10.4 Storage of cleaning equipment

It is likely that your place of work will have a dedicated place for the storage of cleaning agents and equipment. As detailed above, cleaning equipment should be stored in a colour-coded manner, and cleaning agents and chemicals are subject to specific rules under the Control of Substances Hazardous to Health (COSHH) Regulations detailing how they should be stored and what to do in the case of a spill.

3.10.5 PPE for decontamination

A number of chemicals involved in the procedure of decontamination can be harmful to health if you are exposed to them inappropriately or in high doses. Whenever you are decontaminating, you should protect yourself from coming into direct contact with chemicals or any microorganisms that you may be attempting to clean. Be sure to use the appropriate PPE; this is likely to include:

- gloves
- apron
- sleeve protectors
- FFP3 face mask protection – if you are having to scrub something to clean it, there is a high possibility the liquid will become aerosolised, meaning you could inhale associated microorganisms.

3.10.6 Dealing with a biological spillage

Biological spillage refers to the accidental or malicious spilling of bodily fluids, including blood, urine, vomit and faeces. In your place of work, you should have a spill pack immediately available to use.

Although there may be slight differences based on the type of kit, it is likely that their use will follow the below procedure [SWAST, 2016]:

Procedure – Dealing with a biological spillage

1. Isolate the area where the spill has occurred.
2. Select and apply appropriate PPE (gloves, apron and potentially sleeve protectors and face mask).
3. Place an absorbent pad or granules on the spill.
4. Allow fluid to be soaked up into the absorbent material.
5. Remove pad or granules and dispose into the appropriate waste container or bag.
6. Using a disinfectant wipe in the manner described above, clean the areas the spill covered.
7. If the spill is on a floor, mop, using an appropriate cleaning solution.
8. Dispose of all cleaning materials into the appropriate waste bag.

3.11 Handling linen and laundry

All health providers use a large amount of linen on a daily basis and it is important that it is handled in such a way as to help prevent it from contributing to the spread of infection. Fresh linen should be stored in a neat clean environment where it cannot be exposed to potential infection risks. If working on an ambulance, you should carry a stock of clean linen, but you should not carry too much. Ensure that it is neatly stored, away from patient contact, most likely in a cupboard. If linen is visibly dirty, it should not be used, but be replaced with fresh linen.

Following each patient contact, after you have cleaned the ambulance trolley, you should replace the linen with fresh items, ensuring that you follow the procedures below for disposing of the old used linen.

When dealing with used linen, you must segregate and store it according to how it has been used [HSE, 2015d].

3.11.1 Used linen

Most used linen will be placed into a linen bag at hospital or a white plastic bag that can be sealed ready for collection.

3.11.2 Infectious and visibly soiled linen

Linen that has been used by a patient with a known infection or has been visibly soiled with body fluids should be treated as infectious and placed into a red alginate bag, before being placed into a red plastic sack. This signifies that the linen is infected and will be handled and washed in a specific manner to reduce the risk of cross-infection.

3.11.3 Storing linen

If working on an ambulance, it is likely that you will dispose of the majority of your linen at hospital. You should be aware of the procedures for storing used linen and make sure it is stored in such a way that it does not present a cross-infection risk to healthcare workers or patients.

Also be careful when moving linen as full bags can be heavy. Apply safe movement principles to reduce the risk of being injured by the manual handling procedures (see Chapter 7, 'Manual Handling').

3.12 Sharps injury

If handled correctly, there should be minimal risk of a sharps injury occurring. However, accidents do happen, so you should be aware of the action to undertake if you are injured by a sharp object while at work. You should take particular care with any 'used sharps' as these present a risk for transmitting infection. To reduce the risk of sharps injury you should:
- keep sharps covered whenever possible
- immediately dispose of used sharps into approved containers
- know where your sharps are stored and check the integrity of packaging frequently
- ensure that others around you are aware when you are using a sharp item.

If you do receive a sharps injury, then you should [HSE, 2015c]:
- encourage the wound to gently bleed, ideally holding it under running water
- wash the wound using running water and plenty of soap
- don't scrub the wound while you are washing it
- don't suck the wound
- dry the wound and cover with a waterproof plaster or dressing
- seek urgent medical attention as prophylaxis may be required
- report the injury.

Sharps injuries from needles and cannulation equipment are considered to be high risk and can potentially spread infections of blood-borne viruses, including:
- hepatitis B
- hepatitis C
- human immunodeficiency virus (HIV).

You should seek expert medical help as soon as possible after a sharps injury. Your employing organisation will most likely have a procedure in place for doing this, which you should be aware of.

3.13 Splash contamination

There is a risk of diseases being transmitted if blood or other bodily fluids are splashed onto healthcare staff in a location where they can easily enter the body. These locations include:
- open cuts or wounds
- mucosal membranes including the eyes and mouth.

If this happens, you should immediately irrigate the area with copious amounts of tap water. Following this, you should attend an ED or MIU so that a risk assessment can be undertaken and post-exposure prophylaxis administered if it is thought to be necessary, along with gathering blood samples [SWAST, 2016].

3.14 Legionella awareness

Legionella bacteria are commonly found in water and can lead to a deadly form of pneumonia if allowed to multiply [HSE, 2018g]. Your place of work should have a risk assessment for legionella and there may be control measures in place to help reduce the risk. These risk assessments should include strategies to minimise legionella growth, including storing and distributing water above 45°C or below 20°C, and ensuring there are minimal opportunities for water to stagnate: a common breeding ground for legionella.

Local risk assessments may identify that infrequently used water outlets such as shower heads may need flushing on a weekly basis. Where this is the case, it is possible that you will be asked to help achieve this as part of your routine duties and log it in a record on station. You should report any issues that cause standing water to form and remain for long periods of time so that action can be taken to reduce the risk of legionella developing.

3.15 Occupational health

Healthcare is a potentially stressful and physical environment and the hard work, combined with rota shifts, can, in some circumstances, be detrimental to your health. However, occupational health teams are there to work towards keeping staff physically and emotionally well at work [NHS Employers, 2017].

If you become unwell through work or suffer from a work-related condition, it is likely that you will be assessed and receive support from your occupational health team who can refer you for appropriate treatment or make suggestions for reasonable adjustments to be made in order for you to do your job safely and successfully. An example of reasonable adjustments might be the purchasing and supply of different gloves to help with recurrent contact dermatitis, or supplying a different, customised chair for office workers with back problems.

The occupational health team can also support you if you are exposed to infectious diseases at work. For example, if you receive a sharps injury from a hepatitis positive patient, your occupational health team can arrange for appropriate treatment and tests to be undertaken.

It is likely you will be given details of the services your occupational health team provides and how you can contact them when you join your employing organisation.

3.16 Reporting incidents

Any incidents relating to infection prevention and control should be recorded through the usual incident reporting system in place within your organisation.

4 Fire safety

4.1 Learning objectives

By the end of this section, you will be able to:
- describe practices that prevent fires from:
  - starting
  - spreading
- explain emergency procedures to be followed in the event of a fire in the work setting.

4.2 Introduction

Fire is a chemical reaction that requires three elements:
- heat
- oxygen
- fuel.

Together, heat, oxygen and fuel make up the fire triangle (or triangle of combustion; see Figure 6.6). For combustion or burning to occur, oxygen must combine with a fuel. Fuels can be in solid, liquid or gas form to start with, but for flaming combustion to occur, a solid or liquid fuel must be converted into a vapour, which then reacts with oxygen. An oxygen concentration of about 16% is required for combustion to occur and air contains 21%, which is plenty [HMFSIPS, 1998].

4.3 Fire prevention

Prevention is better than cure and there are a number of things you can do to prevent fires from starting [HMG, 2006]:

- Do not smoke in the workplace. The NHS has prohibited smoking in all areas other than those dedicated as smoking zones. Take care with cigarettes and matches; always discard in a suitable place and ensure they are fully extinguished.
- Do not allow the build-up of rubbish or other combustible materials in your work area, corridors or stair enclosures as this is fuel and may create an obstruction to escape routes.
- Do not have fabric, paper or other readily combustible material near electric fires or portable gas heaters.
- Do not leave hotplates or containers, e.g. frying pans, unattended when in use.
- Flammable gases and liquids should be stored in the designated location, e.g. the medical gases store.
- Defective electrical wiring or equipment must be turned off immediately, marked as defective and reported to the Estates Department. If possible, also remove from general access.
- Switch off all electrical and gas appliances when they are not in use.
- Check your working area before you leave for the day.
- Ensure that manual fire-fighting equipment is accessible, undamaged and maintained.

4.4 What to do in the case of fire

If you discover a fire [DoH, 2013a]:
- **Stay safe:** Never compromise your own safety.
- **Raise the alarm:** Press your thumb against the glass of the nearest and safest fire call point (fire break glass). Alternatively, repeatedly shout 'FIRE' to warn others.
- **Phone 999 (or 9 999 from some phones) and request the fire service:** Activation of a building fire alarm does not mean the fire and rescue service is automatically alerted, and you should make the emergency call every time.
- Get out and close the door. Go to the designated fire assembly point immediately.

If you hear the fire alarm, you should [DoH, 2013a]:
- **Leave your place of work:** Close windows and doors behind you if this can be done quickly.
- **Exit calmly:** Make your way to the nearest and safest fire exit. Do not run or stop to collect personal belongings.
- **Encourage others to exit:** Attempt to offer assistance to anyone who appears to be confused or having difficulties, especially people with disabilities. If your usual exit route is blocked by smoke or flames, stop, change direction and find an alternative escape route.

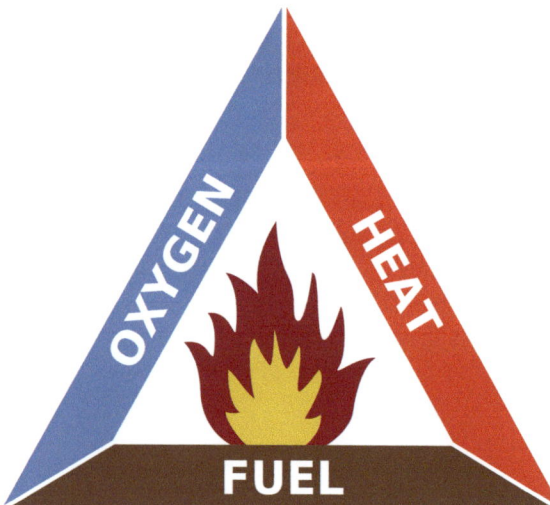

Figure 6.6 Fire triangle.

You should still meet at the normal assembly point for your workplace.
- **Do not use lifts:** Their movement assists fire travel and they may stop suddenly if there is a power failure. They may also take you to the scene of the fire. Use the stairs at all times.
- **Move to your designated assembly point:** Make yourself known to the fire marshal or person who is coordinating the evacuation. Note that fire marshals are typically only appointed in larger premises (i.e. not ambulance stations) and are identified by a yellow tabard.
- **Form an orderly group:** Remain together until a head count is established and until further instructions are given.

4.4.1 Vehicle fires

If a fire breaks out in a vehicle, take the following actions [UK Fire Service Resources, 2019]:
- stop
- switch off the ignition and press the battery isolator button (if the vehicle has one)
- release the bonnet; DO NOT open
- get everyone out of the vehicle
- remove medical gas cylinders if possible
- move any patients, crew and yourself to a place of safety in case the burning vehicle explodes; this may be as much as 200 metres away
- warn oncoming traffic
- summon help by dialling 999 and requesting the fire and rescue service; inform the emergency operations centre
- if and only if you believe it is safe to do so, attempt to put out the fire with the dry powder extinguisher provided. If the fire is in the engine compartment, do not open the bonnet; use the extinguisher through the grill or under the edge of the bonnet. Use with caution, and if in doubt do not attempt to tackle the fire.

5 Stress

5.1 *Learning objectives*

By the end of this section, you will be able to:
- describe common signs and indicators of stress
- compare strategies for managing stress.

5.2 *Introduction*

Stress is the adverse reaction people have to excessive pressures or other types of demand placed on them. There is a clear distinction between pressure, which can create a 'buzz' and be a motivating factor, and stress, which can occur when this pressure becomes excessive [HSE, 2017a].

Six broad areas have been highlighted as being the primary sources of stress at work [HSE, 2017a]:
- **Demands:** This includes issues such as workload, work patterns and the work environment.
- **Control:** How much say the person has in the way they do their work.
- **Support:** This includes the encouragement, sponsorship and resources provided by the organisation, line management and colleagues.
- **Relationships:** This includes promoting positive working to avoid conflict and dealing with unacceptable behaviour.
- **Role:** Whether people understand their role within the organisation and whether the organisation ensures they do not have conflicting roles.
- **Change:** How organisational change (large or small) is managed and communicated in the organisation.

5.3 *Signs of stress*

Stress can cause changes in those experiencing it, making it important for everyone to look out for changes in a person's or a group's behaviour, particularly in NHS ambulance services, where half of employees experience work-related stress [PIE, 2014]. However, in many cases, only you will notice the changes that occur as a result of the stress you experience.

Stress can show itself in many different ways and people will exhibit different signs and symptoms. Some of the well-known signs and symptoms of stress include [HSE, 2018h]:
- behaviour change:
  - difficulty sleeping
  - altered eating habits
  - smoking and/or drinking more
  - avoiding friends and family
  - sexual problems

- physical:
  - tiredness
  - indigestion and nausea
  - headaches
  - aching muscles
  - palpitations
- mental:
  - increased indecision
  - difficulty in concentrating
  - poor memory
  - feeling inadequate
  - low self-esteem
- emotional:
  - mood swings, becoming irritable or angry
  - increased anxiety
  - feeling numb
  - hypersensitivity
  - feeling drained and listless.

5.4 Managing stress

Although stress is not an illness, it can cause serious illness if not identified and managed. The success of coping strategies to help reduce the effects of stress will vary from person to person. Consider some of the strategies that have been recommended [NHS, 2018a]:

- If you're not sure about the trigger for your stress, keep a diary of stressful episodes for 2–4 weeks.
- Take action to help relieve stress:
  - **Exercise:** Physical activity can help remove some of the emotional intensity of stress.
  - **Eat and drink healthily:** Eat a balanced diet and avoid excessive amounts of caffeine and alcohol.
  - **Take control:** This can be easier said than done in the ambulance service, but identify problems and think about possible solutions; having a suggestion adopted by an organisation to help in your daily work, particularly when it is benefiting patients, is very satisfying [Pilbery, 2016].
  - **Talk to someone:** Sharing work troubles can help ease the stress as well as provide an opportunity for others to understand how you are feeling and help you to see things a different way.
  - **Avoid unhealthy habits:** Don't rely on alcohol, smoking and caffeine as a method of coping; the temporary relief they provide can lead to long-term health problems.
  - **Accept the things you can't change:** There are inevitably going to be aspects of the job that you cannot change. Accept those and focus on areas where you can have an impact and take control.

For further information on looking after your own mental well-being and that of your colleagues, refer to the end of Chapter 21, 'Mental Health', later on in this book.

Chapter

7 Manual Handling

1 Principles of manual handling

1.1 Learning objectives
By the end of this section you will be able to:
- define manual handling
- explain principles for safe moving and handling
- describe what action should be taken if the individual's wishes conflict with their plan of care in relation to health and safety and their risk assessment.

1.2 Introduction
Manual handling is a necessary part of your day-to-day work within the ambulance service. However, if not conducted safely, it can lead to injury to yourself, your colleagues and patients. Proportionally, injuries to ambulance staff are much more frequent compared with other professions [HSE, 2019a], so adopting safe manual handling principles is vital.

1.2.1 Definitions
The Health and Safety Executive [HSE, 2016] define manual handling operations as any transporting or supporting of a load (including the lifting, putting down, pushing, pulling, carrying or moving thereof) by hand or bodily force.

A load is defined as a discrete moveable object and may include packages, such as a box of medical stores, bags, including the response bags on an ambulance, and also patients, whether it be carrying them on an orthopaedic stretcher, or guiding them by the arm when they feel unsteady on their feet.

1.3 Consequences of poor manual handling
Moving and handling is an unavoidable part of working for an ambulance service and it is well known that poor moving and handling techniques, as well as repetitive tasks, significantly increase the risk of musculoskeletal injuries, particularly in the back. Musculoskeletal injuries are a significant cause of sickness and the leading cause of back injury for ambulance service staff. One of the most common injuries is a 'slipped disc', also known as a herniated disc (Figure 7.1).

1.3.1 Herniated disc
The spinal column is constructed of vertebrae, with intervertebral discs in between. These discs, which are designed to help take the load through the spine and to cushion the vertebrae, can be damaged by repetitive action or sudden movements, causing the outer layer (the annulus fibrosis) to rupture and protrude out beyond the normal diameter of the vertebrae.

When this happens, it pinches on the nerves, causing significant pain and even potential nerve damage [Nellist, 2013]. Most commonly, due to the natural curvature and the increased weight in this area, this occurs in the lumbar region, meaning that the nerves involved often include the sciatic nerve and lead to sciatic leg and back pain which is very uncomfortable (Figure 7.2).

1.3.2 Consequences to others
You should also consider that it would not just be you who can be injured by poor or inappropriate techniques. It is likely that any inappropriate technique will also lead to injury of your colleagues and even potentially your patient.

It is an unavoidable issue that sometimes you will need to undertake moving and handling procedures in high-pressure emergency environments, but even then you should continue to apply good principles of moving and handling to ensure that nobody is injured by such actions.

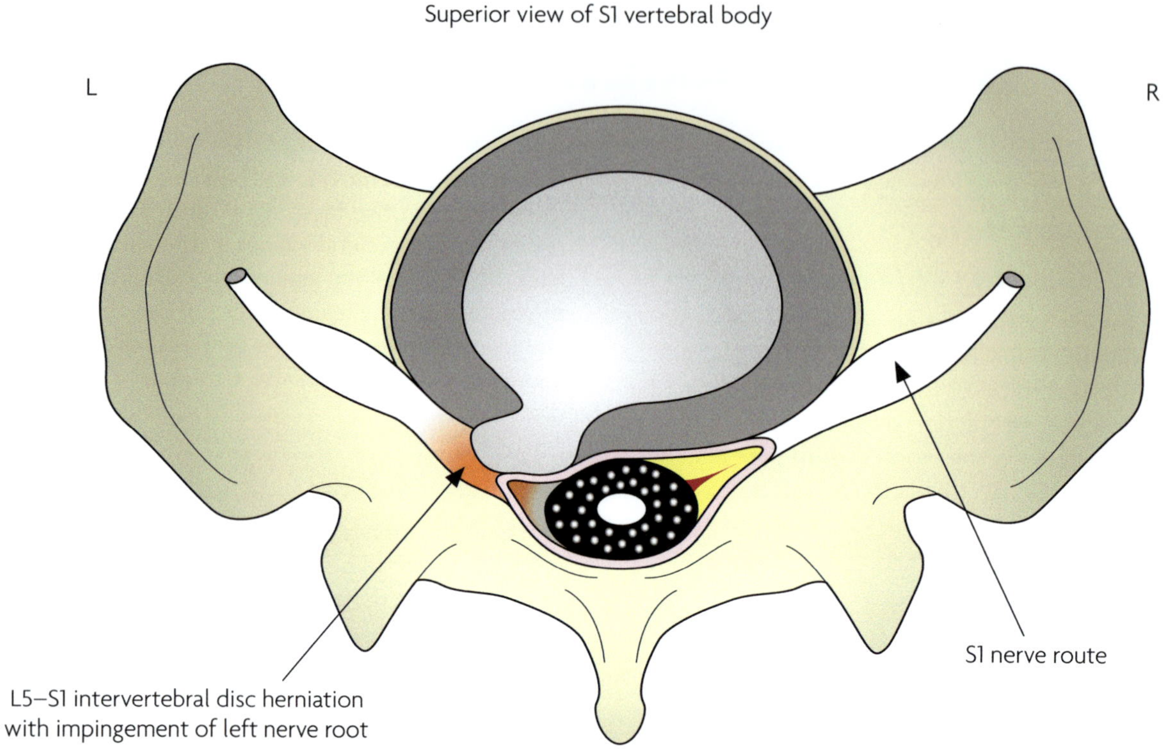

Chapter 7 – Manual Handling

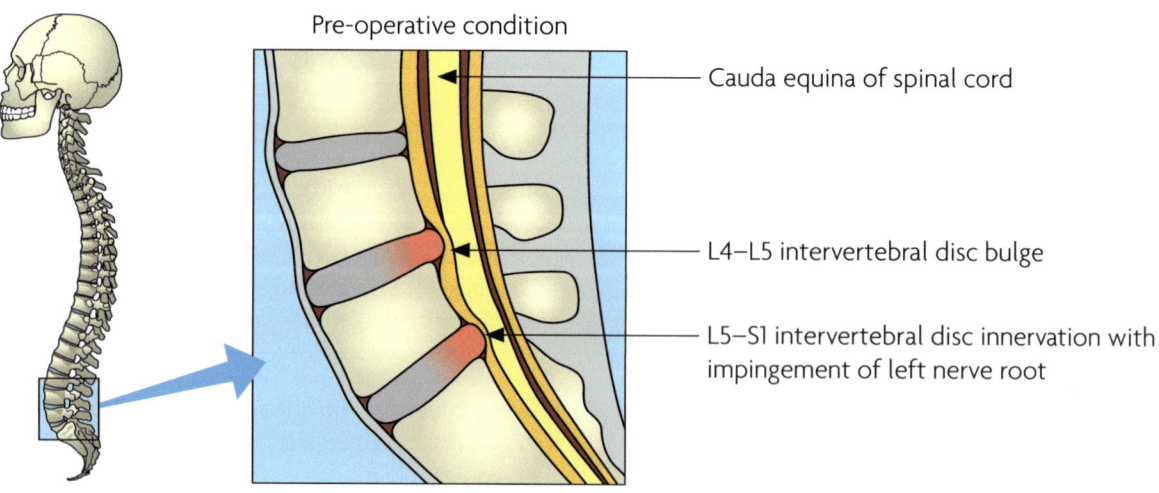

Figure 7.1 Herniated disc.

Figure 7.2 Lumbar spine – herniation.

1.4 Risk assessment

In Chapter 6, 'Health and Safety', you learned about risk assessment; manual handling is a perfect example of a set of actions that need a risk assessment to be undertaken before taking action. The difficulty in emergency situations is that the time available to make this risk assessment may be short.

There are five steps to take [HSE, 2014b]:
1. Identify the hazards.
2. Decide who might be harmed and how.
3. Evaluate the risk and decide on precautions.
4. Record your findings and implement them.
5. Regularly review your assessment and update if necessary.

This is not very user-friendly or specific to manual handling, and so these steps can be encapsulated in the TILEE acronym [HSE, 2011]:
- **Task:** Consider whether the lift:
  - involves holding the load away from the body
  - involves long distances
  - requires strenuous effort or twisting.
- **Individual:** Consider whether the lift:
  - requires specialist training
  - presents a hazard
  - is something you and your colleagues are capable of performing
  - should be undertaken if either you or one of your colleagues are pregnant.
- **Load:** Consider whether the load is:
  - heavy and bulky
  - difficult to get hold of
  - unstable
  - unpredictable
  - harmful
  - likely to grab out when alarmed at being carried down the stairs (if handling a patient).
- **Environment:** Determine the presence of:
  - constraints on posture, e.g. low ceiling, confined spaces
  - poor, uneven flooring
  - hot/cold/wet weather
  - poor lighting
  - noise.
- **Equipment:** Consider what equipment:
  - is available
  - will reduce risk to you and the patient
  - is safe to use
  - you are trained and competent in the use of.

1.4.1 Reducing risk

Legal responsibility

The Manual Handling Operations Regulations 1992, as amended in 2002, bring together European Directive 90/269/EEC on the manual handling of loads, general duties placed on employers by the Health and Safety at Work etc. Act 1974 and the requirements of the Management of Health and Safety at Work Regulations 1999 to detail how employers should reduce the risk from moving and handling injury so far as is reasonably practicable.

This should be done by assessing the risk, reducing the risk so far as is practicable and then regularly reviewing the risk to see if further controls are required.

An example of this is ambulance stretchers. Stretchers used to have to be lifted manually by two people and this led to a large number of injuries. To help reduce the risk, a new generation of ambulance stretchers was introduced that included hydraulic foot pumps, thus reducing the manual handling load. More recently, mechanically powered stretchers have been introduced (Figure 7.3). This further reduces the load and therefore the risk of injury.

Reducing the load in practice

Once you have identified a risk relating to manual handling, you will need to determine how best to manage this. Strategies for managing risk are best considered in advance, for example during your training, or by consulting manuals or guidance provided by your service and the Health and Safety Executive. When you are at the patient's side, however, these approaches are not suitable. You will seldom work alone, so ask colleagues for advice and don't be afraid to ask for additional

Chapter 7 – Manual Handling

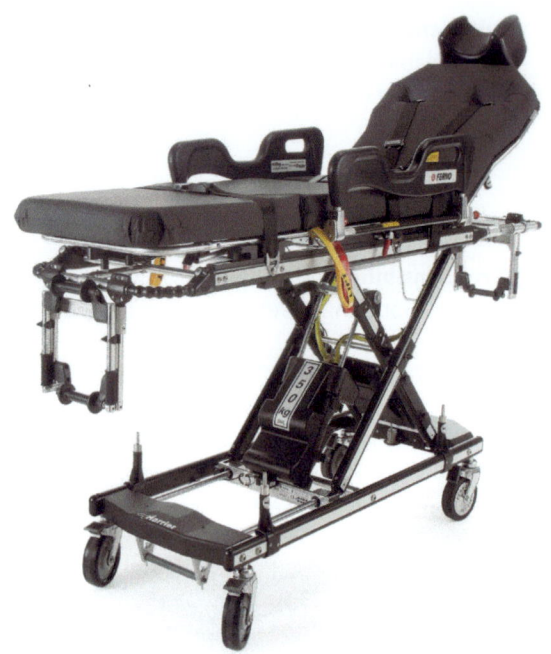

Figure 7.3 A Ferno mechanically powered ambulance stretcher.

help if your risk assessment suggests this would be beneficial. This is especially true for larger patients or where manoeuvres will be difficult due to limited access.

You should not use equipment you are not familiar with. However, some equipment does come with a manual or simple diagrams printed on its surface, which you can use to remind yourself about the correct way round it should be used or the sequence of actions required. Don't forget that other manual handling equipment may be available in your location, such as hoists, which can help reduce the risk to you and the patient. Note that this will usually rely on a trained member of staff being available to help you.

Patients who refuse manual handling aids
It is unlikely during the course of your work that you will encounter patients who refuse to be transferred or lifted using manual handling aids. However, some policies are unlawful in relation to a patient's human rights, such as blanket no-lifting policies, no lifting unless life or limb are at risk, and no lifting if equipment could physically affect the transfer [A & Ors v East Sussex CC].

This does not mean, however, that patients have a right to be manually handled without aids, just that consideration needs to be given to alternatives on a case-by-case basis. For example, a patient who refuses to be hoisted up off the floor does not have a right to be lifted by the ambulance crew, but an alternative, such as a lifting cushion, could be utilised instead [HSE, 2016]. In the event that a compromise cannot be reached, contact your line manager while on scene to assist with decision-making.

1.5   Biomechanics

Biomechanics is the application of the physical laws of mechanics to the human body. In order to reduce the risk of injury and facilitate manual handling, it is important to be aware of the following mechanical principles [Smith, 2011]:

- force
- gravity and equilibrium
- friction
- stress and strain
- pressure
- levers
- moment of force or turning force
- stability and equilibrium.

1.6   General principles

The next section covers specific moving and handling equipment and techniques, but it is helpful to know the basic principles to adopt when approaching a manual handling task [HSE, 2003].

There is no such thing as a completely 'safe' lift, but try to keep the weights for lifting and lowering in the zones shown in Figure 7.4. If you are twisting, reduce weights by 10% if you are required to twist beyond 45°, and by 20% if you must twist beyond 90° [HSE, 2012].

Principles of manual handling

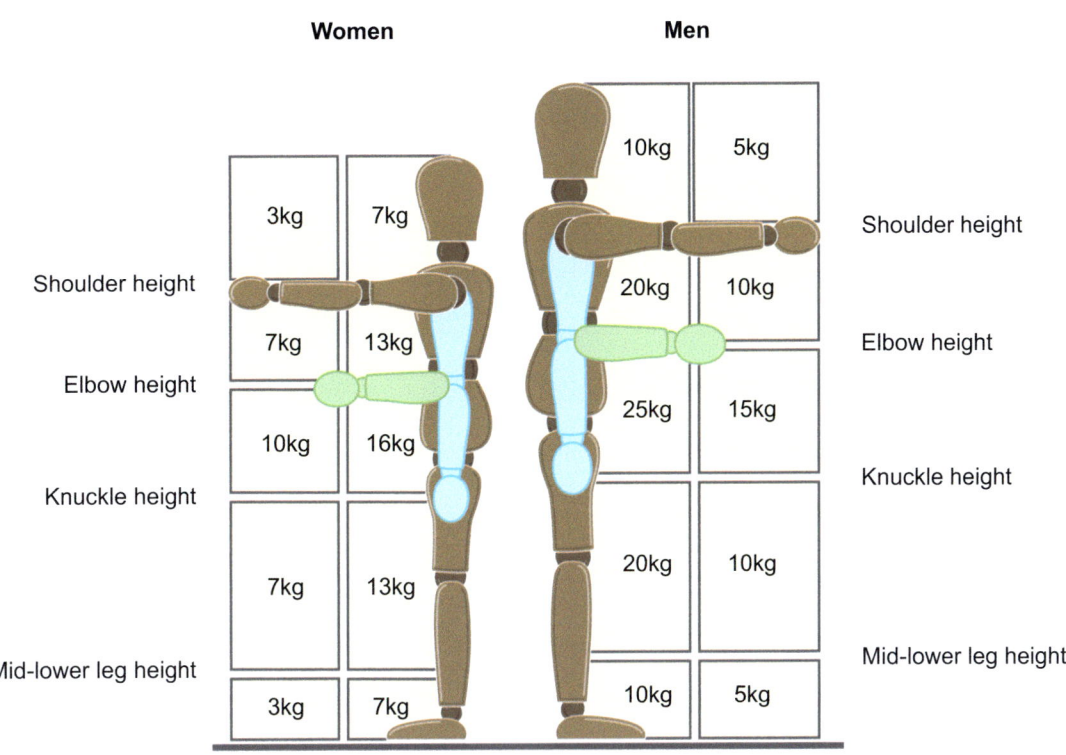

Figure 7.4 Guideline weights for lifting and lowering.

1.7 Handling aids

As you found out in Chapter 6, 'Health and Safety', the Manual Handling Operations Regulations 1992 (as amended in 2002), the Lifting Operations and Lifting Equipment Regulations 1998 and the Provision and Use of Work Equipment Regulations 1998 all require that your employer provides aids to assist in manual handling.

In the ambulance service, this may include:
- patient handling slings
- handling belts
- slide sheets
- transfer (banana) boards
- turntables
- lifting cushions
- a carry chair
- powered ambulance stretcher
- tail-lifts on the back of the ambulance.

Although not typically available on your ambulance, hoists are regularly used in hospitals and nursing homes and you may be able to utilise these if a suitably qualified member of staff is available.

Utilising handling aids appropriately can significantly reduce the likelihood of injury. However, if used incorrectly, they can be a danger to you and to your patient. Make sure you are familiar with the handling aids made available to you and do not try to use anything you are not trained and competent with. Handling aids should be regularly inspected for safety. Be aware of where service dates are marked on items like ambulance trolleys and carry chairs, and check they are in date, not obviously damaged or defective, before using them.

Chapter 7 – Manual Handling

1.8 Procedure

Procedure – Lifting/handling

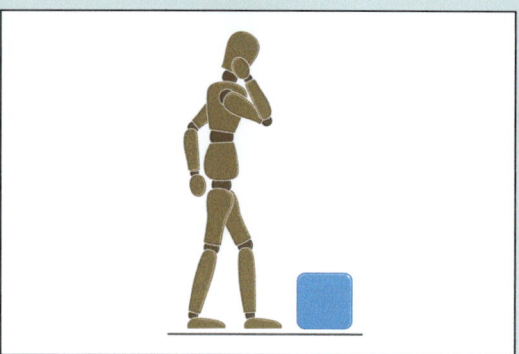

1. **Think before lifting/handling.** Plan the lift. Can handling aids be used? Where is the load going to be placed? Will help be needed with the load? Remove obstructions such as discarded wrapping materials. Can you reduce the moving and handling manoeuvre? For a long lift, consider resting the load midway on a table or bench to change grip.

2. **Prepare the load.** Whatever your load may be, prepare it so that it is as safe as possible to move. This may include securing items if carrying a load of medical stores, or warning a patient what is going to happen and instructing them not to grab out with their hands when on a chair.

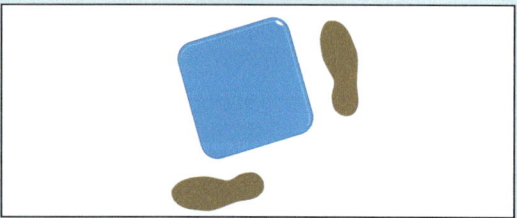

3. **Adopt a stable position.** The feet should be apart with one leg slightly forward to maintain balance (alongside the load if it is on the ground). The worker should be prepared to move their feet during the lift to maintain their stability. Avoid tight clothing or unsuitable footwear, which may make this difficult.

Procedure – Lifting/handling – *cont*

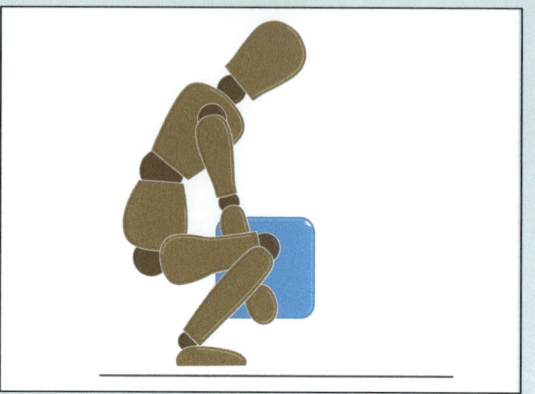

4. **Start in a good posture.** At the start of the lift, slight bending of the back, hips and knees is preferable to fully flexing the back (stooping) or fully flexing the hips and knees (squatting). Don't flex the back any further while lifting. This can happen if the legs begin to straighten before starting to raise the load.

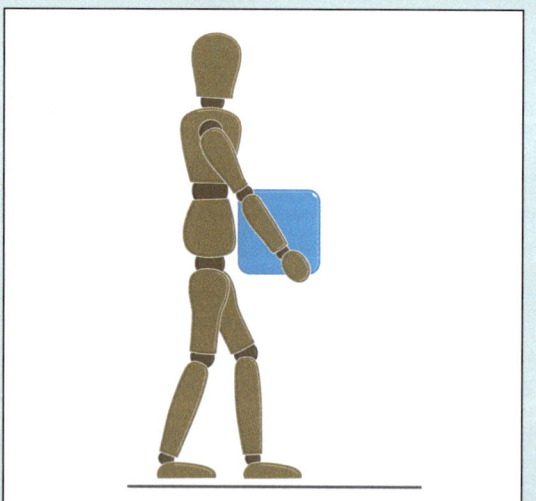

5. **Keep the load close to the waist.** Keep the load close to the body for as long as possible while lifting. Keep the heaviest side of the load next to the body. If a close approach to the load is not possible, try to slide it towards the body before attempting to lift it.

Principles of manual handling

Procedure – Lifting/handling – *cont*

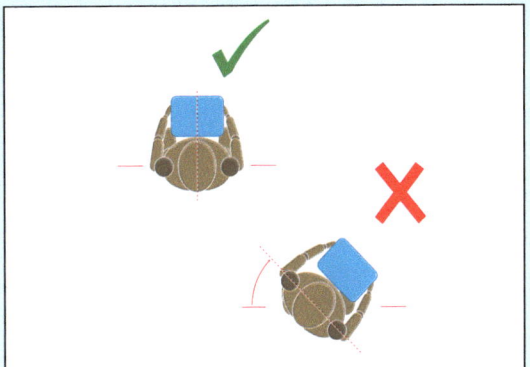

6. **Avoid twisting the back or leaning sideways, especially while the back is bent.** Shoulders should be kept level and facing in the same direction as the hips. Turning by moving the feet is better than twisting and lifting at the same time.

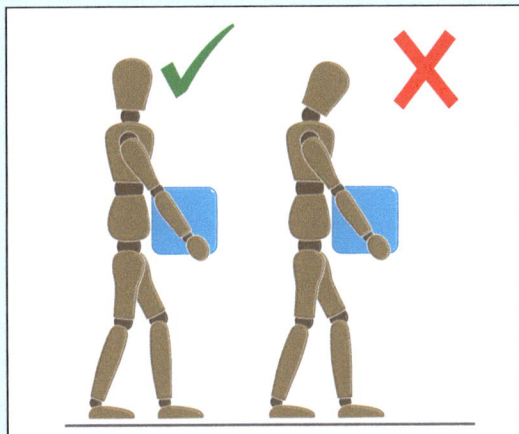

7. **Keep the head up when handling.** Look ahead, not down at the load, once it is held securely. Move smoothly. The load should not be jerked or snatched as this can make it harder to keep control and can increase the risk of injury. Don't lift or handle more than can be easily managed. There is a difference between what people can lift and what they can safely lift. If in doubt, seek advice or get help.

Procedure – Lifting/handling – *cont*

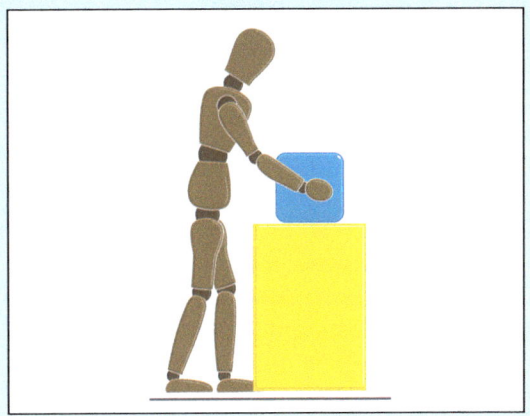

8. **Put down, then adjust.** If precise positioning of the load is necessary, put it down first, then slide it into the desired position.

1.9 Team handling

Working as part of an ambulance crew, you will undertake moving and handling tasks as part of a team, frequently moving a patient in a chair, trolley or on a stretcher with your crew mate. You should try to follow these principles when team handling:
- Try to match those of a similar size, build and strength to appropriate tasks.
- Run through the plan for the entire move in advance so everyone is clear.
- Communicate the command to move clearly: 'Ready, set, move'.
- Ensure that everyone moves and takes other actions at the same time.

Just because you are team handling does not mean that you can double the weight when two people are involved. Each scenario needs an individual risk assessment and you should not try to move loads that are outside of the capabilities of anyone involved in the team.

1.10 Bariatric patients

Bariatric patients are those who are morbidly obese and suffer associated health problems as a result. Definitions of bariatric vary, though most patients who are classed as morbidly obese (BMI >40) are considered to be bariatric. Bariatric patients can be particularly challenging to move due to the extra weight and sometimes reduced mobility as a result. This places both them and you at increased risk of injury if a moving and handling mistake is made.

As with all moving and handling tasks, you should undertake a dynamic risk assessment to determine the appropriate resources required. This may include additional colleagues to assist with moving or specialist equipment. Most ambulance services have specialist bariatric ambulances equipped with handling aids designed for bariatric patients. You should be aware of the weight limits of your handling aids and should not use them if your patient exceeds the limit.

1.11 Further help and support

Moving and handling will be a routine part of your role and you should be familiar with the appropriate techniques to use, and the support and equipment available to you. Should you have any moving and handling queries, you should approach your line manager or an individual appointed with responsibility for manual handling tasks. Most likely this will be a part of the health and safety department.

2 Moving and handling equipment and techniques

2.1 Learning objectives

By the end of this section you will be able to:
- describe the aids and equipment that may be used for moving and positioning
- describe the impact of specific conditions on the correct movement and positioning of an individual.

2.2 Introduction

This section provides guidance on different techniques that can be utilised for moving and handling patients. The choice of technique will depend on the urgency of the move, the number of staff and equipment available as well as the wishes and capabilities of the patient.

2.3 Patients on the floor

The usual advice from a call handler in response to a 999 call is to advise the caller not to move the patient. However, once an assessment has been completed by a crew on scene, the patient may no longer be required to stay immobile and certainly shouldn't remain on the floor.

If they need to remain flat, then an orthopaedic stretcher is helpful, if there is room. In confined spaces, a slide sheet can help to manoeuvre the patient to another location with more space.

If your patient cannot get themselves up off the floor, but is able to sit up, either with or without your support, a lifting cushion such as the Mangar ELK is ideal. However, you may find that your patient can get themselves off the floor, with guidance and assistance from you.

2.3.1 Instructing a patient to get off the floor – one-chair method

In order to undertake this procedure, the patient needs to be able to roll on to their side and be able to kneel, so it may not be suitable for patients with knee and hip problems.

Procedure – Getting off the floor – one-chair method

Take the following steps to instruct a patient to get off the floor using a single chair [Smith, 2011]:

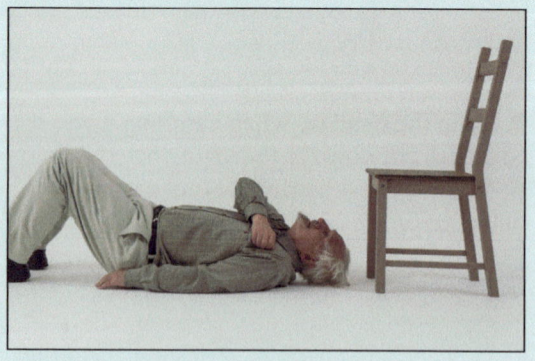

1. Position a chair at the head end of the fallen patient. Instruct them to bend their knees up and to bring one arm across their chest.

Procedure – Getting off the floor – one-chair method – *cont*

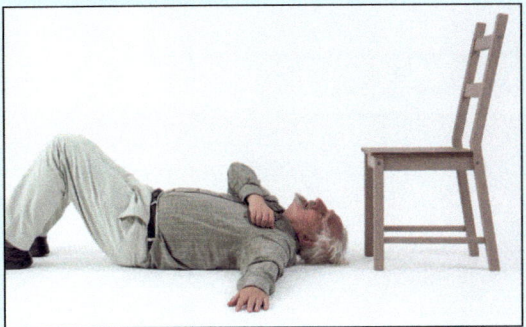

2. Instruct the patient to move their other arm away from the body.

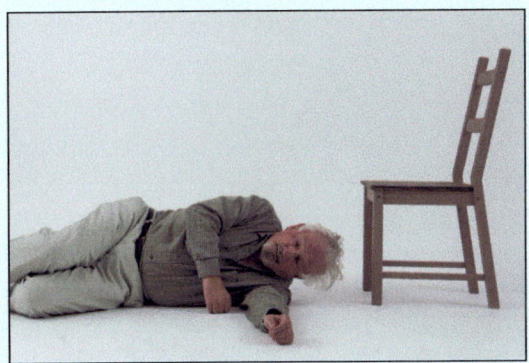

3. Instruct the patient to roll onto their side, and to bring their arm over their body so that it is flat on the floor.

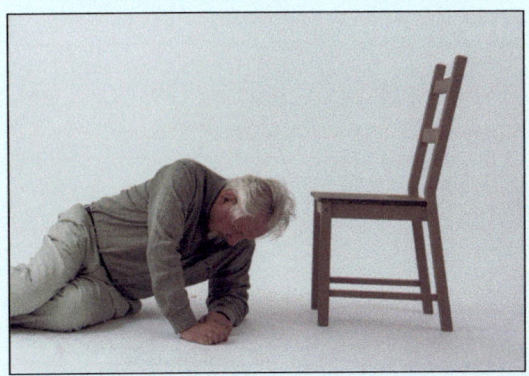

4. Instruct the patient to push up on their hand and at the same time push up on their forearm that is resting on the floor, until they are half-sitting.

Procedure – Getting off the floor – one-chair method – *cont*

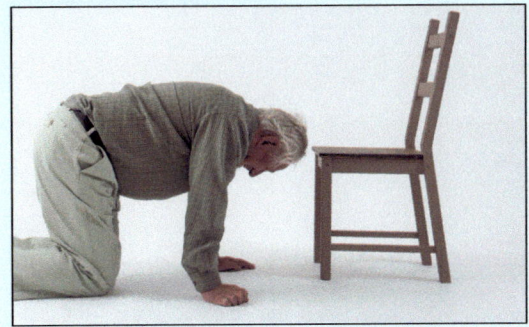

5. Continue to verbally support the patient as they continue to push upwards, until they end up on all fours facing the chair.

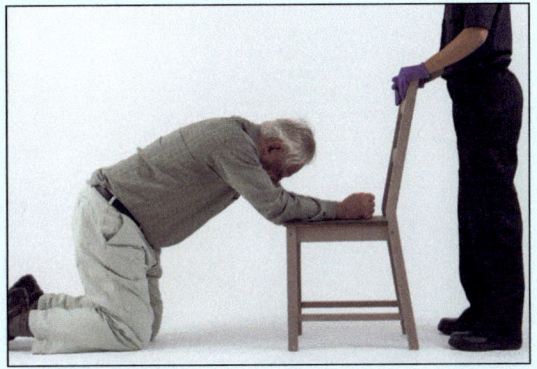

6. While holding the chair steady, instruct the patient to lower their arms onto the chair and ask them to lean on the seat of the chair.

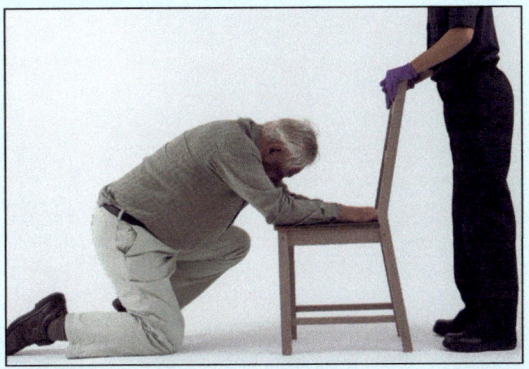

7. Instruct the patient to raise their stronger leg and place the foot of that leg on the floor.

Chapter 7 – *Manual Handling*

Procedure – Getting off the floor – one-chair method – *cont*

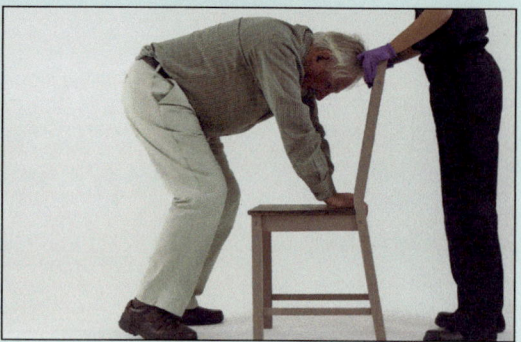

8. Instruct the patient to push up and straighten their legs.

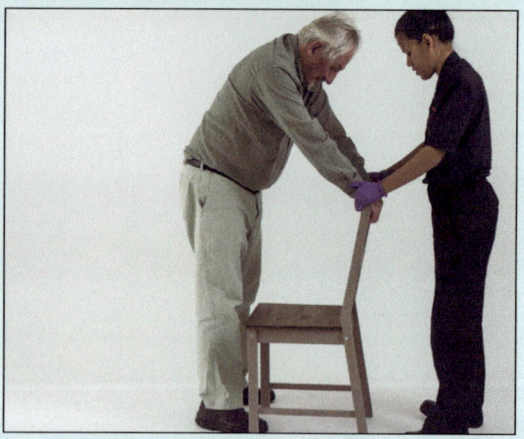

9. Allow the patient time to stabilise themselves and stand up straight, placing their hands on the chair.

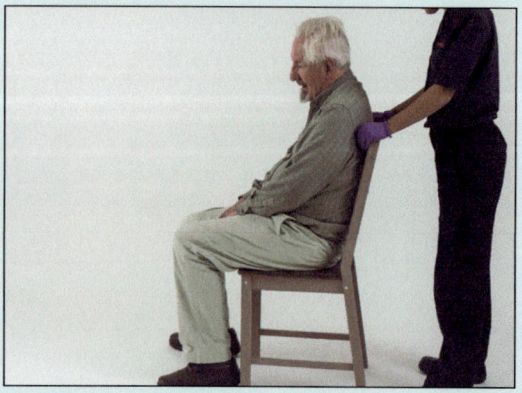

10. Instruct the patient to carefully turn and sit on the chair.

2.3.2 Instructing a patient to get off the floor – two-chair method

Procedure – Getting off the floor – two-chair method

Take the following steps to instruct a patient to get off the floor using two chairs [Smith, 2011]:

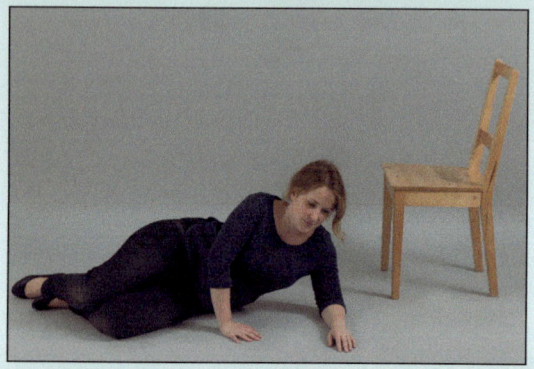

1. Position a chair at the head end of the fallen patient. Instruct them to bend their knees up and roll into side lying. They should then bring one arm over the chest until their hand is flat on the floor. Instruct them to push up with one hand and lower arm into a side sitting position as in the one-chair method.

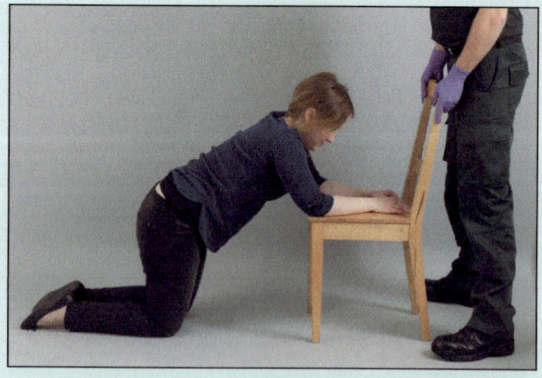

2. Instruct the patient to face the chair and place their forearms on the chair.

Moving and handling equipment and techniques

Procedure – Getting off the floor – two-chair method – *cont*

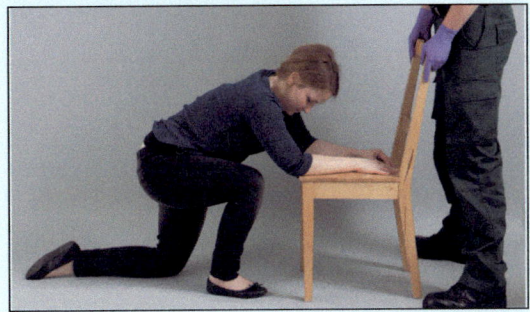

3. Instruct the patient to bend one knee and place the foot of that leg onto the floor, while at the same time pushing up on their forearms and hands.

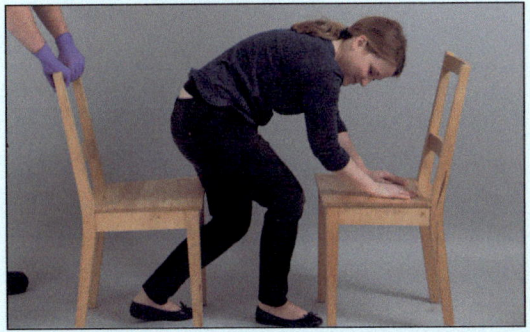

4. Place a second chair behind the patient, ensuring it is under their hips.

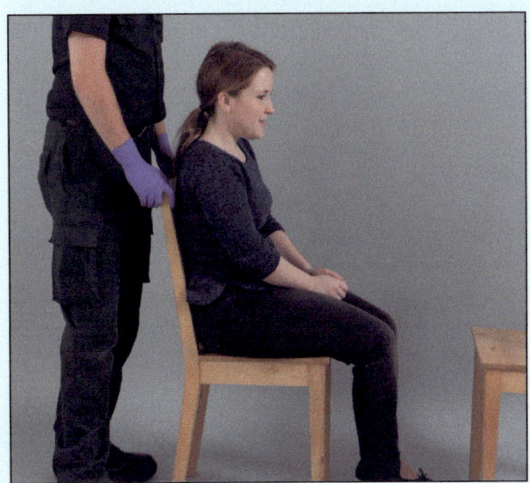

5. Instruct the patient to sit backwards onto the chair.

2.3.3 Lifting cushion

If a patient cannot get themselves off the floor using the one- or two-chair method, a lifting cushion (Figure 7.5) may be helpful. The patient does need to be able to partly assist with a transfer, for example, by shuffling/rolling on to the cushion. They also need to have sitting balance if using a cushion with no back [Smith, 2011].

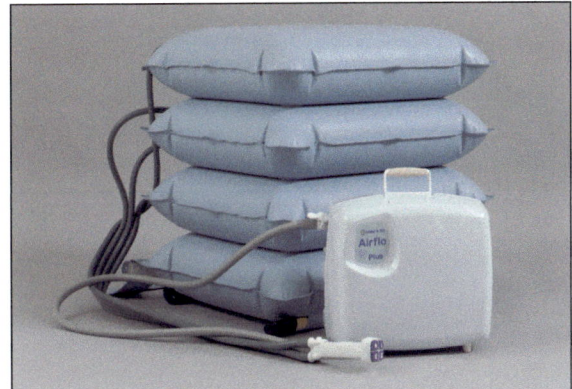

Figure 7.5 The Mangar ELK lifting cushion.

Procedure – Mangar ELK

Take the following steps to assist a patient from the floor using the Mangar ELK [Mangar International, 2016; Smith, 2011]:

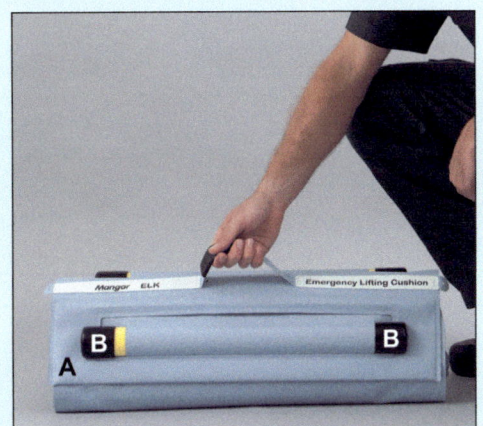

1. Unroll the ELK by unclipping the flap (A) from the ends of the stability bar (B).

Chapter 7 – Manual Handling

Procedure – Mangar ELK – *cont*

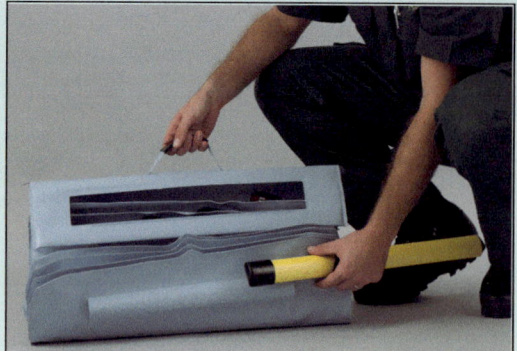

2. Remove the end cap and then the stability bar from its pocket in order to provide a more comfortable transfer for the patient.

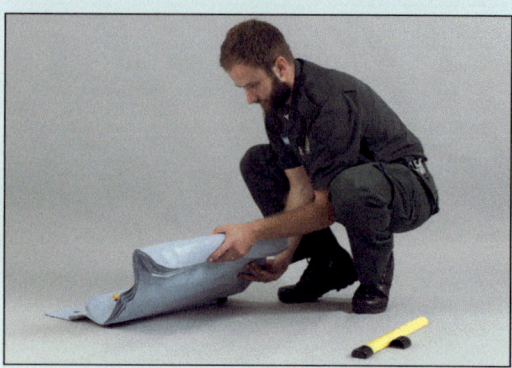

3. Fold the edge of the ELK underneath itself by folding along the line of the stability bar pocket.

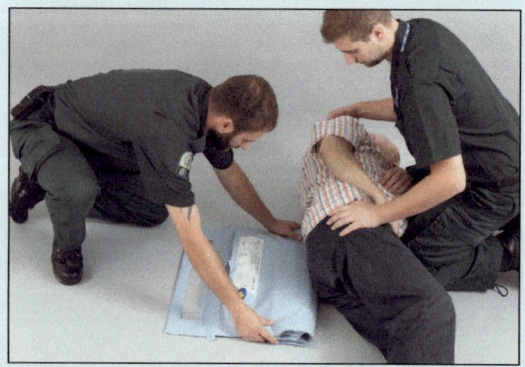

4. One crew member should roll the patient onto their side. A second crew member should position the ELK so that its 'upper' edge is approximately level with and tight

Procedure – Mangar ELK – *cont*

up against the patient's waistband. If the patient cannot sit up on their own, consider inserting a handling sling level with their shoulder blades, so you can assist them to sit up. **Note:** Place a blanket, groundsheet, towel or similar under the ELK if using it on a rough surface.

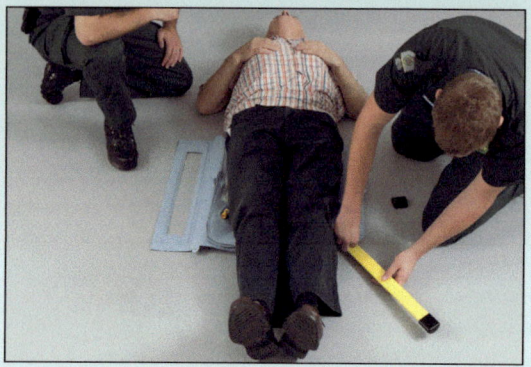

5. Roll the patient over on to the ELK until they are lying fully and squarely on the cushion. Unfurl the edge of the ELK, replace the stability bar and fit the end cap.

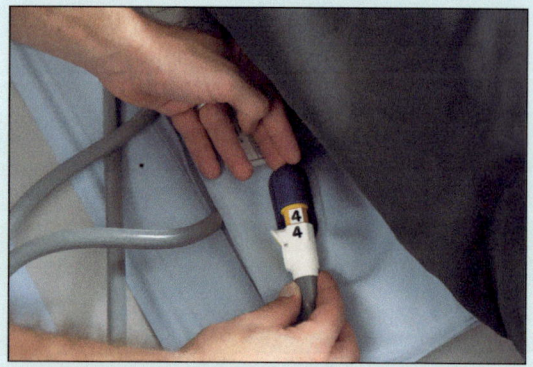

6. Connect the four distribution hoses from the four-way hand control to the four connectors on the ELK. The ends of the hoses are colour-coded and numbered to match the corresponding ELK connectors (No. 4 is the top compartment; No. 1 the bottom). **Note:** If the fallen person is very large, it is recommended to connect the compressor and the hand control before the person is rolled onto the ELK.

Moving and handling equipment and techniques

Procedure – Mangar ELK – *cont*

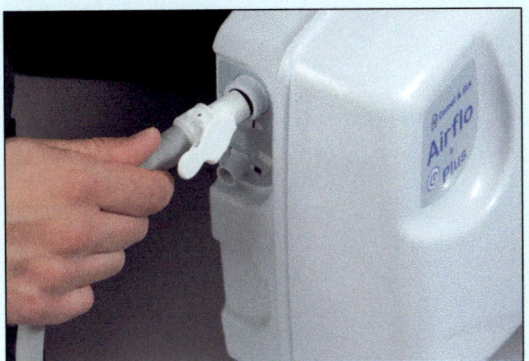

7. Position the Airflo compressor at the side of the ELK, ensuring that it will not be in the way while lifting and supporting the patient. Connect the hose from the four-way hand control to the air outlet socket on the Airflo compressor and select the Auto function on the Airflo compressor by pressing the power button until the LED light comes on.

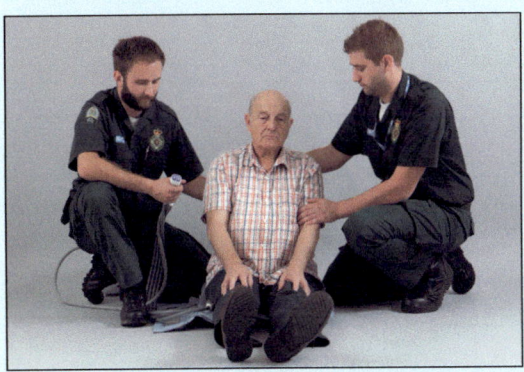

8. Kneeling beside the patient, place them in a seated position on the ELK. If necessary, place a transfer belt (with looped handles) around the patient's waist and adjust to fit. You may find a slide sheet useful. Explain to the patient what to expect when the ELK elevates.

Procedure – Mangar ELK – *cont*

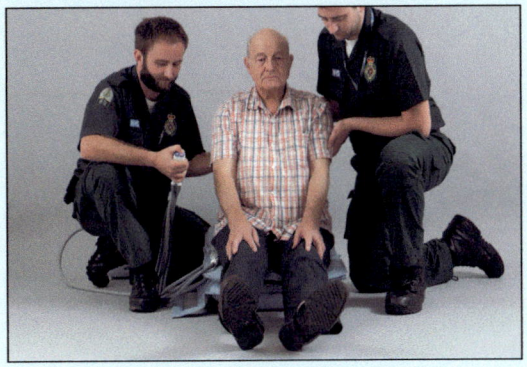

9. Press the No. 1 button on the four-way hand control. Steady the patient as the ELK lifts. Stop inflation when the first (bottom) compartment becomes hard. The compressor will automatically stop as each compartment becomes fully inflated.

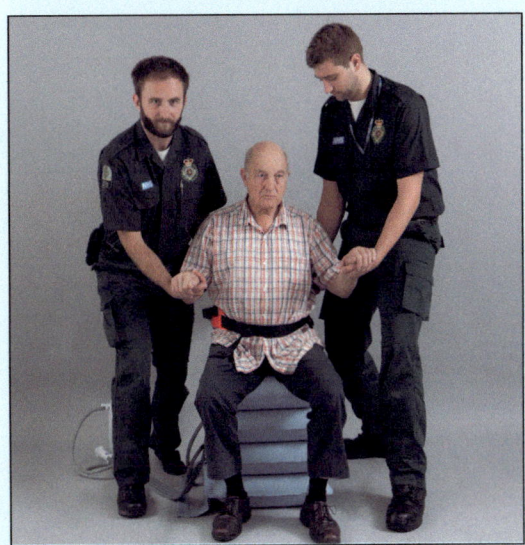

10. Continue to operate buttons 2, 3 and 4, in sequence, in exactly the same manner. Support the patient at all times. Always inflate the ELK sections from the bottom up. When all four compartments are inflated, the patient may be helped to stand or to transfer.

Chapter 7 – *Manual Handling*

Procedure – Mangar ELK – *cont*

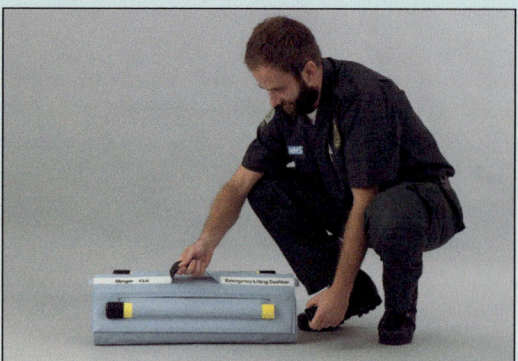

11. To deflate, disconnect each of the air hoses from the ELK. After use, roll the ELK up with the four-way hand control and re-secure the flap around the ends of the stability bar.

Procedure – Mangar Camel

Take the following steps to assist a patient from the floor using the Mangar Camel [Mangar Health, 2016]:

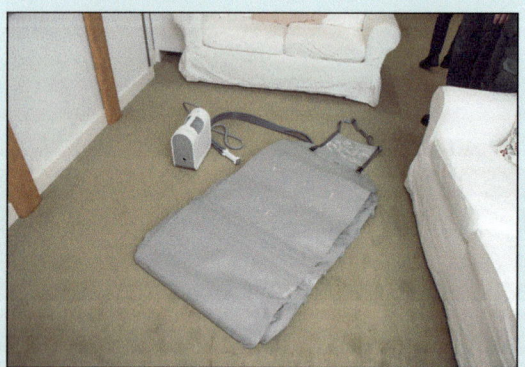

1. Remove the Camel from the carrying bag, unfasten the straps and unroll.

Procedure – Mangar Camel – *cont*

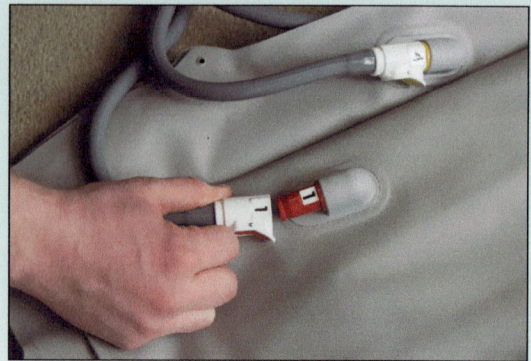

2. Connect the four hoses from the hand control to the corresponding numbered and coloured connectors on the Camel. Then connect the hose from the hand control to the Airflo Plus compressor.

3. Position the Airflo Plus compressor so that it will not be in the way while positioning the patient. Ensure that the hoses are not kinked.

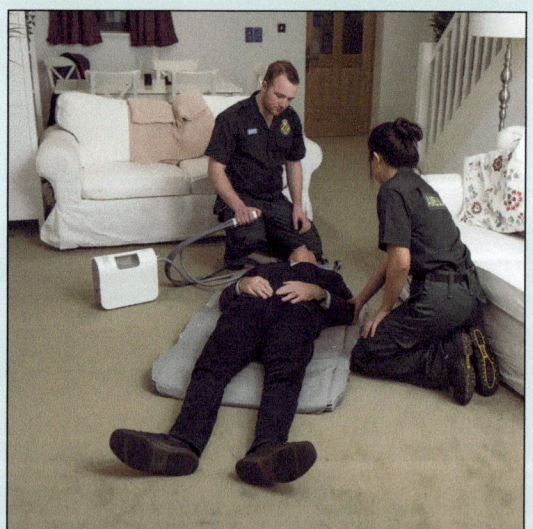

4. Position the Camel at the side of the patient so that the patient's head is level with the Camel badge. **Note:** Place a blanket, groundsheet, towel or similar under the Camel if using it on a rough surface. Transfer the patient onto the Camel. The head should lie on the Camel badge and the body should lie centrally.

Moving and handling equipment and techniques

Procedure – Mangar Camel – *cont*

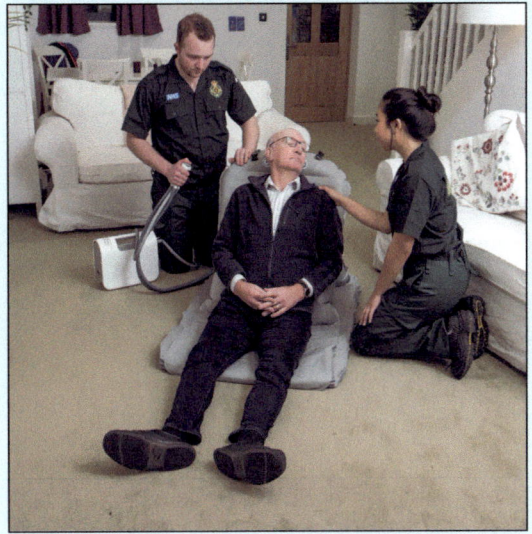

5. Press the No. 1 button on the hand control to partially inflate the backrest section until the patient is in a comfortable position.

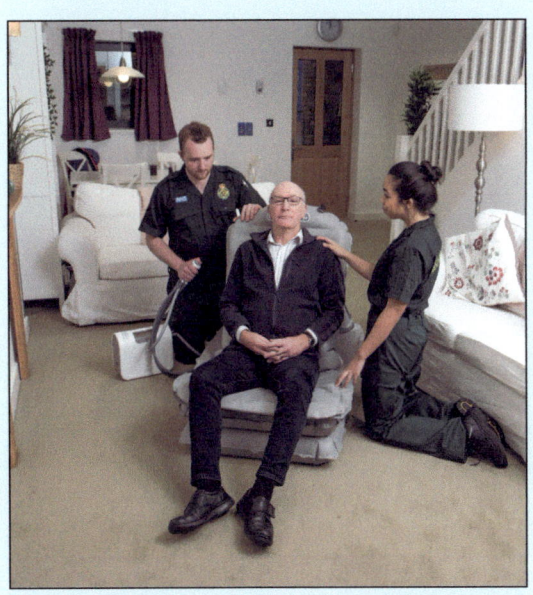

6. Press the No. 2 button to inflate the bottom section until it becomes rigid. Continue to press buttons 3 and 4 in sequence until the sections become rigid, in exactly the same manner.

Procedure – Mangar Camel – *cont*

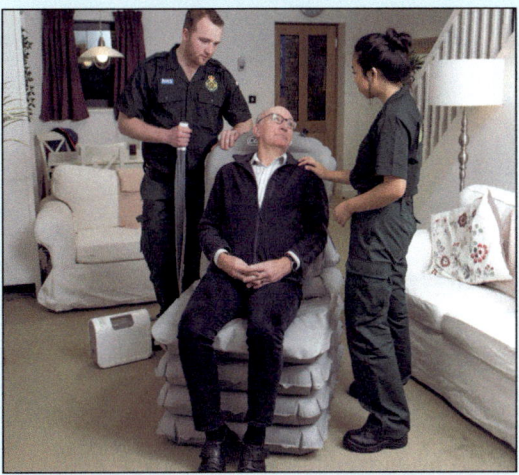

7. Press No. 1 button again to fully raise the backrest and arrive at a sitting position.

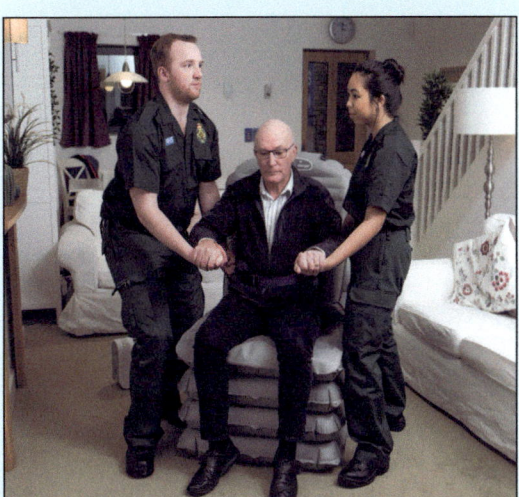

8. Assist the patient to stand if required. To deflate, disconnect each of the air hoses from the Camel. Roll up the Camel with the hand control in the hollow. Secure the straps and place in the carrying bag.

2.3.4 Fall in a confined space

If the patient has fallen in a confined space, such as a bathroom or small bedroom, manual handling is more hazardous. The most practical way to manage these situations is to move the patient to an alternative location while they are still on the floor.

Chapter 7 – *Manual Handling*

Procedure – Fall in confined space

Take the following steps to move a patient in a confined space [Smith, 2011]:

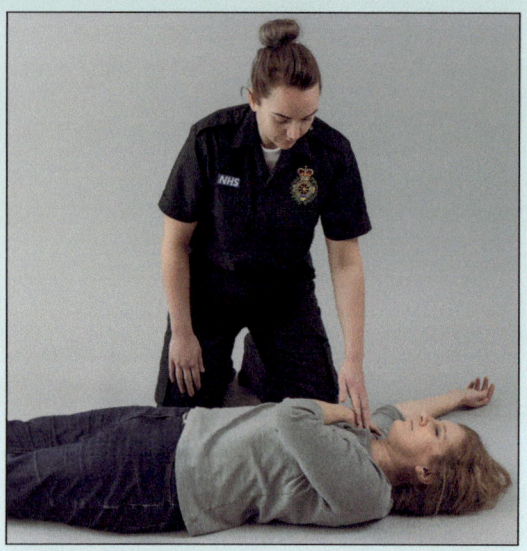

1. Assist the patient to position the arm further away from you across their chest and bring the nearer arm away from the patient's body so that it does not get trapped during rolling.

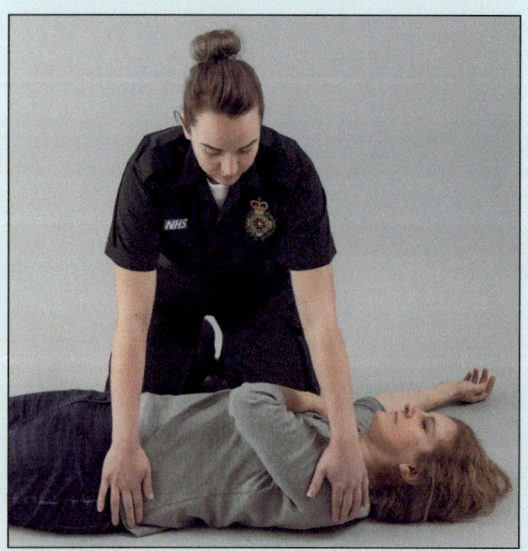

2. Start in a high-kneeling position and support the patient's hip and shoulder.

Procedure – Fall in confined space – *cont*

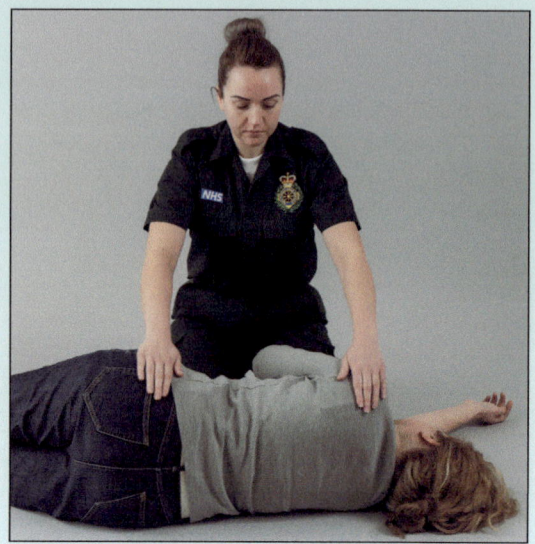

3. Roll the patient onto their side, sitting back into a low-kneeling position as you do so.

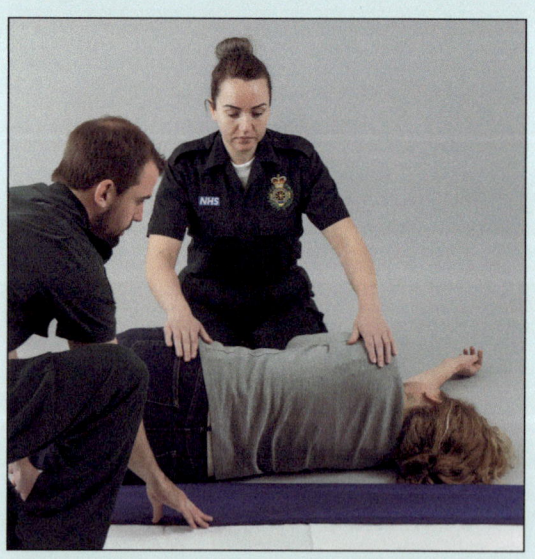

4. Now that the patient is on their side, a second crew member should roll two full-length slide sheets and place them lengthways and half under the patient.

Moving and handling equipment and techniques

Procedure – Fall in confined space – *cont*

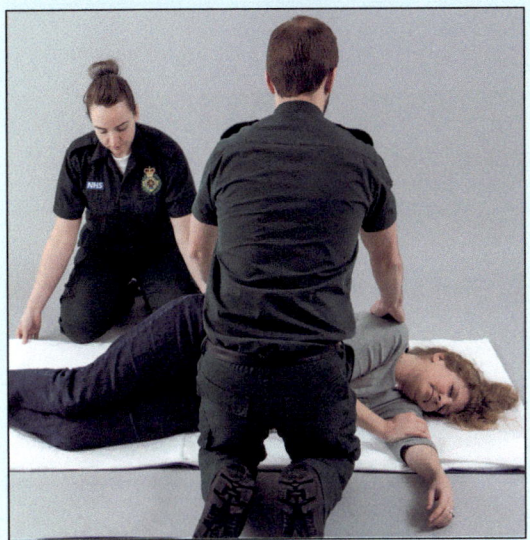

5. Lower the patient and roll them again onto their other side and smooth out the sliding sheets.

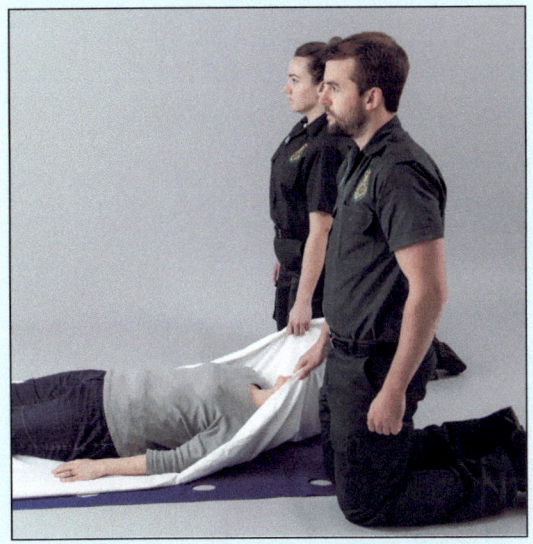

6. Lay the patient flat on their back and position yourself and another crew member, if required, in a high-kneeling position at one end of the patient, whichever is closer to the nearest open space.

Procedure – Fall in confined space – *cont*

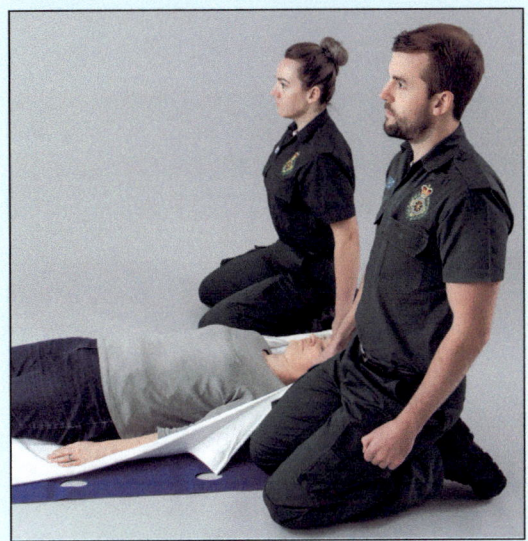

7. Decide which crew member is to issue instructions for the move. Hold the top slide sheet, or the carry sheet, or the top layer of a tubular sheet and transfer your weight so that you end in a low-kneeling position. Repeat until an open space is reached.

2.4 Seated patients

Many patients will be seated, on the toilet, a chair or their bed, when you need to assist them.

2.4.1 Sitting to sitting transfer

A transfer board (also called a banana board on account of the curved shape and yellow colour of some boards!) can enable the patient to transfer from a chair or bed onto the carry chair or vice versa. In order to use this technique, the patient must be able to [Smith, 2011]:
- flex forward and transfer their weight laterally
- place their feet on the floor

Chapter 7 – *Manual Handling*

- use their body strength to assist and understand what is required of them
- place their arm towards the end of the board and assist with movement across it.

A crew member can assist by bringing the patient's feet around (although a turntable can assist with this) and helping to transfer the patient's weight laterally. However, if the patient requires help with their feet and support to sit, then a second crew member should be used, preferably with a handling belt applied.

> **Procedure – Sitting to sitting transfer**
>
> Take the following steps to assist a patient to use a transfer board [Smith, 2011]:
>
>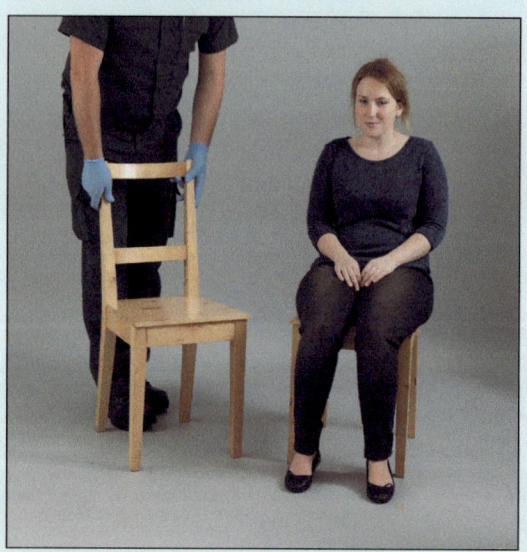
>
> 1. Explain the procedure to the patient and ensure they have suitable footwear. Place the destination chair at the correct angle (this will vary depending on the board used).

> **Procedure – Sitting to sitting transfer** – *cont*
>
>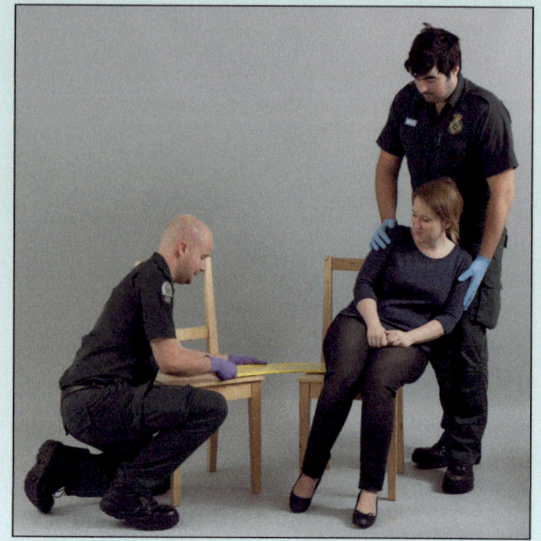
>
> 2. Ask the patient to lean away from the transfer side and insert about a third of the board under the patient's buttock. Ensure that a third of the board rests on the destination chair. Ensure the board is level.
>
>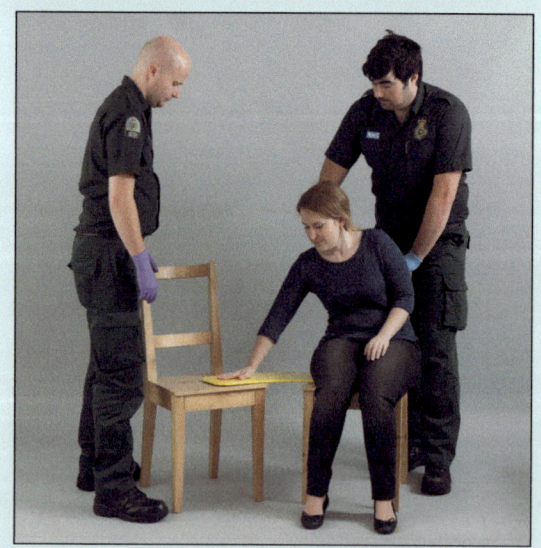
>
> 3. Instruct the patient to place their hand towards the far end of the board and lean towards it. Ensure the patient's fingers are not under the board.

Moving and handling equipment and techniques

Procedure – Sitting to sitting transfer – *cont*

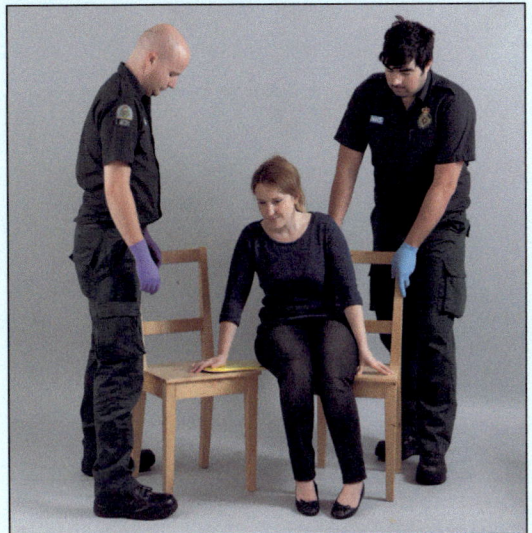

4. The patient should now shuffle across the board, using their other hand and feet to push. If they have reduced ability to push through their legs, use a turntable.

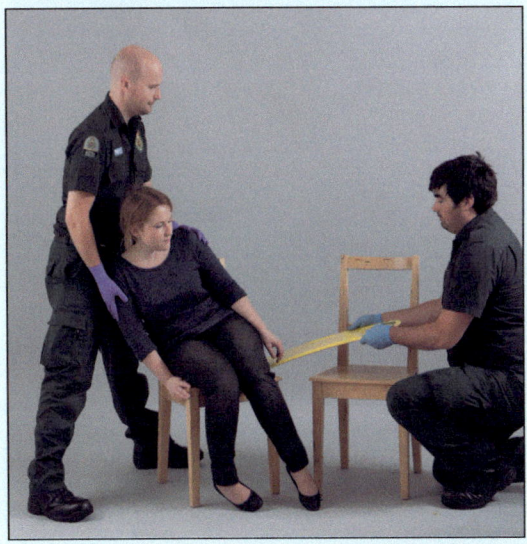

5. Once the patient has transferred onto the destination chair, they should be instructed to lean away from the board to allow its removal. Remove the turntable if used.

2.4.2 Sitting to standing transfer

Standing up out of a chair can be a challenge for some patients, even though they may be able to walk once they are upright.

Procedure – Sitting to standing transfer

Take the following steps to assist a patient to transfer from a sitting position to standing [Smith, 2011]:

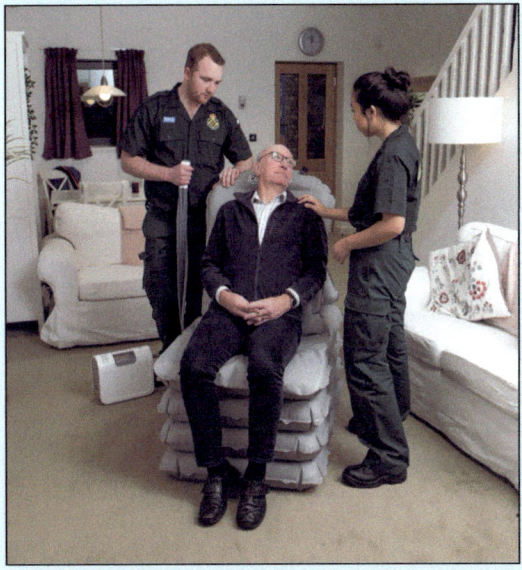

1. Explain the procedure to the patient and ensure they have suitable footwear. Instruct the patient to lean forward so that their back is off the back of the chair. Then instruct them to shuffle their bottom towards the front of the chair/edge of the bed and ensure that both of their feet are firmly on the floor.

2. Instruct the patient to place their hands on the arms of the chair, on their knees, or on the mattress if on a bed. Instruct the patient to lean forward so that their chin is over their knees and encourage them to look up and not at the floor. Instruct them that you will give the command 'Ready, steady, stand', and on 'stand' the patient should push up on the arms of the chair/mattress. The patient should keep their strongest leg close to their body, with the other foot slightly in front.

Chapter 7 – *Manual Handling*

Procedure – Sitting to standing transfer – *cont*

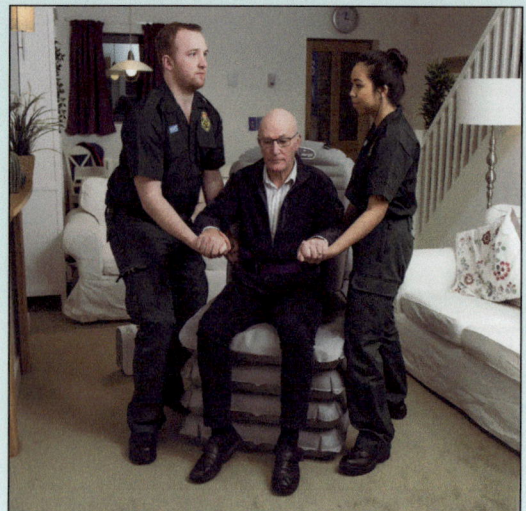

3. Alternatively, if there are no arms on the chair or the patient requires additional assistance, place a handling belt around the patient. Position yourself and another crew member either side of the patient, with your inside hand taking hold of the handling belt and your outer hand in a palm-to-palm hold (Figure 7.6). Instruct the patient as in step 2.

4. Give the command 'Ready, steady, stand'. If you are assisting the patient, a gentle rocking motion can help, and then on 'stand', move forward and then upwards with the patient as they stand.

5a. If the patient normally walks with a frame, provide this to them. It may help the patient's confidence if you walk slightly behind and to one side, with your hands just above the patient's hips.

5b. Alternatively, two crew members can walk with the patient, taking care not to impede the patient's natural step and allowing them to move their feet in their own time.

Procedure – Sitting to standing transfer – *cont*

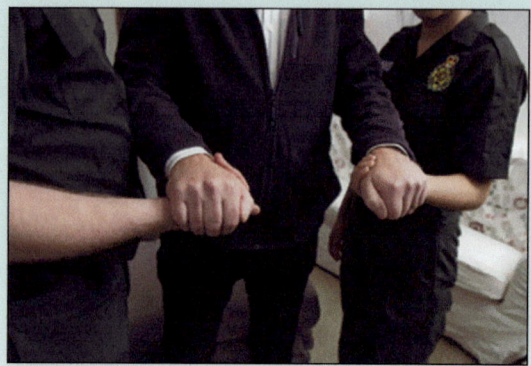

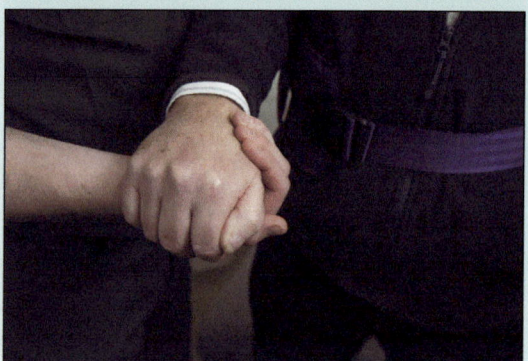

Figure 7.6 Palm-to-palm hold.

2.5 Patients in bed

You will frequently encounter patients in bed or on a hospital trolley who require transferring from either bed to ambulance trolley or bed to chair.

2.5.1 Patient transfer board

A patient transfer board is often available in hospitals and nursing homes to enable the transfer from bed to ambulance trolley and vice versa. An alternative is to use a hoist, if available and patient condition allows.

Procedure – Patient transfer board

Take the following steps to transfer a patient from bed to trolley using a patient transfer board [NEAS, 2014]:

Moving and handling equipment and techniques

Procedure – Patient transfer board – *cont*

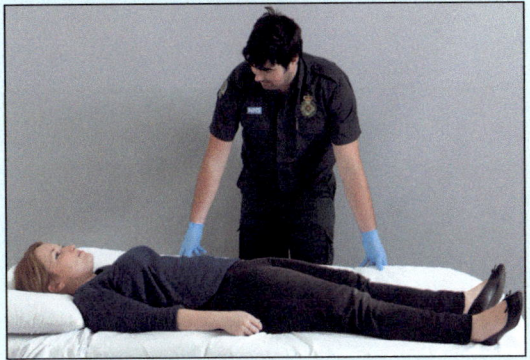

1. Explain the procedure to the patient and gain consent where possible. Place the ambulance trolley next to the bed.

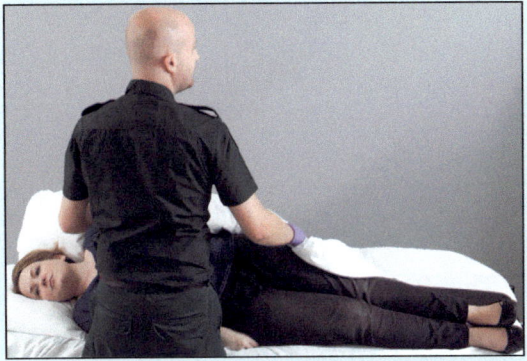

2. Using the sheet on the bed/trolley, one crew member should grip the sheet at the level of the patient's shoulders and roll the patient towards themselves.

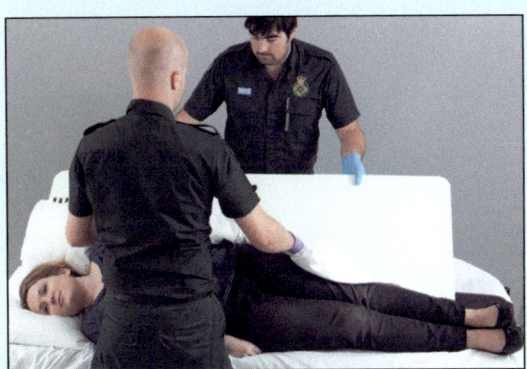

3. A second crew member can then position the board between the patient and the trolley.

Procedure – Patient transfer board – *cont*

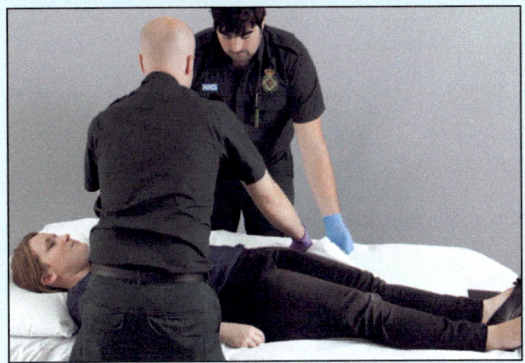

4. The first crew member lowers the patient onto their back while the second maintains the position of the board. The patient's feet should be on the lower end of the sheet.

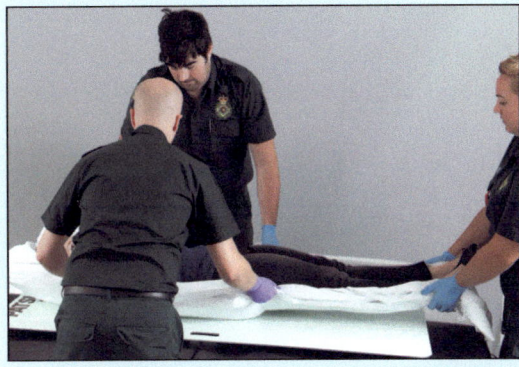

5. With both crew members gripping the sheet at the patient's shoulder and hip, slide the patient across the board and onto the trolley. Additional crew members are helpful to ensure that the patient's legs and feet transfer smoothly. If possible, use a slide sheet.

Chapter 7 – *Manual Handling*

Procedure – Patient transfer board – *cont*

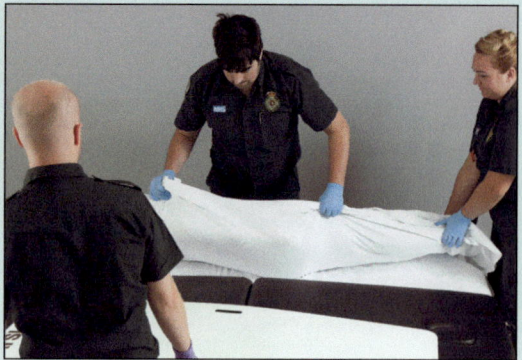

6. After ensuring the patient is centrally positioned, roll them to one side and remove the board.

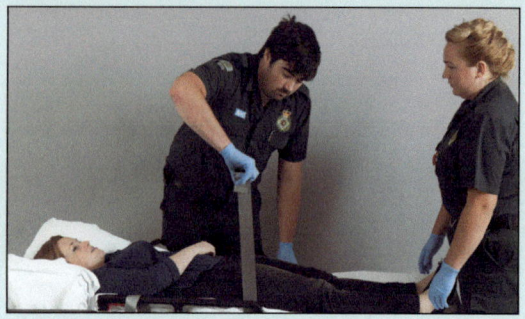

7. Roll the patient on to their back and secure them to the trolley. Don't forget to clean the board.

2.6 Carry chair

The carry chair is an important manual handling aid, used by ambulance services as the primary method for transporting patients up and down stairs and into the ambulance. However, it is associated with a high risk of lower back injury when used to lift patients [Ferreira, 2005]. In addition, the carry chair is not a wheelchair, so plan movements to keep the distance to be travelled to a minimum.

2.6.1 Transporting a patient on a carry chair

The procedure below relates to the Ferno Compact 2 carry chair, commonly found on ambulances. However, there are many models, including those with tracks to assist with descending stairs, so ensure you are appropriately trained, particularly in the lifting techniques required for these chairs, as they are not covered here.

Procedure – Carry chair

Take the following steps to prepare and transport a patient on the Ferno Compact 2 carry chair [EEAST, 2014]:

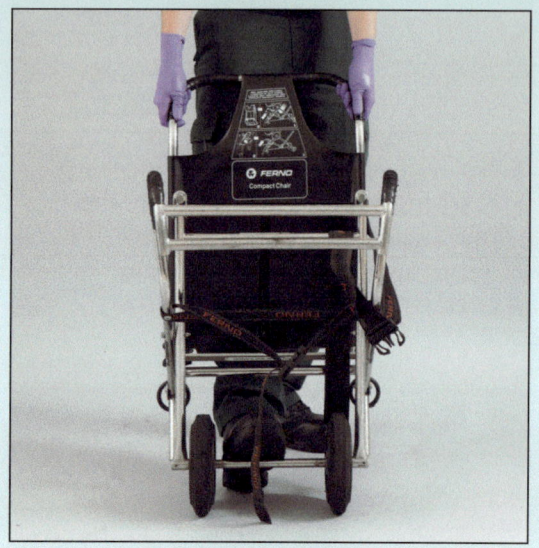

1. Unroll the carry chair by placing it on the ground. With your foot on the chair's foot bar, lift the back up and rearward.

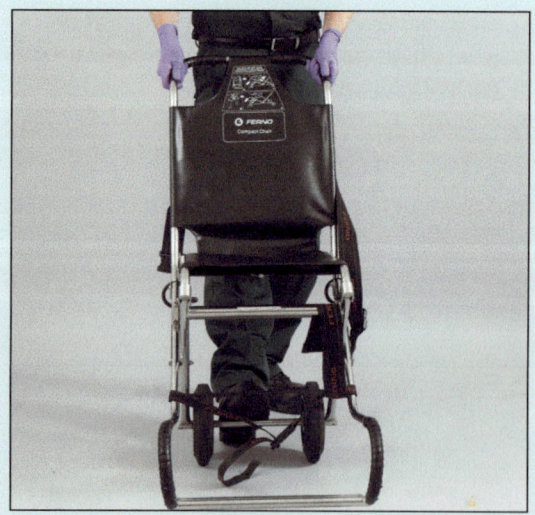

2. Completely unfold by firmly pushing up the back until an audible click is heard.

Moving and handling equipment and techniques

Procedure – Carry chair – *cont*

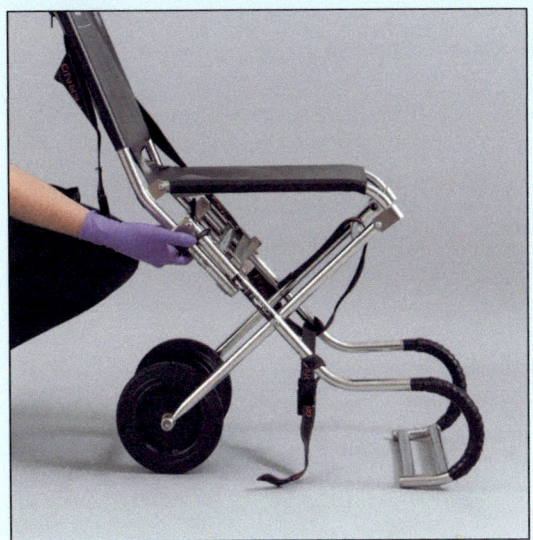

3. Once the chair is locked, move both of the safety rings down over the hinge bracket.

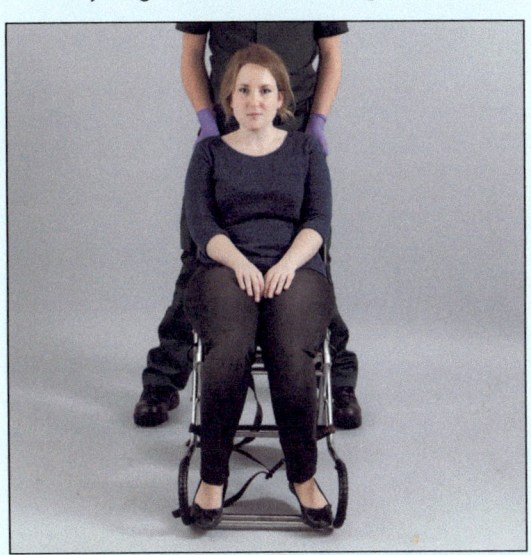

4. When a patient is on the carry chair, ensure that one crew member has a firm grip on the back of the chair at ALL times.

Procedure – Carry chair – *cont*

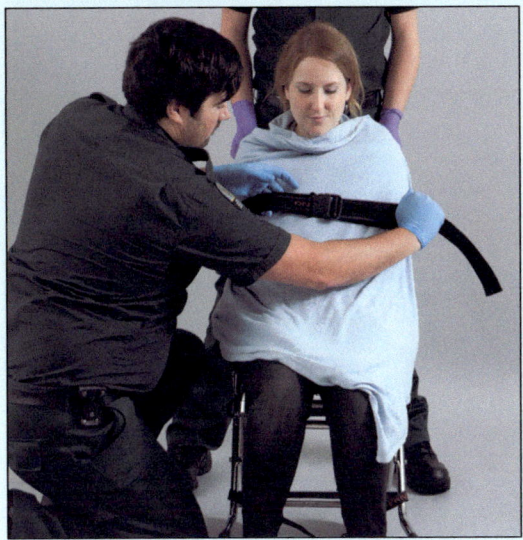

5. Secure the patient onto the chair by using the chest and leg restraints. Blankets can be used with the chair and are helpful for improving patient comfort, but ensure that they are clear of moving parts.

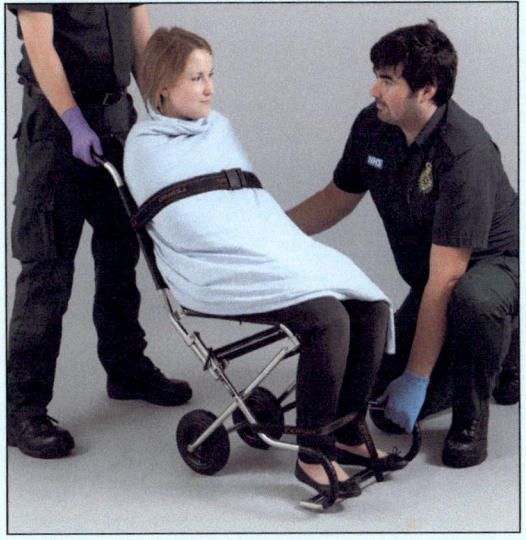

6. Once the patient is secured on the chair, crew members need to position themselves at the back and front of the chair. Instruct the patient not to grab out with their arms during the manoeuvre.

Chapter 7 – Manual Handling

Procedure – Carry chair – *cont*

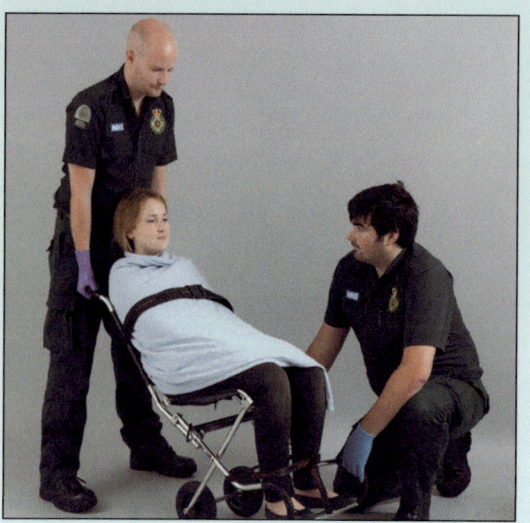

2.6.2 Blanketing on a carry chair

You will move a number of patients around on a carry chair, especially those who are less stable on their feet. If you haven't ever experienced it, then you should sit and be transported in a carry chair to understand what it feels like. They don't feel very stable and can be quite frightening.

One way to make the experience more pleasant is to securely wrap the patient up in blankets before moving them. This is particularly beneficial in cold or wet weather and the patient can stay wrapped in blankets all the way from their house to the emergency department keeping them warm and comfortable.

7. Explain to the patient that you are about to tip them backwards, but reassure them that they will not fall. The crew member at the back of the chair then tilts the chair backwards, until the weight of the chair and patient are balanced on the wheels. The chair can be rolled without lifting, but uneven terrain is likely to require the assistance of one or more additional crew members to ensure the chair does not tip over.

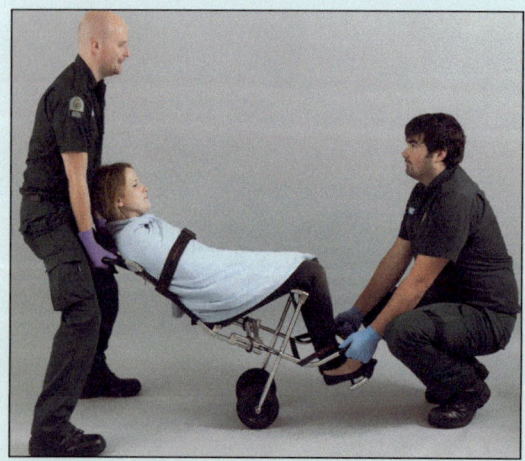

Procedure – Blanketing on a carry chair

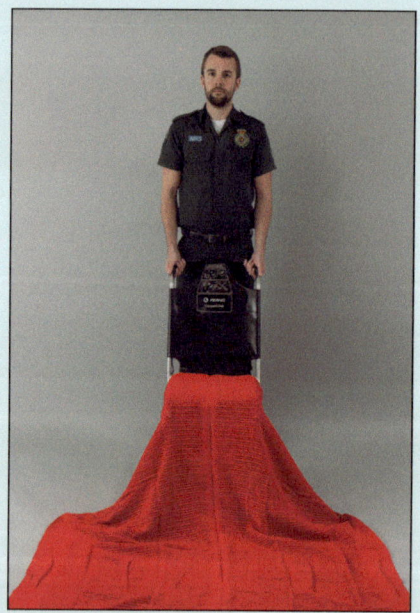

8. To carry the chair, it should be tilted backwards as before, and then crew members should grasp the front and back carrying handles and lift simultaneously.

1. Set up the carry chair and get two blankets and a bed sheet. Place the first blanket on the bottom half of the chair with the longest edge of the blanket running vertically away from the chair.

Procedure – Blanketing on a carry chair – *cont*

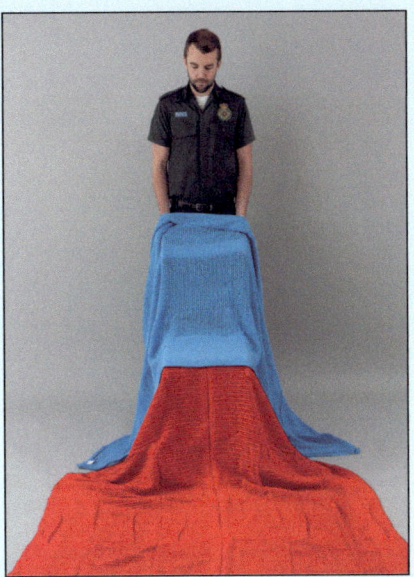

2. Place the next blanket across the top half of the chair with the longest edge running horizontally. The blanket should be slightly to one side so there is a shorter and a longer edge when wrapping them around the front of the patient.

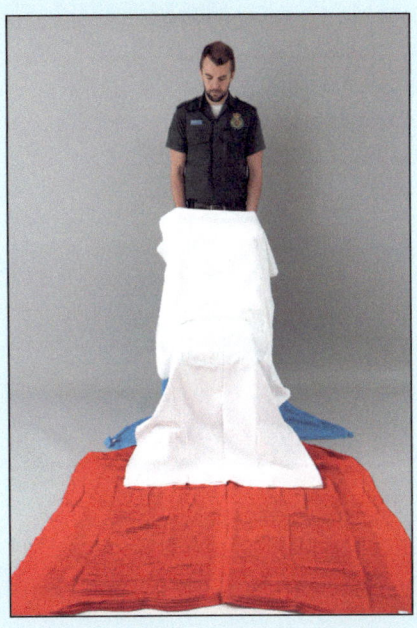

3. Place a bed sheet on top of the blankets.

Procedure – Blanketing on a carry chair – *cont*

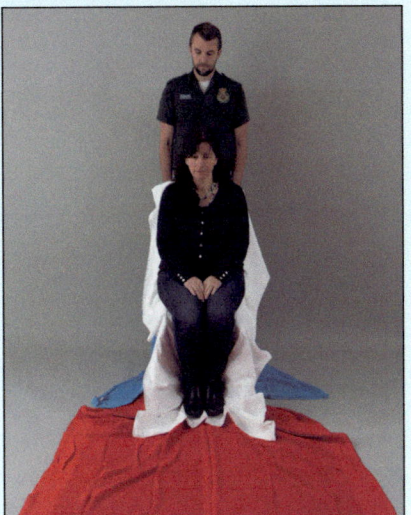

4. Assist the patient to sit in the chair. Make sure someone is holding the top of the chair whenever a patient is sitting in the chair.

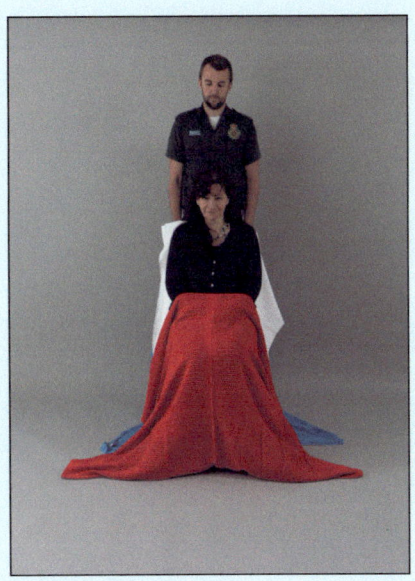

5. Fold the blanket up and over the patient's legs and onto their lap.

Chapter 7 – *Manual Handling*

Procedure – Blanketing on a carry chair – *cont*

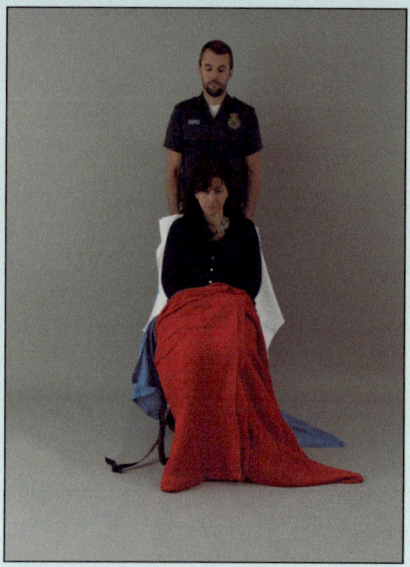

6. Fold the sides of the blanket neatly up into the middle. Make sure no excess blanket is left hanging loose as this can trap in the wheels when it comes to moving the patient.

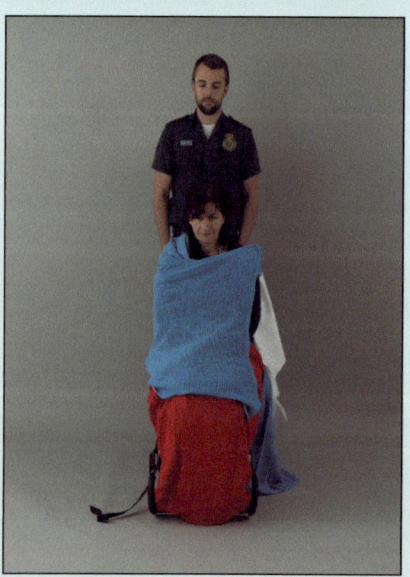

7. Once both sides of the lower blanket have been folded up, cross the upper blanket across the chest of the patient, starting with the shorter edge first.

Procedure – Blanketing on a carry chair – *cont*

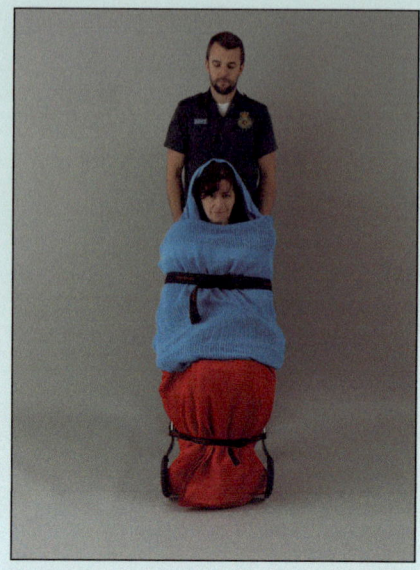

8. There should be enough blanket behind the patient's head to create a hood if needed. Remember to strap the patient in using both the chest and leg straps.

2.7 Ambulance trolley

There are a wide range of ambulance trolleys available, so ensure you are familiar with the one on your ambulance. Basic pre-shift checks common to most trolleys include [EEAST, 2014]:

- Check that the mattress and restraining system are properly installed. Damaged mattresses present an infection control risk and should be replaced.
- Check that the ambulance trolley sides can be raised, lowered and locked in position.
- Check that the ambulance trolley can be raised and lowered satisfactorily.
- Check that the wheels and brakes of the trolley are effective.
- Ensure that the trolley locks properly into the ambulance locking device.
- If the trolley has push/pull handles, check their operation and stow them away.
- If the trolley has a headrest, check that it locks in position when attached to the trolley.

Moving and handling equipment and techniques

2.7.1 Trolley positioning

Ambulance trolleys can be placed in a range of positions to improve patient comfort and clinical condition. The positions may need to be adopted and changed quickly as the patient's condition changes, so ensure you are familiar with how to place the trolley into and out of these positions.

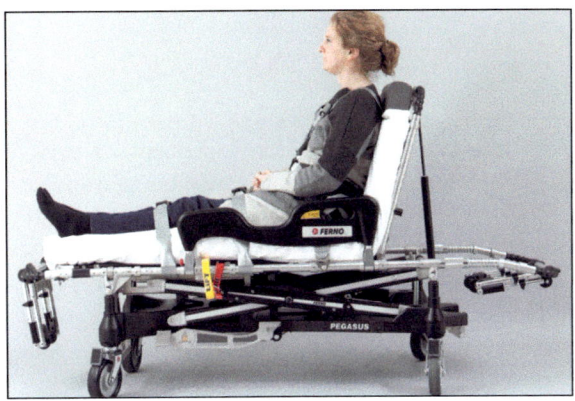

Upright position. This is preferred for patients with breathing problems.

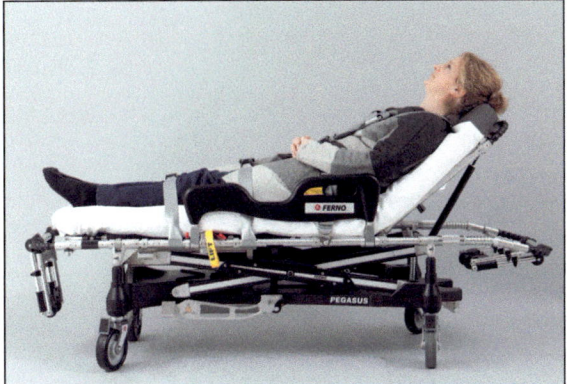

Semi-recumbent position. This consists of placing the patient's head and torso at an angle of 45°.

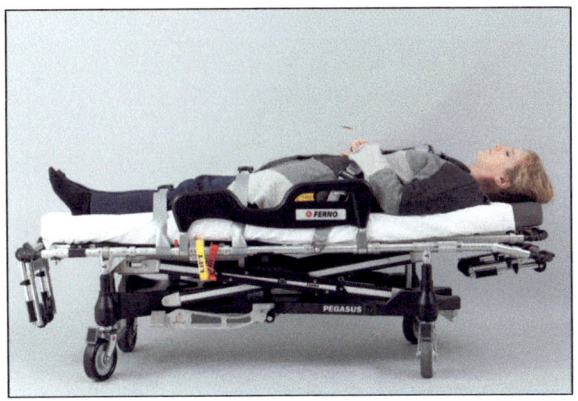

Recumbent position. This is the preferred position for patients with suspected spinal injuries and/or shock.

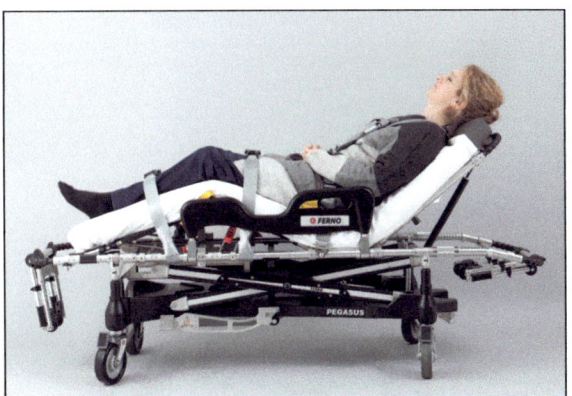

Fowler position. This position can help relieve tension on abdominal muscles, which may make abdominal illness and injuries less painful.

Chapter 7 – Manual Handling

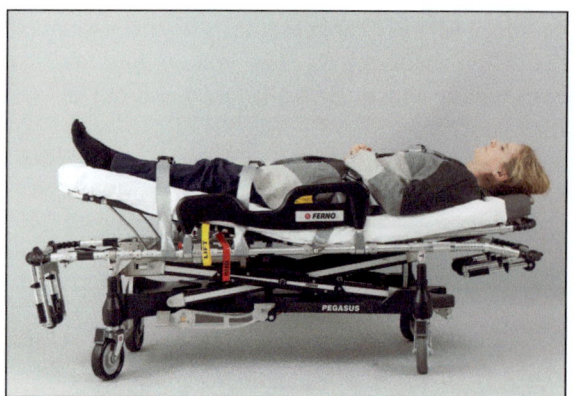 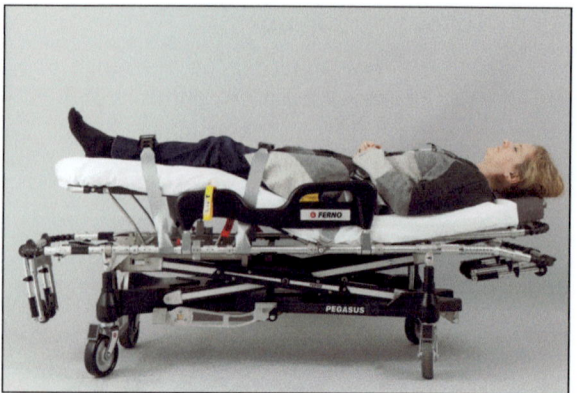

Lower limbs raised. This is helpful for controlling bleeding in lower leg injuries, and will increase cardiac output for several minutes in hypovolaemia [Geerts, 2012].

Trendelenburg. This position is frequently taught as being beneficial for patients with decreased blood volume, but only has a temporary effect on blood pressure and no effect on cardiac output. In addition, this position may aggravate an already impaired ventilatory function due to the weight of the abdominal contents resting on the diaphragm. It may also increase intracranial pressure in patients with a traumatic brain injury [Peña, 2012; Johnson, 2004].

Chapter

8 Drug Administration

1 Drug legislation and guidelines

1.1 Learning objectives

By the end of this section you will be able to:
- identify relevant legislation and clinical guidelines relating to the administration of medication
- list common routes of administration for medication in out-of-hospital practice
- explain your role in the checking and administering of medication.

1.2 Introduction

The administration of drugs to patients is a frequent and important part of an ambulance clinician's practice. Although you are limited in terms of the drugs you personally can administer, you have a responsibility to ensure that the necessary checks are carried out prior to drug administration.

In addition, many of the drugs in use by the ambulance service are given directly into a patient's vein. This intravenous method of administration requires the insertion of a cannula directly into the patient's blood stream; if this is not undertaken correctly, it can result in harm to the patient. Your assistance in these procedures can help reduce the risk of this occurring.

1.3 Legislation and guidelines

The two key pieces of legislation relating to the administration of medicines in the ambulance service are:
- Medicines Act 1968
- Misuse of Drugs Act 1971.

Both have been amended since their introduction. However, other legislation also relevant when discussing medicines includes the Control of Substances Hazardous to Health Regulations 2002 and the Health and Safety at Work, etc. Act 1974, although these are not explored further here.

1.3.1 Medicines Act 1968

Under this Act, medicines are classified into three types [MHRA, 2014]:
- **General sales list medicines (GSL):** These can be sold to the public in original, unopened manufacturers' packs at any lockable premises.
- **Pharmacy medicines (P):** These can only be sold under the supervision of a pharmacist.
- **Prescription-only medicines (POM):** These medicines require a prescription from an appropriate practitioner, such as a doctor or non-medical prescriber.

Many of the drugs (medicines) administered by ambulance service crew members fall into the POM category. However, certain drugs can be administered in emergency situations, such as adrenaline, whereas others can be administered by paramedics in specific circumstances, which are typically the indications given in the UK Ambulance Services Clinical Practice Guidelines [JRCALC, 2019].

Unless you are a paramedic, you are not covered by these exemptions, so it is important that you follow your service guidance about which (if any) drugs you can administer without the direct supervision of a clinician. Typically, drugs such as oxygen can be administered by ambulance associate practitioners (AAPs), but you must be familiar with the medicines management policy of your ambulance service and the scope of practice for your role.

1.3.2 Misuse of Drugs Act 1971

This Act covers drugs that are considered to be dangerous or harmful (because of the risk of dependence and/or misuse) and controls their production, supply and possession, which is why the drugs are known as controlled drugs. Drugs are classified into three types:
- **Part 1:** Class A drugs including cocaine and morphine.

- **Part 2:** Class B drugs including amphetamine and codeine.
- **Part 3:** Class C drugs including diazepam and lorazepam.

The use of these controlled drugs is allowed subject to conditions specified in the Misuse of Drugs Regulations 2001 (and subsequent amendments). These regulations classify controlled drugs into five schedules [Dimond, 2015]:

1. Drugs that cannot be used for medicinal purposes. Their use is typically restricted to research.
2. Drugs with high abuse potential, such as morphine and methadone, and stimulants, such as amphetamines.
3. Drugs that are less likely to lead to physical or psychological dependence.
4. Drugs such as diazepam and anabolic steroids.
5. Typically preparations of controlled drugs with limited risk of abuse.

Both morphine and diazepam are available for paramedics to administer. It is important that you do not prepare or administer any controlled drugs. Only the paramedic is allowed to do this.

1.4 Routes of administration

Drugs can be administered to patients via a number of routes. These are typically divided into two types: parenteral and non-parenteral.

Parenteral routes require the skin or mucous membranes to be breached, such as by an intravenous, intramuscular, intraosseous or subcutaneous injection. Non-parenteral routes rely on passive absorption of the drug, such as by inhalation, nebulisation, oral, rectal, sublingual, buccal, transdermal or intra-nasal administration [JRCALC, 2019].

1.5 Drug administration

Prior to the administration of any drug, check the following [JRCALC, 2019]:
- The patient is not **allergic** to the drug about to be administered.
- It is the **correct** drug.
- The **dose** of drug required.
- The **presentation** of the drug, including its concentration (e.g. 4 mg in 2 ml) and the container it comes in (e.g. ampoule, tablet, prefilled syringe).
- Whether the **packaging** is intact.
- If it is a fluid, the **clarity** (except for intravenous diazemuls (diazepam), which comes as a milky-white emulsion).
- The **expiry** date.

Although it is ultimately the clinician who has the responsibility for the administration of drugs to the patient, you are part of a team, even if you are not personally administering the drug, and spotting and preventing a mistake that can affect patient safety is everyone's responsibility.

2 Administering medication to patients

2.1 Learning objectives

By the end of this section you will be able to:
- explain the procedure for drawing medication from an ampoule
- explain the procedure to prepare and administer medication by the following routes:
  - oral
  - nebuliser
  - intramuscular
  - intranasal.

2.2 Drawing medication from an ampoule

You may be asked to draw up some drugs, but this should not generally include drugs that require mixing. However, follow your employer's guidance on this matter. The most common presentation of a drug that requires drawing up in the ambulance service is an ampoule (Figure 8.1). It is important that you can do this efficiently and safely.

Administering medication to patients

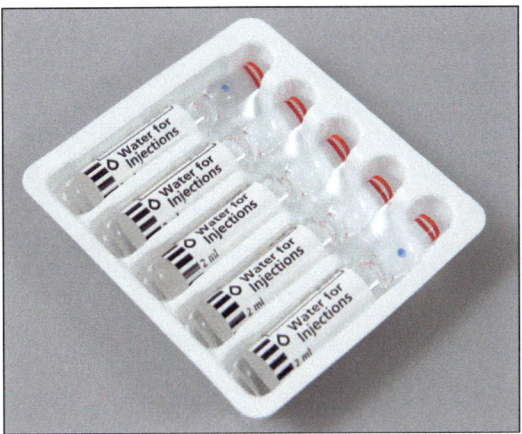

Figure 8.1 Ampoules.

2.2.1 Equipment

You will require the following items:
- appropriately sized syringe
- either blunt filter needle or 23G needle to prevent glass particle contamination [Zabir, 2008; Preston, 2004]
- disposable ampoule breaker
- sharps bin.

2.2.2 Procedure

Take the following steps to draw up drugs from an ampoule [Dougherty, 2015]:

Procedure – Draw up drugs from an ampoule

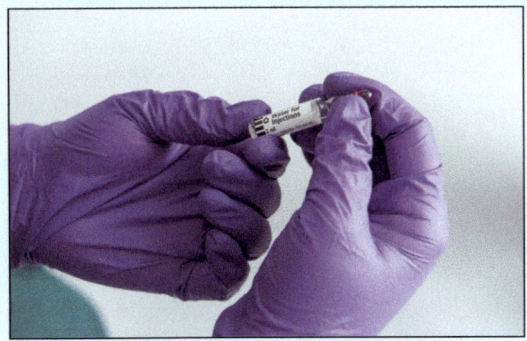

1. Take standard precautions and prepare the equipment. Obtain consent where possible.

   Check the drug:
   - patient not allergic
   - correct drug
   - dose/presentation

Procedure – Draw up drugs from an ampoule – *cont*
   - integrity of the ampoule
   - clarity of contents (if relevant)
   - expiry date

If possible, record the batch number and expiry date of the drug so that the ampoule can be disposed of once the contents have been removed. If any of the drug remains in the top of the ampoule, gently tap the neck.

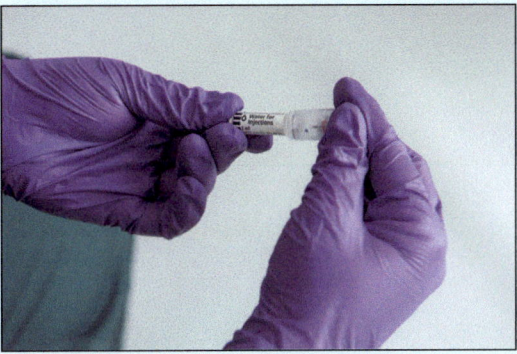

2. Place a disposable ampoule opener over the cone-shaped top of the ampoule. Push it gently downwards until it reaches the neck of the ampoule.

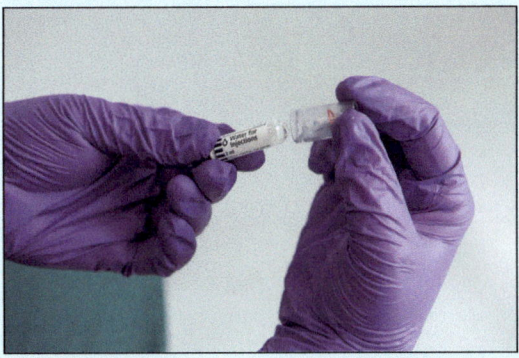

3. With the dot (which signifies where the neck of the ampoule has been scored and so is weaker) facing away from you, snap the neck of the ampoule and dispose of the top of the ampoule in the sharps bin. Check the contents of the ampoule for glass fragments and discard the contents if glass fragments are present.

Chapter 8 – *Drug Administration*

Procedure – Draw up drugs from an ampoule – *cont*

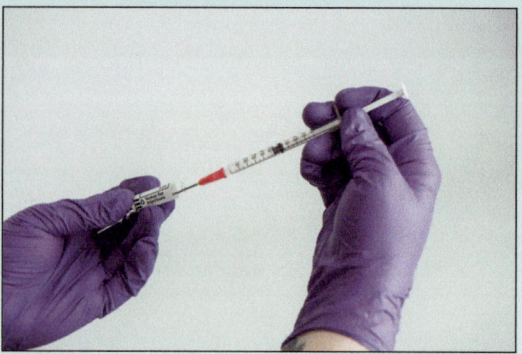

4. Without touching the outer edges of the ampoule (where the ampoule has broken), insert the needle into the medication and draw it into the syringe by pulling back on the plunger.

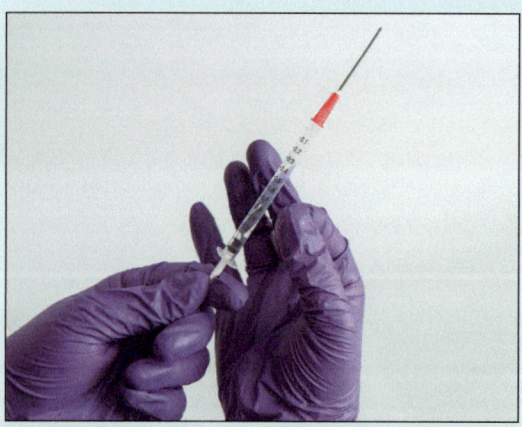

5. Once the ampoule is empty, dispose of it in the sharps bin. Holding the syringe upright, gently tap the barrel to encourage any air bubbles to rise to the top of the syringe.

Procedure – Draw up drugs from an ampoule – *cont*

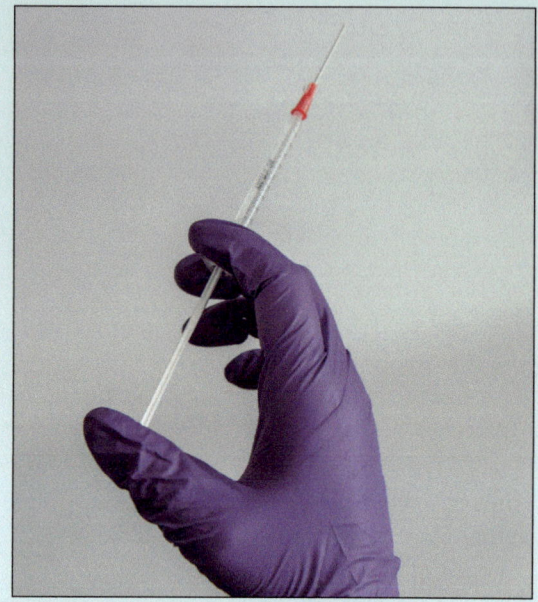

6. Remove the air bubbles by gently pressing on the plunger.

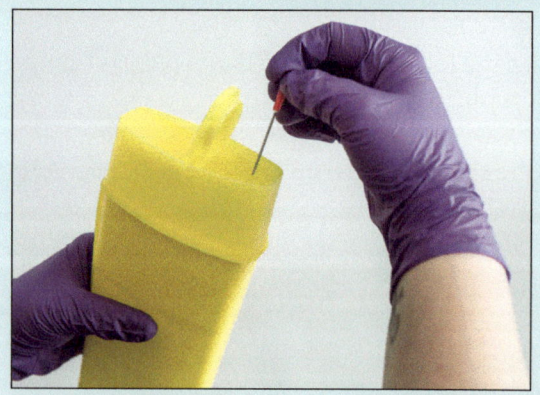

7. Dispose of the needle used to draw up the drug into the sharps bin.

2.3 Administering oral medication

The majority of your patients' medication at home will be taken orally. They come in a variety of forms including tablets, capsules, lozenges and syrups.

2.3.1 Procedure

Take the following steps to administer oral medication [Dougherty, 2015]:

Procedure – To administer oral medication

1. Take standard precautions.
2. Ensure consent has been obtained.
3. Check the drug:
   - correct drug
   - correct dose
   - in date
   - intact packaging.
4. Check that the patient is not allergic to the drug.
5. Avoid touching the medication, unless the patient is not capable of self-administering. Ensure you are wearing gloves in this case.
6. Present it to the patient with clear instructions:
   - most oral medication can be swallowed, except aspirin, which should be chewed or dissolved first
   - sublingual tablets need to be placed under the tongue
   - buccal tablets should be placed between the gum and cheek.
7. Provide water, if indicated and permitted.
8. Ensure the administration is documented.

2.4 Administering nebulised drugs

Nebulisers enable drugs to be inhaled. In the ambulance service, this will usually be salbutamol and ipratropium for patients suffering from asthma, chronic obstructive pulmonary disease and expiratory wheeze due to allergy, anaphylaxis or smoke inhalation, [JRCALC, 2019].

2.4.1 Procedure

Take the following steps to administer drugs via a nebuliser [Dougherty, 2015]:

Procedure – To administer drugs via a nebuliser

1. Adopt standard precautions.
2. Obtain consent if possible.
3. Check the medication:
   - correct drug
   - correct dose
   - expiry date
   - integrity of packaging.
4. Add medication into the chamber (Figure 8.2). This may involve unscrewing the two parts of the nebuliser.
5. Connect the nebuliser to the oxygen source and set the flow rate to 6–8 l/min, or connect to an air-driven nebuliser unit. A fine mist should be generated.

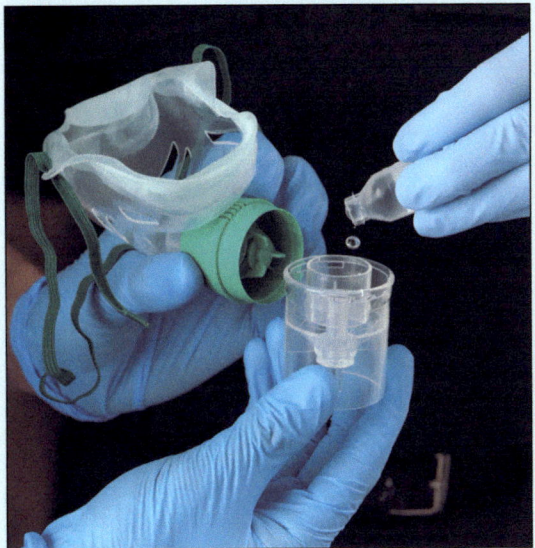

Figure 8.2 Adding medication to the nebuliser chamber.

Chapter 8 – Drug Administration

Procedure – To administer drugs via a nebuliser – *cont*

6. Place the mask over the patient's face and adjust the elastic to make a good seal.
7. Coach the patient's breathing. They should breathe in slowly and deeply and aim to hold their breath for 3–5 seconds before breathing out again.
8. Ensure the administration is documented.

Note: The administration of drugs such as salbutamol with the patient's own inhaler is as effective as a nebuliser if they use a spacer (Figure 8.3). This is particularly true of children [SIGN/BTS, 2016].

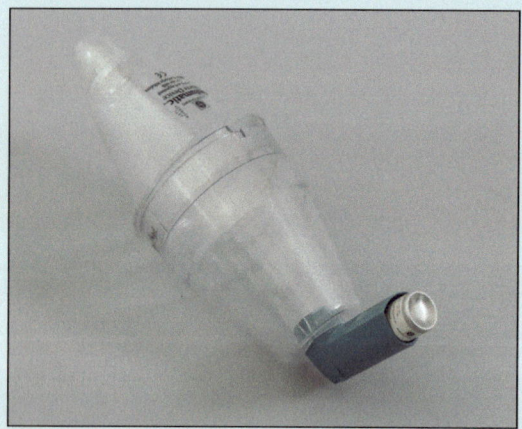

Figure 8.3 An inhaler and spacer.

2.5 Administering intramuscular drugs

Drugs such as adrenaline for anaphylaxis and glucagon for hypoglycaemia can be administered intramuscularly (IM).

2.5.1 Procedure

Take the following steps to administer a drug via the IM route [Gregory, 2010b]:

Procedure – To administer a drug via the IM route

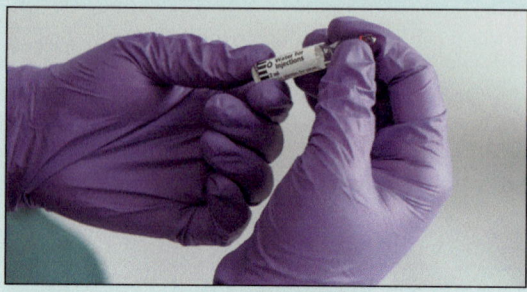

1. Take standard precautions. Explain the procedure to the patient and obtain consent where possible. Advise the patient that it will be uncomfortable. Check the drug:
   - correct drug
   - correct dose
   - in date
   - intact packaging.

   Check that the patient is not allergic to the drug. Draw up the drug if necessary (follow the drawing medication from an ampoule procedure), ensuring that the drawing-up needle is discarded and a 21G needle is connected to the syringe.

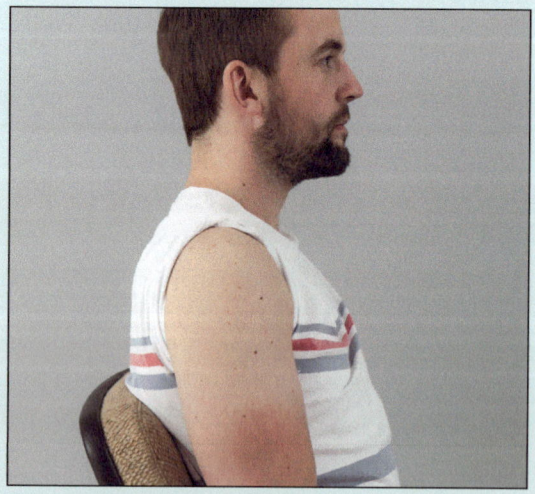

2. Choose an appropriate site. This is most likely to be the deltoid muscle on the upper arm or the anterolateral thigh. Follow local guidance. Ensure the injection site is not infected, bruised or tender.

Administering medication to patients

Procedure – To administer a drug via the IM route – *cont*

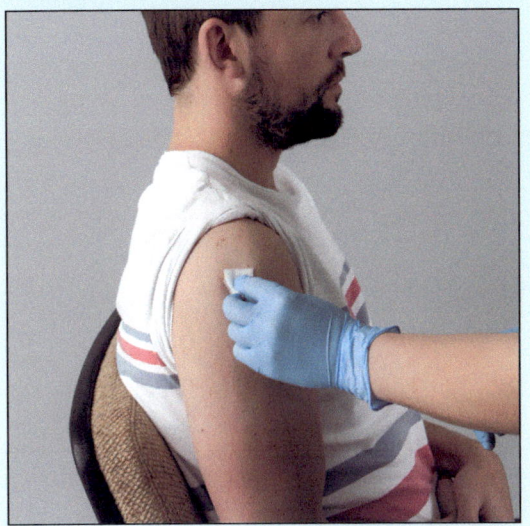

3. Clean the site with ChloraPrep.

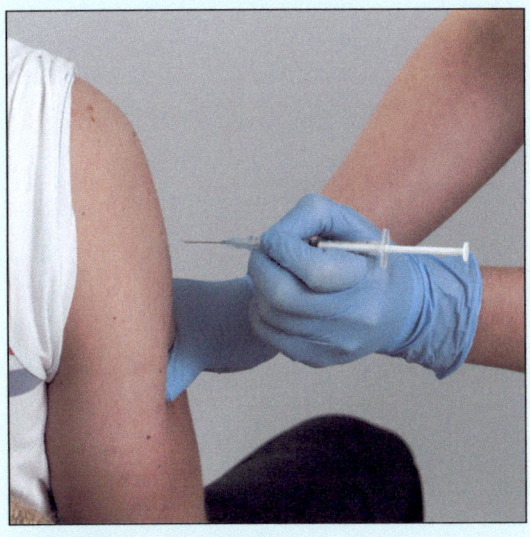

4. Using the hand that is not administering the injection, pull the skin downwards, or sideways, to displace the skin and subcutaneous tissue. Holding the skin taut, insert the needle into the muscle at an angle of 90°.

Procedure – To administer a drug via the IM route – *cont*

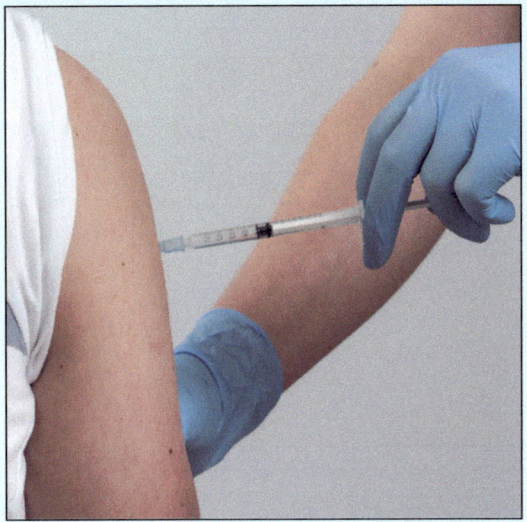

5. Maintaining the tension on the skin, gently pull back on the syringe plunger and ensure that no blood is drawn up into the syringe. If blood does appear, you may be in a blood vessel, and should withdraw needle and syringe and discard. Prepare another dose of the drug for injection.

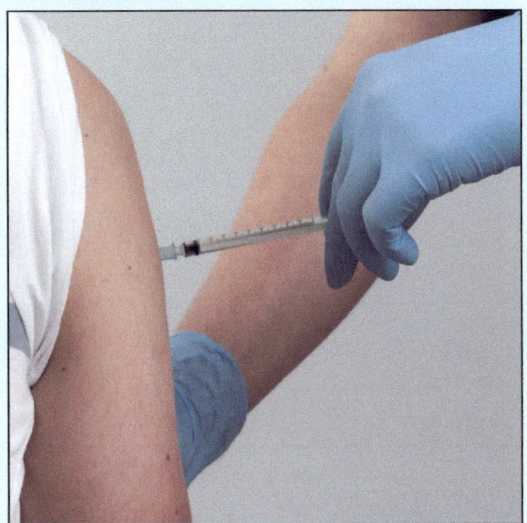

6. Assuming no blood enters the syringe, slowly inject the drug (10 seconds per 1 ml).

Chapter 8 – Drug Administration

Procedure – To administer a drug via the IM route – cont

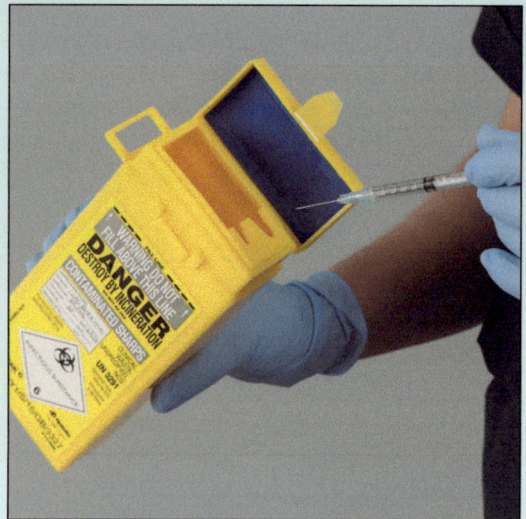

7. Wait ten seconds and withdraw the needle. Dispose of the needle and syringe in a sharps bin.

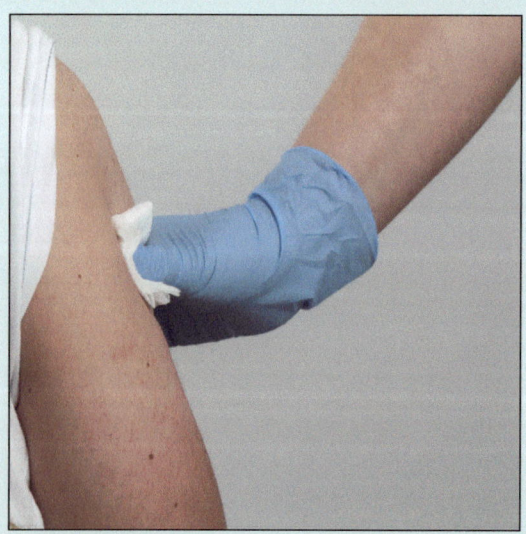

8. Release the tension on the skin and apply gentle pressure with a sterile pad or gauze. Dispose of gloves and cleanse your hands. Document the administration.

2.6 Administering intranasal drugs

Drugs such as naloxone for opiate overdose can be administered via the intranasal (IN) route.

2.6.1 Procedure

Take the following steps to administer a drug via the IN route with a mucosal atomiser device (MAD) [Teleflex, 2013]:

Procedure – To administer a drug via the IN route

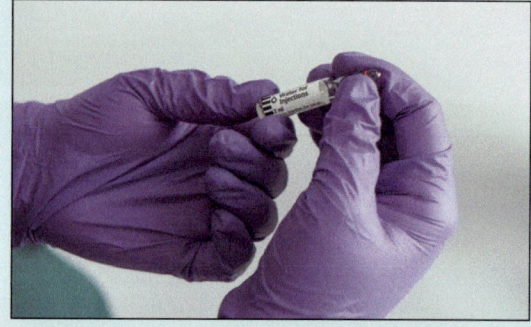

1. Take standard precautions. Explain the procedure to the patient and obtain consent where possible. Check the drug:
   - patient not allergic
   - correct drug
   - dose/presentation
   - integrity of packaging
   - clarity of contents (if relevant)
   - expiry date.

If drawing up the drug from a rubber-topped vial, remove the vial adaptor cap and pierce the medication vial with the syringe vial adaptor. If drawing up the drug from a glass vial, remove the vial adaptor and place in a sharps container. Attach a blunt drawing-up needle to the syringe

Aspirate the proper volume of medication required to treat the patient (an extra 0.1 ml of medication should be drawn up to account for the dead space in the device).

Either remove the vial adaptor or blunt drawing-up needle and dispose of safely in a sharps container.

Administering medication to patients

Procedure – To administer a drug via the IN route – *cont*

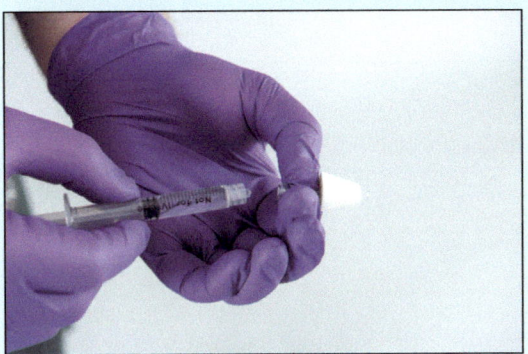

2. Attach the MAD nasal device to the syringe by screwing it into the Luer lock connecter.

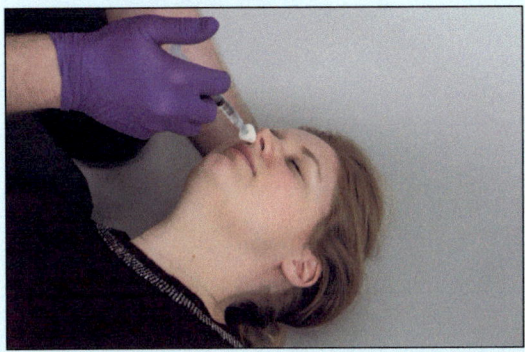

3. Using the free hand to hold the back of the head stable, place the tip of the MAD nasal device snugly against the nostril aiming slightly up and outward (towards the top of the ear). Briskly compress the syringe plunger to deliver half of the medication into the nostril.

Procedure – To administer a drug via the IN route – *cont*

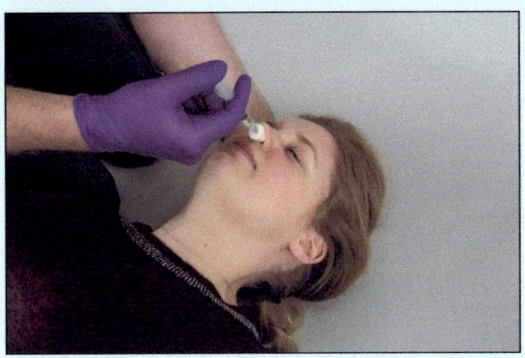

4. Move the device over to the opposite nostril and, repeating step 3, administer the remaining medication into the nostril. Dispose of the MAD and syringe appropriately. Dispose of gloves and cleanse your hands. Document the administration.

Chapter

9 Scene Assessment

1 Scene assessment and safety

1.1 Learning objectives

By the end of this section you will be able to:
- outline and explain the parts of an initial scene assessment
- explain the importance of ensuring scene safety prior to approaching any incident for:
  - patients
  - yourself
  - your colleagues
  - bystanders.
- describe the components of a dynamic risk assessment model.

1.2 Introduction

Despite the name, scene assessment begins before you physically arrive at the patient's location. You will be passed details of the incident, although initially this may only include the address, with further details provided as you respond. The address may be recognised as belonging to a frequent and/or violent caller, having access issues and/or a location prone to high-speed road traffic collisions, for example.

To help you cover the essential aspects of a scene assessment, consider using the SCENE mnemonic [JRCALC, 2019]:
- **S:** Safety
- **C:** Cause including the nature of illness (NOI) or mechanism of injury (MOI)
- **E:** Environment
- **N:** Number of patients
- **E:** Extra resources needed.

1.3 Safety

Maximising the safety of everyone on scene requires risk assessment. The ambulance service has many formal written risk assessments, but these cannot legislate for all eventualities. In order to reduce the risk to you, your colleagues, patients and bystanders, it is necessary to undertake a more fluid and mental (i.e. in your head as opposed to a written down) risk assessment. This is known as a dynamic risk assessment (DRA) and relates to the fact that the environment or situation is dynamic, rather than the risk itself. DRA underpins subsequent decision-making and is focused on thinking before you act, and not the other way around [Asbury, 2014]. The National Ambulance Resilience Unit (NARU) has published a dynamic risk assessment model to assist with risk assessments while on scene (Figure 9.1)

1.4 Cause

Although you are likely to have been passed some details about the incident or call you are attending, you should not be completely led by this. Establishing the presenting complaint from the patient's perspective will come later on in the assessment process, but you may be able to determine what has happened from the scene, particularly in trauma cases, such as when viewing the wreckage of two cars that have collided. However, it is important to keep an open mind even at this stage. For example, although you are attending a road traffic collision, your patient may have suffered from a medical problem, such as a cardiac arrest, which led to their losing control of the car. Conversely, a medical-sounding call, such as a patient with low blood sugar, may also have a traumatic component if, for example, they fell and injured themselves as a result.

In trauma cases, find out about the mechanism of injury (MOI), which you will cover in Chapter 17, 'Trauma'. Knowledge of the MOI can assist in determining what injuries may have been sustained. Equally, for medical patients, establishing the nature of illness (NOI) can assist with the diagnosis, particularly in cases where bystander and/or patient information is limited (for example, if the patient was discovered unresponsive). Clues from

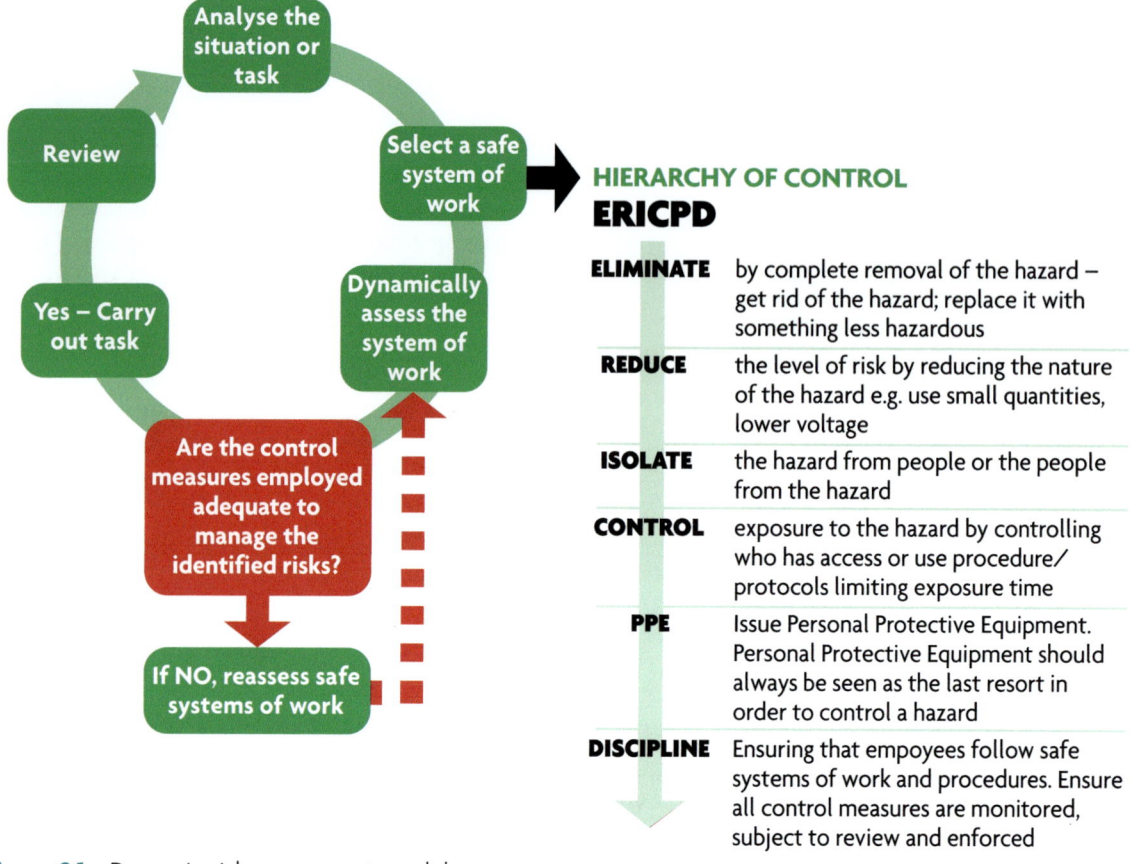

Figure 9.1 Dynamic risk assessment model.
Source: National Ambulance Resilience Unit, National Ambulance Service Command and Control Guidance (October 2015).

the scene (for example, medical equipment such as home oxygen or hoists, medication and/or care notes) may provide clues as to the underlying problem [Bledsoe, 2014].

1.5 Environment

Consider whether there are any environmental factors that need to be taken into account. These may complicate your extrication by affecting access to and from the scene and/or increase the risk of harm to the patient due to the development of hypothermia, for example. Incidents involving water can be hazardous for patient and crew alike. In these cases you must remember to 'call, reach, throw, wade and row' (covered in Chapter 15, 'Exposure/Environment'). The terrain may be an issue, particularly if the patient is located well away from roads that are suitable for an ambulance. In these cases, helicopters and/or mountain rescue teams can prove useful.

Other risky environments include confined spaces, where there may be a risk of low levels of oxygen and/or the presence of toxic/explosive substances, or, in the case of buildings or other structures, further collapse. These require specialist equipment and rescue knowledge that is typically provided by hazardous area response teams (HART) or the fire and rescue service [Bledsoe, 2014].

1.6 Number of patients

Determine the number of patients early on in your assessment to help you decide whether you can manage the scene on your own. It may also help to identify patients who have either wandered off from the scene or who have been ejected from a vehicle, for example, and are currently hidden from view.

In addition, since most acts of terrorism are covert (i.e. there is often no prior knowledge of the time, location or nature of the attack), it is possible that you could be responding first to the aftermath of a terrorist attack. In these cases, the number of patients involved may provide the most important indication that a chemical, biological, radiological, nuclear, explosive (CBRN(e)) event has occurred. In these cases, you should use the STEP 1-2-3 Plus method [Home Office, 2015]:
- **Step 1:** One casualty and no obvious reason. Approach using normal procedures.
- **Step 2:** Two casualties and no obvious reason. Approach with caution, consider all options. Provide a report on arrival to the emergency operations centre (EOC).
- **Step 3:** Three or more casualties in close proximity and no obvious reason. Use caution and follow Plus.
- **Plus**: Follow the CBRN(e) First Responder Flow Chart (Figure 9.2) to consider what actions can be undertaken to save life using the following principles:
  - **Evacuate:** Get people away from the scene of contamination.
  - **Communicate and advise:** Immediate medical advice and reassurance that help is on its way.
  - **Disrobe:** Remove clothing.
  - **Decontaminate:** Improvised decontamination – dry decontamination when a non-caustic agent is suspected and wet decontamination when a caustic agent is suspected.

1.7 Extra resources

Depending on the number of patients, the severity of their injuries and the nature of the incident, you may need additional help and/or equipment from other emergency services. For example, you may require the police to keep a scene safe, or additional ambulances, including the air ambulance, for patient transport, or the fire and rescue service to stabilise a car that has rolled. Don't forget others, such as the coastguard, mountain rescue, utility and public transport companies. Request help early as it may take time for messages to be passed on and the relevant staff to arrive on scene.

2 Major incidents

2.1 Learning objectives

By the end of this section you will be able to:
- explain the term 'emergency preparedness, resilience and response'
- define the terms 'major incident' and 'interoperability'
- describe the Joint Decision Model
- state ambulance service responsibilities with regard to a major incident
- state who can declare a major incident
- state the roles of the attendant and driver of the first crew on scene
- list the responsibilities of subsequent ambulance crews on scene
- describe the potential roles for ambulance officers on scene
- state the role of strategic, tactical and operational commanders
- explain the principles of triage sieve and sort.

2.2 Introduction

2.2.1 Emergency

According to the Civil Contingencies Act 2004 an emergency is defined as:
- an event or situation which threatens serious damage to human welfare in a place in the UK
- an event or situation which threatens serious damage to the environment of a place in the UK
- war, or terrorism, which threatens serious damage to the security of the UK.

To distinguish this definition of emergency from the regular emergency work of the ambulance service, the term used most often is 'major incident'.

NHS ambulance services are classed as category 1 (primary) responders under the Civil Contingencies Act [2004]. As such, these organisations are expected to have plans in place to prevent emergencies, and to reduce, control

Chapter 9 – Scene Assessment

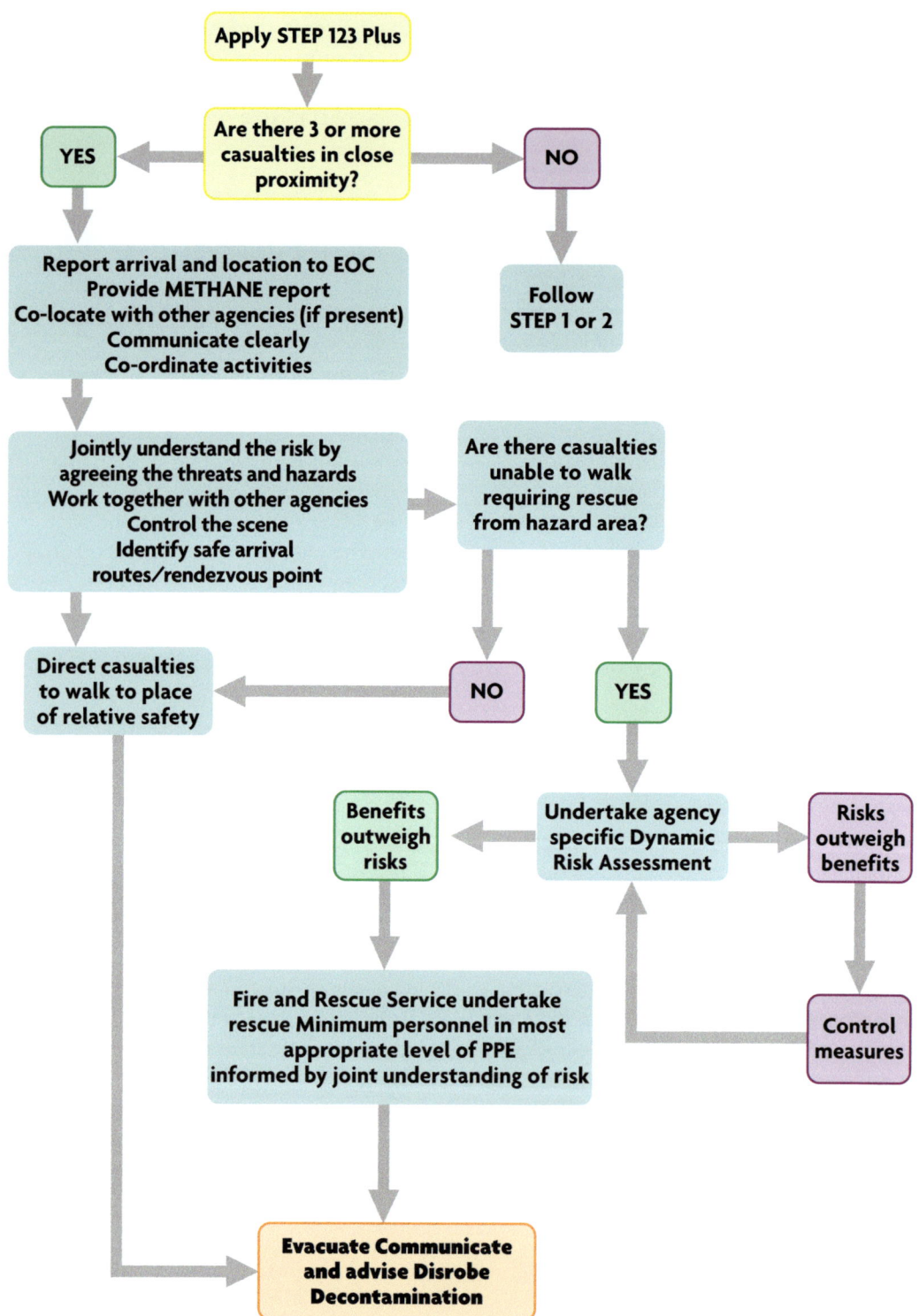

Figure 9.2 CBRN(e) first responder flowchart.
Source: Joint Emergency Services Interoperability Programme. Available at: https://www.jesip.org.uk/uploads/media/pdf/CBRN%20JOPs/IOR_Guidance_V2_July_2015.pdf.

and mitigate emergencies once they occur [NARU, 2015a]. In addition, business continuity arrangements need to be in place to ensure services are maintained to patients even in the event of disruptions, such as severe weather or an IT failure, for example. Collectively, all these activities fall under the umbrella term 'emergency preparedness, resilience and response' (EPRR) [NHS England, 2017].

2.3 Interoperability and JESIP

2.3.1 Interoperability

Interoperability is the extent to which organisations can work together effectively to achieve a joint aim. This requires planning that anticipates emergency management and incident response contingencies and challenges, but is essential if emergency service personnel are to work effectively with colleagues within their own service and other services [NARU, 2015a].

To support this, in 2012 the Joint Emergency Services Interoperability Programme (JESIP) was launched to improve the way emergency services work together at multi-agency incidents [JESIP, 2016].

2.3.2 The JESIP principles

Under the interoperability framework, there are five main working principles of improving interoperability [JESIP, 2016]:

- **Co-locate:** Commanders of each service should be brought together to a single, safe and easily identified location near the scene.
- **Communicate:** Clear communication in plain English (avoiding jargon and service-specific terms).
- **Co-ordinate:** Commanders need to agree on the lead service, identify priorities, resources and capabilities in order to mount an effective response to the incident.
- **Jointly understand risk:** Share information about the likelihood and impact of threats and hazards and agree measures to control risk.
- **Shared situational awareness:** Use tools such as the joint decision model and METHANE.

2.3.3 The joint decision model

The joint decision model is a standard decision-making process used by commanders from different agencies to bring together available information, reconcile objectives and make effective decisions (Figure 9.3).

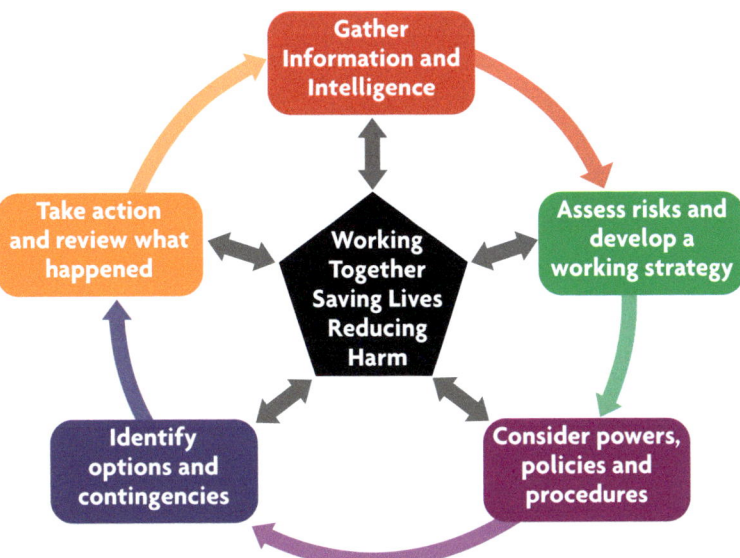

Figure 9.3 JESIP joint decision model. This tool is used to support the decision-making of commanders throughout the chain of command at an emergency incident.

Source: Joint Emergency Services Interoperability Programme. Available at: https://www.jesip.org.uk/joint-decision-model.

2.3.4 METHANE communication model

Historically, different emergency services used differing models to communicate key information at the scene of a major incident. However, all emergency personnel are now encouraged to use the same communication model: METHANE [JESIP, 2016].

The mnemonic METHANE is designed to provide the initial communication surrounding details of the major incident. It consists of [NARU, 2015a]:
- **M**ajor incident declared or standby. The person making the report should be explicit whether this is a major incident declaration or a standby in anticipation of the occurrence of a major incident.
- **E**xact location of the incident. Where possible the grid reference or GPS co-ordinates should be included, along with any landmarks or iconic sites.
- **T**ype of incident. What is the exact nature of the incident (for example, rail, chemical, road or terrorist)?
- **H**azards. What hazards are known to be present or could potentially manifest themselves?
- **A**ccess and egress. What are the agreed or best routes to and from the scene?
- **N**umber of casualties. How many casualties are there and, if possible to determine, what triage priority are they? i.e. 10 P1, 4 P2.
- **E**mergency services. Which emergency services are present and which are required? Include specialist resource request if known.

2.4 Classification of incidents

2.4.1 Major, mass and catastrophic incidents

NHS organisations are required to develop emergency preparedness arrangements for three levels of incident [DoH, 2007]:
- **Major:** Involving tens of patients and handled by individual trusts. An example is the London Bridge attack on 3 June 2017.
- **Mass:** Involving hundreds of patients and requiring mutual aid response from neighbouring trusts. An example would be the 7 July 2005 London bombings.
- **Catastrophic:** Involving thousands of patients and severely disrupting health and social care and other support functions. An example would be the Great East Japan Earthquake on 11 March 2011.

2.4.2 Causes of major incidents

Major incidents can arise from a number of causes [Blom, 2014]:
- **Big bang:** A serious transport accident, explosion or series of smaller incidents.
- **Rising tide:** A developing infectious disease epidemic, or a capacity/staffing crisis.
- **Cloud on the horizon:** A serious threat such as a major chemical or nuclear release developing elsewhere and needing preparatory action.
- **Headline news:** Public or media alarm about a personal threat.
- **Internal incidents:** Fire, breakdown of utilities, major equipment failure, hospital-acquired infections, violent crime and internal security issues.
- **Deliberate:** Release of chemical, biological, radiological, nuclear and explosive (CBRN(e)) materials.
- **Mass casualties:** Involving hundreds of patients and requiring mutual aid response from neighbouring trusts
- **Pre-planned major events:** Demonstrations, sports fixtures, air shows.
- **Marauding terrorist attack (MTA):** An act of terrorism, typically utilising firearms and/or explosives (known as a marauding terrorist firearms attack, MTFA), although less sophisticated weapons such as knives and vehicles can also be used. As the name implies, the location of the incident can change over time as the terrorists are often mobile, sometimes striking multiple locations simultaneously [Chauhan, 2018].

2.5 Role of the ambulance service

NHS ambulance trusts have the responsibility for alerting, mobilising and co-ordinating the NHS response to short-notice or sudden-impact emergencies. This includes [NARU, 2015a]:
- initiating and maintaining a command and control system to provide appropriate support

and guidance to all NHS responders and other agencies
- co-ordinating all NHS communications on scene
- managing the health, safety and welfare of all NHS responders
- providing casualty triage, treatment and transport, including the selection of appropriate receiving hospitals
- provision of specialist incident response capabilities, including hazardous area working, decontamination of casualties and active shooter incidents.

During a major incident, the response of the ambulance service revolves around seven key principles, sometimes referred to by the mnemonic, CSCATTT [Mackway-Jones, 2012]:
- **Command and control:** Each emergency service on scene has an incident commander, but the police usually take overall command.
- **Safety:** Personal safety is paramount and the appropriate personal protective equipment (PPE) must be worn. This does not always happen when crews are faced with a major incident. Of particular concern are hazardous materials or CBRN(e) incidents.
- **Communication:** This is the most common failing at major incidents [Mackway-Jones, 2012]. Modern radio networks used by the ambulance service should in theory alleviate some of the problems that have occurred in the past, but the use of runners should be considered if required.
- **Assessment:** A rapid initial assessment of the scene can provide an estimate of the number of those injured and the severity of their injuries. This can be refined as the incident unfolds.
- **Triage:** The dynamic process by which casualties are sorted into priorities for treatment. It needs to be repeated frequently.
- **Treatment:** 'Do the most for the most' is the standard mantra. This depends on the skills of the providers, severity of injuries and time on scene. The nature of the environment and casualty load may restrict the ability of the providers to give 'gold standard' care.
- **Transport:** Most patients will probably be transported to hospital by ambulance, but alternative methods of transport can be used.

The aim is to get the right patient to the right place at the right time.

2.6 Incident command and control

The ambulance service employs a three-tier command system comprising a strategic commander, a tactical commander and an operational commander. This is a hierarchical system whereby individuals are empowered through their role within the structure, which provides them with specific authority over others for the duration of the event [NARU, 2015a].

2.6.1 Strategic

The strategic commander is in overall charge of each service, and is responsible for formulating the strategy for the incident. Each strategic commander has overall command of the resources of their own organisation, but delegates tactical decisions to their respective tactical commander(s).

During major incidents, the strategic commander's responsibilities include [NARU, 2015a]:
- Establish a framework for the overall management of the incident.
- Assess and assure the effectiveness of the response.
- Determine strategic objectives and priorities.
- Rapidly formulate and implement an integrated media and communications plan.
- Ensure clear lines of communication with the tactical commander and external agencies.
- Instigate further contingency and recovery planning as required.
- Ensure the long-term resourcing and expertise for command resilience.
- Decide on what resources or expertise can be made available (mutual aid).
- Undertake liaison with strategic commanders in other agencies.
- Plan beyond the immediate response phase from recovering from the emergency to returning to or towards a new state of normality.

2.6.2 Tactical

The tactical commander works at the tactical level and is also known as the ambulance incident

commander (AIC). Their responsibilities include [NARU, 2015a]:
- Obtain sufficient information to determine the current status of the response. This should include ensuring that a detailed and formal handover is received from the acting ambulance incident commander (AIC) and that the whole command chain is aware that such a handover has taken place and appropriate log entries are made.
- Formulate a tactical plan that takes account of all available information, including any pre-determined emergency plans, and anticipated risks.
- Implement tactics in a timely manner, confirming roles, responsibilities, tasks and communication channels.
- Conduct ongoing risk assessment and management in response to the dynamic nature of emergencies.
- Review tactics with relevant others including key personnel involved in command, control and co-ordination.
- Ensure actions to implement tactics are carried out, taking into account the impact on individuals, communities and the environment.
- Determine priorities for allocating available resources.
- Anticipate likely future resource needs, taking account of the possible escalation of emergencies.
- Work in co-operation and communicate effectively with other responders.
- Liaise with relevant organisations to address the longer-term priorities of restoring essential services and helping to facilitate the recovery of affected communities.
- Obtain and provide technical and professional advice from suitable sources to inform decision-making where required.
- Provide accurate and timely information to inform and protect communities, working with the media where relevant.
- Monitor and maintain the health, safety and welfare of individuals during the response.
- Review actions taken at operational level.
- Identify where circumstances warrant a strategic level of management and engage with the strategic level as required.
- Ensure that any individuals under their area of authority are fully briefed and debriefed.
- Evaluate the effectiveness of tactics and use this information to inform future practice.
- Fully record decisions, actions, options and rationale in accordance with current information, policy and legislation.
- Ensure engagement with multi-agency responders, providing a joined-up and proportionate response.
- Request Airwave interoperability where appropriate.
- Ensure appropriate control measures are employed to manage all identified risks, reviewing and updating logs and risk assessments as appropriate.
- Follow any action cards specific to the tactical commander role as issued by the host ambulance trust.

2.6.3 Operational

The operational commander has responsibility for the activities undertaken at the scene. They are usually located at the incident scene, ideally alongside the operational commanders of the other responding agencies at the forward command post.

Responsibilities of the operational commander include [NARU, 2015a]:
- Make an initial assessment of the situation and report this to other responders in accordance with established procedures.
- Ensure a METHANE message is communicated to the relevant EOC.
- Prepare and implement an initial plan of action.
- Ensure actions are carried out, taking into account the impact on individuals, communities and the environment.
- Conduct ongoing risk assessment and management in response to the dynamic nature of emergencies.
- Work in co-operation and communicate effectively with other responders.
- Confirm the availability and location of relevant services and facilities.
- Identify any resources required and deploy them to meet the demands of the response.

Major incidents

- Ensure the establishment of the functional roles required to manage the incident and that appropriately trained individuals undertake each role.
- Communicate any resource constraints to the relevant person, or find suitable alternatives.
- Monitor and protect the health, safety and welfare of individuals during the response.
- Deal with individuals in a manner that is supportive and sensitive to their needs.
- Liaise with relevant organisations as required for an effective response.
- Identify where circumstances warrant a tactical level of management and engage with the tactical level as required.
- Implement the tactical plan where applicable, within a geographical area or functional area of responsibility.
- Ensure that any individuals under their area of authority are fully briefed and debriefed.
- Fully record decisions, actions, options and rationale in accordance with current information, policy and legislation.
- Follow any action cards specific to the operational role as issued by the host ambulance trust.

2.6.4 Additional roles

A key principle of any command system is limiting how much responsibility a single person has to contend with. In order to achieve this at a major incident, commanders will often delegate responsibilities for tasks to others. There are a number of roles and responsibilities that can be delegated by operational commanders; these are shown in Figure 9.4 and explained in further detail below.

Additional support roles are not always required and/or may be undertaken by a single officer, depending on workload. They include [NARU, 2015a]:

- **Safety officer:** Responsible for the health and safety of all NHS responders entering and working within the cordons of the incident.
- **Parking officer:** Responsible for creating and maintaining a clear and functional parking area. They will ensure vehicles and crews are logged into the area and direct resources to the casualty clearing station (CCS) when casualties need to be removed from the incident.
- **Loading officer:** Responsible for keeping a log of the number and destinations of casualties transported from the CCS.
- **Primary triage officer:** Responsible for co-ordinating the triage of all casualties at the incident.
- **Casualty clearing officer (CCO):** Responsible for the management of the CCS. Works closely with the triage, parking and loading officers to ensure an efficient triage and treatment of all casualties and the appropriate use of available transport resources.
- **Equipment officer:** Responsible for ensuring the supply and re-supply of equipment to all responding NHS resources.
- **Hazardous area response team (HART) leader:** Provides direct line management for all HART resources.
- **National inter-agency liaison officer (NILO):** Ensures a co-ordinated response and safe systems of work are maintained between emergency services, particularly when commanders cannot be co-located.

2.7 First crew on scene

Your role as first on scene is laid out in your organisation's major incident plan and you should familiarise yourself with it **before** you are called to a major incident. However, initial action cards should be available in your major incident packs on your vehicle.

The first vehicle on scene needs to park up close to police control, if present, and as close to the incident as possible upwind and uphill. As part of a double-crewed ambulance (DCA), the driver will assume the role of communications officer until relieved. They will remain with their vehicle, securing the doors to prevent the ambulance from being inadvertently loaded with casualties.

Gathering appropriate resources to cope with a major incident takes time, so it's important to request help early. You do not have to wait until an officer arrives on scene to declare a major incident. It is likely that your senior colleague will make the decision, but, as the communications officer, you will relay the message.

Chapter 9 – *Scene Assessment*

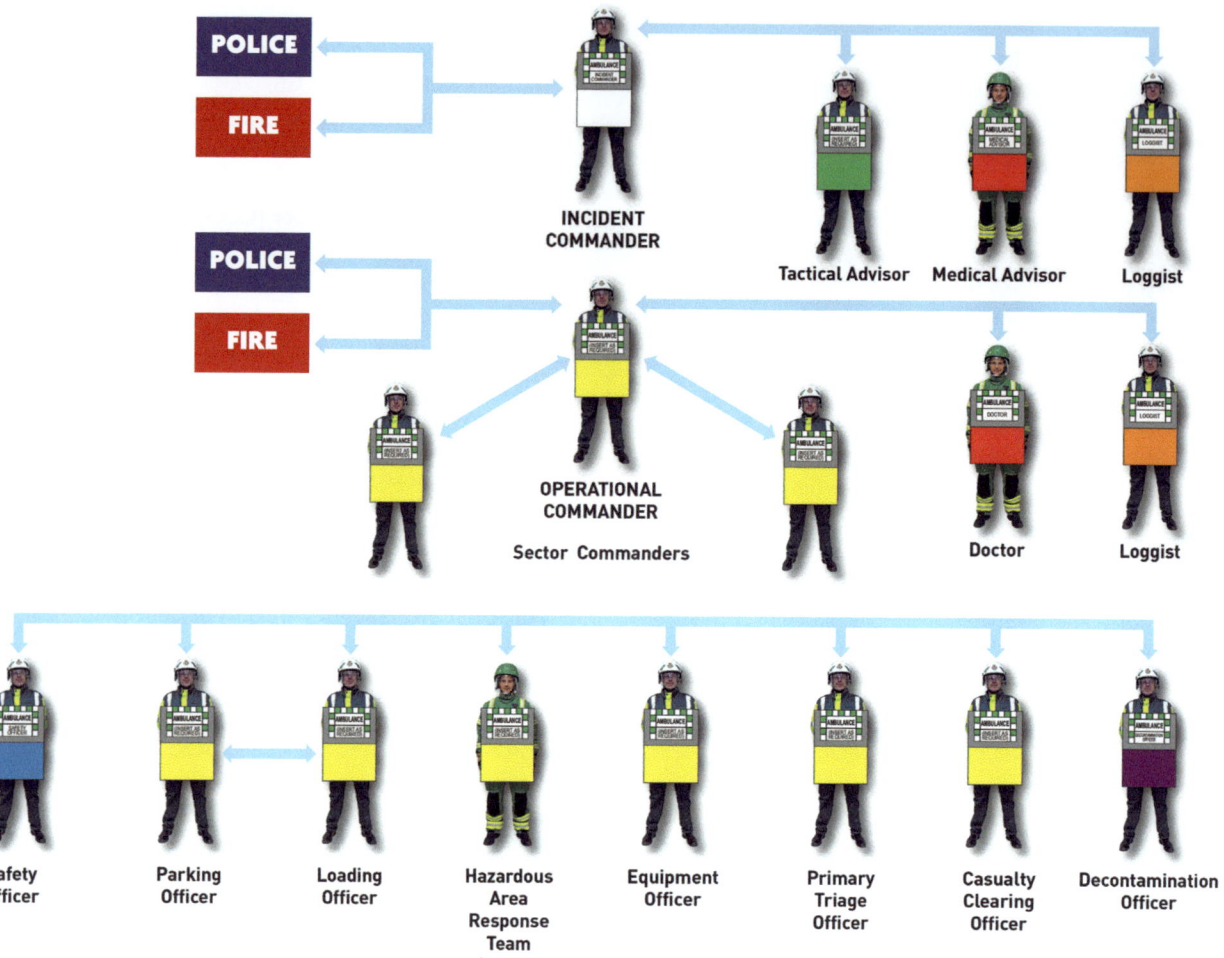

Figure 9.4 An incident command structure showing examples of the additional support roles that may be required.

Source: Reproduced by kind permission of the National Ambulance Resilience Unit (NARU).

2.7.1 Attendant's role

The attendant will be the ambulance incident commander until relieved. If there is one on the ambulance, they should put on a green-and-white chequered tabard and wear appropriate personal protective equipment (PPE). They must not get involved in the treatment of any casualties.

Actions they will take include [NARU, 2015b]:
- Assess the scene and, if determined safe to enter, carry out a reconnaissance of the incident, using the mnemonic METHANE to collate the information necessary for the driver to report back to the emergency operations centre (EOC).
- Assess the need for specialist teams e.g. HART, air ambulance.
- Working with other services to establish:
  - access to and egress from the incident
  - an initial rendezvous point
  - an ambulance parking point
  - a casualty clearing station.
- Briefing the senior officer on arrival and complying with their requests.

2.7.2 Driver's role

Your actions as driver are as follows [NARU, 2015b]:
- Stay with the vehicle.
- Do not attempt to treat casualties.

Major incidents

- Leave the rooftop blue lights illuminated and the engine running.
- Don your personal protective equipment (PPE).
- Secure the doors of your vehicle to ensure patients are not inadvertently loaded.
- Maintain contact with the emergency operations centre (EOC).
- Start a log.
- Relay a METHANE report to the EOC once the attendant has provided you with the necessary details.
- Compile a debrief report of the incident

2.8 Subsequent crews on scene

Additional crews should report their presence to the communications officer once on scene. In addition, they will be required to do the following [NARU, 2015b]:

- Change to the designated radio talk group for the incident if advised to by the EOC.
- Don appropriate PPE.
- Turn off the ambulance blue lights and ensure keys are left in the ignition.
- Proceed as instructed to the parking officer for tasking (operational commander if role not established).
- Take a functional role as allocated by the operational commander and don the appropriate tabard.
- Do not deviate from this assigned role unless otherwise directed by the operational commander.
- On leaving the scene:
  - advise the ambulance loading officer of your departure
  - confirm the receiving hospital.

2.9 Triage

The aim of triage is to do the most for the most and it should be used any time that the number of casualties exceeds the number of skilled rescuers. It is a dynamic process and therefore needs to be repeated many times during the care of each casualty.

2.9.1 Triage sieve and sort

There are two phases to triage. The first, the triage sieve (Figure 9.5), takes place where the casualty is found [NARU, 2013]. This is a fast, physiological assessment of the casualty.

The second, more in-depth assessment is called the triage sort and generally takes place at the casualty clearing station. The triage sort usually adopts the Triage Revised Trauma System [Champion, 1989], which utilises respiratory rate, systolic blood pressure and Glasgow Coma Scale (GCS), with scores attached to ranges of values. The total score identifies the patient category. You are only likely to perform a triage sort if you are tasked to assist in the casualty clearing station at a major incident.

The triage sieve and sort are not the only primary and secondary tools that have been developed.

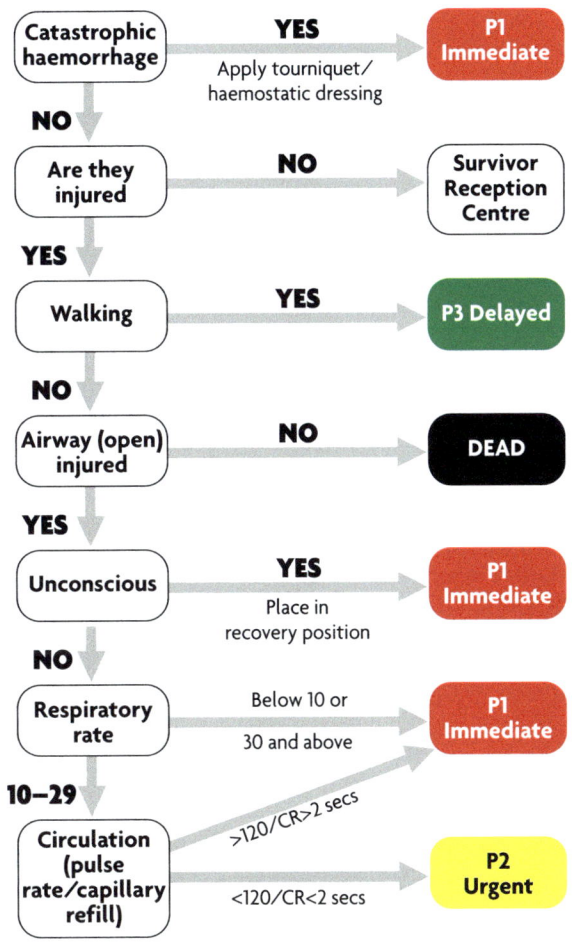

Figure 9.5 The triage sieve.
Source: National Ambulance Resilience Unit, 2014.

Although they are not evidence-based, this has not stopped their widespread use in civilian and military major incident management [Jenkins, 2008]. Whatever method you use in your organisation for triaging patients, it is important to appreciate that triage is a dynamic process that must be frequently repeated, since a patient's clinical condition can change.

2.9.2 Over- and under-triaging

A key aspect of triaging is not under- or over-triaging, i.e. making sure that the right priority is identified for any casualty. An example of over-triage would be a patient who is not breathing, even with airway opened, but has a pulse. This patient should be triaged as dead, but this can be difficult to reconcile with ambulance crews, who ordinarily would attempt to resuscitate this patient [JCO, 2010; Kilner, 2002].

Another cause of over-triaging is to use the adult triage sieve on children. This can be avoided by use of a specific children's triage sieve. The most common in the UK is probably the paediatric triage tape (PTT), but there are other systems in use worldwide [Wallis, 2006]. However, if this is not available, children should be triaged using the adult triage sieve, as this will avoid under-triage.

Over-triage is dangerous as it puts pressure on already scarce resources and has been adversely linked to critical mortality (the number of deaths in critically injured survivors) [Frykberg, 1988].

Under-triage can occur when triaging casualties with normal physiological observations (i.e. respiratory rate of 10–29 breaths per minute and heart rate less than 120 beats per minute or capillary refill time less than two seconds), but who are unable to walk. The triage sieve makes no allowance for patients who cannot normally walk, for example casualties who require a wheelchair to mobilise or babies who have not yet learned how to walk.

Under-triage can also occur when the casualty has a normal respiratory rate and is triaged without consideration given to their pulse rate or capillary refill time, which are abnormal. This results in the casualty being triaged as Urgent instead of the correct category, Immediate [Kilner, 2002].

2.9.3 Treating and triaging

Treatment in the triage sieve should be limited to simple interventions such as the insertion of basic airway adjuncts or turning an unconscious patient into the recovery position. Catastrophic haemorrhage should also be controlled.

2.9.4 Recording your findings

There are various triage tagging systems in use. The simplest are 'slapper bands', which are in use by several ambulance services in the UK. More commonly, you will find triage labels, with space to allow the recording of findings and to provide a means to identify the patient (Figure 9.6). It doesn't matter which system your service uses as long as you know where the tags are and how to use them!

2.9.5 Vulnerable populations

The Civil Contingencies Act 2004 identified vulnerable persons as a priority in emergencies. Therefore, major incident plans need to take account of specific groups such as children, non-English speakers and people with learning difficulties and mental illness [DoH, 2005].

Children

The injured casualties in a major incident may be children only, a mixture of adults and children, or adults only with children who need caring for. As

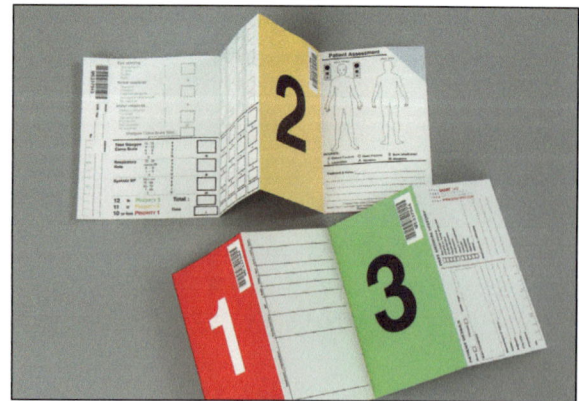

Figure 9.6 A triage label.

far as is practically possible, families should be kept together, but this may not be possible depending on resources and the severity of injuries.

Section 11 of the Children Act 2004 requires ambulance services to safeguard the well-being of children. When children are unaccompanied but uninjured, the local authority is responsible for the child. Since social workers may not be immediately available, children may need to be cared for by the ambulance service or police. Children should not be entrusted to adults with no connection with the child, however well-meaning.

Check with your service to find out exactly what procedures are in place for children at a major incident.

3 Hazardous materials

3.1 Learning objectives

By the end of this section you will be able to:
- describe the systems for labelling hazardous substances
- describe how to find out information about a hazardous substance
- describe the risks when attending a hazardous substance incident
- describe actions that need to be undertaken when attending a hazardous substance or CBRN(e) incident.

3.2 Introduction

There's a good chance if you have a look in the cupboard under your kitchen sink or shed/garage that you will find a hazardous/dangerous substance. Since the key component of scene assessment is safety for yourself, your colleagues, patients and bystanders, it is important that you appreciate how readily available hazardous substances are. Patients who are contaminated with a hazardous substance can easily contaminate others. On a grander scale are incidents involving transport vehicles, most commonly on the road, but also by rail, sea and air. You are unlikely to become heavily involved with these types of incidents as you will not have the training or equipment to be able to safely do so. These are incidents for the fire and rescue service and the hazardous area response team (HART) to deal with. However, if you can identify the hazardous substance early on, this can assist commanders in determining what resources are required.

Information about the hazardous material can be obtained from a number of sources [HSE, 2017b]:
- The packaging and associated warning labels.
- Emergency telephone advice from services such as Chemsafe or TOXBASE (typically accessed through the emergency operations centre).
- The driver and the documentation being carried in the case of vehicular incidents.

3.3 Labelling hazardous substances

In June 2015, the Classification, Labelling and Packaging of Substances and Mixtures (CLP) Regulations came into force, which define what information must be provided on the label of a hazardous substance or mixture (Figure 9.7). This includes [ECA, 2017]:
- name, address and telephone number of the supplier(s)
- the nominal quantity of the substance or mixture in the package where this is being made available to the general public, unless this quantity is specified elsewhere on the package
- product identifiers
- hazard pictograms, where applicable
- the relevant signal word, where applicable
- hazard statements, where applicable
- appropriate precautionary statements, where applicable
- a section for supplemental information, where applicable.

This replaced the former regulations, the Dangerous Substances Directive (DSD) and Dangerous Preparations Directive (DPD). However, it is likely that you will encounter packaging with both, so it is important that you are familiar with them.

Chapter 9 – Scene Assessment

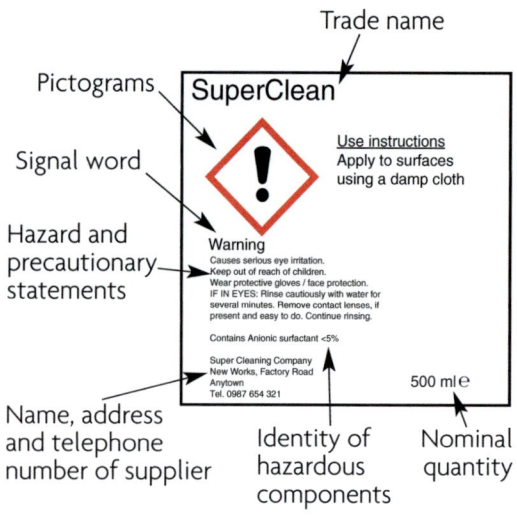

Figure 9.7 An example label for a hazardous mixture [EC, 2013].

3.3.1 CLP pictograms

The CLP has introduced nine pictograms, which have replaced the older orange square warning symbols (Table 9.1). In addition, there are two signal words that accompany the pictograms [EC, 2013]:

- **Danger:** Substances and mixtures with the most severe hazards.
- **Warning:** Substances and mixtures with less serious hazards.

3.4 Transporting hazardous substances

Road and rail vehicles registered in Great Britain on domestic journeys are required to display a hazard warning panel with an Emergency Action ('Hazchem') Code, United Nations (UN) number, danger label, contact number and (optionally) company name or logo (Figures 9.8 and 9.9) [NCEC, 2017].

3.4.1 International journeys

Vehicles on international journeys must display the Hazard Identification Number (HIN) on an orange-coloured plate. This also contains information about the hazardous properties of the substance, as well as its UN number (Figure 9.10).

3.5 Danger labels

Danger labels are displayed on vehicles and packaging/containers of dangerous goods that are to be transported (Figure 9.11).

3.6 Ambulance crew actions at scene

In the event that an 'ordinary' emergency call turns out to involve hazardous substances, or you come across an incident that appears to involve hazardous substances, previous guidance for unprotected ambulance staff was to withdraw and await specialist teams, such as the hazardous area response team (HART) [HPA, 2009a].

However, following research conducted as part of the Optimisation through Research of Chemical Incident Decontamination Systems project, it has become apparent that additional lives can be saved by the rapid (within 15 minutes of exposure) implementation of a number of measures, including the removal of the patient's outer clothing [HPA, 2009b]. This has led to a change in the guidance for all emergency service personnel who are the first response to a CBRN(e) incident.

3.6.1 Arrival

It is possible that the emergency operations centre (EOC) will have made you aware that you are attending a CBRN(e) incident, but in the early stages, this may be hard to determine.

Signs of a CBRN(e) release include [JESIP, 2016]:
- dead or distressed people, birds and animals
- multiple individuals showing unexplained signs of:
  - skin, eye or airway irritation
  - vomiting
  - sweating
  - pin-point pupils

Hazardous materials

Table 9.1 CLP pictograms and sample hazard statements.

CLP pictogram	Example hazard statement	Old DSD/DPD symbol	CLP pictogram	Example hazard statement	Old DSD/DPD symbol
💥	Explosive; mass explosion hazard	💥	❗	Causes skin irritation	✖
🔥	Extremely flammable gases/aerosols/liquids/solids	🔥	🫁	May cause allergy or asthma symptoms or breathing difficulties if inhaled	✖
🔥⭕	May cause or intensify fire; oxidiser	🔥⭕	🐟	Toxic to aquatic life with long-lasting effects	🌳🐟
☠	Fatal if swallowed	☠			
🧪	Causes severe skin burns and eye damage	🧪	🛢	Contains gas under pressure; may explode if heated	

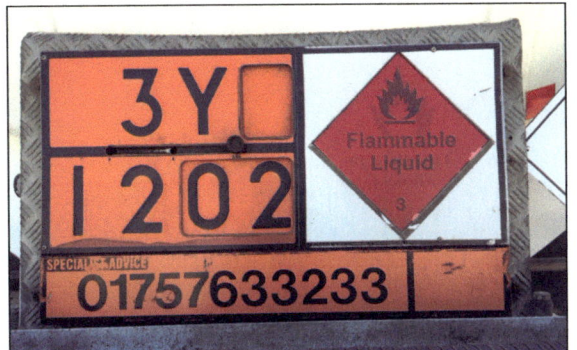

Figure 9.8 A hazard warning panel from a diesel tanker.

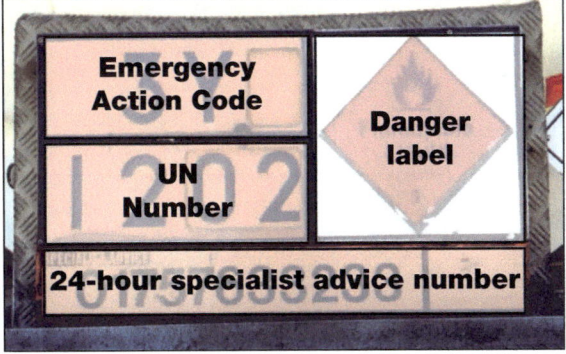

Figure 9.9 Annotated hazard warning panel.

137

Chapter 9 – Scene Assessment

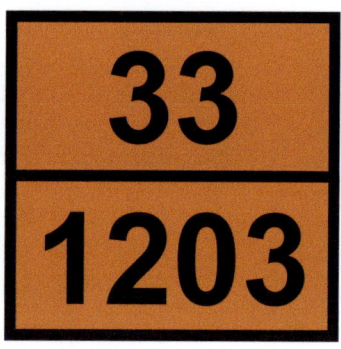

Figure 9.10 Orange plate with HIN (top) and UN number (bottom).

- runny nose
- disorientation
- breathing difficulties
- seizures
- presence of hazardous or unusual materials/equipment
- unexplained vapour/mist clouds and/or oily droplets or film on surfaces of water
- withered plant life or vegetation.

Provide a situation report to the EOC using the METHANE mnemonic.

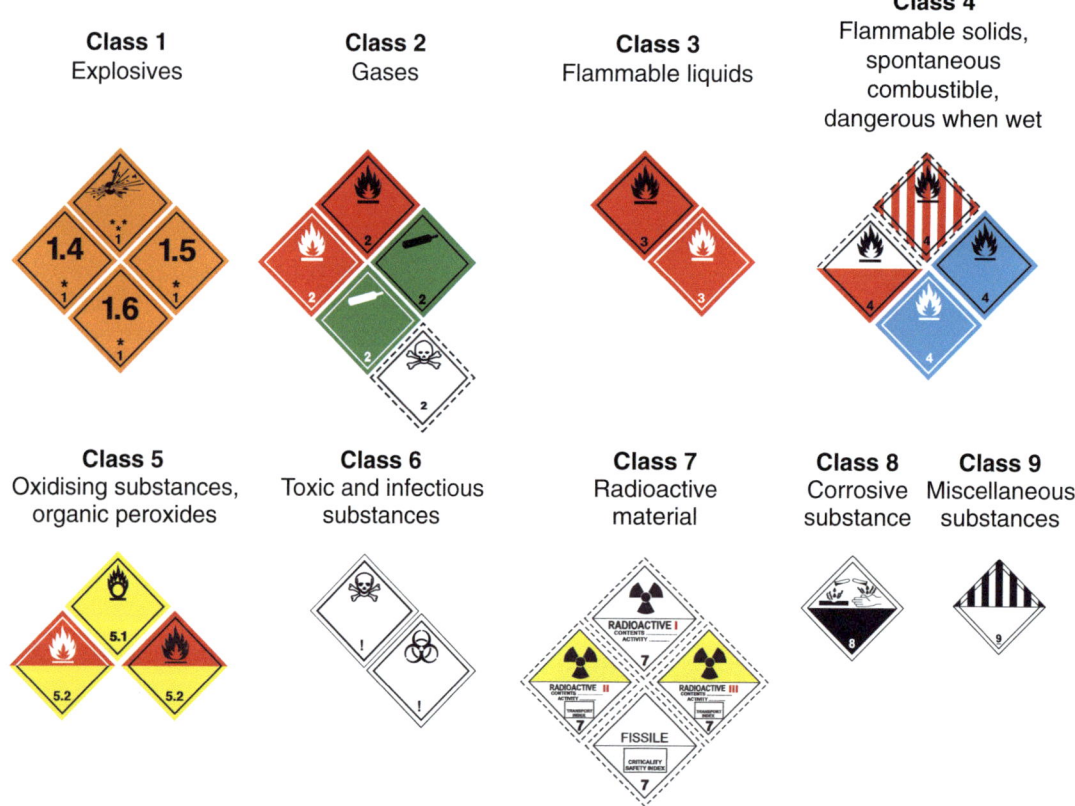

Figure 9.11 Danger labels.

3.6.2 Hazard assessment

If there are three or more patients in close proximity with no obvious cause, you should conduct a hazard assessment, preferably with other emergency services if they are on scene. This hazard assessment should include:
- CBRN(e) release indicators
- patient numbers (walking and non-walking)
- signs and symptoms of casualties
- weather conditions
- hazards present or suspected
- location: is it a likely target for terrorists or a hazardous material incident?
- built environment: is it a city centre, open space, underground?
- presence of perpetrators.

This will enable a decision to be made on the hazard area and on the safe working area, and enable a joint operational plan.

3.6.3 Evacuate, disrobe and decontaminate (remove, remove, remove)

Encourage patients to move away from the main area of contamination (hot zone, remove themselves) into an area that, ideally, should be uphill and upwind (warm zone). However, you should avoid physical contact where possible. Once in the warm zone, patients need to undress to their underwear (remove outer clothing). Skin, hair, clothing and items such as jewellery are all likely to be contaminated and need to be removed. Advise patients that they should not remove clothing over their heads, but cut them off if necessary. Absorbent materials such as paper towels, towels and medical dressings can be used to remove contaminants from exposed skin. If you have disrobing packs, distribute them to patients, but alternative clothing or blankets can be used to protect patients from hypothermia and maintain dignity. However, patients must leave all items removed during the disrobing procedure where they are removed. Finally, patients should remove the substance from their skin using a dry absorbent material to either soak up the substance or brush it off [NARU, 2017a].

Communication

Asking patients to remove their clothes, particularly in public, requires trust. One method to achieve this is to communicate clearly with patients. You should ensure that you tell patients [JESIP, 2016]:
- why and how they need to be undressed and decontaminated
- to assist others if they can
- that additional help and resources are on the way
- that they should not eat, drink or smoke and they should avoid touching their face.

Chapter

10 Patient Assessment

1 Patient assessment process

1.1 Learning objectives

By the end of this section you will be able to:
- state the components of the patient assessment process
- describe the <C>ABCDE approach to initial patient assessment including:
  - catastrophic haemorrhage
  - airway
  - breathing
  - circulation
  - disability
  - exposure
- state the components of the AVPU tool to assess level of consciousness
- outline how to obtain a patient history using the acronyms SAMPLE and SOCRATES
- describe the steps in a 'head-to-toe' assessment
- explain the components of the National Early Warning Score (NEWS2).

1.2 Introduction

Once you have completed your scene assessment, the next step is to conduct a patient assessment. This chapter will break down the patient assessment process into its separate parts so you can explore them further. Figure 10.1 shows the patient assessment process from start to finish. This chapter and some of the subsequent chapters are going to cover this in some detail, so just concentrate on the order of the assessment process, rather than on what it is you are expected to do during each stage [Nolan, 2016; JRCALC, 2019].

1.3 Primary survey

The primary survey (Figure 10.2) is a swift patient assessment and management process, which can be completed within 60–90 seconds [JRCALC, 2019]. It is designed to be a step-wise approach, meaning that any abnormalities identified in one step

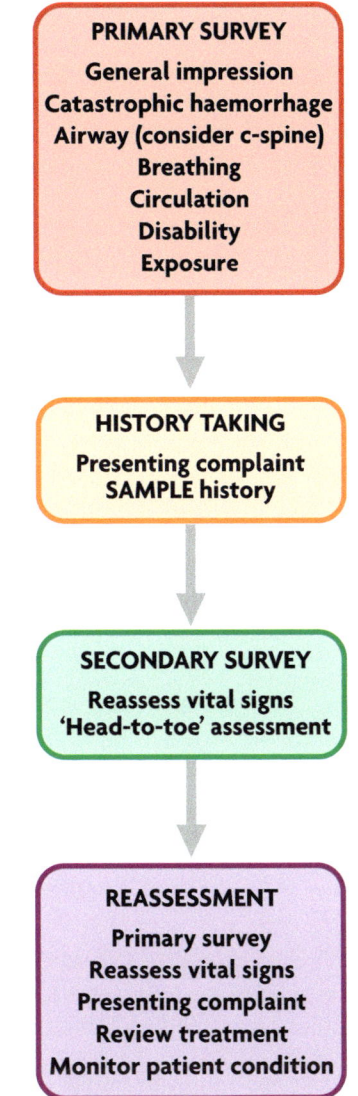

Figure 10.1 The patient assessment process.

should be addressed before moving on to the next. Patients who have suffered traumatic injuries should have a check for life-threatening (or catastrophic) haemorrhage, before you check the patient's airway. In addition, in this group of patients you should give consideration to the patient's cervical spine and avoid unnecessary movement of the head and neck. This is covered in more detail in Chapter 17, 'Trauma'.

Chapter 10 – Patient Assessment

> **PRIMARY SURVEY**
> General impression
> Catastrophic haemorrhage
> Airway (consider c-spine)
> Breathing
> Circulation
> Disability
> Exposure

Figure 10.2 The primary survey.

1.3.1 General impression

The general impression is your first and immediate assessment of the patient and their current location, which will give you an early indication as to how sick and/or injured your patient is. Some of this information you will have already gathered from your scene assessment. As you approach a patient ensure that you are wearing appropriate personal protective equipment (PPE). Note the patient's approximate age, and signs of obvious frailty, injury or disability, as your management and expectations of what the patient can do will vary. For example, a one-year-old child will not present in the same way as an adult. In addition, patient positioning can give you early clues. Is the patient sitting up and smiling (Figure 10.3a) or are they lying apparently lifeless on the floor (Figure 10.3b)? This step relies heavily on experience and intuition and can be challenging [NAEMT, 2019].

This is also your chance to assess how responsive the patient is. If the patient is awake, introduce yourself with 'Hello, my name is…' and identify yourself as being from the ambulance service. Ask how they would prefer to be addressed.

If the patient appears not to be awake or is unconscious, check for responsiveness by asking them if they are all right, or try giving them a command such as 'Open your eyes'. If they do not respond, gently shake the patient's shoulders. Patients who fail to respond are critically ill until proven otherwise [Nolan, 2016].

1.3.2 Catastrophic haemorrhage

Bleeding that is likely to cause death in minutes is referred to as a catastrophic haemorrhage.

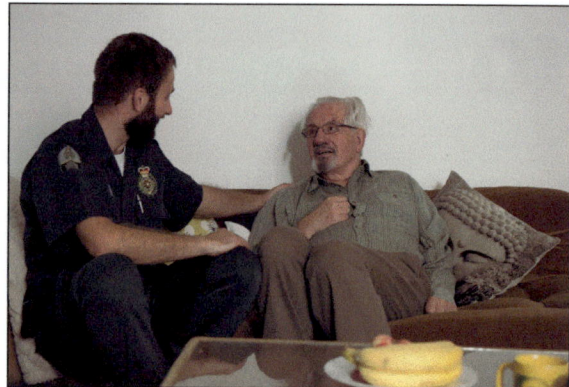

Figure 10.3a General impression. Patient sitting up and smiling.

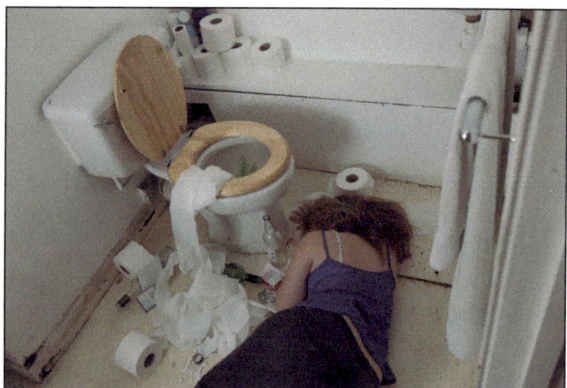

Figure 10.3b General impression. Patient lying apparently lifeless on the floor.

This bleeding needs to be stopped, even before assessing the airway, to prevent the patient from bleeding to death. This is covered in Chapter 17, 'Trauma'.

1.3.3 Airway

Assessment of the airway involves three steps:
- **Look** for signs of airway obstruction.
- **Listen** for noisy or absent breathing.
- **Feel** for air movement as the patient breathes.

Remember, the primary assessment proceeds in a step-wise manner. Any signs of obstruction such as snoring or gurgling sounds need to be addressed now before moving on to breathing. You will learn how to deal with airway problems in Chapter 11, 'Airway'.

1.3.4 Breathing

Once you have a patent (open) airway, you are ready to move on to breathing. As with the airway, you will adopt a look, listen, feel approach.

The first question you should ask is whether the patient is breathing. If they aren't, then you will have to provide breaths for the patient, i.e. ventilate them. If they are breathing, you will need to decide whether it is adequate. You can start with the respiratory rate and depth of breathing (indicated by chest movement), but Chapter 12, 'Breathing', will also explain about other methods of assessing breathing that can be recorded at this stage, including pulse oximetry, accessory muscle use and auscultation (using a stethoscope to listen for sounds from the lungs and other organs).

1.3.5 Circulation

You can obtain a good idea of the patient's circulation by looking at the colour of their limbs (usually the hands as they are the most accessible and normally visible). Feeling for a pulse is a skill that you will cover in Chapter 13, 'Circulation'. The pulse can tell you the heart rate and adequacy of the cardiac output, particularly if distal pulses such as the wrist are absent when a central pulse (such as found in the neck) is palpable. Clearly, a patient who does not have a pulse needs CPR immediately! This is covered in Chapter 24, 'Cardiac Arrest'. Since you will typically be working as part of a crew, it may be possible to undertake a blood pressure or electrocardiogram (ECG) while you or your colleague are identifying potential life-threats that affect circulation.

1.3.6 Disability

Disability in the primary assessment refers to the patient's level of consciousness, or how awake they are. There are many causes of unconsciousness and these are covered in Chapter 14, 'Disability'. During the primary assessment, you will need to check three things to assess the patient's disability [JRCALC, 2019]:
- level of consciousness
- pupils
- blood sugar.

Level of consciousness

A rapid assessment of the patient's level of consciousness (LOC) can be undertaken using the acronym AVPU:

A: Alert
V: Responds to verbal stimulus
P: Responds to pain
U: Unresponsive.

Pupils

When looking at a patient's pupils, you are interested in whether they are of equal size and react to light. There are a number of reasons why this may not be the case and you'll find out about these in Chapter 14, 'Disability'.

Blood sugar

Hypoglycaemia, or low blood sugar, is a cause of reduced level of consciousness, which can usually be corrected by the administration of glucose, either orally (by mouth) or intravenously. In addition, there are drugs that can mobilise the body's own glucose stores and you will learn about these in Chapter 16, 'Medical and Surgical Emergencies'.

1.3.7 Exposure

You will undertake a full 'head-to-toe' assessment later on in the patient assessment process, but a quick look early on will provide you with clues to obvious illness/injury that needs to be managed quickly. For example, some types of rashes (e.g. non-blanching) signal serious illness such as sepsis. It also provides a chance to identify sites of hidden bleeding that you did not pick up on earlier on in your assessment.

Working out of hospital, however, you do need to be mindful about maintaining patient privacy by not unnecessarily exposing them in public as well as ensuring that they do not lose body heat. This is particularly important in trauma as patients are three times more likely to die if they are hypothermic (their body temperature is below 35°C) [Ireland, 2011].

1.4 *History taking*

1.4.1 Presenting complaint

The presenting complaint is usually the reason you have been called to the patient (Figure 10.4).

> **HISTORY TAKING**
> **Presenting complaint**
> **SAMPLE history**

Figure 10.4 History taking.

The majority of presenting complaints fall into the categories of pain, discomfort and/or abnormal body function. Sometimes this is explicit ('I have terrible chest pain') but can be vague, particularly in the elderly ('I just don't feel right today'). Avoid using words like 'problem' or 'complaint' when finding out the reason for the emergency call from the patient (despite the fact that it is referred to as the 'presenting complaint' within medical circles!) [Innes, 2018].

1.4.2 SAMPLE history

Once you know the presenting complaint, you will need to ask further questions. At the bare minimum, this should include the parts of the SAMPLE acronym:

- **S:** Signs and symptoms of the presenting complaint
- **A:** Allergies (particularly to medication or food)
- **M:** Medications
- **P:** Past medical history
- **L:** Last oral intake
- **E:** Events that led to the current illness or injury.

Note that when you are working with a paramedic, you may find that they use and document a different method, made up of the following components [Innes, 2018]:

- history of presenting complaint
- past medical history
- drug history including allergies
- family history
- social history
- systematic enquiry.

Signs and symptoms of the presenting complaint

To help you organise the signs and symptoms of the presenting complaint, you can use the SOCRATES acronym. This was originally designed with assessment of pain in mind, but can be helpful for other presenting complaints.

SOCRATES:

- **S:** Site
- **O:** Onset
- **C:** Character
- **R:** Radiation
- **A:** Association (are there any other signs and symptoms associated with the presenting complaint?)
- **T:** Timing
- **E:** Exacerbating/relieving factors
- **S:** Severity.

1.4.3 Allergies and medication

Allergies

The range of drugs that you can administer is limited, but there is still scope for patient harm if administered inappropriately. You should always ask the patient about any allergic reactions to medication they have received in the past. It is also a good idea to ask about other allergies, such as those caused by food, animals, pollen or metal [Innes, 2018].

Medication

Write down all of the patient's medication including the dose and frequency of administration. Just writing 'drugs with patient' or similar is not acceptable.

It is also a good idea to ask about any over-the-counter medicines (i.e. those not prescribed by a doctor, but obtained from a pharmacist or supermarket), as well as herbal and homeopathic remedies. Don't forget to consider whether illicit drugs have been taken by patients. In addition, there are cases where patients take medication prescribed for other family members or friends!

1.4.4 Past medical history

You will probably cover some of the patient's medical history while obtaining the history of the presenting complaint, but the following questions will help you uncover other medical illnesses or previous surgery that may prove helpful [Innes, 2018; Gregory, 2010b]:

- Have you had any illnesses that you have seen your GP about?

- Have you had to take any time off work because of ill health?
- Have you had any operations?
- Have you been admitted to hospital and, if so, why?
- Have you suffered any injuries?

1.4.5 Last oral intake and events leading to illness/injury

Last oral intake

Find out when the patient last had anything to eat or drink. This information is useful for patients who are unconscious or deteriorate on the way to hospital, or who may require surgery, as patients with a full stomach are at risk of aspiration. Also, you may be able to identify the onset of food poisoning and/or food allergies [Gregory, 2010b].

Events leading to the illness or injury

This is also known as the history of the presenting complaint and if you have used the SOCRATES acronym, you will have already obtained most of the information required.

Additional information that is useful to obtain includes [Gregory, 2010b]:

- **Associated symptoms:** For example, does the patient have shortness of breath and nausea with their chest pain?
- **Previous episodes:** Find out what happened last time, including any diagnoses made or hospital admissions.
- **Effect on daily living:** Does the presenting complaint interfere with getting to the toilet or making a cup of tea, for example?

1.5 Secondary survey

The secondary survey is often tailored to your findings from the primary survey and history (Figure 10.5). For example, if the presenting complaint is shortness of breath, then you are going to ensure that you obtain a respiratory rate and oxygen saturations, and auscultate (examine using a stethoscope) the lungs.

1.5.1 Reassess vital signs

Your ambulance service may have a specified minimum set of observations to obtain, but this will generally include:

- respiratory rate
- oxygen saturations
- pulse rate
- blood pressure
- level of consciousness (AVPU or Glasgow Coma Scale score, GCS)
- blood sugar
- temperature
- National Early Warning Score (NEWS2).

Depending on the patient's presenting complaint and the management plan, you may also obtain an electrocardiogram (ECG), if you haven't already.

Being able to record vital signs accurately is a fundamental skill and these will be explored in depth in the relevant chapters later in the book.

1.5.2 National Early Warning Score

In order to standardise the initial assessment of an acute illness, the Royal College of Physicians, in conjunction with other healthcare professions, have developed the National Early Warning Score (NEWS, now in its second revision and known as NEWS2) (Figure 10.6). It is aimed at improving [RCP, 2017]:

- the assessment of acute illness
- the detection of clinical deterioration
- initiation of a timely and competent clinical response.

Once you have recorded the patient's clinical observations, you simply add up the score awarded to each of the physiological parameters. For example, consider a patient with the following observations:

- respiratory rate: 10 breaths/minute
- oxygen saturations on air: 93%
- air or oxygen: Air
- systolic blood pressure: 108 mmHg
- heart rate: 110 beats/min
- consciousness: alert
- temperature: 38.1°C.

SECONDARY SURVEY
Reassess vital signs
'Head-to-toe' assessment

Figure 10.5 The secondary survey.

Chapter 10 – Patient Assessment

National Early Warning Score (NEWS2)

Physiological parameter	3	2	1	0	1	2	3
Respiration rate (per minute)	≤8		9–11	12–20		21–24	≥25
SpO₂ Scale 1 (%)	≤91	92–93	94–95	≥96			
SpO₂ Scale 2 (%)	≤83	84–85	86–87	88–92 ≥93 on air	93–94 on oxygen	95–96 on oxygen	≥97 on oxygen
Air or oxygen?		Oxygen		Air			
Systolic blood pressure (mmHg)	≤90	91–100	101–110	111–219			≥220
Pulse (per minute)	≤40		41–50	51–90	91–110	111–130	≥131
Consciousness				Alert			CVPU
Temperature (°C)	≤35.0		35.1–36.0	36.1–38.0	38.1–39.0	≥39.1	

Figure 10.6 National Early Warning Score version 2.
Source: Royal College of Physicians, 2017. Available at: https://www.rcplondon.ac.uk/projects/outputs/national-early-warning-score-news-2.

Note: NEWS2 is not suitable for children under 16 years or women who are pregnant, as physiological responses to acute illness can be modified in these groups [RCP, 2017]. When calculating the NEWS2 score, use the SpO2 Scale 1, unless directed to use Scale 2 by a clinician or local policy. Under consciousness, there is an addition 'C', which stands for new onset of confusion, disorientation or reduction in level of consciousness.

This patient's NEWS2 is calculated as: 1 + 2 + 0 + 1 + 1 + 0 + 1 = 6.

Trigger scores
Patients are categorised into three broad groups:
- Low score: NEWS 1–4.
- Medium score: NEWS 5–6 or a single RED score i.e. physiological parameter that scores a 3.
- High score: NEWS of 7 or more.

Follow local guidance as to the appropriate actions to be taken with patients who have low, medium and high scores. If you are with your patient for a long time, don't forget to reassess and monitor the trend in score. A rising NEWS, for example, is cause for concern.

1.5.3 'Head-to-toe' assessment

It is not always appropriate to perform a 'head-to-toe' or full-body examination for every patient, but in cases of multiple injury, or in cases when the patient is found collapsed and the history is limited or non-existent, it can be helpful to identify signs of injury or illness. The assessment outlined here is a rapid full-body assessment. Clinicians that you work with are likely to perform more thorough assessments on specific areas of the body depending on the presenting complaint.

Procedure

Take the following steps to perform a 'head-to-toe' assessment [JRCALC, 2019]:

1. Look at the face for obvious injuries such as lacerations, bruising, fluid leakage from the nose and ears, and deformities.
2. Inspect the area around the eyes.
3. Check the eyes for redness and the presence of contact lenses.
4. Assess the pupils with a pen torch, to ensure that they react to light.
5. Look behind the ears for bruising and in the ear for signs of fluid or blood leaking out.
6. Look for bruising, lacerations and deformity around the head and then gently feel for tenderness and depressions of the skull.
7. Feel the cheekbones for tenderness, symmetry and instability.
8. Feel the maxilla (the bone just below the nose).
9. Check the nose for blood and fluid leaking out.
10. Feel the jaw.
11. Assess the mouth and nose for cyanosis (blue-tinged skin), foreign bodies (including loose teeth and/or dentures), bleeding, lacerations and deformities.
12. Smell the patient's breath for specific odours (such as pear drops, which can be present in some diabetic patients).
13. Look at the neck and note any obvious lacerations, bruises and/or deformity. Look for bulging veins in the neck and feel the trachea to ensure it is centrally located.
14. Feel the back of the neck for tenderness and deformity.
15. Look at the chest for any obvious injury and watch the chest rise and fall as the patient breathes.
16. Gently feel the ribs to ensure they are intact and to identify if they are tender. Don't press over any obvious bruising or fractures.
17. Listen for breath sounds.
18. If safe to do so, roll the patient and listen to the back of the chest. Also, look for injuries and feel for deformities and tenderness.
19. Check the abdomen and pelvis for obvious injury and gently feel the abdomen, which should be soft and non-tender.
20. Look at the pelvis for signs of injury, then gently feel the iliac crests for signs of instability, tenderness or crepitus. Do not compress the pelvis (sometimes called 'springing').
21. Check the extremities (arms and legs) for lacerations, bruises, swelling, deformities and the presence of medical bracelets. Feel for distal pulses and check motor and sensory function. Compare the right and left sides.

1.6 *Reassessment*

The first thing you'll probably notice about reassessment is that it contains many of the things you have already undertaken as part of the patient assessment process (Figure 10.7). As with scene safety, a patient's clinical condition is dynamic and frequently changes, either due to the illness and/or injury they have acquired, or as a result of an intervention you have performed, such as defibrillation or drug administration. Frequent reassessment will mean that you will not miss these changes.

REASSESSMENT
Primary survey
Reassess vital signs
Presenting complaint
Review treatment
Monitor patient condition

Figure 10.7 Reassessment.

Chapter 11 Airway

1 Airway anatomy

1.1 Learning objective

By the end of this section you will be able to:
- identify and describe the structures of the upper and lower airway.

1.2 Introduction

The respiratory system is made up of a number of structures (Figure 11.1):
- nose
- mouth
- pharynx (throat)
- larynx (voicebox)
- trachea (windpipe)
- bronchi
- lungs.

Structurally, the respiratory system is split into two halves: the upper and lower respiratory systems. The upper consists of everything above the cricoid cartilage, and the lower comprises the cricoid cartilage and lower structures.

1.3 Nose

The nose is mostly constructed from cartilage and is external to the skull. Its orifices (nostrils, or nares) open into the nasal cavity of the skull, which is divided by the nasal septum. The nasal cavity contains the superior, middle and inferior turbinates (Figure 11.2), which increase the internal surface area of the nasal cavity, which in turn increases the temperature and humidity of air that passes through during breathing [Drake, 2015].

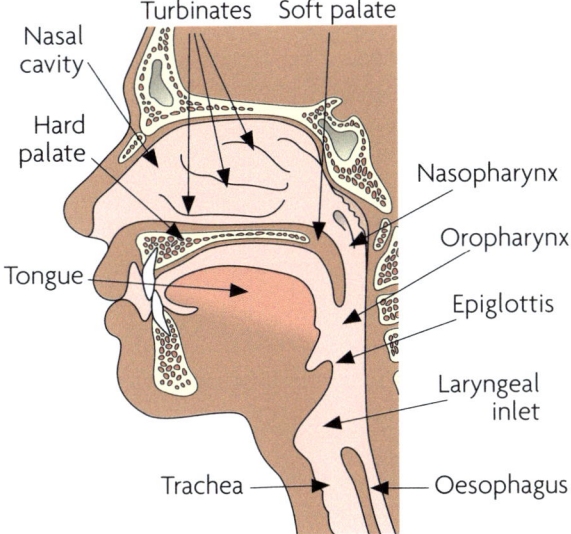

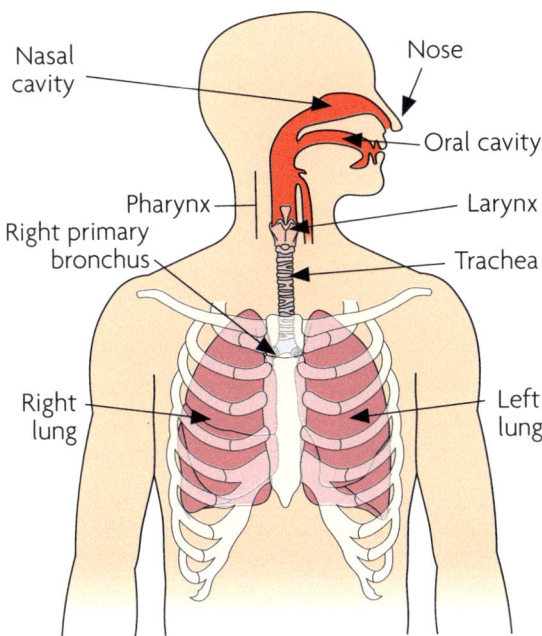

Figure 11.1 The structures of the respiratory system.

Figure 11.2 The upper airway.

1.4 Mouth

The mouth (or oral cavity) starts at the lips and is continuous with the oropharynx posteriorly. The roof of the mouth is made up of the hard and soft palates, with the floor made up of mostly soft tissue, including the tongue. The tongue is a muscular, non-compressible tissue that attaches to the mandible,

Chapter 11 – Airway

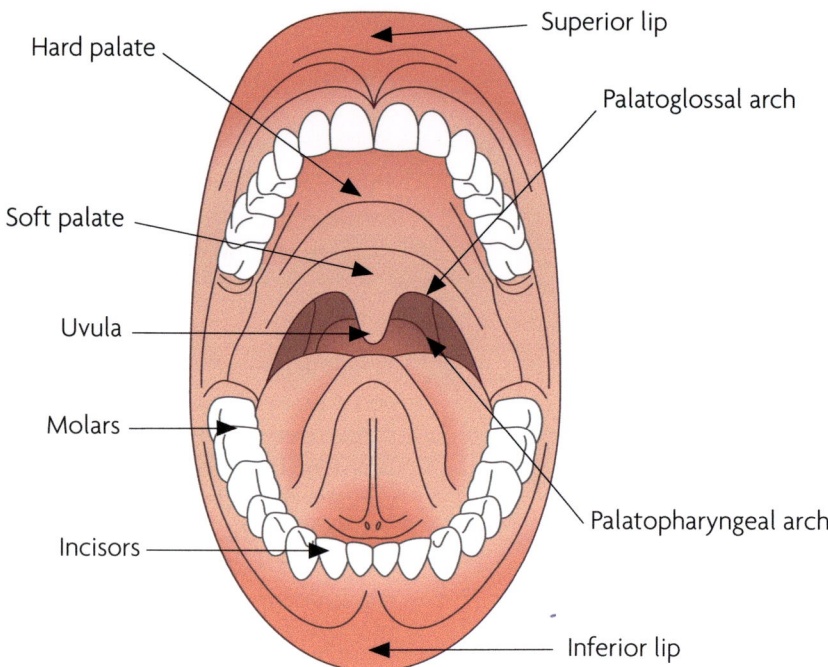

Figure 11.3 The oral cavity.

stylohyoid process and hyoid bone (Figure 11.3). The tongue, in the past, has been accused of being the most common cause of obstruction. However, research conducted on adult anaesthetised patients has demonstrated that it is usually the soft palate and epiglottis that cause obstruction of the airway, not the tongue [Nolan, 2016].

1.5 Pharynx

The pharynx is a funnel-shaped tube extending from the back of the nasal cavity to the top of the oesophagus. Although a continuous structure, it is typically divided into three sections anatomically (Figure 11.2):
- nasopharynx
- oropharynx
- laryngopharynx.

1.5.1 Nasopharynx

This is the area at the back of the nasal cavity, above the level of the soft palate. It is bordered by the sloping base of the skull above and mostly skeletal muscle on either side, forming a domed vault at the top of the pharyngeal cavity. Elevation of the soft palate during swallowing helps to ensure that food does not rise up into the nasal cavity. The tissues that cover the top of the nasopharynx contain the pharyngeal tonsil. In severe cases, enlargement of this can block the nasopharynx.

1.5.2 Oropharynx

This is the area posterior to the oral cavity, below the level of the soft palate but continuous with the nasopharynx, and above the margin of the epiglottis (which marks the start of the laryngopharynx). Anteriorly, the palatoglossal folds mark the boundary between the oral cavity and oropharynx.

1.5.3 Laryngopharynx

This is continuous with the oropharynx, running from the superior margins of the epiglottis to the top of the oesophagus around the level of the sixth cervical vertebra (spinal bone) in adults. Just anterior to the laryngopharynx are a pair of mucosal pouches called valleculae (where the tip of a curved laryngoscope blade goes) (Figure 11.4).

Airway anatomy

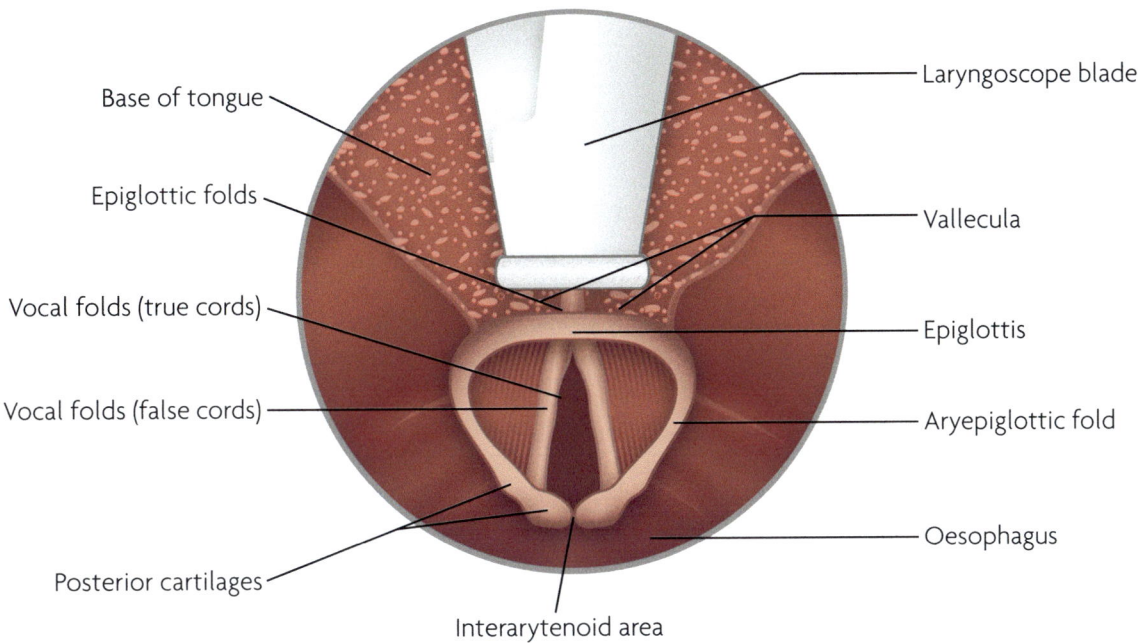

Figure 11.4 View of the laryngopharynx during laryngoscopy.

1.6 Lower airway

1.6.1 Larynx

The larynx is a hollow structure made up of muscles and ligaments, and marks the start of the lower respiratory tract. In adults, it is cylindrical in shape, with the narrowest part of the airway at the level of the vocal cords. It is continuous with the trachea below and opens into the laryngopharynx posteriorly.

The larynx is suspended from the hyoid bone above, and trachea below, by a series of membranes and ligaments, which makes it very mobile within the neck (Figure 11.5). During swallowing, it moves upwards and forwards causing the epiglottis to swing downwards, effectively closing the laryngeal inlet while at the same time opening the oesophagus.

As well as acting as a valve to close off the respiratory tract during swallowing, the larynx also produces sound for speech, singing, etc. It is the most heavily innervated sensory structure and stimulation (by a laryngoscope, for example)

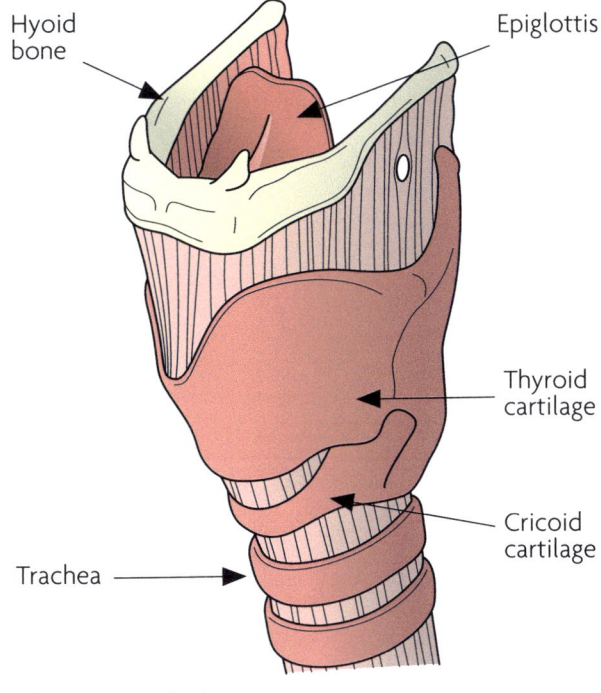

Figure 11.5 The larynx.

can result in a doubling of heart rate and blood pressure. However, in children, stimulation can sometimes cause bradycardia, which, if severe, results in asystole [Walls, 2012].

1.7 Trachea

The trachea extends from the cricoid cartilage to the level of the sixth thoracic vertebra where it splits into the left main bronchus and right main bronchus (together, the bronchi) at the carina (Figure 11.6). In an adult, the trachea is approximately 12–15 cm long and consists of C-shaped cartilages, which are completed posteriorly by the trachealis muscle [Kovacs, 2011].

1.8 Bronchi

The left and right main bronchi split into secondary bronchi, tertiary bronchi, the bronchioles, and finally the terminal bronchioles. The right main bronchus is more vertical, wider and shorter than the left, which explains why objects that are inhaled (foreign bodies) tend to end up here. In a similar design to the trachea, the main bronchi are incomplete rings of cartilage.

1.9 Lungs

The lungs are a pair of spongy, cone-shaped organs located in the thoracic (chest) cavity. They are separated by the mediastinum, a region in the thoracic cavity that contains the heart, major vessels, oesophagus and trachea, among others. This means that in the event that one lung collapses, due to air entering the thoracic cavity after a traumatic injury, for example, the other lung may remain inflated.

The lungs are covered by the pleura, which consists of two layers: the parietal pleura, which covers the wall of the thoracic cavity, and the visceral pleura, which covers the lungs. In between is the pleural cavity, a potential space filled with a fluid to prevent friction and allow the pleura to slide over each other during breathing. It also helps the membranes stick together due to the surface tension of the fluid, in a similar way that a glass with a wet bottom lifts the coaster it was sitting on.

The lungs extend from the diaphragm to just above the clavicles. The left lung is smaller than the right due to the space taken up by the heart. It also has only two lobes, the upper and lower, whereas the right lung has three, the upper, lower and middle lobes [Tortora, 2017] (Figure 11.6).

2 Assessing and managing the airway

2.1 Learning objectives

By the end of this section you will be able to:
- identify clinical signs that indicate a need to manage the airway
- explain factors that affect airway patency and the step-wise approach to airway management
- explain how to perform a range of manual airway manoeuvres
- describe the equipment required for suction and its safe use.

2.2 Introduction

More often than not, your patient will be conscious and able to talk, scream or cry, indicating that they have a patent airway. For some, however, you will need to assist them in opening and maintaining

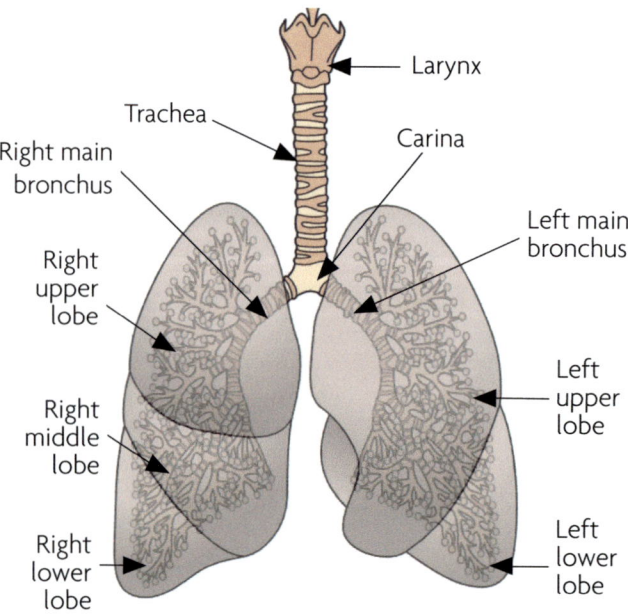

Figure 11.6 The lower airway.

their airway. Basic manoeuvres with nothing more than your hands are often enough to open and keep a patient's airway open but things can change and it is important that you frequently reassess airway patency, i.e. perform a dynamic airway assessment.

In this section, you will review the clinical signs of airway compromise and the step-wise approach to airway management that is recommended by ambulance clinical practice guidelines to address them [JRCALC, 2019]. This will be followed by an explanation of the following basic airway manoeuvres, which may be familiar to you if you have undertaken a first aid course:
- head tilt–chin lift
- jaw thrust
- triple airway manoeuvre
- recovery position.

Once the manual manoeuvres have been covered, the following more advanced procedures will be described:
- suction
- oropharyngeal airways
- nasopharyngeal airways
- supraglottic airway devices
- laryngoscopy for choking patients.

Endotracheal intubation is covered in Chapter 18, 'Assisting the Paramedic'. Children and infants also have a chapter all to themselves (Chapter 20, 'Children and Infants'), since the management of a child's airway requires modification based on their age.

2.3 Assessing the airway

In Chapter 10, 'Patient Assessment', you were introduced to the three-step approach to airway assessment:
- **Look:** As you approach the patient, note their position as it can give you an indication of the patency of the airway. Conscious patients who have adopted a tripod position (Figure 11.7) or who are showing other signs of increased work to breathe may have a partially obstructed airway.
- **Listen:** Even without a stethoscope, you can sometimes hear sounds that indicate a potential

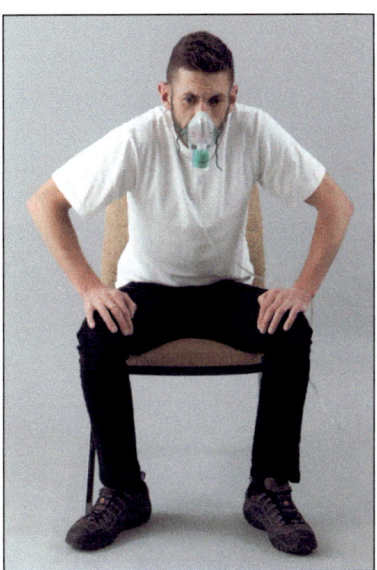

Figure 11.7 A patient in the tripod position.

airway obstruction. High-pitched inspiratory (although sometimes can be expiratory, too) sounds can be a sign of upper airway narrowing (known as stridor). Lower pitch sounds usually heard on expiration (wheeze) are a sign of lower airway partial obstruction, particularly in acute exacerbations of conditions such as asthma or chronic obstructive pulmonary disease (COPD). Other sounds include snoring, typically due to the soft tissues of the pharynx relaxing, and gurgling, due to fluid, secretions and vomit, etc. Snoring can usually be remedied with manual airway manoeuvres or an adjunct such as an oropharyngeal airway, whereas gurgling is an indication that the patient's airway requires suction.
- **Feel:** You will not always need to place your ear close enough to your patients to feel their breath on your cheek! However, in unresponsive patients it is important to determine if there is airflow and not just rely on chest movement.

The chest can move even in complete airway obstruction and is sometimes associated with a see-saw, paradoxical movement of the abdomen with the chest. So, as the chest expands, the abdomen sinks and vice versa.

Chapter 11 – Airway

2.4 Step-wise approach to the airway

In general, you will start with basic manoeuvres, such as the head tilt–chin lift or recovery position for patients who have an obstructed airway. Depending on the patient's condition and potential threats to their airway, you may elect to escalate their management to include airway adjuncts, such as oropharyngeal airways (OPAs) and nasopharyngeal airways (NPAs). If these are insufficient, you may elect to insert a supraglottic airway device (SAD) instead. Finally, if you are working with a paramedic, they may decide to intubate the patient. Depending on the patient's condition, it may be necessary to rapidly escalate airway management. Figure 11.8 shows a recommended step-wise approach to the airway [JRCALC, 2019].

2.5 Manual airway manoeuvres

Manual airway manoeuvres can be achieved with just your (or a colleague's) hands. They are great for the initial management of the airway, and in some cases may be all that is required.

2.5.1 Head tilt–chin lift

When to do it (indication)
- An unresponsive patient who has an airway obstruction caused by loss of pharyngeal muscle tone.

When not to do it (contra-indication)
- If the patient has a suspected spinal injury.

Advantages
- No equipment is required.
- Technique is simple and non-invasive.

Disadvantages
- Does not protect the airway from aspiration.
- Not suitable for patients with cervical spinal injury.

Procedure – Head tilt–chin lift

Take the following steps to perform a head tilt–chin lift [Nolan, 2016]:

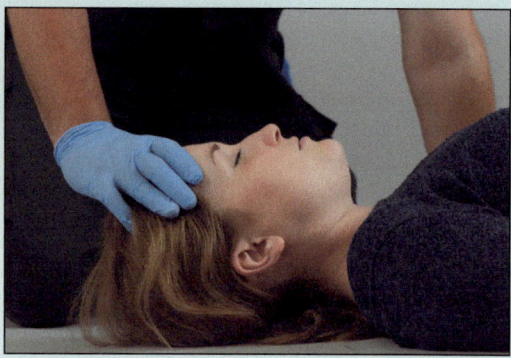

1. With your patient lying on their back (supine), position yourself at the patient's side. Place the hand closer to the patient's head on their forehead and gently tilt the head backwards.

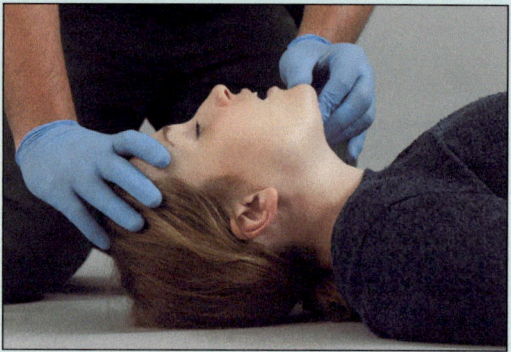

2. Place two fingers on the bony part of the chin and gently lift upwards.

2.5.2 Jaw thrust

When to do it (indication)
- An unresponsive patient who has an airway obstruction caused by loss of pharyngeal muscle tone.

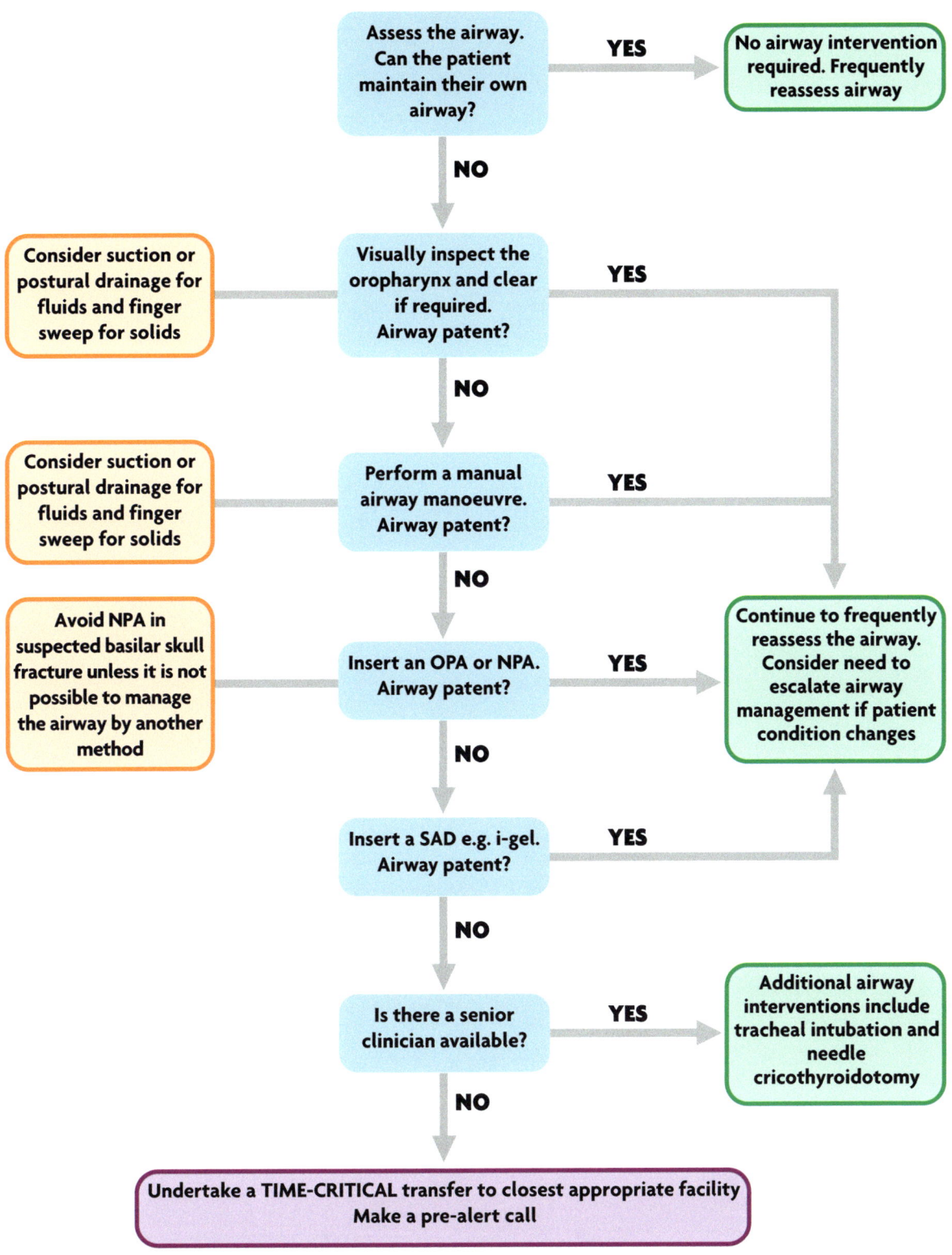

Figure 11.8 Step-wise approach to airway assessment and management.

When not to do it (contra-indication)
- A responsive patient.

Advantages
- No equipment is required.
- Technique is simple and non-invasive.
- Maintains neutral alignment of the head when cervical spinal injury suspected.

Disadvantages
- Does not protect the airway from aspiration
- Difficult to maintain for prolonged periods
- Requires second person to provide ventilations, if required.

When not to do it (contra-indication)
- A responsive patient.

Advantages
- No equipment is required.
- Technique is simple and non-invasive.

Disadvantages
- Does not protect the airway from aspiration.
- Difficult to maintain for prolonged periods.
- Requires second person to provide ventilations, if required.

> **Procedure – Jaw thrust**
>
> Take the following steps to perform a jaw thrust [Nolan, 2016]:
> - With your patient lying on their back (supine), position yourself at the patient's head.
> - Identify the angle of the mandible.
> - Place your fingers behind the mandible and lift in an upwards and forwards direction (Figure 11.9).
> - Using your thumbs, open the patient's mouth.
>
>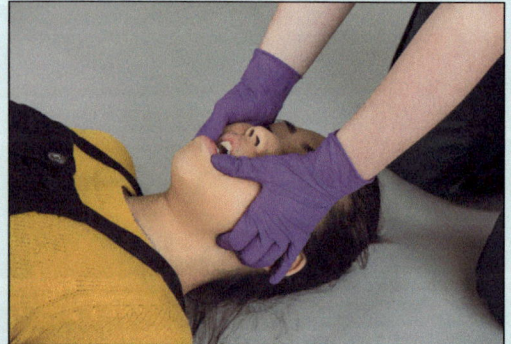
>
> **Figure 11.9** Lifting the mandible.

> **Procedure – Triple airway manoeuvre**
>
> Take the following steps to perform a jaw thrust with head tilt [QAS, 2018a]:
> - With your patient lying on their back (supine), position yourself at the patient's head.
> - Identify the angle of the mandible.
> - Place your fingers behind the mandible and lift in an upwards and forwards direction.
> - Using your thumbs, open the patient's mouth.
> - Tilt the head backwards.

2.5.4 Recovery position

When to do it (indication)
- A spontaneously breathing but unconscious patient who does not have a spinal injury.

When not to do it (contra-indications)
- Patients with spinal injuries.
- Patients who require assisted ventilation or insertion of an advanced airway.

2.5.3 Triple airway manoeuvre

When to do it (indication)
- An unresponsive patient who has an airway obstruction caused by loss of pharyngeal muscle tone and jaw thrust alone is not sufficient to open the airway.

Advantages
- Simple and quick to perform, even for a single rescuer,
- Does not require equipment,
- Encourages postural drainage of secretions or vomit from the patient's mouth.

Assessing and managing the airway

Disadvantages
- Not a definitive airway maintenance technique, i.e. the patient may still aspirate,
- Can make assessment of patient's breathing difficult.

There are a number of variations of the recovery position. This is the method that the European Resuscitation Council recommend [Zideman, 2015]:

Procedure – Recovery position

Take the following steps to place a patient in the recovery position:

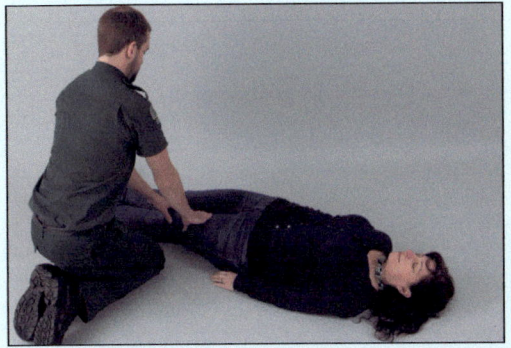

1. Kneel beside the patient and straighten both of their legs. Quickly check if they have any items in their pockets that should be removed before rolling them.

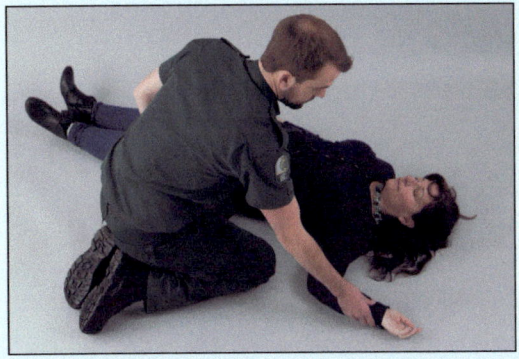

2. Place the arm nearer to you at right angles to their body, with the arm bent at the elbow and palm of the hand facing upwards.

Procedure – Recovery position – *cont*

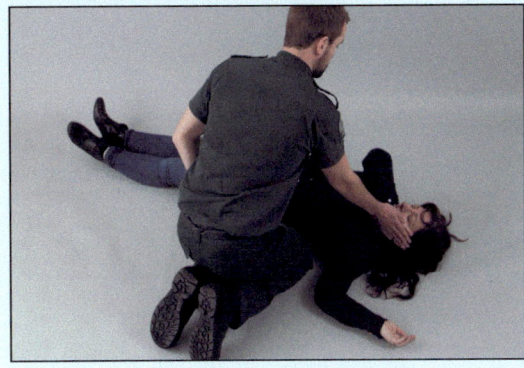

3. Bring the other arm across the chest and hold the back of their hand against the cheek that is nearer to you. Don't let go.

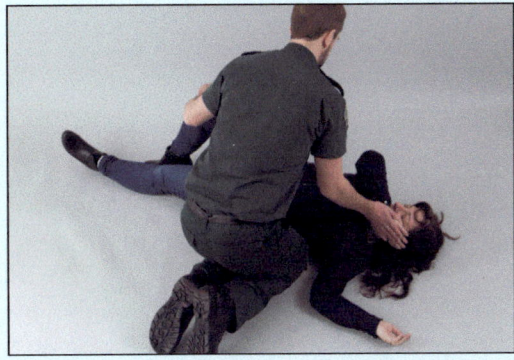

4. With your other hand, grasp the leg further away from you just above the knee and lift upwards so the leg flexes. Keep the foot on the ground.

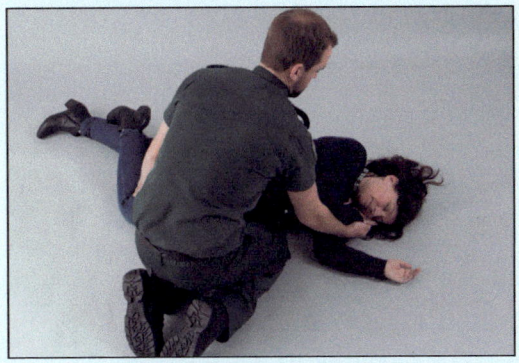

5. While supporting the head, pull the leg towards you, so that the patient rolls to face you.

Chapter 11 – Airway

Procedure – Recovery position – *cont*

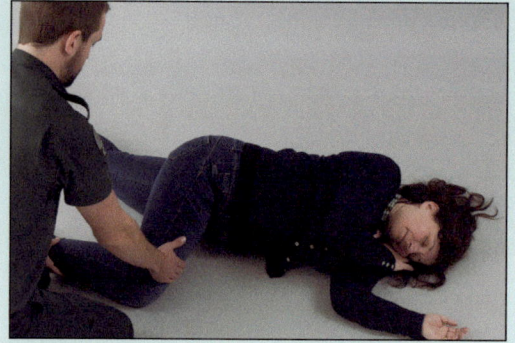

6. Adjust the uppermost leg so that the patient's hip and knee are bent at right angles.

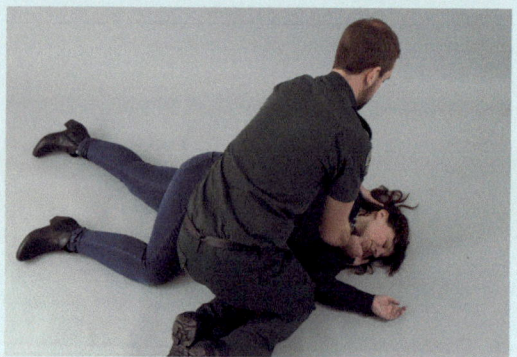

7. Tilt the head back to ensure the airway remains open. Adjust the patient's hand that is under their cheek, if required, to maintain head tilt and keep the patient facing slightly downwards, to allow free drainage of secretions from the mouth. Reassess frequently.

2.6 Suction

If you can hear gurgling in the airway, you should think about suction. Suctioning an airway involves removing vomit, blood and secretions with suctioning equipment. On your ambulance, you will usually have a mains-operated/battery-powered suction unit (Figure 11.10) and a hand-operated device (Figure 11.11). Make sure you are familiar with the operating instructions for the devices you carry.

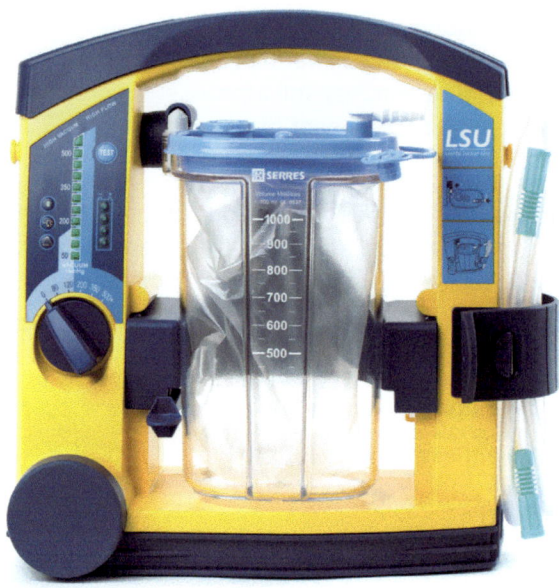

Figure 11.10 Mechanical suction device.
Source: Image reproduced by the kind permission of Laerdal Medical.

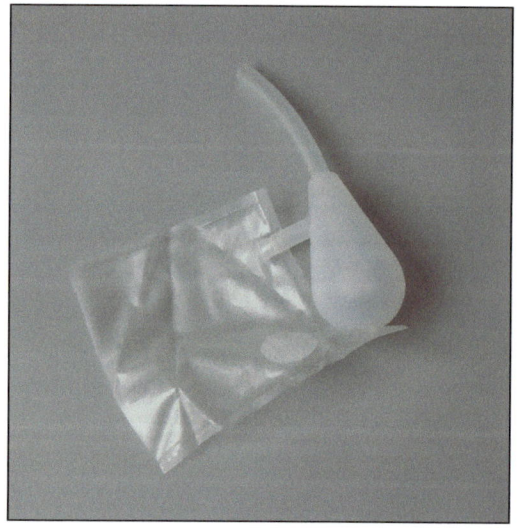

Figure 11.11 Hand-operated suction device.

2.6.1 Suction catheters

You are likely to have two types of suction catheters on the ambulance: a rigid, wide-bore catheter and a smaller, flexible catheter that can fit down an oropharyngeal or nasopharyngeal airway, but is limited by its small size and is unsuitable for blood and vomit (Figure 11.12).

Assessing and managing the airway

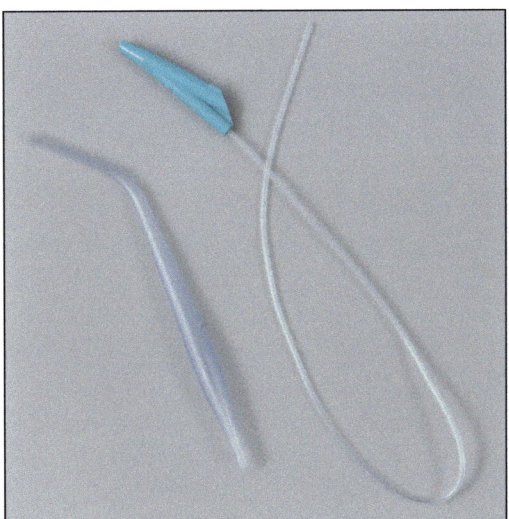

Figure 11.12 Suction catheters. Rigid, wide-bore (left) and flexible (right).

When to do it (indication)
- In patients who cannot maintain and clear their own airway and in whom vomit, blood or secretions are at risk of entering the lower respiratory tract.

When not to do it (contra-indication)
- In patients who can maintain and clear their own airway.

Advantage
- Prevents aspiration of vomit, blood and secretions.

Disadvantage
- Suctioning removes air as well as secretions. Keeps suction times short.

Procedure – Suction using a mechanical suction device

Take the following steps to perform suction using a mechanical suction device [Randle, 2009; Roberts, 2014]:

1. Prepare your equipment. You will need:
   - suction unit
   - rigid wide-bore and soft-tip catheters and suction tubing
   - gloves
   - protective eyewear
   - oxygen.
2. Explain the procedure to the patient and obtain consent if conscious.
3. Pre-oxygenate if possible.
4. Put on gloves and eyewear.
5. Attach suction tubing and catheter and switch on suction unit
6. Open the patient's mouth and insert the catheter into their mouth without suctioning. Make sure you can visualise the end of the suction catheter at all times.
7. Apply suction by occluding the control vent on the catheter (mechanical device) or squeezing the handle (hand-operated device) and gently withdraw the catheter. Suction for no more than 15 seconds.
8. Re-oxygenate the patient and reassess the airway. Further suction attempts may be required.

Notes:
If you only need to clear small amounts of saliva, then a suction pressure of 150–200 mmHg is sufficient [Randle, 2009]. However, in cases where there is a large amount of blood or vomit, turn the suction up to maximum initially and adjust downwards, as required.

In cases of severe bleeding or active vomiting, positioning the patient to allow for postural drainage is more important; for example, turning a patient on to their side when they are immobilised on an orthopaedic stretcher [Nutbeam, 2013].

Although prolonged suctioning will cause hypoxia (which is why suctioning for no more than 15 seconds is suggested), an airway obstructed by blood or vomit will not allow any air exchange and is likely to result in aspiration. In this case, patient positioning and aggressive suctioning will be required until the airway is at least partially clear. Re-oxygenation can then be performed and suctioning repeated as required. Follow the guidance of the senior clinician on scene [NAEMT, 2020].

2.7 Airway adjuncts

Airway adjuncts are devices that assist in airway management. Probably the most commonly used airway adjunct is the oropharyngeal airway (Figure 11.13), but there are others, including the nasopharyngeal airway.

2.7.1 Oropharyngeal airway (OPA)

When to do it (indication)
- An unresponsive patient with an absent gag reflex.

When not to do it (contra-indication)
- Any patient who has a gag reflex.

Advantages
- Easy to place.
- Technique is simple.

Disadvantages
- Tongue can be pushed back during insertion, making obstruction worse.
- Does not protect against vomiting.

Procedure – Insert an oropharyngeal airway

Take the following steps to insert an oropharyngeal airway [Nolan, 2016]:

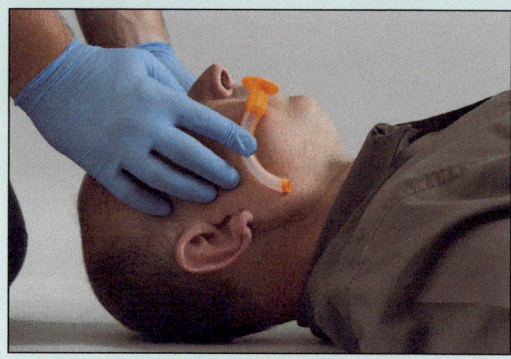

1. Select the correct size OPA by measuring the vertical distance between the patient's incisors and the angle of the jaw.

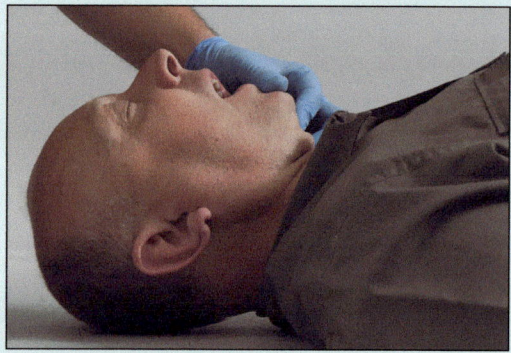

2. Open the patient's mouth and check it is clear of foreign bodies, vomit, blood or secretions. Suction if required.

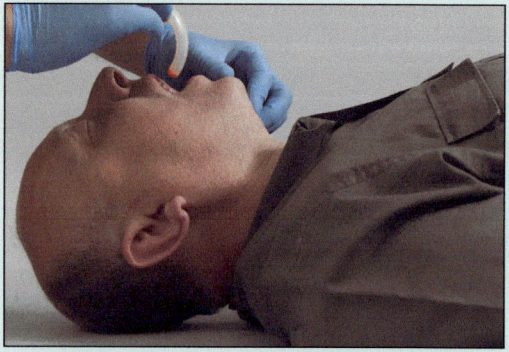

3. Insert the airway 'upside down' along the roof of the mouth until it reaches the soft palate.

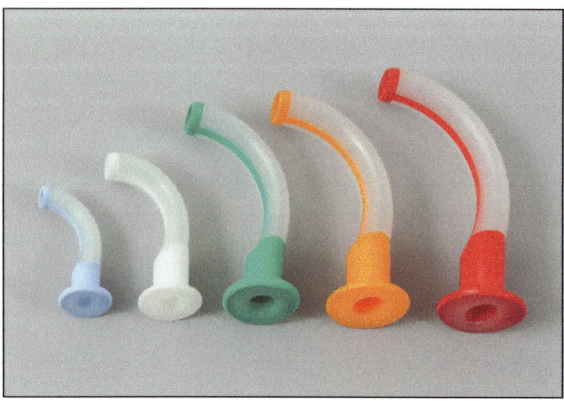

Figure 11.13 A collection of oropharyngeal airways.

Assessing and managing the airway

Procedure – Insert an oropharyngeal airway – *cont*

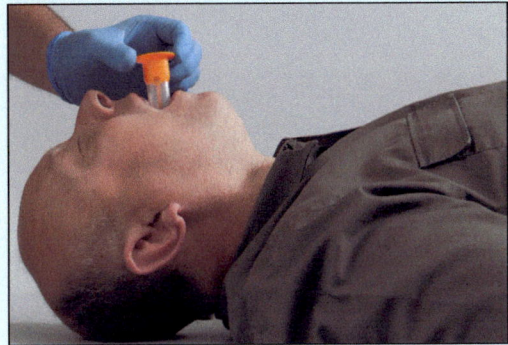

4. Rotate the OPA through 180°.

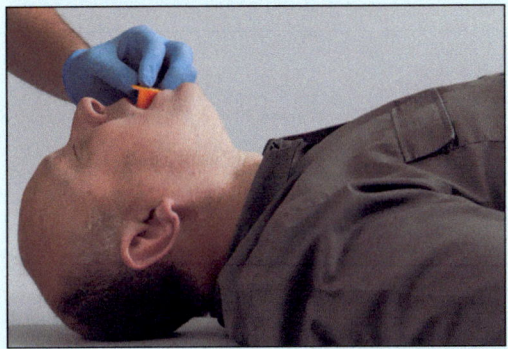

5. Advance the OPA until it rests in the pharynx. Remove immediately if the patient gags. Continue to provide manual manoeuvres such as head tilt–chin lift or jaw thrust as appropriate.

2.7.2 Nasopharyngeal airway (NPA)

When to do it (indication)
- An unresponsive patient, or a patient with a reduced level of consciousness who has an intact gag reflex.

When not to do it (contra-indication)
- Patients who do not tolerate the procedure.

Cautions
- Patients who have a basal skull fracture.
- Patients with nasal polyps.

Advantages
- Can be suctioned through.
- Can be tolerated by patients who are not unconscious.
- Does not require the mouth to open.

Disadvantages
- Poor technique can cause bleeding.
- Does not protect against aspiration.

Procedure – Insert a nasopharyngeal airway

Take the following steps to insert a nasopharyngeal airway (NPA) [Nolan, 2016; Roberts, 2003b]:

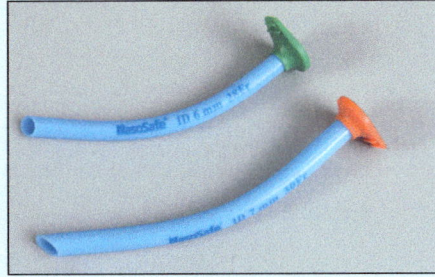

1. Adopt standard precautions. Prepare equipment. You will need the following:
  - an appropriately sized NPA, which is generally considered to be a 7.0 for an average adult male and 6.0 for an average adult female
  - water-soluble gel
  - suction.

If the NPA you are using comes with a safety pin, insert it through the non-bevelled end to avoid accidentally inserting the NPA too far.

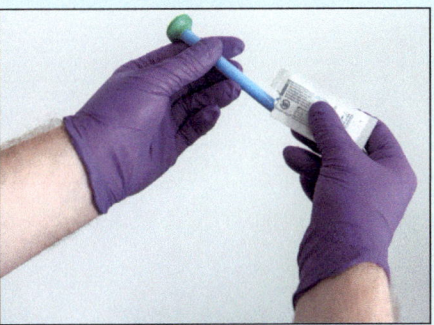

2. Lubricate the NPA ensuring that the gel does not go over the open ends of the airway.

Procedure – Insert a nasopharyngeal airway – *cont*

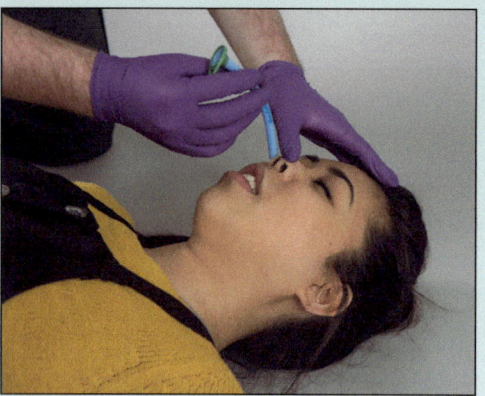

3. The NPA will be inserted with the bevel facing the nasal septum. This means that the right nostril is usually used, although if the left is clearly larger, then this can be used instead. If the left nostril is used, the NPA should be initially inserted 'upside down' and then rotated through 180° once it enters the nasopharynx.

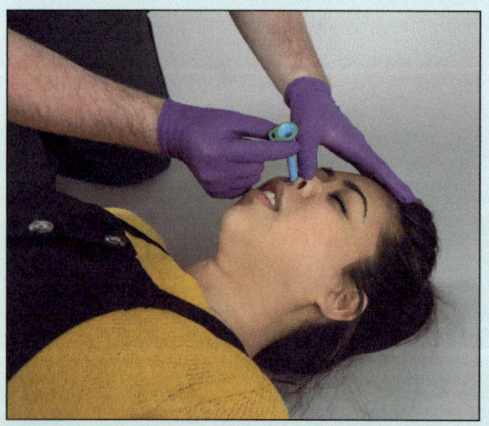

4. If resistance is felt when inserting the NPA, twist the device a little; if it still cannot be advanced, consider changing nostrils or using a smaller size NPA. Check for blanching of the patient's nostrils. If this occurs, the NPA should be removed and a smaller diameter NPA inserted instead. The correct technique will minimise the risk of bleeding, but if this occurs, have suction ready.

Procedure – Insert a nasopharyngeal airway – *cont*

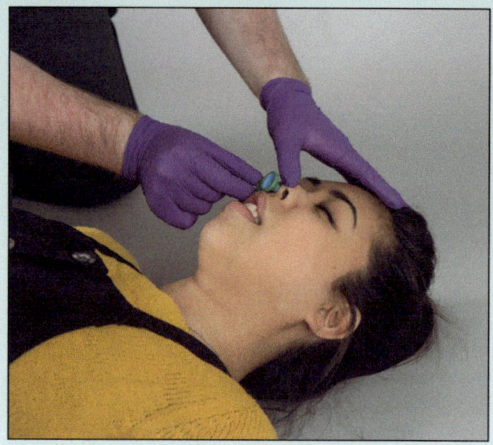

5. Confirm position by listening for breath sounds and ensuring the chest rises and falls.

2.8 Supraglottic airway device (SAD)

Supraglottic airway devices (SADs) have been used by anaesthetists in operating theatres for over 20 years and have proven to be safe and reliable. SADs generally lead to better ventilation and less air entering the stomach than bag-valve-mask (BVM) ventilation, particularly in the hands of the inexperienced [Nolan, 2016].

When to do it (indications)
- When BVM ventilation is not effective, is unable to be performed by an experienced person and/or prolonged ventilation is required.
- When intubation fails and BVM ventilation is not possible (can't intubate, can't ventilate).

When not to do it (contra-indications)
- Any patient who has a gag reflex.
- Any patient who is not deeply unconscious.

Advantages
- Better oxygenation than BVM with an oropharyngeal airway (OPA) [Cook, 2006; Dixon, 2009].
- No need to maintain continuous manual airway seal.
- Easier than tracheal intubation and does not require laryngoscopy.
- Provides protection from airway secretions.

Assessing and managing the airway

Disadvantages
- Does not protect against vomiting.
- May leak when high ventilatory pressures are required, such as in obese, asthmatic and chronic obstructive pulmonary disease (COPD) patients.

A common SAD in use in ambulance services is the i-gel and the technique for insertion is described here. However, there are others in use and you should be familiar with the devices relevant to your service.

2.8.1 i-gel insertion technique

When to do it (indications)
- An unresponsive patient with an absent gag reflex in whom more basic airway manoeuvres are inadequate.
- Airway of choice in cardiac arrest as it is easy to insert.

When not to do it (contra-indications)
- Trismus.
- Patients with limited mouth opening.

Advantages
- Easy to place.
- Straightforward insertion without needing to interrupt chest compressions.
- Small suction catheter can be placed down side-port to drain oesophageal secretions.

Disadvantages
- May leak, particularly if high inflation pressures are required.
- Does not protect against vomiting.

Figure 11.14 shows the equipment you will require in order to insert an i-gel.

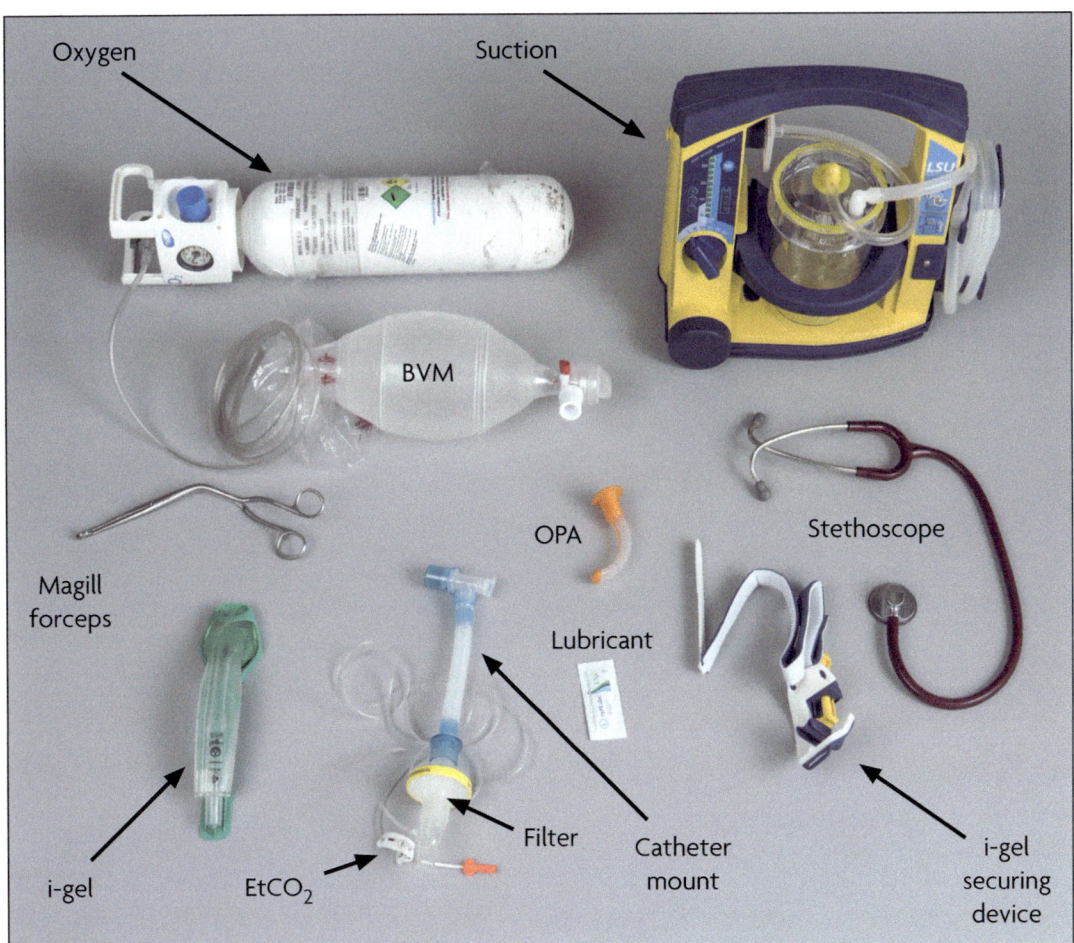

Figure 11.14 Equipment for i-gel insertion.

Chapter 11 – *Airway*

Procedure – Insert an i-gel

Take the following steps to insert an i-gel [Intersurgical, 2017]:

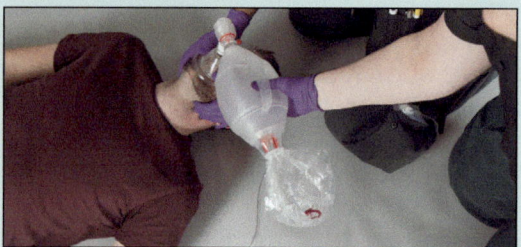

1. Pre-oxygenate the patient while preparing your equipment.

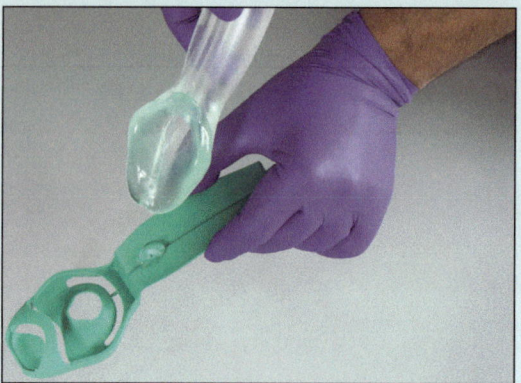

2. Choose the correct size i-gel: 3 for small adults, 4 for medium adults and 5 for large adults. Weight ranges are provided on the i-gel. Open the packaging and remove the i-gel from its cradle. Place a small amount of water-based lubricant on to the back, sides and front tip of the i-gel.

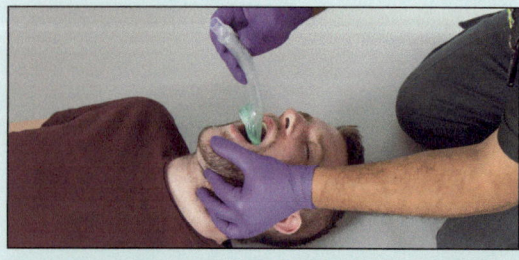

3. With the patient in the 'sniffing the morning air' position, hold the i-gel by the integrated bite block, gently pull down on the patient's chin and introduce the green tip into the patient's mouth, directed at the hard palate.

Procedure – Insert an i-gel – *cont*

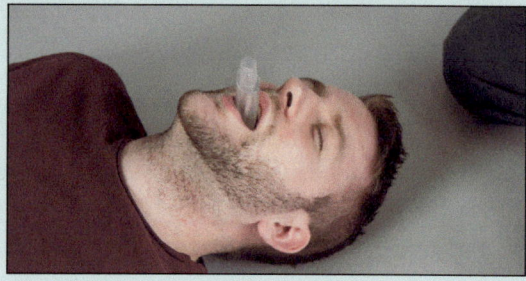

4. Glide the device downwards and backwards along the hard palate with a continuous but gentle push until a definitive resistance is felt. As a rough guide, the bite block should end up at the level of the incisors at the hard palate.

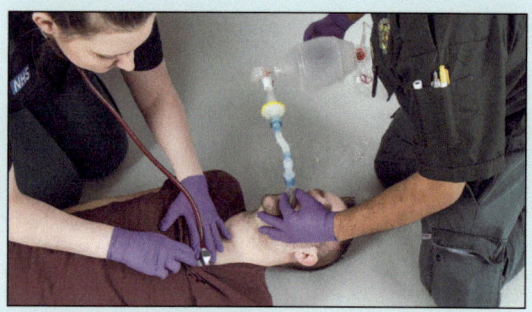

5. Connect the i-gel to waveform capnography, catheter mount and bag-valve-mask. Check for end-tidal carbon dioxide and bilateral chest air entry and movement on ventilating the patient.

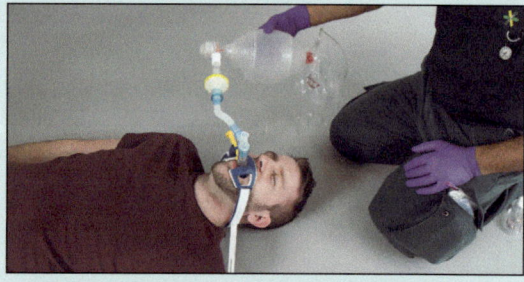

6. Secure the device appropriately.

2.9 Removal of foreign bodies with laryngoscopy in adults

For unconscious patients with a definite history of airway obstruction, in addition to performing chest compressions and ventilations at a rate of

Assessing and managing the airway

30:2, and only if you are trained to do so, you may attempt to remove the obstruction under direct vision. However, if the obstruction is not obviously visible in the anterior oropharynx, you will need to use laryngoscopy to view the deeper and lower structures of the airway.

When to do it (indication)
- To facilitate removal of foreign bodies located in the pharynx in the unconscious patient.

When not to do it (contra-indications)
- Any patient who has an effective cough.
- Any patient who is not unconscious.

Advantage
- May be more effective at removing foreign bodies than more basic manoeuvres (although evidence is weak) [Sakai, 2014; Soroudi, 2007].

Disadvantages
- Aggressive or careless laryngoscopy can damage tissues of the pharynx.
- Manipulating a foreign body can cause a partial obstruction to become a complete obstruction.

Procedure – Remove a foreign body with laryngoscopy in adults

Take the following steps to remove a foreign body with laryngoscopy in adults [QAS, 2018a]:

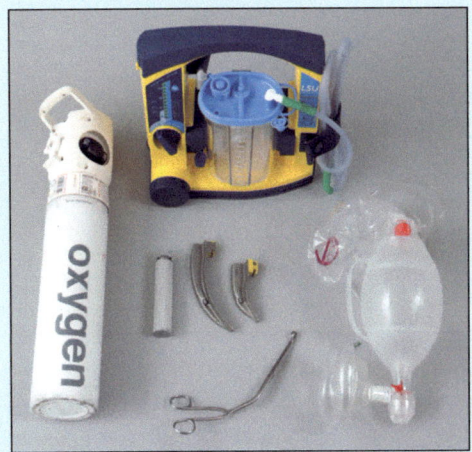

1. Prepare your equipment. You will need:
   - suction
   - laryngoscope and blade (size MAC 4)

Procedure – Remove a foreign body with laryngoscopy in adults – *cont*
   - magill forceps
   - oxygen
   - BVM.

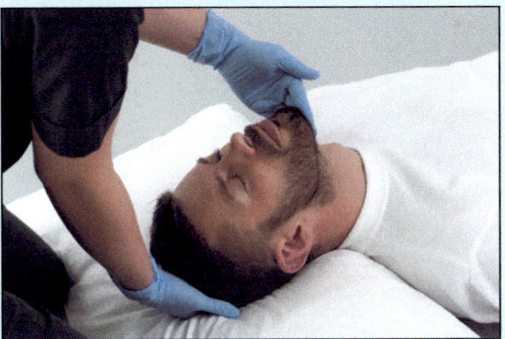

2. Position your patient. Ideally, your patient will be on a bed or ambulance trolley where you can adjust the height so that the patient's head is your focal length away (usually 12–18 cm or the distance you would hold a book to read). However, most of your patients are likely to be on the floor, but you can still at least place the patient in the supine position and perhaps move them so that you have more space to work. It is a misconception that a 'sniffing' position is simply an extension of the head and neck. To obtain the best view, the head should be extended but the neck should be flexed. A good measurement to determine whether you have achieved a good position is to check whether the external auditory meatus ('earhole') is at the same level as the sternal notch ('neck hole'). In an adult, the vertical height from the floor to their occiput is likely to be around 8–10 cm [Levitan, 2000]. Use pillows/cushions/towels/books or anything else in the vicinity of your patient to maintain this position.

Procedure – Remove a foreign body with laryngoscopy in adults – *cont*

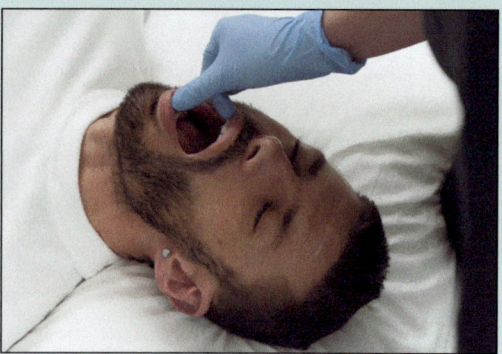

3. Open the patient's mouth and inspect the oral cavity. Some patients, when placed in an appropriate head position, will have a jaw that opens to reveal a gaping chasm, preferably without teeth. However, for the remainder, you will need to achieve mouth opening by using a 'scissor technique'. This is achieved by placing the thumb of your right hand on the lower incisors and middle finger on the upper incisors and scissoring the jaw open. Remove dentures, if present, to give yourself more room to work.

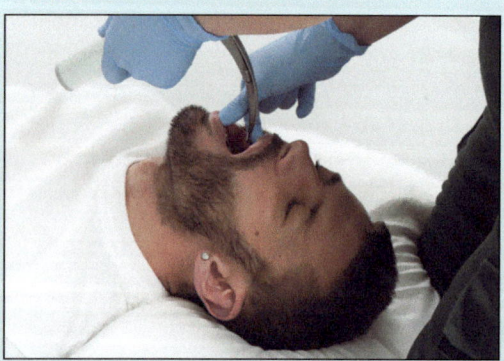

4. Insert the laryngoscope. With the mouth open, check to see whether suction is required, but take care only to suction the oropharynx that you can see. Check to see whether the foreign body is visible, too. If it is, you may be able to remove it with the Magill forceps without using the laryngoscope. Assuming this is not possible, take hold of the laryngoscope. You should

Procedure – Remove a foreign body with laryngoscopy in adults – *cont*

grip low down on the handle, such that the proximal end of the blade pushes into the thenar or hypothenar eminence of your left hand. Insert the blade along the right mandibular (lower) molars and gently sweep the tongue to the left. With the blade now in the midline, slowly advance the blade down the tongue until the foreign body or epiglottis comes into view, as the epiglottis is reliably located at the base of the tongue [Levitan, 2000]. If you cannot locate the epiglottis, consider using suction if the airway is soiled. Alternatively, you may have inserted the blade too far and it is easy to become 'lost' in a sea of soft tissue that makes up the posterior pharynx and oesophagus. In this case withdraw, pre-oxygenate and try again.

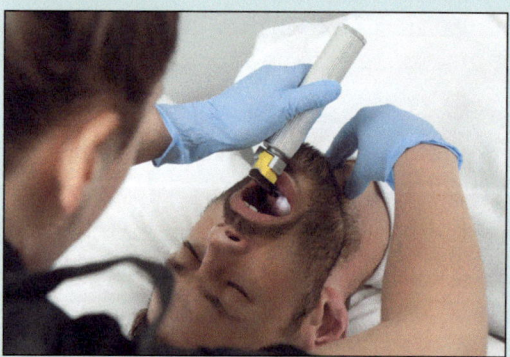

5. Perform bimanual laryngoscopy. With the epiglottis located, you need to convert the potential space of the vallecula into an actual space. This is best achieved by placing your right hand on to the thyroid cartilage and pressing down (posteriorly) in a similar technique that an assistant might use during the backwards-upwards-rightwards pressure (BURP) manoeuvre (see Chapter 18, 'Assisting the Paramedic') [Levitan, 2006]. This should make it straightforward to insert the tip of the blade into the vallecula. Now lift the blade at an angle of 45° (or parallel to the handle). Do not lever backwards

Procedure – Remove a foreign body with laryngoscopy in adults – *cont*

on the handle (think pulling a pint) as this can not only damage the upper teeth, but also worsen the view. At the same time as lifting the laryngoscope, press down on the thyroid (bimanual laryngoscopy). Keep lifting until you can see the foreign body [Schmitt, 2002].

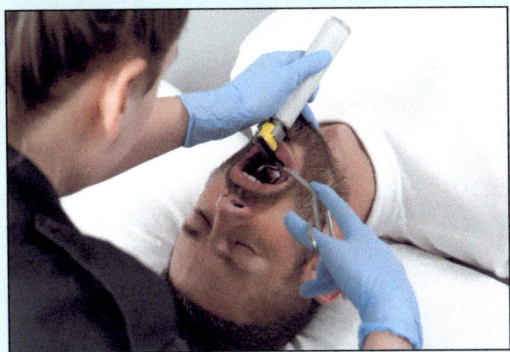

6. **Insert Magill forceps.** Grasp the forceps in your right hand, inserting your thumb and either ring or middle finger into the ring handles. You can use your index finger to guide the forceps by resting it on the shaft of the forceps. Insert the closed forceps into the patient's mouth.

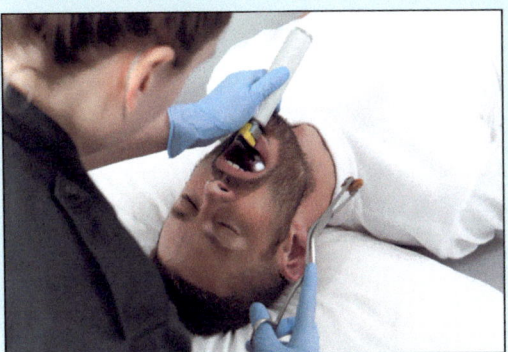

7. **Retrieve foreign body.** Under direct vision, open the forceps to grasp the foreign body, taking care not to grab any pharyngeal structures or the epiglottis in the process.

8. **Oxygenate your patient,** with assisted ventilations, if required.

Note: You are likely to have to repeat this procedure in order to retrieve a foreign body. However, if you cannot remove the foreign body after two attempts, concentrate on chest compressions instead. As always, follow local guidance.

3 Tracheostomies

3.1 Learning objectives

By the end of this section you will be able to:
- explain the difference between laryngectomy and tracheostomy
- describe how to manage the airway of a patient with a laryngectomy or a tracheostomy.

3.2 Introduction

A tracheostomy is an artificial opening made into the trachea through the neck (Figure 11.15). Patients have them inserted for a number of reasons including [Feber, 2006; Bowers, 2007]:
- following trauma or surgery to the head and neck, which leads to an airway obstruction
- bypassing a tumour that obstructs the upper airway
- for prolonged ventilation
- for some types of chronic disease where minimising the anatomical dead space is beneficial
- to provide access to chest secretions in the event of respiratory insufficiency
- to protect from aspiration in the event of impaired swallow reflex (for example, neuromuscular disorders).

As the name suggests, a laryngectomy is the removal of the larynx. This is typically due to the involvement of the larynx in oral, pharyngeal and laryngeal cancers. If the patient requires a total laryngectomy, the larynx is removed and the trachea cut and stitched to the front of the neck [NTSP, 2014]. This is important for subsequent management, because these patients cannot be ventilated from the mouth and/or nose (Figure 11.15).

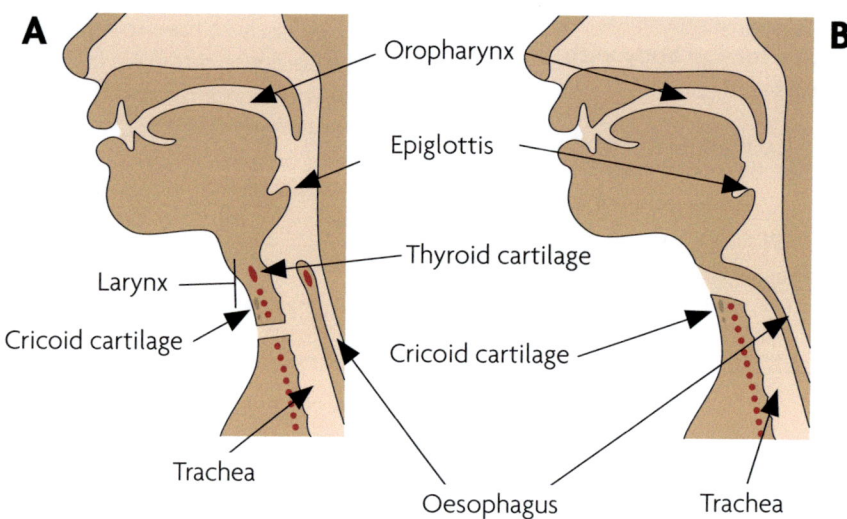

Figure 11.15 The anatomical differences between (A) tracheostomy and (B) laryngectomy.

3.3 Tracheostomy tubes

There are a wide variety of tracheostomy tubes, which can seem rather overwhelming. However, tubes are broadly classified into the following categories [NTSP, 2014]:
- cuffed/uncuffed
- with/without inner cannula
- fenestrated/unfenestrated.

3.3.1 Cuffed/uncuffed tubes

As with adult endotracheal tubes, a cuffed tracheostomy tube has a soft balloon around the distal end, which is inflated by injecting air into the pilot balloon via the injection port (Figure 11.16). These are used when patients require positive pressure ventilation (PPV) and/or when the patient cannot protect their own airway from secretions. Note that if the cuffed tube is inflated and the lumen becomes blocked or occluded, the patient will not be able to breathe!

Uncuffed tubes tend to be used in longer-term patients, but since they lack the cuff, it is important that these patients have an effective cough and gag reflex to minimise the chance of aspiration. These tubes are not suitable for positive pressure ventilation.

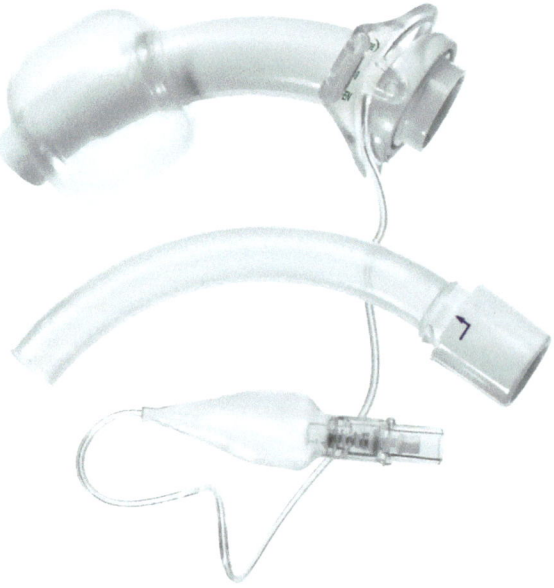

Figure 11.16 A cuffed, unfenestrated tracheostomy tube (*top*). Inner cannula with no fenestrations (*middle*). Pilot balloon and inflation valve for tracheostomy cuff (*bottom*).

3.3.2 Inner cannulas

Tracheostomy tubes with an inner cannula (sometimes called double-cannula or double-lumen tubes) consist of an outer tube or cannula which maintains airway patency, and an inner cannula, which can be removed for cleaning and/or disposed of and replaced (Figure 11.17). Uncuffed, double-cannula tracheostomy tubes are the safest type to use in the community [NTSP, 2014].

3.3.3 Fenestrated tubes

These tracheostomy tubes have an opening in the outer cannula that allows air to pass through the patient's oropharynx and nasopharynx. This is helpful because it allows the patient to talk and produce an effective cough. However, fenestrations increase the risk of aspiration and prevent positive pressure ventilation unless a non-fenestrated inner cannula is used. Non-fenestrated inner cannulas should also be used if the patient requires suction (Figure 11.17).

3.4 Management of the tracheostomy patient

Patients with tracheostomies have a potentially patent upper airway, since the upper airway and trachea are anatomically connected. However, it is quite possible that the reason the patient had a tracheostomy in the first place is that their upper airway is difficult or impossible to manage [McGrath, 2012].

3.4.1 Help and equipment

You will not be able to manage on your own and assistance is vital. If a relative or carer is present, it is quite possible that they know more about tracheostomy management than you do, so listen to their advice and encourage them to help.

Patients may well have equipment to hand, such as replacement tubes, but you can manage with the equipment from your vehicle:
- airway adjuncts such as oropharyngeal and nasopharyngeal airways
- bag-valve-mask
- supraglottic airway devices
- laryngoscope and endotracheal tubes
- bougie
- monitor capable of waveform capnography.

3.4.2 Airway and breathing

Check and open the upper airway as normal. Look, listen and feel for breathing at the face and tracheostomy site for no more than ten seconds. Apply waveform capnography to the tracheostomy tube as soon as possible [Whitaker, 2011].

If the patient is breathing, apply high-flow oxygen to both face and tracheostomy. This may require two cylinders, or the addition of a flowmeter to the Schrader valve of the oxygen cylinder. If the patient is not breathing, making agonal gasps or there are no signs of life, start chest compressions and follow the basic life support (BLS) algorithm while continuing to troubleshoot the tracheostomy, since this may be the cause of the cardiac arrest [Perkins, 2015].

3.4.3 Tracheostomy patency

Start by checking for and removing the following:
- decannulation caps (used when removing tracheostomies), which can block the end of the tracheostomy
- obturators (inserted inside the tracheostomy when first inserting a tube into the patient; see Figure 11.18)

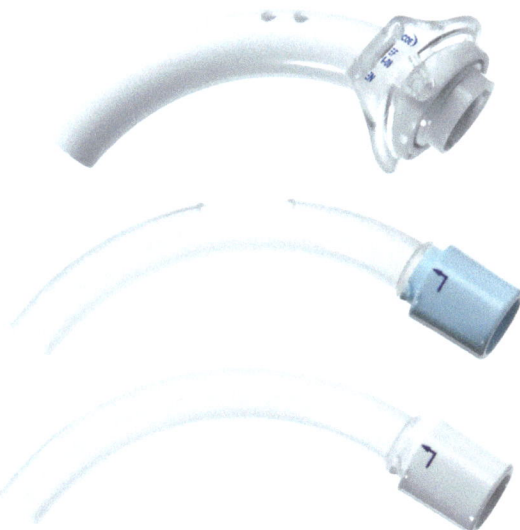

Figure 11.17 An uncuffed, fenestrated tracheostomy tube (*top*). Inner cannula with opening for fenestrations (*middle*). Inner cannula with no fenestrations (*bottom*).

Chapter 11 – Airway

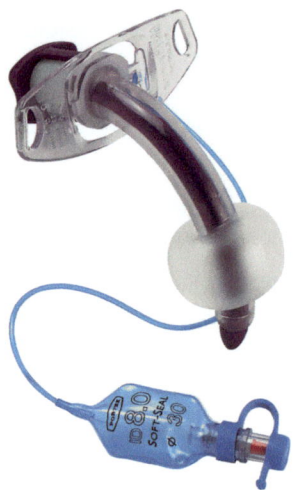

Figure 11.18 A tracheostomy tube with an obturator inside.

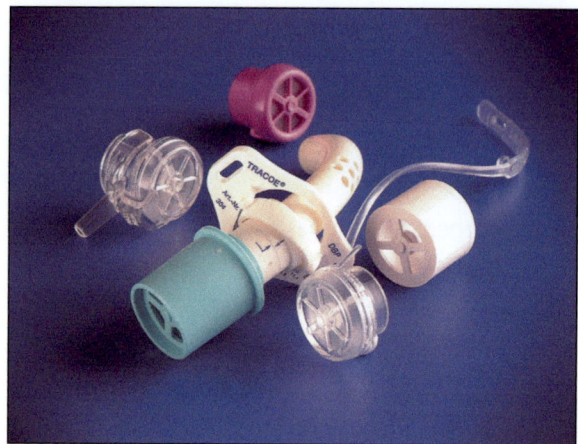

Figure 11.19 A selection of speaking valves. These should be fitted to uncuffed tubes.

- speaking valves, which should not be used with an inflated cuffed tube (Figure 11.19)
- blocked humidification devices such as Swedish noses.

If the tracheostomy tube is a double-cannula design, remove the inner cannula, but remember that with some types of tubes the connector required for bag-mask ventilation is mounted on the inner cannula. Pass a suction catheter through the tube and into the trachea to check patency. It should pass easily through the tube. Don't use a bougie at this stage as it is more rigid than a suction catheter and might create a false passage in cases where the tube is misplaced. If the suction catheter passes through the tube, suction the tube and attempt to ventilate the patient. If this fails and the tube has a cuff, deflate it and reassess the patient using the same look, listen and feel technique as before at both the face and the stoma site.

3.4.4 Next steps

If everything attempted thus far has failed to improve the patient's condition, remove the tube. Reassess the patient again and hopefully they will be breathing. If the patient is in cardiac arrest, continue with BLS. Attempt to oxygenate the patient via the oral route, but don't forget to cover the stoma site with swabs or a gloved hand.

Use standard airway adjuncts to achieve effective ventilation. Alternatively, a paediatric face mask or supraglottic airway device (SAD) can be placed over the stoma and the patient ventilated. If there is a large air leak from the mouth and/or nose, occlude them both during PPV.

If it is not possible to effectively ventilate the patient, then a suitable clinician will need to attempt endotracheal intubation. This may be possible via the oral route, although they should expect it to be difficult. Use an uncut tube as it will need to be inserted further than normal in order to bypass the stoma.

In patients with an established tracheostomy or who have a known upper airway problem that is going to make intubation difficult, it can actually be more straightforward to simply insert another, smaller diameter tracheostomy or endotracheal tube into the stoma. Always use capnography and auscultation as well as bilateral chest rise to confirm correct placement [Whitaker, 2011; Kodali, 2013].

3.5 Management of the laryngectomy patient

Unlike patients with a tracheostomy, laryngectomy patients do not have any connection between the upper airway and their lungs. Do not attempt to ventilate via the mouth/nose. Laryngectomy patients do not normally have tracheostomy tubes either, but may have a tracheo-oesophageal puncture (TEP) valve fitted to allow for speech. This may be visible inside the stoma, but should not be removed. They are usually fitted with a one-way valve to prevent aspiration [NTSP, 2014].

Since these patients have, in effect, no upper airway, it cannot be obstructed by an inappropriate head position. Due to the reduction in anatomical dead space, chest compressions typically generate sufficient tidal volume to negate the need for PPV if this proves difficult to administer. Instead, just provide a supply of high-flow oxygen to the stoma site.

Tracheostomies are ten times more commonly performed than laryngectomies, so in the event that there is any uncertainty about whether the stoma is a laryngectomy or tracheostomy site, it is better to apply oxygen to both face and stoma.

3.5.1 Help and equipment

As with tracheostomy patients, these are not patients that you can manage alone, and assistance is vital. If a relative or carer is present, it is quite possible that they know more about laryngectomy management than you do, so listen to their advice and encourage them to help.

Patients may well have equipment to hand such as replacement tubes, but you can manage with the equipment from your vehicle:
- airway adjuncts such as oropharyngeal and nasopharyngeal airways
- bag-valve-mask
- supraglottic airway devices
- laryngoscope and endotracheal tubes
- bougie
- monitor capable of waveform capnography.

3.5.2 Airway and breathing

Check and open the upper airway as normal. Look, listen and feel for breathing at the stoma site for no more than ten seconds. If the patient is breathing, apply high-flow oxygen to the stoma site. If the patient is not breathing, making agonal gasps or if there are no signs of life, start chest compressions and follow the BLS algorithm while continuing to troubleshoot the laryngectomy stoma, since this may be the cause of the cardiac arrest.

3.5.3 Laryngectomy stoma patency

Most patients will not have a tube in place, but you should remove any stoma cover (sometimes called a 'button') if in place. If a tracheostomy tube is in place and is of a double-cannula design, remove the inner cannula, but remember that with some types of tubes the connector required for bag-mask ventilation is mounted on the inner cannula.

Pass a suction catheter through the stoma and into the trachea to check patency. It should pass easily into the trachea. If it does, the stoma is patent, so suction the trachea and attempt to ventilate the patient if they are not breathing. If this fails and there is a cuffed tracheostomy tube in place, deflate it and reassess the patient, preferably with capnography.

3.5.4 Next steps

If everything attempted thus far has failed to improve the patient's condition, remove any tracheostomy tubes, if present. Reassess the patient again and hopefully they will be breathing. If the patient is in cardiac arrest, continue with BLS.

Attempt to ventilate the patient using a paediatric face mask or SAD placed over the stoma. If this fails, a suitably qualified clinician will need to intubate the stoma with either a smaller diameter tracheostomy or endotracheal tube. Capnography, auscultation and the presence of bilateral chest rise should be used to confirm correct placement.

4 Choking in adults

4.1 *Learning objectives*

By the end of this section you will be able to:
- define choking and list some common causes
- state the signs that an adult is choking
- describe the procedure for managing the choking adult.

4.2 Introduction

Choking is a mechanical obstruction of the airway occurring anywhere between the mouth and carina (where the left and right bronchi split from the trachea). Common causes include [Walls, 2012]:
- foreign bodies
- blood
- secretions
- teeth
- vomit.

It is not known how common choking is in adults. Death from choking is thankfully rare, mostly because choking episodes are witnessed [Perkins, 2015]. In England and Wales, around 380 people die each year as a result of a foreign body in the respiratory tract. Most of these are over 65 years of age [ONS, 2017].

4.3 Recognition

The signs of choking in an adult depend on the severity of the airway obstruction that has occurred. Typically, the episode will have occurred while eating. If the patient is still conscious, they may clutch their neck (Figure 11.20).

In the case of a mild airway obstruction, if you ask the patient if they are choking, they will still be able to speak and confirm that this is the case. They will also be able to breathe and cough.

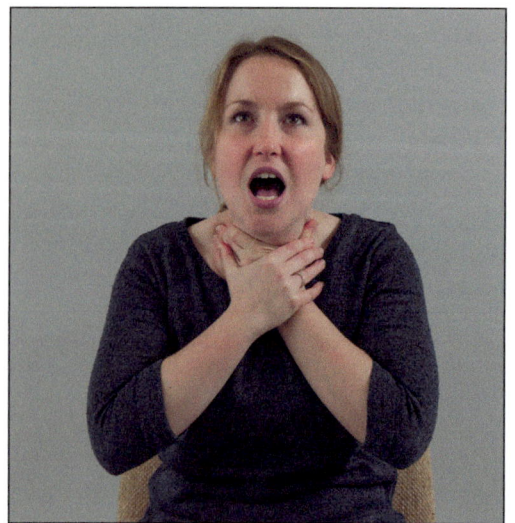

Figure 11.20 A choking victim clutching her neck.

However, in cases of severe airway obstruction, the patient will be unable to speak, so may only be able to respond to you by nodding their head in response to your question about whether they are choking. Any attempts at coughing will be silent, and if this continues the patient will lose consciousness, possibly before your arrival [Nolan, 2016].

4.4 Management

Start by determining the severity of the obstruction. In adults, this is typically determined by the patient's response to the question 'Are you choking?' A patient who can reply 'Yes', i.e. can speak, cough and breathe, is classified as mild, whereas the patient who is clutching their throat, is unable to speak and who cannot breathe falls into the severe category.

4.4.1 Conscious and choking

If the patient is coughing effectively, do not perform any interventions other than encouraging the patient to continue coughing.

If the obstruction is severe, administer up to five back blows, by standing just to the side and slightly behind the patient, leaning them forward, and then administering sharp blows between the shoulder blades with the heel of one hand.

If this fails, move on to abdominal thrusts. Position yourself behind the patient and place a clenched fist just under the xiphisternum. Grasp the fist with your other hand and pull sharply upwards and inwards up to five times.

Repeat the back blows/abdominal thrusts until the obstruction is relieved, or the patient becomes unconscious [Nolan, 2016].

4.4.2 Unconscious and choking

Lay the patient on their back and start chest compressions and ventilations at a rate of 30:2. If you are competent to do so, attempt laryngoscopy in order to directly view the obstruction and clear it with forceps or suction (Figure 11.21).

Before each set of ventilations, check the mouth to see whether the chest compressions have expelled the foreign body, enabling you to remove it.

Choking in the paediatric patient

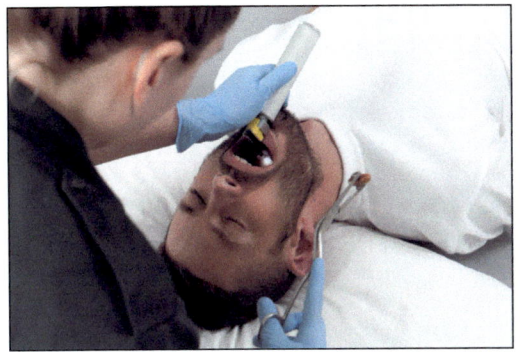

Figure 11.21 Removal of a foreign body by direct laryngoscopy.

4.4.3 Adult choking management algorithm

Figure 11.22 shows the choking management algorithm, which summarises the explanation provided in the previous section.

5 Choking in the paediatric patient

5.1 *Learning objective*

By the end of this section you will be able to:
- demonstrate how to manage a choking paediatric patient.

5.2 *Introduction*

It is estimated that around 20 children aged 0–14 years of age per 100,000 population will experience at least one food-related choking episode each year. It is more common in boys and children under one year of age [Chapin, 2013]. Since most choking episodes involving infants and children are witnessed by an adult, intervention can commence straight away, as long as the adult knows the correct action to take [Skellett, 2016].

5.3 *The paediatric airway*

Children's airways more readily obstruct than those of adults, and they are particularly sensitive to soft tissue swelling. With a tracheal diameter of around 4 mm in infants compared with 8 mm in the adult, small amounts of swelling dramatically increase airflow resistance and the work of breathing required to maintain adequate ventilation.

The most dramatic differences are found in infants. By the age of 10–12 years, children have mostly adult anatomy, albeit smaller in size [Walls, 2012; Benger, 2009]. Other differences include [ALSG, 2010; AAP, 2018]:
- Infants have a large, prominent occiput, which results in neck flexion if they are laid supine on

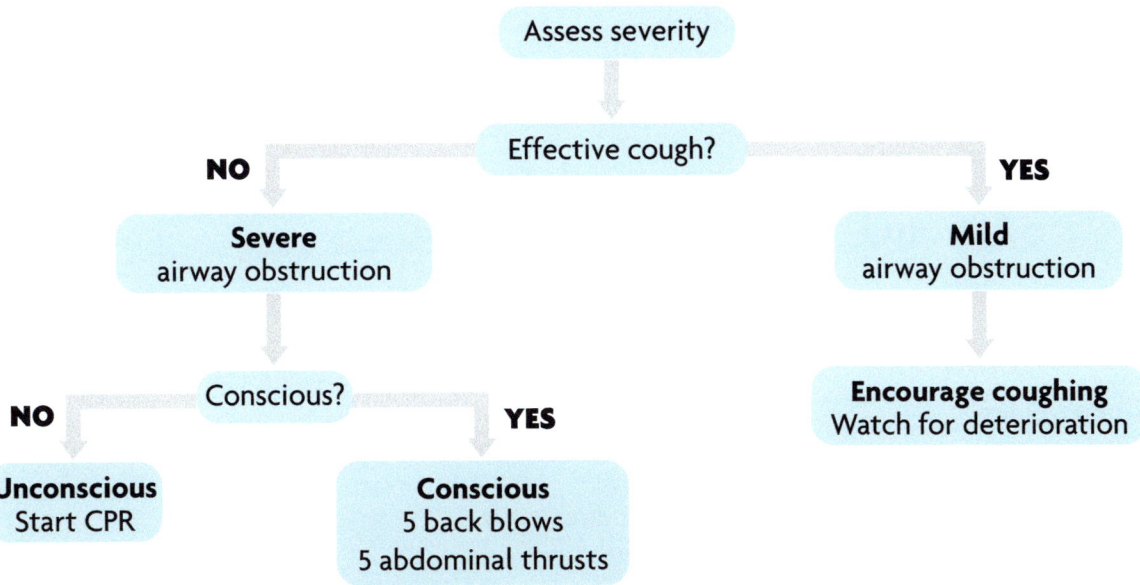

Figure 11.22 The choking algorithm for adults.

a flat surface. Use padding under the torso to maintain a neutral alignment.
- The glottic opening is at the level of the first cervical vertebra (C1) in infants, descending to C3–C4 by the age of five, resulting in a high, anterior larynx
- The epiglottis is horseshoe (or omega) shaped, floppy and proportionally larger than that of an adult.
- The tongue is proportionally larger than that of adults, occupying more of the mouth.
- Children possess a small cricothyroid membrane, and in children under 3–4 years of age it is virtually non-existent, making needle cricothyroidotomy very difficult.
- The narrowest portion of the airway in children is at the level of the cricoid ring due to their funnel-shaped larynx compared to the more cylindrical shape of the adult larynx.

5.4 Recognition

Major choking episodes in children and infants usually occur during feeding or playing and are often witnessed by a carer. However, remember to ask about any recent history of playing with or eating small objects and consider choking in any child with a sudden onset of breathing problems.

The severity of the obstruction can be determined by the effectiveness of the patient's ability to cough. An effective cough is better than external manoeuvres, so an actively coughing child should be encouraged to continue to do so. Other signs of a mild obstruction include [Maconochie, 2015]:
- crying/verbal response to questions
- long cough
- able to take breaths before coughing
- fully alert.

Contrast this with signs of a severe airway obstruction and an ineffective cough:
- unable to verbalise
- quiet/silent cough
- unable to breathe
- cyanosis
- decreasing level of consciousness.

5.5 Management

The management of the choking paediatric patient depends on their ability to effectively cough and on whether they are conscious or unconscious (Figure 11.23) [Skellett, 2016].

5.5.1 Conscious and choking

Infants
Start with back blows. If your patient is an infant, sit on a chair or kneel on the floor and place the infant across your lap in a prone (face-down) position. Support their head with the thumb and fingers of

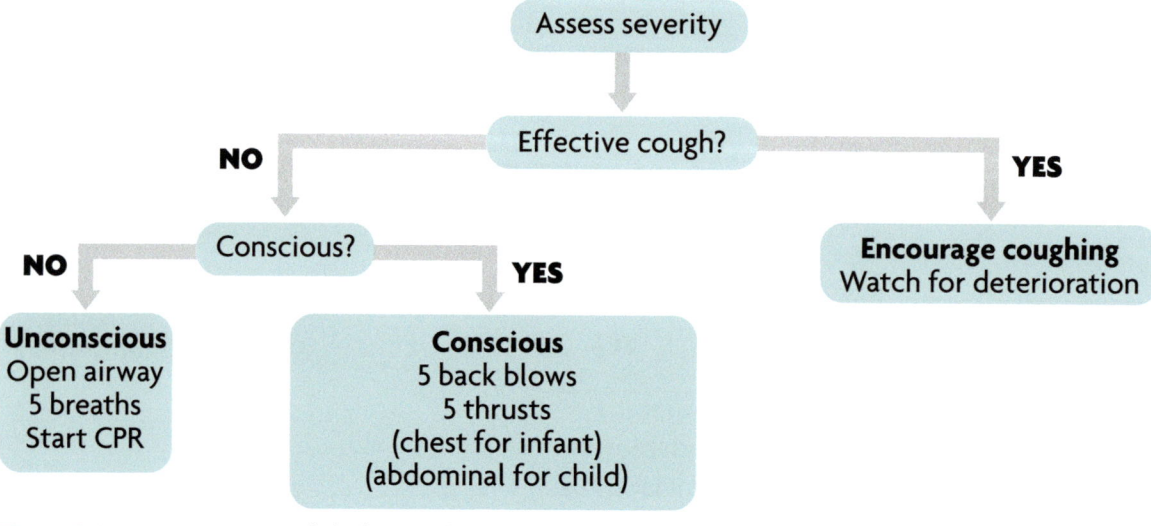

Figure 11.23 Management of choking in the paediatric patient.

one hand at the angle of their jaw, taking care not to compress the soft tissues. Administer up to five sharp blows between their scapulae with the heel of your other hand.

If these fail, turn the infant on to their back with their head downwards. Locate the landmarks for chest compression (i.e. one finger width above the xiphisternum) and administer up to five chest compressions, making them sharper and slower than those administered during cardiac arrest.

Children (over one year of age)
If the patient is a child, support them in a head-down position and administer up to five inter-scapular blows. If this does not clear the obstruction, administer abdominal thrusts by standing behind the child and leaning them forward. Place a clenched fist midway between the xiphisternum and belly button. Grasp the fist with your other hand and pull inwards and upwards, up to five times.

Frequently reassess and alternate between back blows and chest thrusts in the infant, and back blows and abdominal thrusts in the child.

5.5.2 Unconscious and choking

If a child or infant becomes, or is, unconscious, place them on their back with appropriate padding to maintain an open airway. Check the mouth for a visible obstruction and make a single attempt to remove it if a foreign body (FB) is visible.

Attempt to ventilate, but if this does not cause chest expansion try repositioning the head and try again. If after five attempts you still cannot ventilate the child, move on to chest compressions and alternate with further ventilations using a ratio of 15:2. Don't forget to check the airway for a dislodged FB after re-opening the airway prior to ventilating.

Chapter

12 Breathing

1 Respiratory system physiology

1.1 Learning objective

By the end of this section you will be able to:
- describe and explain the function of the respiratory system.

1.2 Introduction

In Chapter 11, 'Airway', you learnt about the structure (or anatomy) of the respiratory system, but it is also important to understand the function (physiology) of the respiratory system. Functionally, the respiratory system is split into two portions [Tortora, 2017]:
- **Conducting portion:** This is made up of the interconnecting cavities and tubes starting at the mouth and nose and ending at the terminal bronchioles. These filter, warm and moisten the air and transfer it to the lungs and out again.
- **Respiratory portion:** This is made up of the tissues inside the lungs that exchange the gas. It consists of the respiratory bronchioles, alveolar ducts and sacs, and the alveoli. This is where gas exchange between the air and blood occurs.

These portions combined enable the respiratory system to perform its functions:
- gas exchange, which imports oxygen (which is taken up into the blood and delivered to the body's cells) and expires the waste gas, carbon dioxide
- assists in the regulation of blood acidity levels
- removes small amounts of heat and water
- filters inspired air, produces vocal sounds and contains receptors providing a sense of smell.

1.3 Respiration

Respiration is the process of gas exchange in the body (mainly of oxygen and carbon dioxide). It consists of three steps [Tortora, 2017]:

- **Pulmonary ventilation:** The process of moving air into and out of the lungs. It is divided into inspiration (inhalation), when air is moved into the lungs, and expiration (exhalation), when air is moved out of the lungs.
- **External respiration:** The exchange of gases between the alveoli of the lungs and the blood inside the pulmonary capillaries.
- **Internal respiration:** The exchange of gases between the blood in capillaries around the body and tissue cells.

1.4 The lungs

In order to understand ventilation and external respiration, we just need to cover a little more anatomy. Recall from section 1, 'Anatomy', in Chapter 11, 'Airway', that the lungs extend from the diaphragm to just above the clavicles. The left lung is smaller than the right due to the space taken up by the heart. It also has only two lobes, the upper and lower lobes, whereas the right lung has three: the upper, lower and middle lobes [Tortora, 2017].

The lungs are divided into lobes by deep grooves known as fissures. Both lungs have an oblique fissure, but the right lung also has a horizontal fissure (Figures 12.1, 12.2 and 12.3).

1.4.1 Lobes, lobules and alveoli

Each lobe of the lung has its own secondary branch (bronchus), branching from the right and left primary bronchi (Figure 12.4).

These in turn divide into tertiary bronchi, each supplying a segment of lung called a bronchopulmonary segment. Within these are many much smaller components known as lobules, within which are contained three to five respiratory units, which is where the gas exchange occurs. Respiratory units (or acini) emerge from the terminal bronchioles and consist of several respiratory bronchioles, which subdivide into alveolar ducts and, finally, the alveoli [Hickin, 2015].

Chapter 12 – Breathing

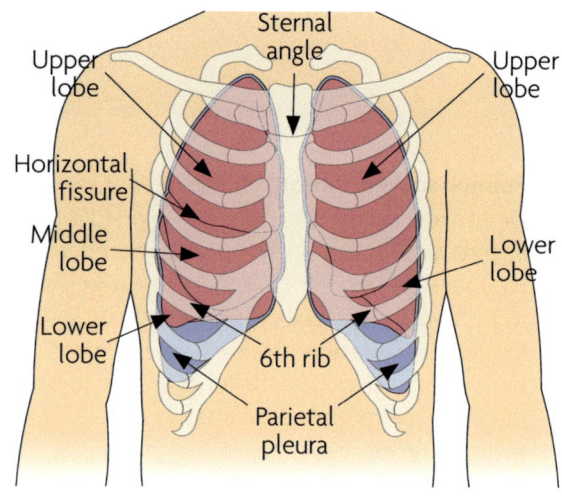

Figure 12.1 Anterior view of the lungs in relation to surface anatomy.

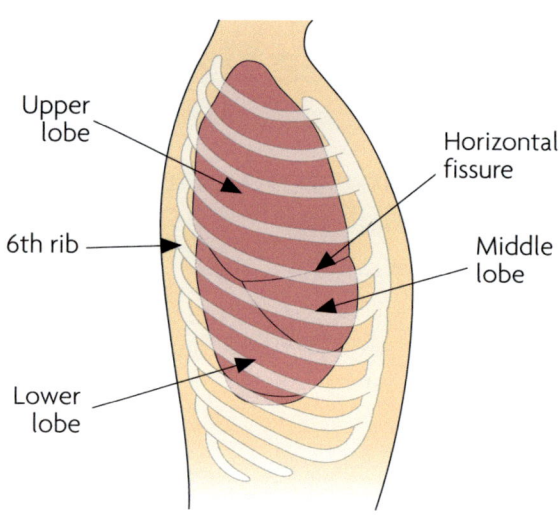

Figure 12.3 Lateral view of the lungs in relation to surface anatomy.

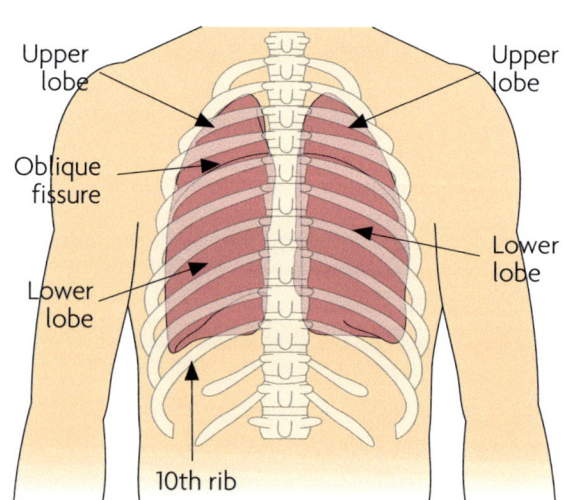

Figure 12.2 Posterior view of the lungs in relation to surface anatomy.

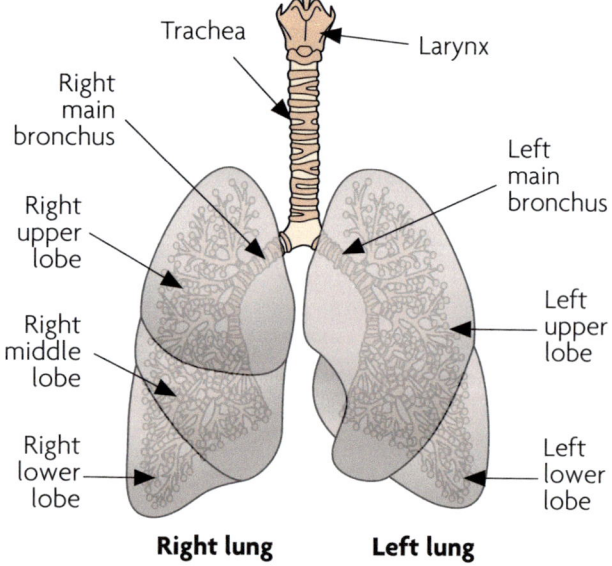

Figure 12.4 The lower respiratory tract showing the left and right bronchi.

Alveoli

The alveoli are cup-shaped pouches with very thin walls that enable the exchange of oxygen and carbon dioxide with the pulmonary capillaries that surround them. There are around 150–400 million in each normal lung, creating a large surface area for gaseous exchange (approximately 50–100 m^2) [Hickin, 2015].

1.5 Mechanics of breathing

1.5.1 Air pressure

Air moves into and out of the lungs because ventilation changes the pressure inside the alveoli. This is achieved by changing the volume of the thoracic cavity (the contents of the body surrounded by the ribs and diaphragm). As the volume inside this cavity increases, the pressure inside decreases (a relationship known as Boyle's Law). This causes the lungs to expand, increasing their volume and so decreasing the alveolar pressure.

Since air moves from areas of high pressure to low pressure, once the pressure inside the alveoli drops below that outside the body, i.e. atmospheric pressure, air enters the lungs. At the end of inspiration, the volume of the thoracic cavity decreases, and the pressure rises; once it becomes higher than that of atmospheric pressure, air leaves the lungs [Hickin, 2015].

1.5.2 Inspiration

During normal, quiet respiration, most of the work of respiration is undertaken by the diaphragm. This is a dome-shaped muscle that seals the thoracic cavity from the abdomen. When it contracts, it flattens and descends, increasing the volume inside the thoracic cavity, and is responsible for about 75% of the air entering the lungs.

The remaining 25% of air entering the lungs is the result of the external intercostal muscles contracting, which pulls the ribs upwards and outwards like a bucket handle [Tortora, 2017].

1.5.3 Expiration

During normal, quiet respiration, breathing out (expiration) is a passive process as no muscles are involved. This is because of elastic recoil, a property of the thoracic wall and the lungs to 'spring back' to their original position when they are stretched by the muscles of inspiration.

1.5.4 Forceful breathing

When exercising and in other instances when the body requires more oxygen, additional, accessory, muscles can be used to aid inspiration and expiration (Figure 12.5). These can often be seen in use by patients with respiratory distress.

1.6 Gas exchange

You have already read that gas moves from areas of high pressure to low, and it turns out that this is the

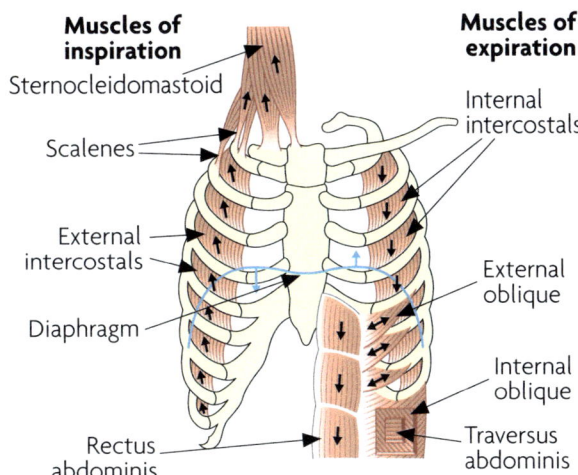

Figure 12.5 Muscles of inspiration and expiration.

case even for a mixture of gases. Take room air, which you are breathing in. It is made up of the following (percentages are approximate) [Tortora, 2017]:
- oxygen (O_2): 20.9%
- nitrogen (N_2): 78.6%
- carbon dioxide (CO_2): 0.04%
- other gases/water vapour: 0.46%.

The pressure each of the gases exerts to make up the pressure of air is known as the gas' partial pressure. For example, the partial pressure of oxygen (PO_2) in the air is 21 kilopascals (kPa).

Each gas acts independently of the others, so in the alveoli, oxygen moves from an area of higher pressure (the alveoli) to an area of lower oxygen pressure (the pulmonary circulation), by a process known as diffusion.

1.6.1 Diffusion

Diffusion is a process by which molecules (such as oxygen and carbon dioxide) move around. It has two key characteristics [Hickins, 2015]:
- Diffusion occurs from areas of high concentration to areas of low concentration.
- Diffusion continues until both areas have the same concentration of molecules.

Oxygen diffuses from the alveoli into the pulmonary circulation, whereas carbon dioxide has a higher partial pressure inside the pulmonary circulation so moves across into the alveoli, where it can be expired. In this way, oxygen is taken up by the body and the waste gas, carbon dioxide, is removed [Tortora, 2017].

1.7 Control of breathing

The muscles of respiration are dependent on the nervous system to tell them to contract and relax. This is achieved through two types of nervous system control [Tortora, 2017]:

- **Voluntary (or conscious) control:** This originates in the cerebral cortex and is the way you can control your breathing by holding your breath or controlling the flow of air in order to play a wind instrument, for example. In addition, other centres in the brain, such as the hypothalamus and limbic system, can stimulate respiration, allowing laughing and crying to affect the breathing pattern.
- **Automatic control:** This originates from groups of nerve cells (neurons) in the brain stem (mainly the pons and medulla). The neurons in the medulla are responsible for the basic rhythm of breathing and send impulses to the inspiratory muscles via the phrenic and intercostal nerves. Expiratory neurons generally become active only during forceful breathing, such as when exercising.

The respiratory centres containing these inspiratory and expiratory neurons are influenced by sensory input from nerves around the body. For example, stretch receptors prevent the lungs from being overinflated and others are linked to receptors that can detect movement, stimulating the respiratory centres to increase ventilation during exercise.

Breathing is also regulated by the partial pressures of oxygen (PaO_2) and carbon dioxide ($PaCO_2$), and hydrogen ion concentration (pH) in the blood. $PaCO_2$ is the most important and has the most profound effect on respiration. Special sensory neurons called chemoreceptors are located close to the medulla (central chemoreceptors) and in the walls of the aortic and carotid arteries [Tortora, 2017].

Note: The extra 'a' in PaO_2 and $PaCO_2$ denotes the partial pressure of oxygen and carbon dioxide in arterial blood.

1.7.1 Chemical control

The central chemoreceptors are sensitive to $PaCO_2$, not PaO_2, and are responsible for 80% of the drive to breathe. They are also affected by drugs such as opiates (like morphine). Regulatory mechanisms are very sensitive and precise, keeping the $PaCO_2$ levels stable even when exercising. For example, once $PaCO_2$ levels begin to rise, ventilation is rapidly increased to expire more CO_2. Conversely, when the $PaCO_2$ level falls, ventilation is slowed, allowing the $PaCO_2$ level to increase.

The peripheral chemoreceptors are sensitive to PaO_2, $PaCO_2$, pH, blood flow and temperature. However, they are particularly sensitive to hypoxaemia (low PaO_2). Once this drops below 6.7 kPa, ventilation is dramatically increased. When this was first discovered, it was suggested that if low levels of oxygen could increase ventilation, then giving too much might decrease ventilation. This is known as the hypoxic drive theory. In fact, when the PaO_2 rises above 8 kPa there is no significant reduction in ventilation, and when PaO_2 is above 13 kPa there is no further reduction in ventilation at all [O'Driscoll, 2017].

1.8 Oxygen physiology

Oxygen is vital for cell metabolism, but tissues in the body have no mechanism for storing it. Instead, cells rely on a constant supply that can vary depending on cell metabolism.

The arterial oxygen tension (also known as the partial pressure of oxygen, PaO_2) is a measure of the oxygen dissolved in blood plasma. It is not very soluble and, as a result, only 1.5% of oxygen is transported in this way.

Most oxygen is carried in the blood (about 98.5%) bound to haemoglobin inside the red blood cells. This makes global oxygen delivery dependent on cardiac output and the oxygen content of the blood. The oxygen content of the blood is, in turn, dependent on arterial oxygen saturation (oxygen bound to haemoglobin, SaO_2) and the amount of haemoglobin in the blood.

Normal daily activities consume around 25% of the oxygen delivered to the cells. The remainder is returned to the lungs as a mixed venous saturation and is usually 65% saturated with oxygen. As oxygen consumption increases or supply decreases, the amount of oxygen extracted by the tissue cells increases to maintain aerobic metabolism. This can continue until around 60–70% of oxygen is extracted. If consumption continues to increase or supply decreases, tissue hypoxia will occur [Tortora, 2017].

1.8.1 Oxygen transport

Only dissolved oxygen can diffuse into cells, so the process of binding and dissociating oxygen from haemoglobin is carefully managed, thanks to the design of haemoglobin, which can accept up to four oxygen molecules.

There are a number of factors that control this process, the most critical of which is the partial pressure of arterial oxygen. This relationship between the saturation of haemoglobin (SaO_2) and the partial pressure of arterial oxygen (PaO_2) is shown in the oxyhaemoglobin dissociation curve (blue line in Figure 12.6).

At a very low PaO_2, haemoglobin binds few oxygen molecules because the haemoglobin subunits are held together tightly. However, once a single oxygen molecule binds to haemoglobin, it becomes progressively easier for subsequent oxygen molecules to come aboard as the haemoglobin changes shape. This explains why the curve is so steep between a PaO_2 of approximately 2 kPa and 5 kPa.

At the typical PaO_2 found in a healthy lung (13 kPa), the total SaO_2 is around 97%. Other factors affecting haemoglobin's affinity for oxygen include: acidity, the partial pressure of arterial carbon dioxide ($PaCO_2$) and temperature.

An increase in any of these decreases haemoglobin's affinity for oxygen, resulting in a shift of the oxyhaemoglobin curve to the right (the red line in Figure 12.6), known as the Bohr effect. Thus, for any given PaO_2, the saturation of haemoglobin will be lower. In the tissues, there are increased levels of hydrogen ions (H^+) and carbon dioxide and so oxygen is released thanks to the Bohr effect [Tortora, 2017].

2 Using medical gases safely

2.1 *Learning objectives*

By the end of this section you will be able to:
- describe the dangers of using compressed gas
- outline the safe use, storage and handling of medical gases
- state the guidelines for the use of oxygen therapy including:
  - indications
  - contra-indications
- outline the safe use of Entonox including:
  - the properties of Entonox
  - complications of environmental temperature with regards to Entonox
  - the benefits of Entonox therapy
  - indications
  - cautions and contra-indications
- explain the use of facial barriers, the bag-valve-mask and mechanical ventilators.

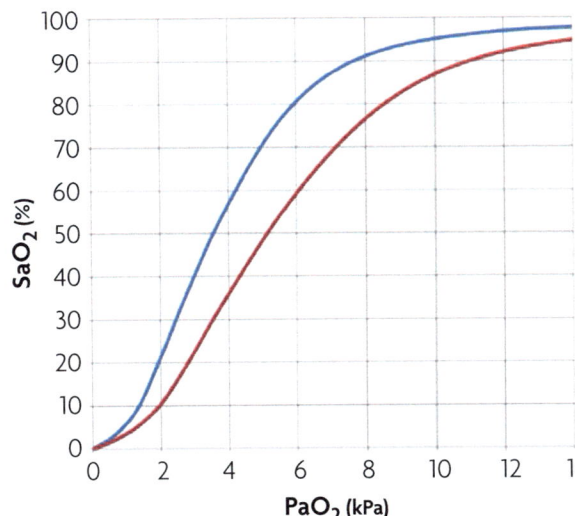

Figure 12.6 Oxyhaemoglobin dissociation curve.

2.2 Introduction

There are two main medical gases in use by ambulance services: oxygen and Entonox (Figure 12.7). These gases are compressed into cylinders of varying sizes. Typically, you will have a small, portable cylinder for carrying into a patient's house or for transporting on the ambulance trolley, for example, and a larger, heavier cylinder that is fitted to the ambulance and is generally removed only when it is empty and needs replacing.

Note: Entonox is usually only provided as the smaller, portable cylinder.

Oxygen behaves differently to air, compressed air, nitrogen and other inert gases. It is very reactive. Pure oxygen, at high pressure, such as from a cylinder, can react violently with common materials such as oil and grease. Other materials may catch fire spontaneously. Nearly all materials including textiles, rubber and even metals will burn vigorously in oxygen [HSE, 2013a].

Even a small increase in the oxygen level in the air to 24% can create a dangerous situation. It becomes easier to start a fire, which will then burn hotter and more fiercely than in normal air. It may be almost impossible to put the fire out. A leaking valve or hose in a poorly ventilated room or confined space can quickly increase the oxygen concentration to a dangerous level.

The main causes of fires and explosions when using oxygen are [HSE, 2013f]:
- oxygen enrichment from leaking equipment
- use of materials not compatible with oxygen
- use of oxygen in equipment not designed for oxygen service
- incorrect or careless operation of oxygen equipment.

2.3 Medical gas cylinder storage

Somewhere on your ambulance station is a medical gas cylinder store (Figure 12.8). It should meet all of the following requirements [DoH, 2006]:
- On ground level, as close as possible to delivery point.
- Clearly identifiable, so it can easily be located in an emergency.
- Not close to any installation that may cause a fire risk (such as the fuel pump).
- Have a level floor, made of concrete or other non-combustible material.
- Well-ventilated.
- Contain only medical gases.
- Adequate means of securing large cylinders to prevent falling.
- Clear and separate areas for full and empty cylinders.
- Kept free from naked flames and marked with signage such as 'No smoking'.
- Not prone to excessively hot or cold temperatures.

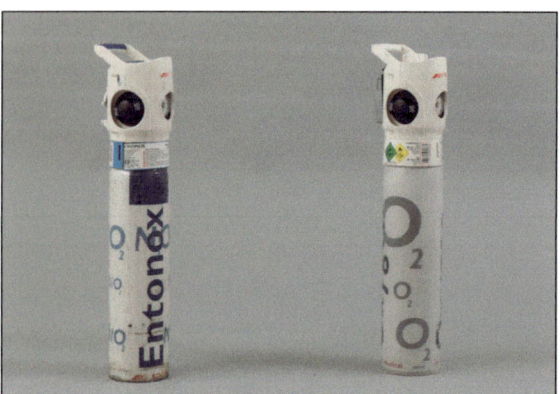

Figure 12.7 Medical gases. Entonox on the left, oxygen on the right.

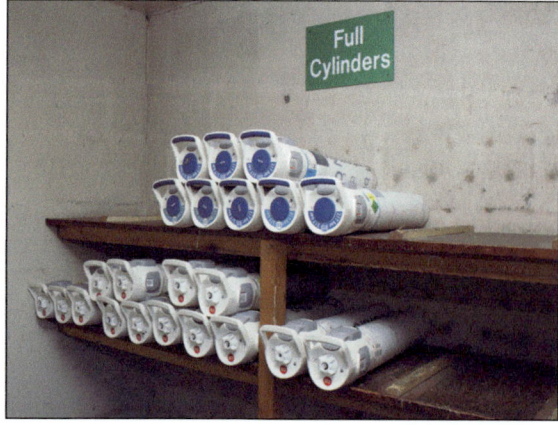

Figure 12.8 An ambulance station medical gas cylinder store.

Using medical gases safely

- Contain shelving to store smaller cylinders horizontally.
- Be secure enough to prevent theft and misuse.

2.4 Anatomy of a medical gas cylinder

Integrated valve cylinders (Figure 12.9) are the most common type found in UK ambulance services and are covered in this section. You may find, however, that your service still uses the older-style cylinders, which require a regulator head to be fitted before they can be used, and you should seek guidance on their use.

There is a British Standard (BS EN 1089-3:2011) relating to the labelling of medical gases to ensure that they are easy to identify and so avoid inappropriate administration [BSI, 2011]. Medical gases always have a white body, but have different-coloured collars to indicate the type of gas. The most commonly encountered gases that you will find on an ambulance are oxygen (white collar), Entonox (blue and white collar) and air (black and white collar).

Important components of the cylinder are [BOC, 2013a]:
- flow selector
  - desired flow rate can be selected by rotating the dial
  - positive 'click' between flow rates to ensure correct setting is chosen
- 'live' contents gauge
  - shows contents of cylinder, even when turned off
  - green = full
  - red = low/empty
- handwheel
  - simple on/off dial; no spanner required
  - turn anti-clockwise to open
  - turn clockwise to close

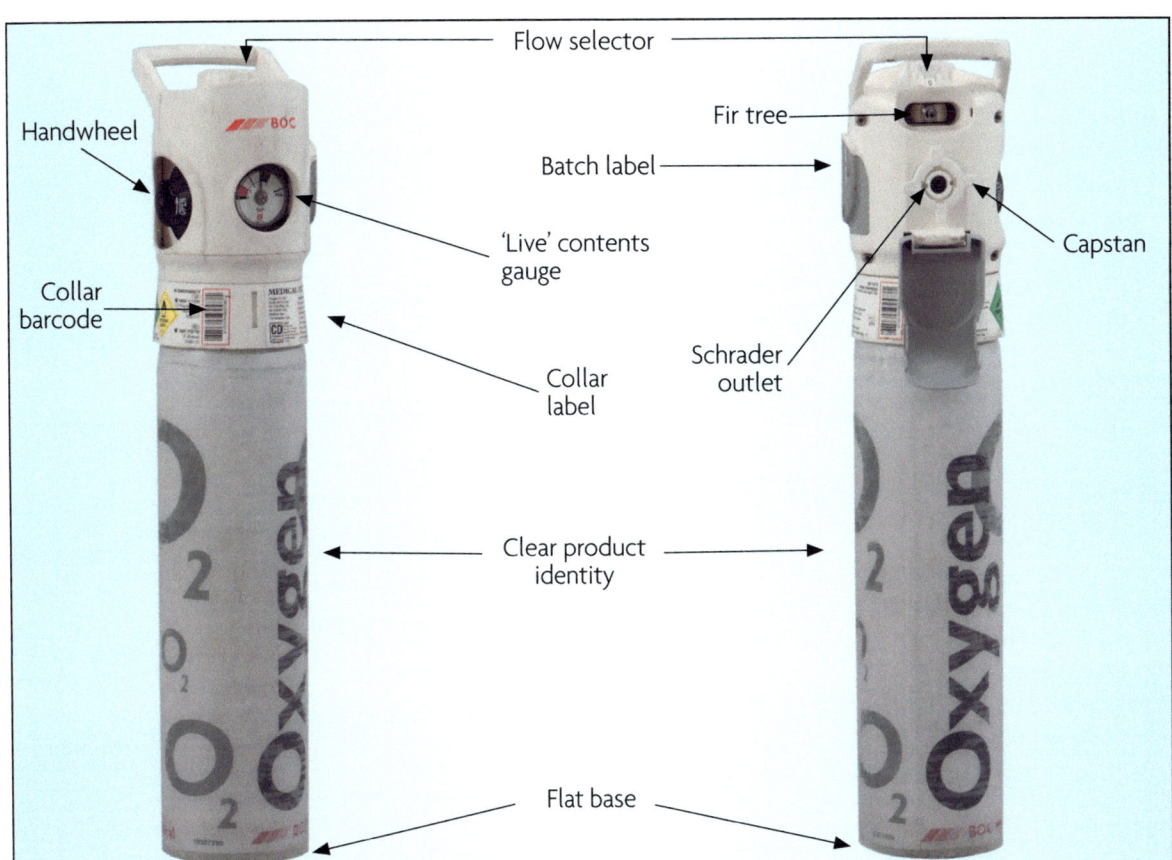

Figure 12.9 CD-sized integrated valve oxygen cylinder.

Chapter 12 – Breathing

- clear product identity
  - name of gas is written on cylinder collar and body
- flat base
  - easier to handle
  - improves stability
- fir tree
  - attachment point for oxygen tubing
- batch label
  - located on guard or collar
  - shows expiry date
  - required when reporting cylinder defect
- Schrader outlet
  - push-fit connector for other methods of administration/connection to artificial ventilators
  - gas-specific to avoid inadvertent inappropriate administration
  - out sleeve (capstan) can be twisted to release.

2.5 Safety first

Prior to using a medical gas, there are a number of safety checks required [BOC, 2013a]:

- Make sure your hands are clean. If you have used an alcohol-based handrub, ensure that it has evaporated completely.
- Check the cylinder to ensure it is clean and free from damage.
- Ensure the cylinder is free from oil and grease, especially around the Schrader and fir tree outlets.
- Both oxygen and Entonox are non-flammable, but strongly support combustion. Keep away from naked flames, sources of ignition and combustible materials.

If the medical gas is Entonox, check that it has not been allowed to get too cold. Below -6°C the nitrous oxide will separate from the gas mixture. To prevent this, it should be stored above 10°C for at least 24 hours prior to use. If this is not possible and the bottle is of a portable size, warm the bottle to 10°C and then invert three times prior to use to mix the gases.

2.6 Preparing a new cylinder for use

Procedure – Preparing a new cylinder for use

The following steps apply to both oxygen and Entonox cylinders [BOC, 2013a; BOC, 2013b]:

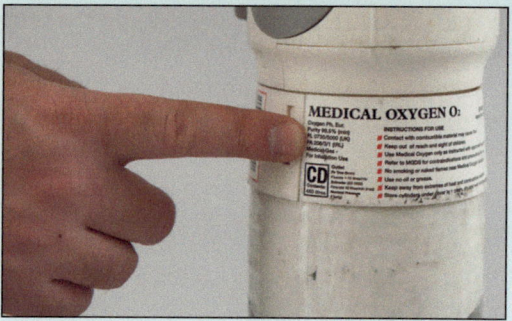

1. Ensure you have the correct medical gas by checking the cylinder label.

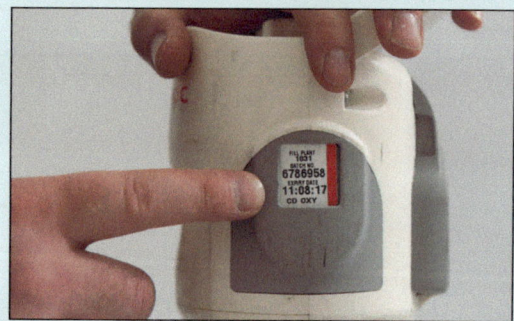

2. Check the expiry date on the batch label fitted to the cylinder.

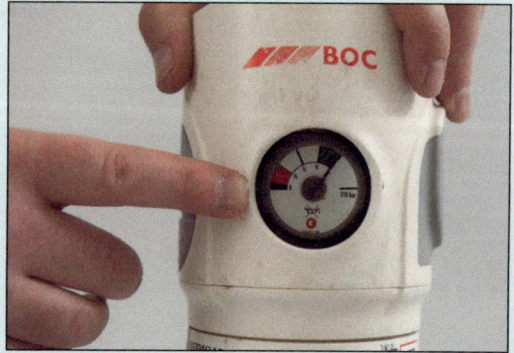

3. Make sure the contents gauge is in the green zone. This indicates that the cylinder is full.

2.7 Oxygen delivery devices

The fir tree connector (Figure 12.10) is used to connect oxygen tubing to the cylinder, which in turn can provide oxygen to a bag-valve-mask (BVM), oxygen-driven nebuliser, oxygen masks and nasal cannulae (Figure 12.11).

Note: The masks and nasal cannulae all require the patient to be spontaneously breathing in order to work. If the patient is not breathing effectively, they require assisted and artificial ventilation, most commonly with a BVM.

Procedure – Preparing a new cylinder for use – *cont*

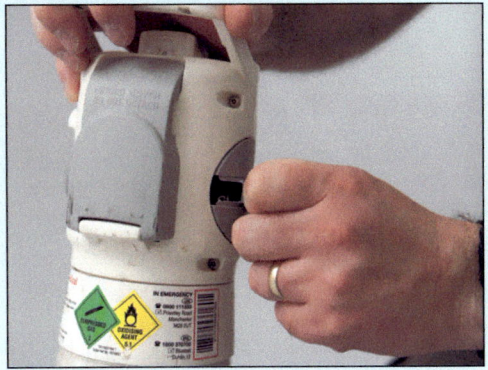

4. Remove the tamper-evident handwheel cover by pulling the tear ring.

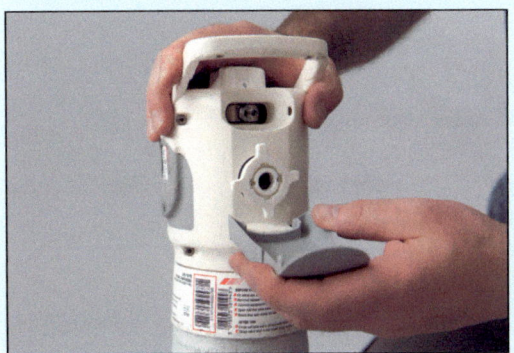

5. Remove the valve outlet cover. Pull the grey cover downwards. It stays attached to the cylinder.

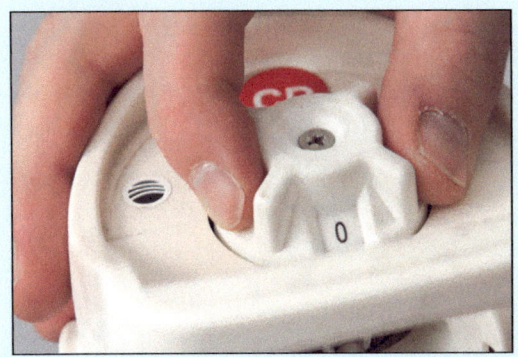

6. Ensure the flow selector on top of the cylinder is set to zero and the handwheel is turned off before connecting equipment.

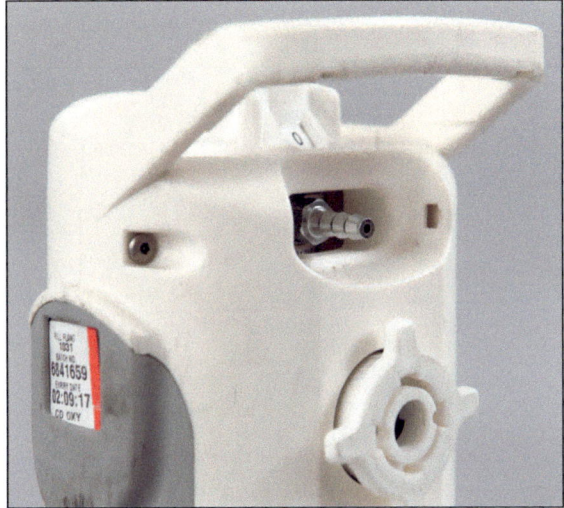

Figure 12.10 Oxygen fir tree connector.

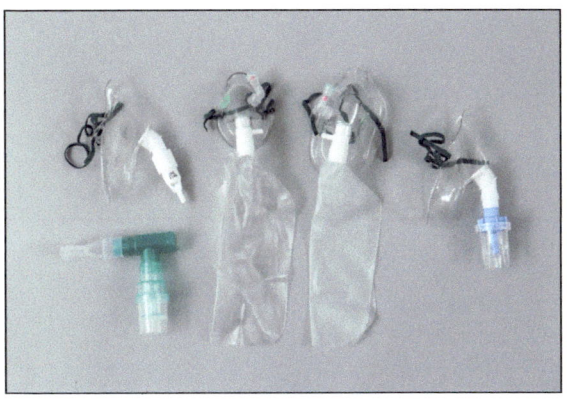

Figure 12.11 A variety of devices to administer oxygen.

2.7.1 Procedure

Procedure – Administer oxygen

Follow the steps below to provide oxygen from the appropriate oxygen delivery device [BOC, 2013a]:

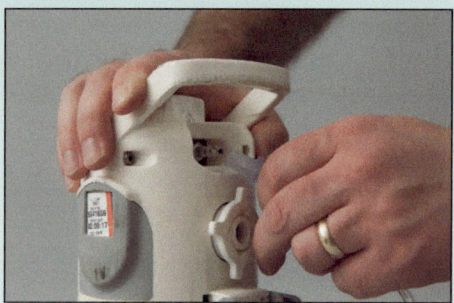

1. Attach tubing from mask or nasal cannulae to the fir tree outlet. Ensure the tubing is pushed on securely.

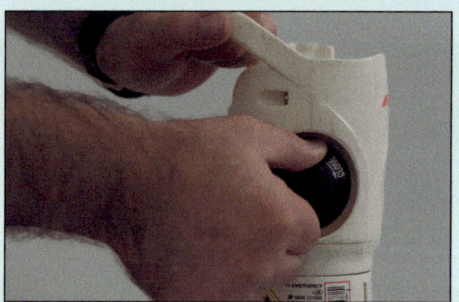

2. Slowly turn on the cylinder by rotating the handwheel anti-clockwise until it comes to a complete stop. Do not use excessive force.

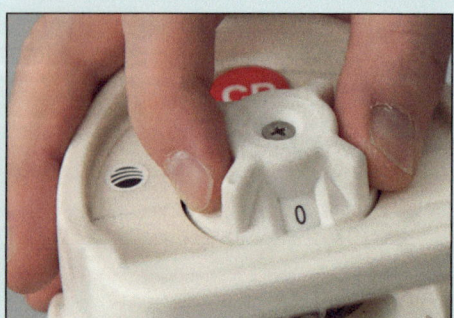

3. Set the prescribed flow by rotating the flow selector dial. Ensure that the correct flow rate number is clearly visible in the flow selector window. Check the gas is flowing.

Procedure – Administer oxygen – *cont*

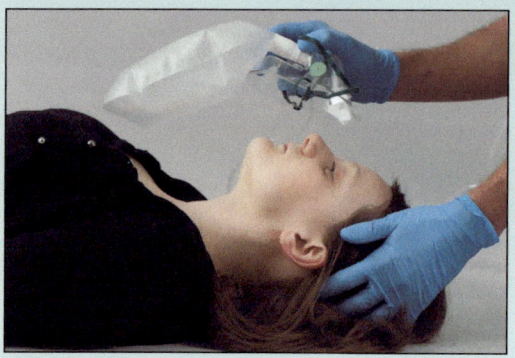

4. Place oxygen mask or nasal cannulae on the patient.

2.7.2 Supplemental oxygen delivery devices

Non-rebreathe mask

This mask is used when the patient requires a high concentration of oxygen. At 15 l/minute, the mask can deliver up to 85% inspired oxygen. It consists of a mask and reservoir bag that is fitted with a one-way valve, ensuring that the patient can only inhale oxygen from it and not exhale into the bag. The bag must be inflated in order to ensure maximum inspired oxygen.

Medium concentration mask (simple face mask)

This face mask has ports on either side to allow room air to be drawn inside. At 10 l/minute, it will deliver around 40% oxygen, but this is variable depending on how well fitting the mask is.

Venturi mask

This mask also draws in (or entrains) room air, but allows for more accurate oxygen delivery than the medium concentration face mask. It comes with a variety of spigots, which are capable of delivering a variety of oxygen concentrations. The percentage of oxygen and flow rate required are usually clearly marked on the spigot. They are particularly useful when providing oxygen to patients with chronic obstructive pulmonary disease (COPD).

Using medical gases safely

Nasal cannulae
These deliver oxygen via two nasal prongs, which sit just inside the patient's nostrils. Oxygen flow rates are typically limited to 1–4 l/minute as higher rates lead to irritation of the nasal lining. They are often used by patients on long-term oxygen therapy and may be preferred by patients who do not tolerate a face mask.

Nebuliser
This is used to deliver aerosolised drugs. The pressurised chamber when powered by oxygen turns the liquid drug inside (usually salbutamol or ipratropium) into a mist (i.e. aerosolises the drug), which is then inhaled by the patient. Some nebulisers (particularly if the patient has one at home) are powered using compressed room air.

Firesafe
You may notice a small device inserted into a patient's tubing if they are on home oxygen (Figure 12.12). This is a Firesafe, a cannula valve that is designed to cut the oxygen supply to the patient in the event of a fire. It will not affect the oxygen flow to the patient as long as it is inserted the correct way around (the arrow shows the direction of gas flow).

2.8 Assisted ventilation

Patients who are breathing inadequately (for example, because they have a slow respiratory rate or an irregular pattern of respiration) and patients whose breathing is too shallow or who are not breathing at all require assisted ventilation. Assisted ventilation can be provided with a pocket mask, BVM or oxygen-powered ventilation device. In most circumstances, you will be using a BVM.

2.8.1 Gastric distension

In contrast to the normal way we breathe (i.e. the negative pressure inside the chest cavity draws air into the chest), assisted and artificial ventilation require the use of positive-pressure ventilation i.e. actively blowing air into the lungs. This has some disadvantages as high inflation pressures can result in air going into the stomach instead of the lungs, leading to gastric distension and ultimately vomiting. This is more likely if:
- high inflation pressures are used
- ventilations are performed too fast
- the airway is partially obstructed.

A distended stomach is bad for the patient as vomit can rise up into the airway and be inhaled (aspirated). It also pushes up the diaphragm, reducing the amount of space for lung expansion.

2.8.2 Mouth-to-mouth

The most basic ventilation device is your mouth and lungs, using mouth-to-mouth ventilation. However, healthcare professionals and members of the public are sometimes reluctant to perform mouth-to-mouth on people they do not know. In addition, there are risks relating to exposure to blood and other body fluids through direct contact with the patient's mouth and nose. In certain cases, direct mouth-to-mouth contact is not appropriate, such as in cases of poisoning [Nolan, 2016].

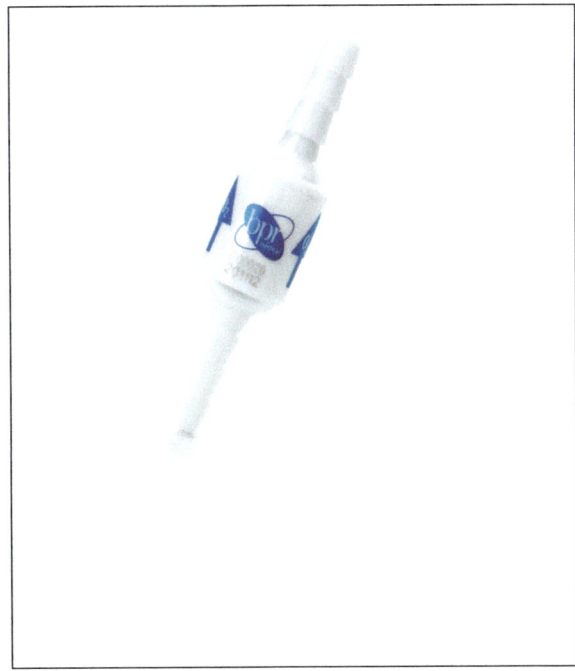

Figure 12.12 A Firesafe.

Chapter 12 – *Breathing*

Procedure – Mouth-to-mouth ventilation

Take the following steps to perform mouth-to-mouth ventilation [SJA, SAA, BRC, 2016]:

1. Place the patient on their back (supine).
2. Open the airway using a head tilt–chin lift, or jaw thrust if cervical spine injury is suspected.
3. Pinch the patient's nose to close the nostrils.
4. Take a breath and seal your lips over the patient's mouth.
5. Blow steadily for about one second, just enough to make the chest rise.
6. While maintaining the head tilt–chin lift, take your mouth away from the patient and watch the chest fall.
7. Repeat, aiming to provide a breath to an adult every six seconds.

Note: If the patient is not breathing and has no signs of life, commence chest compressions, not ventilations (this will be covered in Chapter 24, 'Cardiac Arrest').

2.8.3 Facial shields

To provide some protection for yourself, it may be possible to use a face shield, which provides a plastic barrier between you and the patient. Face shields are also fitted with a filter that fits over the patient's mouth. As with mouth-to-mouth ventilation, this method does not allow for the administration of supplemental oxygen. The technique is the same for mouth-to-mouth ventilation.

2.8.4 Mouth-to-mask ventilation

Using a pocket mask to provide mouth-to-mask ventilation uses your lungs as before, but does not require direct contact with the patient's mouth. The one-way valve also prevents you coming into contact with blood and secretions from the

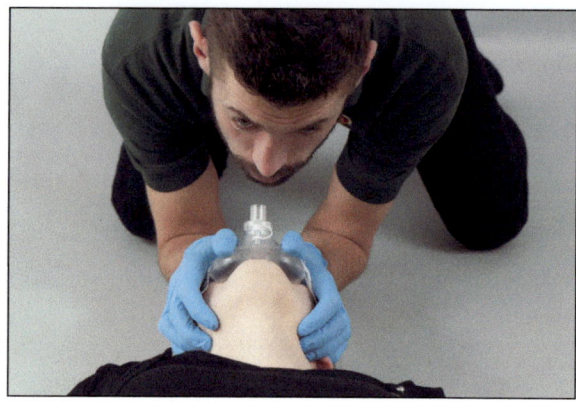

Figure 12.13 Mouth-to-mask ventilation.

patient's mouth. You use both hands to hold the mask to the patient's face, which makes it easier to get a good seal and deliver effective ventilations (Figure 12.13).

Some pocket masks also have an oxygen port, allowing administration of supplemental oxygen. Even with pocket masks without an oxygen port, oxygen tubing can be placed under one side of the mask.

Procedure – Mouth-to-mask ventilation

Take the following steps to perform mouth-to-mouth ventilation [SJA, SAA, BRC, 2016]:

1. Place the patient supine with their head in the sniffing position (neck slightly flexed and head extended).
2. Apply the mask to the patient's face using the thumbs of both hands.
3. Grip the jaw and perform a jaw thrust, while pressing down with the thumbs to make a tight seal.
4. Blow gently for one second through the valve and watch the chest rise.
5. Stop inflation and watch the chest fall.
6. Repeat every six seconds or as instructed by the senior clinician.

Using medical gases safely

> **Procedure – Mouth-to-mask ventilation** – *cont*
>
> Leaks between the face and pocket mask can be reduced by increasing the jaw thrust, or changing finger position and pressure being applied. Oxygen, if available, should run at 10 l/minute.

2.8.5 Bag-valve-mask ventilation

The bag-valve-mask (BVM) consists of a self-inflating bag, one-way valve and mask. Optionally, the mask can be removed and the bag-valve attached to other airway devices such as catheter mounts, supraglottic airway devices (SADs) and endotracheal tubes (see Chapter 18, 'Assisting the Paramedic').

When used without oxygen, it delivers room air (21% oxygen). This can be increased to 45% when high-flow oxygen is attached, but it should generally be used with a reservoir bag attached, as this can result in oxygen concentrations of around 85% (Figure 12.14) with oxygen supplied at 10 l/minute [Nolan, 2016].

The BVM can be used by one person, but this requires considerable skill. Where possible, a two-person technique is generally recommended [Monsieurs, 2015]. Whenever possible, an oropharyngeal airway should be inserted prior to using a BVM.

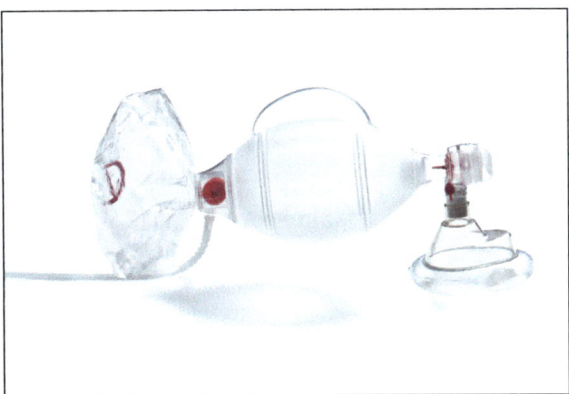

Figure 12.14 Bag-valve-mask with oxygen reservoir bag attached and inflated.

> **Procedure – One-person ventilation**
>
> Take the following steps to perform BVM ventilation with one person [Walls, 2012]:
>
> 1. Use appropriate personal protective equipment (PPE).
> 2. Choose the correct mask size, which should cover the area from the bridge of the nose to the chin.
> 3. Prepare the BVM by connecting the mask and high-flow oxygen. Ensure the reservoir bag is inflated.
> 4. Position the mask on the patient's face and ensure an adequate seal.
> 5. Form a 'C' shape with the thumb and index finger and rest this on top of the mask; place the middle and ring fingers on the ridge of the jaw and the little finger behind the angle of the jaw (Figure 12.15).
> 6. Gently squeeze the bag just enough to see the chest rise.
>
>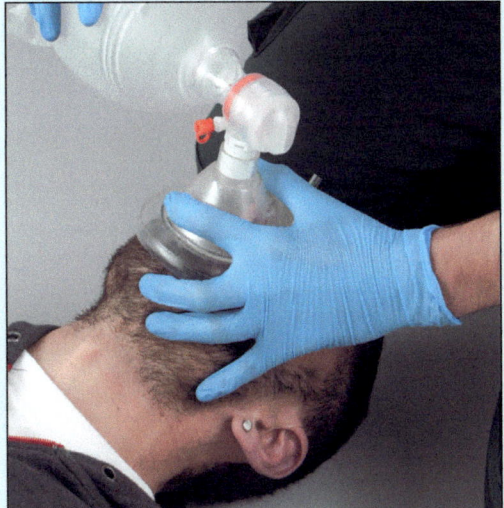
>
> **Figure 12.15** Correct hand position for one-person BVM use.

Chapter 12 – Breathing

Procedure – Two-person ventilation

This is the same as the one-person technique, with the exception that another person holds the mask to the patient's face using the same method as for the pocket mask (Figure 12.16). This is the preferred technique when enough personnel are available [Nolan 2016].

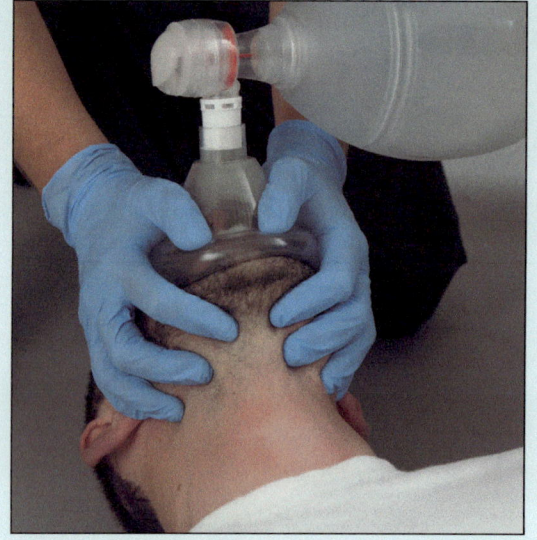

Figure 12.16 Two-person BVM technique.

2.9 Mechanical ventilation

There are a wide variety of portable mechanical ventilators, so ensure that you are familiar with the one used by your ambulance service. One of the most commonly used ventilators in UK ambulance services is the Pneupac ParaPAC ventilator (Figure 12.17). The instructions listed here apply to this ventilator, although the steps are likely to be similar with other ventilators.

Indications for the use of the ventilator will also depend on the service, but use will typically be restricted to patients who have a supraglottic device or endotracheal (ET) tube inserted, who are in respiratory or cardiac arrest and are being transported to hospital [NEAS, 2014].

Getting the setting correct on a ventilator can be challenging and if done incorrectly can be harmful to your patient. Normally your senior clinician will set up the ventilator, but if in any doubt use a BVM rather than the ventilator.

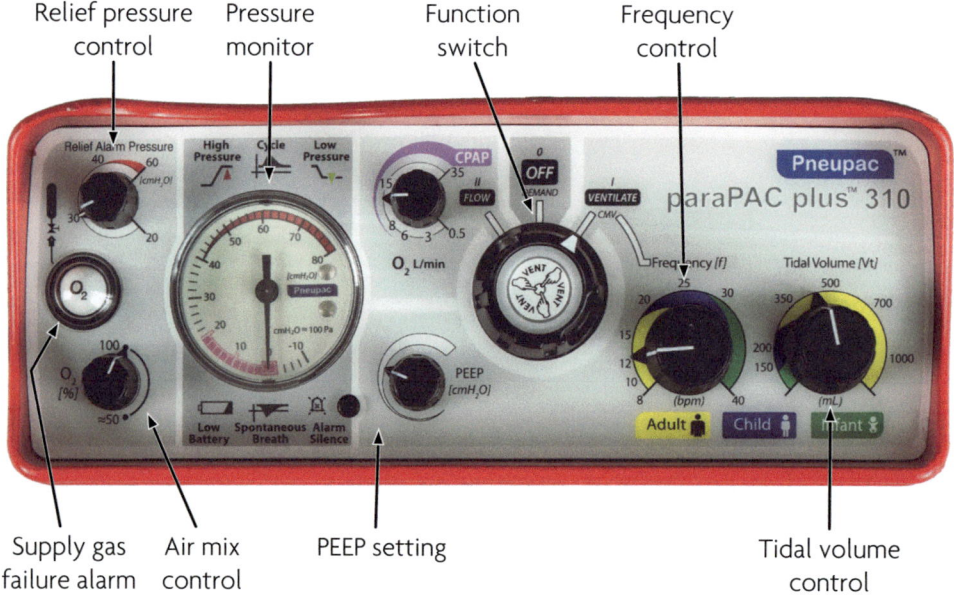

Figure 12.17 The Pneupac ParaPAC® plus 310.

Using medical gases safely

2.9.1 Procedure

Procedure – To prepare a mechanical ventilator for use

Take the following steps to prepare a mechanical ventilator for use [Smiths Medical, 2014]:

1. Connect supply hose probe to oxygen supply.
2. Check oxygen supply is turned on.
3. Check that the visual alarm for supply gas failure has changed from red to white.
4. Turn Function switch to VENTILATE.
5. Check that the alarm indicators flash in sequence, to indicate correct function.
6. Set the frequency control and tidal volume to match the patient's requirements; typically a volume of 6 ml/kg of body weight and a starting rate of 14/min for adults.
7. Briefly occlude the patient connection port of the patient valve with the thumb. Check that the peak inflation pressure reading on the pressure monitor is appropriate for the patient and that the pneumatic audible alarm sounds and the high inflation pressure indicator shows red.
8. Connect the ventilator to the catheter mount/i-gel/tracheal tube.
9. Check chest movement and pressure monitor to ensure correct ventilation.
10. Check that the green cycle indicator light flashes when inflation pressure rises above 10cmH$_2$O.
11. Check for air-tightness and adequate chest movement, and adjust the tidal volume as appropriate.
12. Check the correctness of the indicated air pressure:
    - a high-pressure alarm may indicate an excessive tidal volume, incorrect airway position or kinked ET tube
    - a low-pressure alarm may indicate a leakage or insufficient tidal volume.

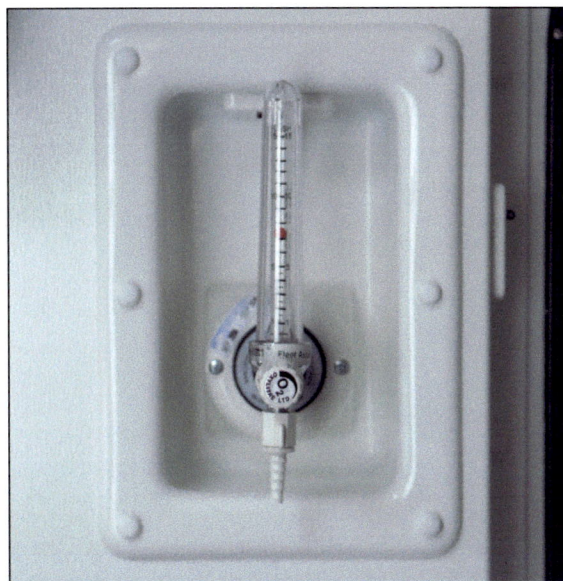

Figure 12.18 Pressure-compensated flowmeter attached to a Schrader outlet.

2.9.2 Schrader outlet

In order to connect a mechanical ventilator to the oxygen supply, you will need to use the Schrader outlet. In addition to being present on the integrated valve cylinders, there are usually several wall outlets on ambulances, though they may have a pressure-compensated flowmeter in place already (Figure 12.18). These flowmeters have a small ball inside a tube that rises or falls depending on the oxygen flow rate. Because they are affected by gravity, it is important that they remain upright.

Procedure – To prepare a pressure-compensated flowmeter for use

Take the following steps to prepare a pressure-compensated flowmeter for use [BOC, 2013a]:

1. Insert the oxygen probe into the Schrader outlet. Ensure the probe clicks securely into place.
2. Slowly turn on the cylinder by rotating the handwheel anti-clockwise until it comes to a stop. Do not use excessive force.
3. Check for leaks, which may be indicated by a hissing sound. If you suspect that you have

Chapter 12 – Breathing

> **Procedure – To prepare a pressure-compensated flowmeter for use –** *cont*
>
> a leak, turn off the cylinder and check the equipment is properly connected. Turn on the cylinder and recheck for leaks. If the leak continues, turn off and remove the cylinder from service. Report it using your ambulance service equipment defect procedure.

2.10 Oxygen administration

The UK Ambulance Services Clinical Practice Guidelines [JRCALC, 2019] have divided oxygen administration for adults into four categories.

Note: Children are not included here. They should always receive high-concentration oxygen if they have a significant illness or injury. Follow local guidance.

Indications
- Critical illnesses requiring high levels of supplemental oxygen.
- Serious illnesses requiring moderate levels of supplemental oxygen if the patient is hypoxaemic.
- COPD and other conditions requiring controlled or low-dose oxygen therapy.
- Conditions for which patients should be monitored closely but oxygen therapy is not required unless the patient is hypoxaemic.

Contra-indication (when not to administer the drug)
- Explosive environments.

Cautions
- Oxygen increases the fire hazard at the scene of an incident.
- Defibrillation: Ensure pads are firmly applied to reduce spark hazard.

Side-effects
- Non-humidified oxygen is drying and irritating to mucous membranes over a period of time.
- In patients with COPD there is a risk that even moderately high doses of inspired oxygen can produce increased carbon dioxide levels, which may cause respiratory depression, and this may lead to respiratory arrest.

Dosage and administration
- Measure oxygen saturation (SpO_2) in all patients using pulse oximetry.
- For the administration of moderate levels of supplemental oxygen, nasal cannulae are recommended in preference to simple face masks as they offer a more flexible dose range.
- Administer the initial oxygen dose until a reliable oxygen saturation reading is obtained.
- If the desired oxygen saturation cannot be maintained with a simple face mask, change to a reservoir (non-rebreathe) mask.
- For dosage and administration of supplemental oxygen, refer to Table 12.1 for patients with critical illnesses, Table 12.2 for serious illnesses and Table 12.3 for patients who need controlled or low-dose oxygen therapy.
- For conditions where no supplemental oxygen is required unless the patient is hypoxaemic, refer to Table 12.4.

Table 12.1 High levels of supplemental oxygen for adults with critical illnesses.

Administer the initial oxygen dose until the vital signs are normal, then reduce oxygen dose and aim for target saturation within the range of 94–98%.		
Condition	**Initial dose**	**Method of administration**

- Cardiac arrest or resuscitation:
  – basic life support
  – advanced life support
  – foreign body airway obstruction
  – traumatic cardiac arrest
  – maternal resuscitation
- Carbon monoxide poisoning
	Maximum dose until vital signs are normal.	Bag-valve-mask (BVM)

Using medical gases safely

Condition	Initial dose	Method of administration
• Major trauma: 　– abdominal trauma 　– burns and scalds 　– electrocution 　– head trauma 　– limb trauma 　– spinal injury and spinal cord 　– pelvic trauma 　– immersion 　– thoracic trauma 　– trauma in pregnancy • Anaphylaxis • Major pulmonary haemorrhage • Sepsis e.g. meningococcal septicaemia • Shock • Drowning	15 l/min	Non-rebreathe mask
• Active convulsion • Hypothermia	Administer 15 l/minute until a reliable SpO$_2$ measurement can be obtained and then adjust oxygen flow to aim for target saturation within the range of 94–98%	Non-rebreathe mask

Table 12.2 Moderate levels of supplemental oxygen for adults with serious illnesses if the patient is hypoxaemic.

Administer the initial oxygen dose until a reliable SpO$_2$ measurement is available, then adjust oxygen flow to aim for target saturation within the range of 94–98%.

Condition	Initial dose	Method of administration
• Acute hypoxaemia (cause not yet diagnosed) • Deterioration of lung fibrosis or other interstitial lung disease • Acute asthma • Acute heart failure • Pneumonia • Lung cancer • Post-operative breathlessness • Pulmonary embolism • Pleural effusions • Pneumothorax • Severe anaemia • Sickle cell crisis	**SpO$_2$ < 85%** 10–15 l/minute **SpO$_2$ 85–93%** 2–6 l/minute **SpO$_2$ 85–93%** 5–10 l/minute	Non-rebreathe mask Nasal cannulae Simple face mask

Chapter 12 – Breathing

Table 12.3 Controlled or low-dose supplemental oxygen for adults with COPD and other conditions.

\multicolumn{3}{l}{Administer the initial oxygen dose until a reliable SpO$_2$ measurement is available, then adjust oxygen flow to aim for target saturation within the range of 88–92% or pre-specified range as detailed on the patient's alert card.}
Condition	Initial dose	Method of administration
• Chronic obstructive pulmonary disease (COPD) • Exacerbation of cystic fibrosis	4 l/minute Increase flow rate to 6 l/minute if respiratory rate is > 30 breaths/minute (i.e. 50% above minimum specified for the mask)	28% Venturi mask (or patient's own)
• Chronic neuromuscular disorders • Chest wall disorders • Morbid obesity	4 l/minute	28% Venturi mask (or patient's own)
Note: If the oxygen saturation remains below 88%, change to simple face mask	5–10 l/minute	Simple face mask
Note: Critical illness AND COPD or other risk factors for hypercapnia	As for Table 12.1	As for Table 12.1

Table 12.4 No supplemental oxygen required for adults with these conditions unless the patient is hypoxaemic but patients should be monitored closely.

\multicolumn{3}{l}{If hypoxaemic (SpO$_2$ <94%), administer the initial oxygen dose, then adjust oxygen flow to aim for target saturation within the range of 94–98% as per the table below.}
Condition	Initial dose	Method of administration

• Myocardial infarction and acute coronary syndromes
• Stroke
• Cardiac rhythm disturbance
• Non-traumatic chest pain/discomfort
• Implantable cardioverter defibrillator firing
• Pregnancy and obstetric emergencies:
  – birth imminent
  – haemorrhage during pregnancy
  – pregnancy-induced hypertension
  – vaginal bleeding
• Abdominal pain
• Headache
• Hyperventilation syndrome or dysfunctional breathing
• Most poisonings and drug overdoses (see Table 12.1 for carbon monoxide poisoning and special cases below for paraquat poisoning)
• Metabolic and renal disorders
	SpO$_2$ < 85%
	10–15 l/minute
	
	SpO$_2$ 85–93%
	2–6 l/minute
	
	SpO$_2$ 85–93%
	5–10 l/minute
		Non-rebreathe mask
		
		Nasal cannulae
		
		Simple face mask

Condition	Initial dose	Method of administration
• Acute and sub-acute neurological and muscular conditions producing muscle weakness (assess the need for assisted ventilation if SpO$_2$ < 94%) • Post-convulsion • Gastrointestinal bleeds • Glycaemic emergencies • Heat exhaustion/heat stroke **SPECIAL CASES** • Poisoning with paraquat • Poisoning with bleomycin Patients with paraquat or bleomycin poisoning may be harmed by supplemental oxygen so avoid oxygen unless the patient is hypoxaemic Target saturation 85–88%		

2.11 After use

Procedure – After administering oxygen

Once you have finished administering oxygen to a patient, take the following steps [BOC, 2013a]:

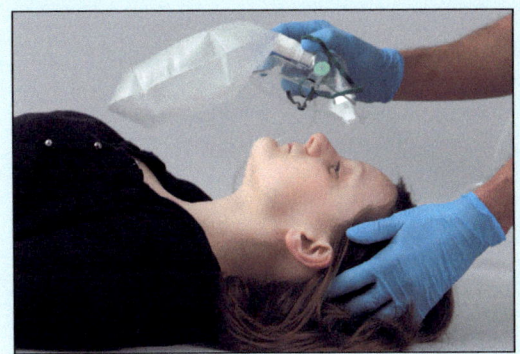

1. Remove the mask or nasal cannulae from the patient.

Procedure – After administering oxygen – *cont*

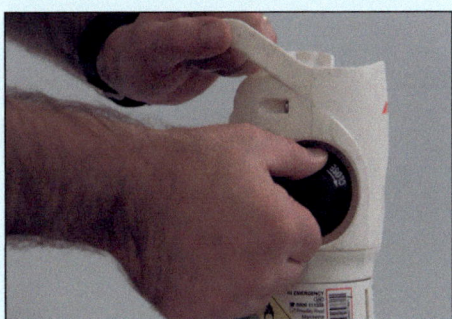

2. Turn off the cylinder by rotating the handwheel clockwise until it comes to a stop. Do not use excessive force.

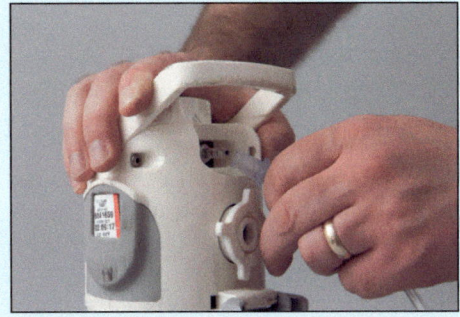

3a. Disconnect equipment. Remove the tubing by firmly pulling the tube while holding the cylinder handle.

Chapter 12 – Breathing

Procedure – After administering oxygen – *cont*

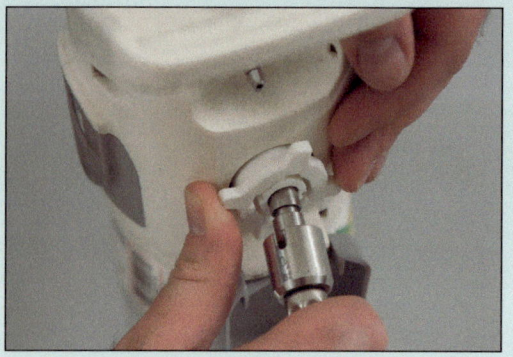

3b. If you have used the Schrader valve, release by twisting the capstan clockwise.

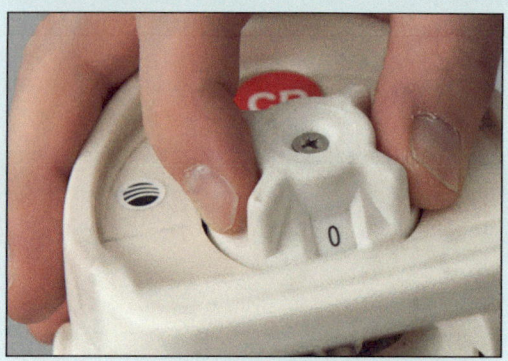

4. Turn the flow selector to zero.

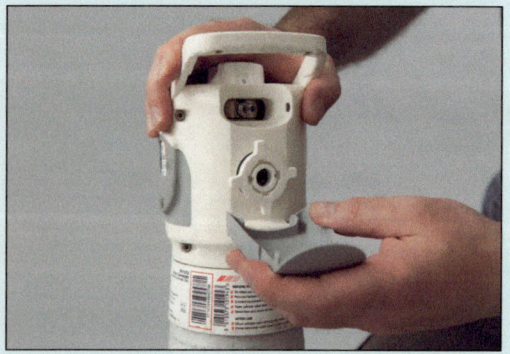

5. Replace the outlet cover by pulling up the hinged grey cover.

Procedure – After administering oxygen – *cont*

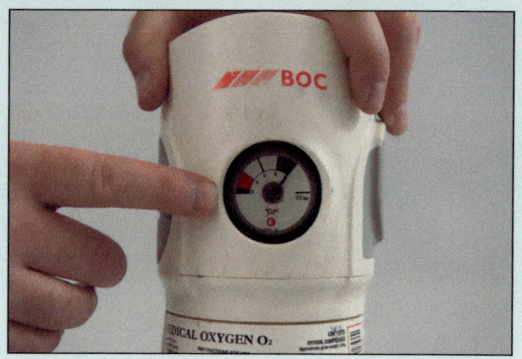

6. Check the cylinder gauge and replace if necessary.

2.12 Entonox

Entonox is a combination of 50% nitrous oxide and 50% oxygen. The cylinders that contain Entonox have a blue and white collar (Figure 12.19).

2.12.1 Procedure

Procedure – Preparing Entonox for administration

Take the following steps to prepare Entonox for administration [BOC, 2013b]:

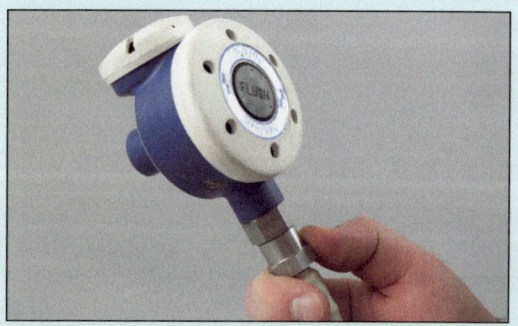

1. Ensure the demand valve is clean and ready for use.

Using medical gases safely

Procedure – Preparing Entonox for administration – *cont*

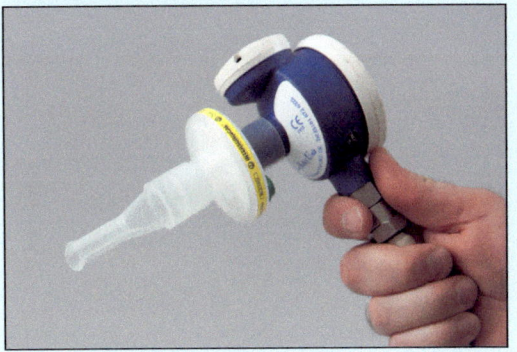

2. Fit a new microbial filter and mouthpiece to the demand valve. They are single use.

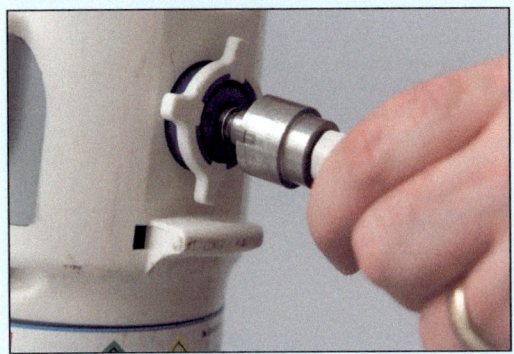

3. Insert the probe on the hose connected to the demand valve into the Schrader outlet on the Entonox cylinder. Push firmly to ensure the probe clicks into place.

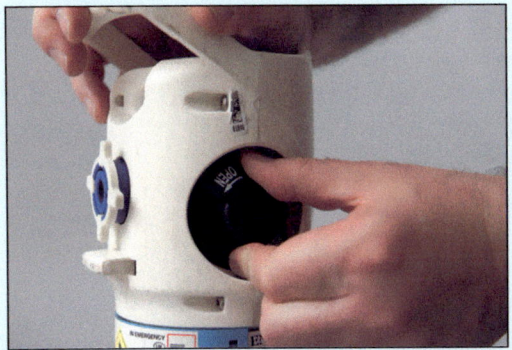

4. Slowly turn the cylinder on by rotating the handwheel anti-clockwise until fully open. Do not use excessive force.

Procedure – Preparing Entonox for administration – *cont*

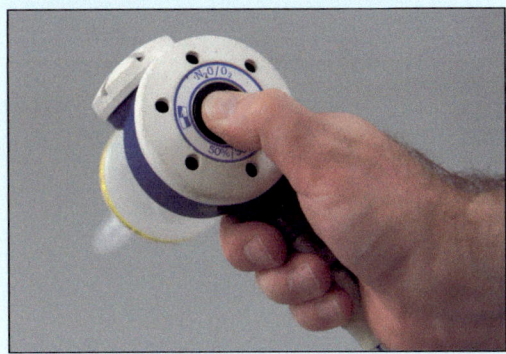

5. Check the demand valve is operative by pushing the 'test button'. You should hear the gas flowing.

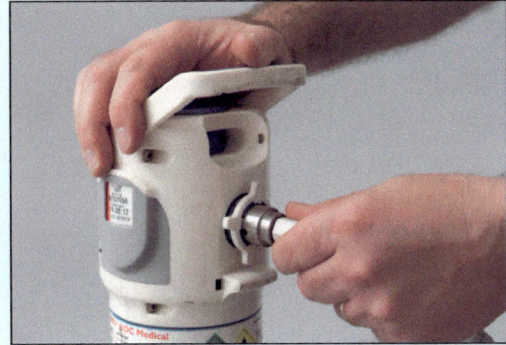

6. Check for leaks, which may be indicated by a hissing sound. If you suspect that you have a leak, turn off the cylinder and check the equipment is properly connected. Turn on the cylinder and recheck for leaks. If the leak continues, turn off and remove the cylinder from service. Report it using your ambulance service equipment defect procedure.

Chapter 12 – Breathing

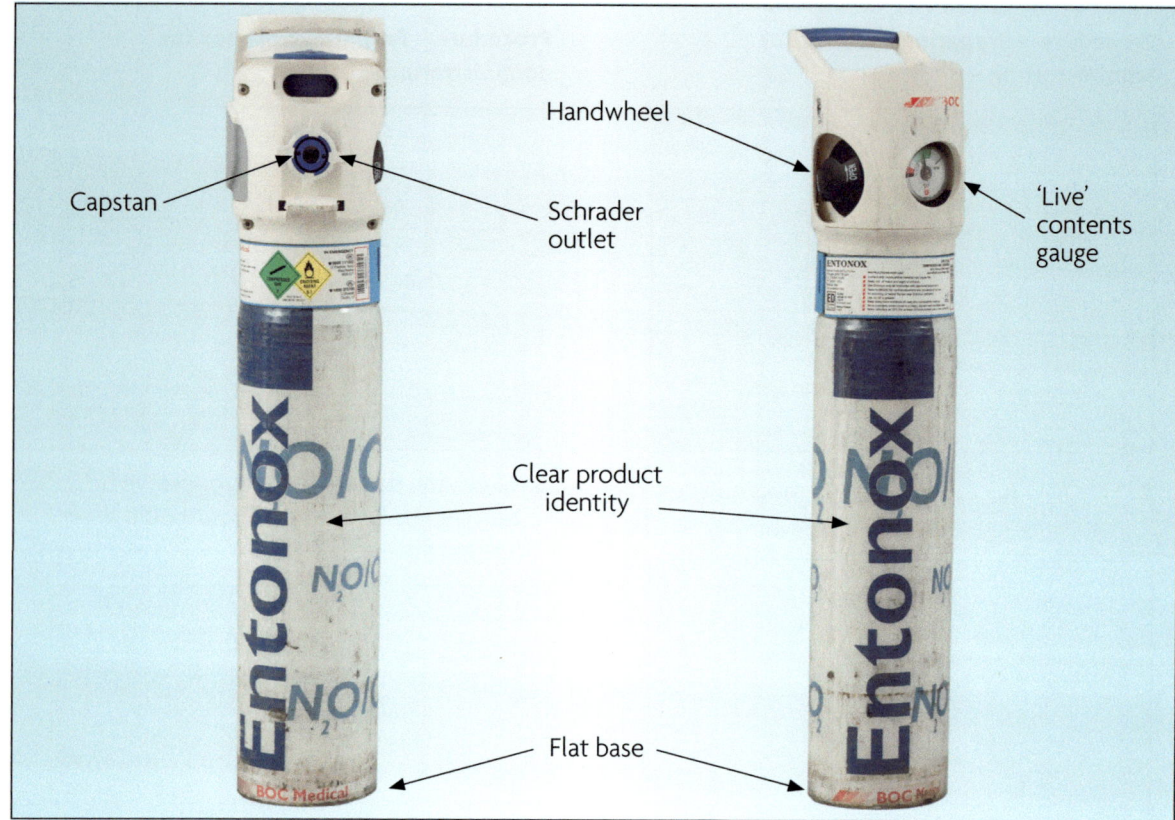

Figure 12.19 An Entonox cylinder.

2.12.2 Entonox administration

The UK Ambulance Services Clinical Practice Guidelines [JRCALC, 2019] for Entonox administration are as follows:

Indications
- Moderate to severe pain.
- Labour pains.

Action
- Inhaled analgesic agent.

Contra-indications
- Severe head injuries with impaired consciousness.
- Decompression sickness (the bends) where Entonox can cause nitrogen bubbles within the bloodstream to expand, aggravating the problem further. Consider anyone who has been diving within the previous 24 hours to be at risk.
- Violently disturbed psychiatric patients.
- Intraocular injection of gas within the last four weeks.
- Abdominal pain where intestinal obstruction is suspected.

Caution
- Any patient at risk of having a pneumothorax, pneumomediastinum and/or a pneumo-peritoneum, e.g. polytrauma, penetrating torso injury.

Side-effects
- Minimal side-effects.

Dosage and administration
Adults:
- Entonox should be self-administered via a face mask or mouthpiece, after suitable instruction. It takes about 3–5 minutes to be effective, but it may be 5–10 minutes before maximum effect is achieved.

Children:
- Entonox is effective in children provided they are capable of following the administration instructions and can activate the demand valve.

Additional information
- Prolonged use for more than 24 hours, or more frequently than every four days, can lead to vitamin B12 deficiency.
- Administration of Entonox should be in conjunction with pain score monitoring.
- Entonox's advantages include:
  - rapid analgesic effect with minimal side-effects
  - no cardio-respiratory depression
  - self-administered
  - analgesic effect rapidly wears off
  - the 50% oxygen concentration is valuable in many medical and trauma conditions.
- Entonox can be administered while preparing to deliver other analgesics.

2.12.3 After use

Procedure – Finishing using Entonox

Take the following steps once the patient has finished using the Entonox [BOC, 2013b]:

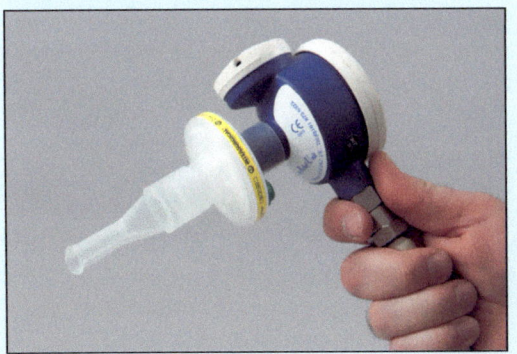

1. Remove the demand valve from the patient. Dispose of the filter and mouthpiece.

Procedure – Finishing using Entonox – *cont*

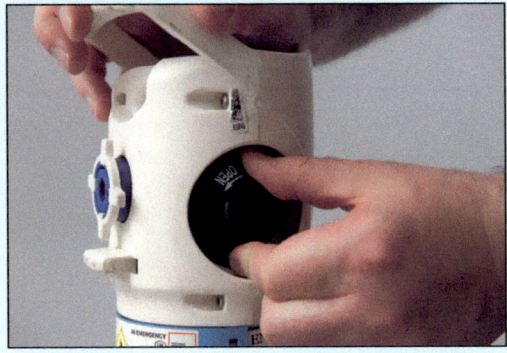

2. Turn off the cylinder by rotating the handwheel clockwise until it comes to a stop. Do not use excessive force.

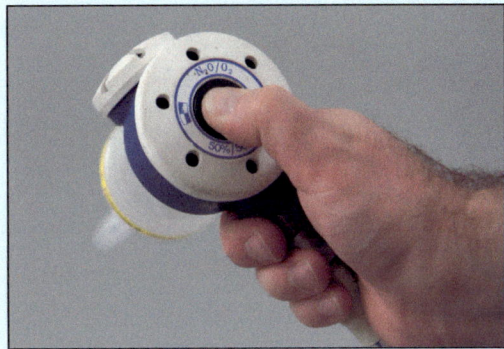

3. Vent any residual gas in the hose by pressing the test button on the demand valve. Keep pressing until the gas has stopped venting.

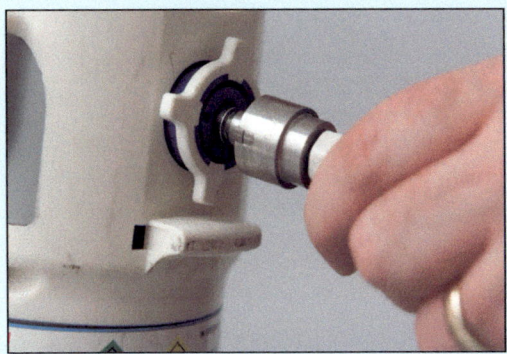

4. Disconnect the probe from the cylinder outlet. Holding the probe, twist the capstan and withdraw the probe from the Schrader outlet.

Chapter 12 – Breathing

Procedure – Finishing using Entonox – *cont*

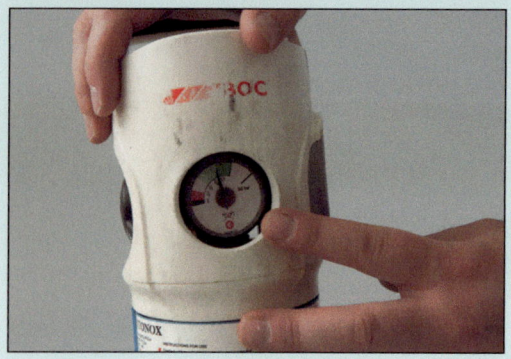

5. Replace the outlet cover by pulling up the hinged grey cover. Check the cylinder gauge and replace if empty.

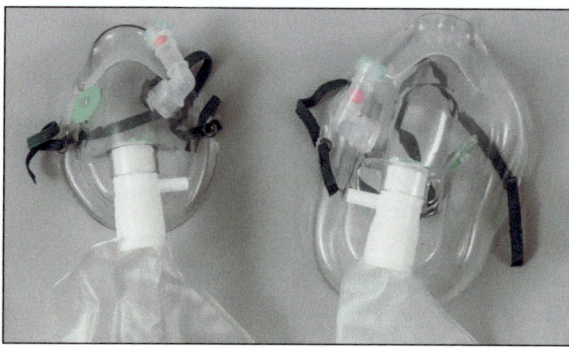

Figure 12.20 Non-rebreathe masks with integral respiratory rate indicator.

Ideally, you want to measure your patient's respiratory rate for a full minute using one of the following techniques [Gregory, 2010b]:
- Watching the chest rise and fall.
- Counting the respiratory rate while listening to the chest with a stethoscope.
- Using an oxygen mask with an integral respiratory rate indicator (Figure 12.20).
- Monitor the end-tidal CO_2 trace.

3 Assessment of breathing

3.1 Learning objectives

By the end of this section you will be able to:
- record the following observations:
  - respiratory rate
  - oxygen saturations
  - peak flow
  - capnography
- describe how to auscultate the chest.

3.2 Respiratory rate

A normal adult respiratory rate is 12–20 breaths per minute (breaths/minute) [Nolan, 2016].

Patients with a respiratory rate of less than 10 breaths/minute or more than 30 breaths/minute may need assisted ventilation, so inform your senior clinician immediately [JRCALC, 2019].

3.2.1 Measuring respiratory rate

How fast are you breathing now? Before considering this question, it is likely that you weren't even thinking about your respiratory rate. So it is with patients. Don't tell them that you are going to record their respiratory rate!

3.3 Oxygen saturations

Most oxygen is transported around the body bound to haemoglobin in the blood (oxyhaemoglobin), as it travels from the lungs to the body's tissues. Oxygen saturation is the ratio of oxyhaemoglobin to the total amount of haemoglobin and is usually shown as a percentage [Tortora, 2017].

Oxygen saturations are measured in two ways: invasively and non-invasively. In hospital, it is common for patients to have an arterial blood gas sample taken, whereby a small amount of blood from an artery (often the radial) is taken and the arterial oxygen saturation measured (SaO_2). However, this is not practical to undertake outside of hospital, so oxygen saturations are measured non-invasively using a technique known as pulse oximetry (SpO_2) [O'Driscoll, 2017].

3.3.1 Pulse oximetry

Pulse oximetry works by shining red and infrared light through a part of the body that is relatively translucent and has an arterial pulse, such as a finger, toe or earlobe. The amount of light transmitted through the tissue depends on the amount of oxyhaemoglobin present; this enables the pulse oximeter to calculate the oxygen saturation and will also provide the pulse rate. The target oxygen saturation for most patients is 94–98%.

3.3.2 Indications and limitations

Indications

Pulse oximetry is useful for [Gregory, 2010b; Walls, 2012]:
- assessing severity of respiratory illness or injury
- providing early warning of a patient who is deteriorating
- providing feedback about the effectiveness of oxygen therapy
- detecting pulses in limbs that have been fractured.

Limitations

Like any tool, the pulse oximeter can produce inaccurate results, particularly in the presence of the following [Walls, 2012]:
- **Bright ambient light:** Simple to solve with a towel over the probe.
- **Excessive patient motion:** Such as shivering, convulsions or a bumpy ambulance ride.
- **Poor perfusion:** Since the pulse oximeter requires an arterial pulse to work, conditions that result in poor peripheral perfusion can lead to problems. Examples include patients in shock, cardiac arrest and those who are cold.
- **Nail varnish/polish:** Some dark-coloured nail varnish can affect the accuracy of pulse oximeters, although this is not likely to be too serious. Finger probes can be rotated 90° if this is a worry, but if a reliable and consistent reading is being obtained through nail varnish, then the reading is probably accurate [Chan, 2003; Hinkelbein, 2007].
- **Low blood pressure:** Pulse oximetry becomes more inaccurate as the systolic blood pressure drops below 80 mmHg.
- **Abnormal haemoglobin:** Other molecules can attach themselves to haemoglobin and create an artificially high oxygen saturation reading. Carbon monoxide is probably the most well-known, so don't be reassured by a high oxygen saturation in a patient who is a victim of smoke inhalation, for example.
- **Response time:** Pulse oximetry is not instantaneous; typically, a reading can take up to 20 seconds depending upon the patient's physiological state. Probes closer to the heart (such as one sited on an earlobe) usually respond faster than probes on fingers and toes.

3.3.3 Recording oxygen saturations

Procedure – To record a patient's oxygen saturations

Take the following steps to record a patient's oxygen saturations [WHO, 2011]:

1. Turn the pulse oximeter on.
2. Select the appropriate probe with particular attention to correct sizing and where it will go (usually the finger, toe or ear). If used on a finger or toe, make sure the area is clean. Consider removing nail varnish, or rotate the probe 90°.
3. Connect the probe to the pulse oximeter.
4. Position the probe carefully; make sure it fits easily without being too loose or too tight. If possible, avoid the arm being used for blood pressure monitoring as cuff inflation will interrupt the pulse oximeter signal.
5. Allow several seconds for the pulse oximeter to detect the pulse and calculate the oxygen saturation.
6. Look for the displayed pulse indicator that shows that the machine has detected a pulse. Without a pulse signal, any readings are not reliable.

Chapter 12 – Breathing

> **Procedure – To record a patient's oxygen saturations –** *cont*
>
> 7. Once the unit has detected a good pulse, the oxygen saturation and pulse rate will be displayed.
> 8. Like all machines, oximeters may occasionally give a false reading – if in doubt, rely on clinical judgement rather than the machine
> 9. If in doubt, check the pulse oximeter is working properly by placing it on your own finger.

3.4 Peak flow

The measurement of the peak expiratory flow rate (PEFR or PEF), or peak flow, is common in patients with obstructive airways diseases such as asthma and chronic obstructive pulmonary disease (COPD). You should record an asthmatic patient's peak flow before and after treatment, assuming they are capable of undertaking the technique (Figure 12.21) [JRCALC, 2019].

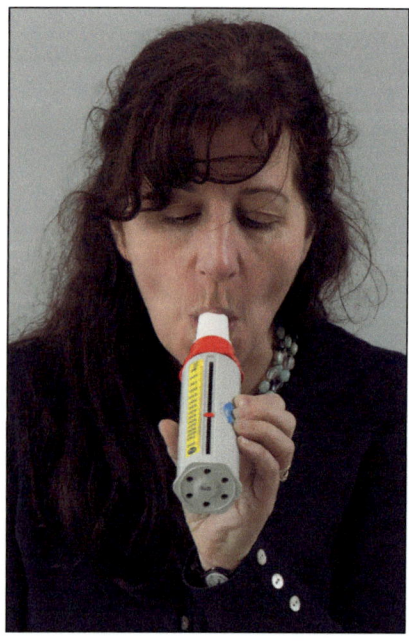

Figure 12.21 A patient providing a peak flow reading.

3.4.1 Procedure

> **Procedure – To record a peak flow**
>
> Take the following steps to record a peak flow [CCI, 2017; Booker, 2007]:
>
> 1. Explain the procedure to the patient before starting and ask if they know what their normal or best peak flow value is. You can use the normal value chart (Figure 12.22), but a comparison with the patient's usual value is better.
> 2. Insert the mouthpiece into the meter (these are single patient use).
> 3. Ask the patient to hold the peak flow meter with their fingers clear of the scale and slot. Ensure that the holes at the end of the meter are not blocked.
> 4. With the patient in a standing, or upright sitting, position, ask them to take a deep breath.
> 5. Ask them to place the peak flow meter in their mouth and hold horizontally, closing their lips around the mouthpiece before blowing as hard and fast as they can. This should be a short, sharp 'huff'.
> 6. Note the number on the scale indicated by the pointer.
> 7. Return the pointer to zero and repeat steps 3–6 twice to obtain three readings.
> 8. The patient's peak flow is the highest of the three readings.

Common errors in recording a peak flow measurement
- Failure to take a deep breath.
- The patient holding their breath and not expiring into the flow meter straight a.way.
- Blocking the mouthpiece with the teeth or tongue
- Air leaking around the mouthpiece due to blowing the cheeks out, loose-fitting teeth or facial palsy.

Assessment of breathing

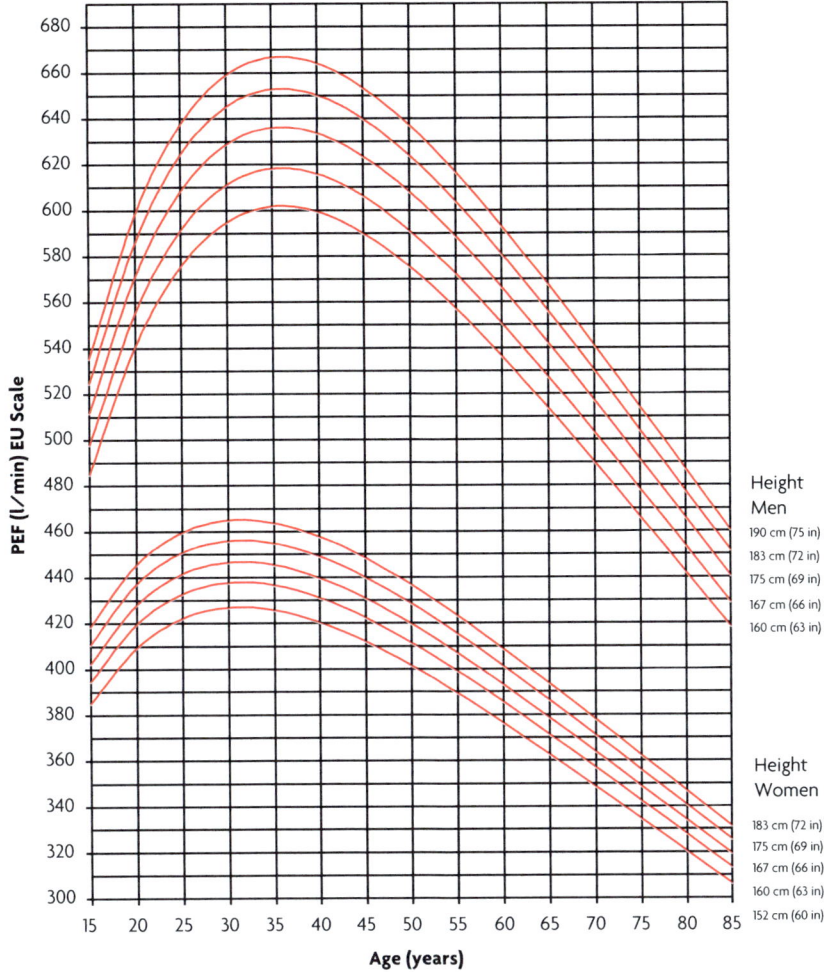

Figure 12.22 Normal peak flow values.
Source: Adapted by Clement Clarke for use with EN13826/EU scale peak flow meters from Nunn AJ Gregg I, *Br Med J* 1989:298;1068–70.

3.5 Capnography

Carbon dioxide (CO_2) is a waste gas that is expired. It is a normal by-product of body metabolism and the quantity expired is dependent on metabolism, venous return to the heart and the pulmonary circulation (carrying blood to, from and around the lungs). Expired CO_2 can provide an insight into all three of these.

3.5.1 Terminology

A number of terms are related to expired CO_2 monitoring, and these are sometimes used incorrectly, which can cause confusion. These are:

- **Capnography:** The measurement of carbon dioxide in exhaled breath.
- **Capnometry:** A numerical measurement of exhaled carbon dioxide. Usually this is the amount of expired CO_2 at the end of expiration and is known as the end-tidal CO_2 (EtCO_2).
- **Capnogram:** A waveform illustrating the measurement of carbon dioxide across time and with a height corresponding to the quantity of carbon dioxide exhaled.

3.5.2 Uses for capnography

The ability to measure EtCO_2 has a number of uses in the ambulance service including [Helm, 2003; Burton, 2006; Pokorná, 2010]:

- preventing hyper- and hypoventilation of head-injured patients

- giving early warning of respiratory distress or failure in patients who have received sedative drugs (such as epileptic patients who have been given diazepam by paramedics)
- helping to confirm the correct positioning of an endotracheal tube or supraglottic airway device
- indicating a return of spontaneous circulation (ROSC) of a patient who has been in cardiac arrest.

Note: A normal $EtCO_2$ measurement is usually in the range of 35–45 mmHg (4.7–6.0 kPa) although is likely to be lower during CPR.

3.5.3 The capnogram

Figure 12.23 shows a typical, normal waveform that appears during a patient's respiratory cycle. $EtCO_2$ waveforms have two axes, with the x-axis representing time and the y-axis CO_2 concentration. Examples of abnormal capnograms can be seen in Table 12.5.

3.6 Auscultation

Auscultation is the technique of listening to the sounds inside the body, most commonly with the help of a stethoscope.

3.6.1 The stethoscope

In 1816, René-Théophile-Hyacinthe Laennec (a French doctor) needed to examine the chest of a young woman. At the time, the technique of listening for breath sounds was placing your ear on the patient's chest, a practice that is now generally frowned upon. In respect of his patient being a young woman, he rolled up some paper into a tube and discovered that he could hear the woman's heart sounds much more clearly than by direct auscultation [Thadepalli, 2002].

With experimentation, he developed his discovery into a wooden cylinder, which he called a stethoscope. Many of the terms in use today in relation to breath sounds come from Laennec,

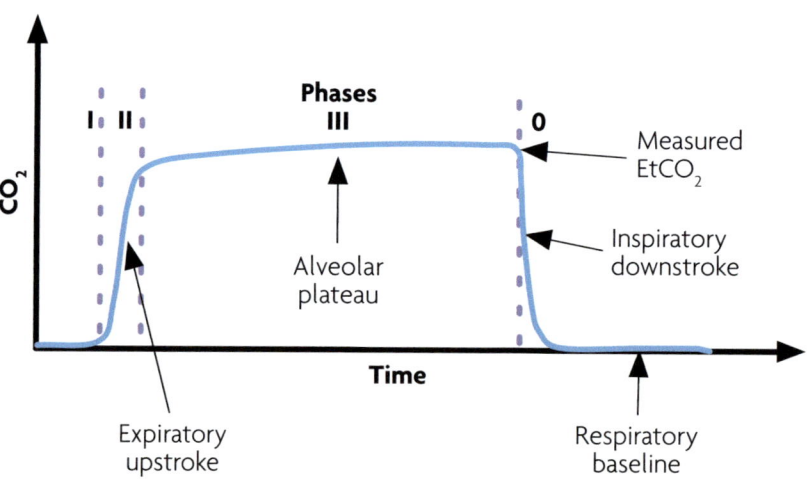

Figure 12.23 A normal capnogram.

Key:
- **I** The flat baseline represents exhalation and so should not contain any CO_2 (i.e. should be at 0 mmHg). It is the gas from the dead air space of the bronchiole tree.
- **II** Expiratory upstroke. This represents the mixing of dead air space and exhaled CO_2 from the lungs.
- **III** Plateau phase. The exhalation of alveolar gas is represented as a slow rise until the sudden descent in the waveform that marks inspiration. It is just prior to the sudden descent that the $EtCO_2$ is measured, as this is the end of alveolar emptying and closely mirrors the partial pressure of pulmonary CO_2.
- **0** Inspiratory downstroke. This represents gaseous mixing and levels of CO_2 decline as a new breath is taken with fresh air.

Assessment of breathing

Table 12.5 Abnormal capnograms.

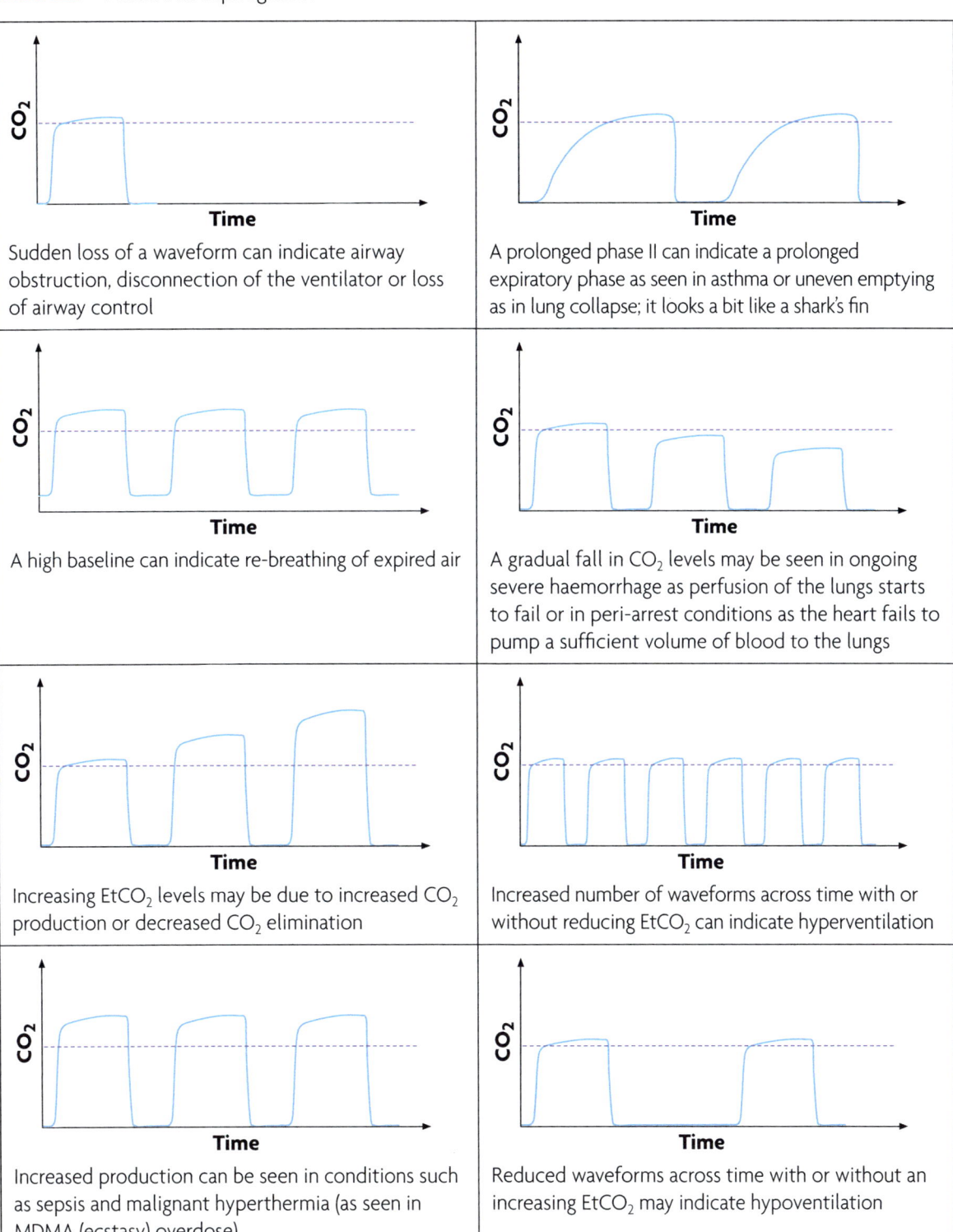

Chapter 12 – Breathing

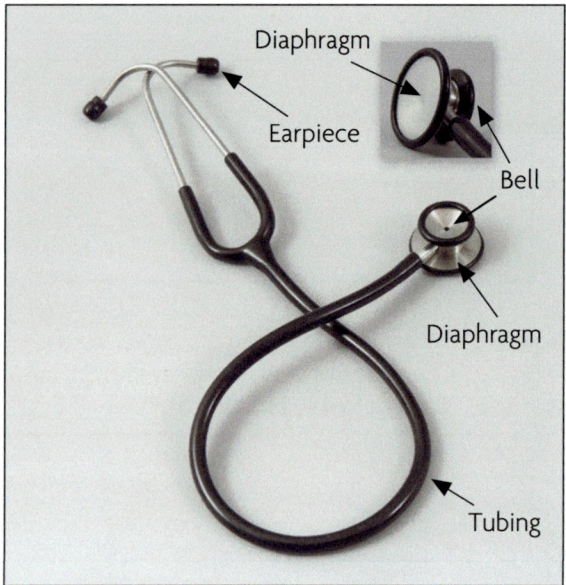

Figure 12.24   A stethoscope.

including pectoriloquy, crepitation (now more commonly called crackles) and rub. Laennec's wooden stethoscope design continued to be used until the mid-19th century, when rubber tubing was developed. However, not until 1925 did the bell and diaphragm design, typically found in modern stethoscopes, come into use after being developed by Bowles and Sprague (Figure 12.24) [Roguin, 2006].

3.6.2 Breath sounds

There are broadly two types of breath sounds you will hear on auscultation: normal and added (or adventitious).

Normal breath sounds

These sounds are caused by turbulent airflow in large airways and are loudest at the trachea at the start of inspiration, and quietest at the end of inspiration, as airflow decreases. If you auscultate elsewhere on the chest, the sound diminishes as it passes through the lung tissue and the chest wall itself [Macleod, 2005]. Normal breath sounds are often split into three sub-types:

- **Vesicular:** These are soft and low-pitched and can be heard throughout inspiration and the first third of expiration [Bickley, 2006]. They have been described as the sound of wind rustling through leaves [Talley, 2006].
- **Bronchial:** These breath sounds have a high-pitched and hollow or blowing quality, similar to the sound you hear by placing a stethoscope over the trachea. Bronchial breath sounds are similar in duration during both inspiration and expiration, with a gap in between as airflow slows prior to changing direction [Macleod, 2005].
- **Bronchovesicular:** These breath sounds are louder than vesicular, but quieter than bronchial sounds. Inspiratory and expiratory duration are typically the same, but unlike bronchial sounds, there may not be a gap between the two.

Added (adventitious) sounds

There are two types of added sounds: crackles and wheezes.

- **Crackles:** These are interrupted, non-musical sounds, formerly called rales or crepitations [Talley, 2006]. Usually, they are caused by the re-opening of collapsed alveoli and small bronchi. The timing and pitch of crackles can provide clues as to the cause. For example, early inspiratory crackles that are rather coarse in quality suggest small airways disease and are common in chronic obstructive pulmonary disease (COPD) [Piirilä, 1995].
  - Fine crackles that occur late in inspiration are typically caused by pulmonary fibrosis, whereas coarser crackles late in inspiration are more suggestive of left-sided heart failure.
  - Crackles can also be heard when air bubbles through secretions in the major bronchi, or the dilated bronchi of bronchiectasis. These are usually very coarse, may be heard without a stethoscope and will typically resolve or change location on coughing [Buss, 2010].
- **Wheezes:** These are continuous, musical sounds that are caused by air passing through partially obstructed bronchi and are normally only heard on expiration. They can be localised (e.g. in cancer of the lung) or diffuse, as is typical in asthma. Note that wheeze on inspiration is generally taken to be a significant sign of airway

narrowing [Macleod, 2005]. Wheezes can be monophasic, that is at a single pitch (which used to be called rhonchi), or polyphonic, i.e. more musical, due to the sound being produced at different pitches.

- One type of loud monophasic (and usually) inspiratory wheeze that can be heard without a stethoscope is stridor. This is caused by laryngeal spasm and mucosal swelling, which causes vocal cord contraction and airway narrowing [Buss, 2010].

Absent sounds

Breath sounds are decreased or absent when airflow is limited. This can be due to low inspiratory airflow rates, which generate less turbulent flow required to produce sound. Air or fluid in the pleural space (due to a pneumothorax or pleural effusion, for example) can increase the acoustic impedance and filter or stop transmission of breath sounds to the chest wall. This also occurs at the chest wall itself if there is an excessive amount of adipose tissue [Buss, 2010].

3.6.3 Auscultating the chest

Procedure – Auscultating the chest

Ideally, you should expose the patient's chest to perform auscultation, but this will depend on whether you can ensure privacy and adequate environmental heating (such as a warm ambulance). Ensure that you inform the patient about what the procedure involves and obtain consent.

Then take the following steps [Gregory, 2010b]:

1. Ask the patient to take deep breaths in and out through their mouth.
2. Place the diaphragm on the chest, starting above the clavicle. If the patient is very slim or has a hairy chest, use the bell instead.
3. Listen during inspiration and expiration, before moving the stethoscope to another area of the chest.
4. After each breath, move the stethoscope to the opposite side of the chest to compare each part of the lung fields. Listen to the

Procedure – Auscultating the chest – *cont*

anterior (Figure 12.25), posterior (Figure 12.26) and lateral (Figure 12.27) aspects of the chest for normal and adventitious breath sounds.

Hints

It may be helpful to coach the patient to breathe using 'in... and out'.

Avoid long periods of deep breathing as it may cause dizziness. Patients who are short of breath may not be able to comply with your instructions.

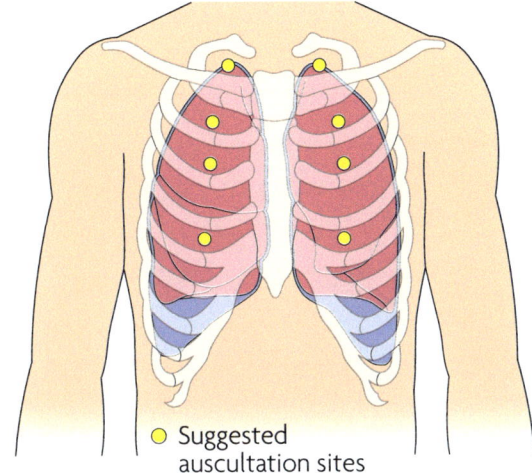

○ Suggested auscultation sites

Figure 12.25 Auscultation sites of the anterior chest.

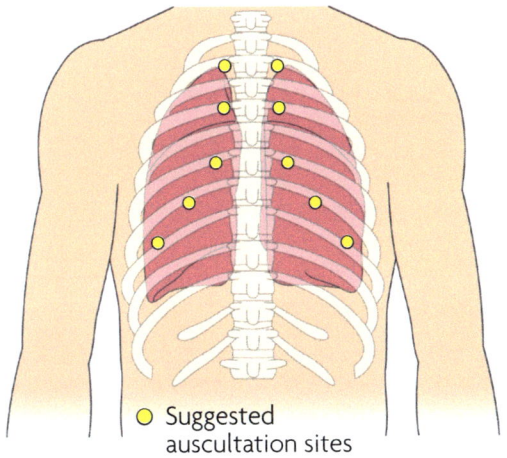

○ Suggested auscultation sites

Figure 12.26 Auscultation sites of the posterior chest.

Chapter 12 – Breathing

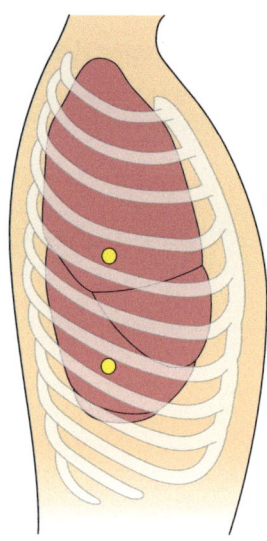

○ Suggested auscultation sites

Figure 12.27 Auscultation sites of the lateral chest.

4 Common respiratory conditions

4.1 Learning objectives

By the end of this section you will be able to:
- describe the following conditions of the respiratory system:
    - asthma
    - chronic obstructive pulmonary disease (COPD)
    - pneumonia
    - pulmonary embolism.

4.2 Asthma

4.2.1 Definition

Asthma is a condition characterised by intermittent, reversible airway obstruction [Simon, 2010].

4.2.2 Pathophysiology

Asthma is caused by a chronic inflammation of the bronchi, making them narrower. The muscles around the bronchi become irritated and contract, causing sudden worsening of the symptoms. The inflammation can also cause the mucous glands to produce excessive sputum which further blocks the air passages.

The obstruction and subsequent wheezing are caused by three factors within the bronchial tree:
- increased production of bronchial mucus
- swelling of the mucosal cells that line the bronchi and bronchioles
- spasm and constriction of bronchial muscles.

These three factors combine to cause blockage and narrowing of the small airways in the lung. Because inspiration is an active process involving the muscles of respiration, the obstruction of the airways is overcome on breathing in. Expiration occurs with muscle relaxation and is severely delayed by the narrowing of the airways in asthma. This generates the wheezing on expiration that is characteristic of this condition.

4.2.3 Medication

Asthma is managed with a variety of inhaled and tablet medications. Inhalers are divided into two broad categories: preventer and reliever.

Preventer
The preventer inhalers are normally anti-inflammatory drugs. These include steroids and other milder anti-inflammatories such as Tilade. The common steroid inhalers are beclomethasone (Becotide), budesonide (Pulmicort) and fluticasone propionate (Flixotide). These drugs act on the smooth muscles of the bronchi and bronchioles over a period of time to reduce the inflammatory reaction that causes the asthma. Regular use of these inhalers often eradicates all symptoms of asthma and allows for a normal lifestyle.

Reliever
The reliever inhalers include salbutamol (Ventolin), terbutaline (Bricanyl), tiotropium bromide (Spiriva) and ipratropium bromide (Atrovent). These inhalers work rapidly on the bronchi and bronchioles to relax the smooth muscle spasm when the patient feels wheezy or tight-chested. They are used in conjunction with preventer inhalers. Inhalers are often used through large plastic spacer devices

Common respiratory conditions

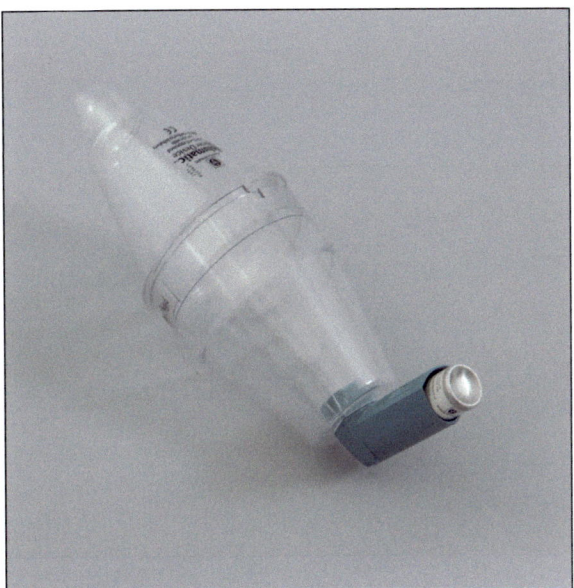

Figure 12.28   An inhaler with a spacer device.

(Figure 12.28). This allows the drug to spread into a larger volume and enables the patient to inhale it more effectively. In mild and moderate asthma attacks some patients may be treated with high doses of 'relievers' through a spacer device [SIGN/BTS, 2016].

4.2.4 Signs and symptoms

History
Patients will typically tell you about increasing shortness of breath with wheezing over the past 6–48 hours, with increasing inhaler use. The reliever inhalers may also be proving less effective than normal.

Ask specifically about:
- repeated attendances at ED for asthma care in the past year
- previous admissions for asthma
- previous near-fatal asthma, e.g. previously required ventilation/intensive care
- heavy use of reliever inhalers
- brittle asthma.

Assessment of severity
The signs and symptoms of asthma are organised according to their severity [SIGN/BTS, 2016]. Table 12.6 shows the broad categories of asthma severity, which in turn will determine the most appropriate interventions for your patient [JRCALC, 2019].

4.2.5 Medication
The indications and contra-indications listed below are taken from the UK Ambulance Services Clinical Practice Guidelines [JRCALC, 2019]. However, you should be familiar with your own service guidelines as restrictions on administration may exist.

Salbutamol

Presentation
- Nebules containing either salbutamol 2.5 mg in 2.5 ml or 5 mg in 2.5 ml.

Actions
- Salbutamol is a selective beta-2 adrenoreceptor stimulant drug. This has a relaxant effect on the smooth muscle in the medium and smaller airways, which are in spasm in acute asthma attacks. If given by nebuliser, especially if oxygen-powered, its smooth muscle-relaxing action, combined with the airway-moistening effect of nebulisation, can relieve the attack rapidly.

Indications
- Acute asthma attack where normal inhaler therapy has failed to relieve symptoms.
- Expiratory wheeze associated with allergy, anaphylaxis, smoke inhalation or other lower airway cause.
- Exacerbation of chronic obstructive pulmonary disease (COPD).

Contra-indications
- None in the emergency situation.

Cautions
- Salbutamol should be used with care in patients with:
  - hypertension
  - angina
  - overactive thyroid
  - late pregnancy (can relax uterus).
- Severe hypertension may occur in patients on beta-blockers and half doses should be used unless there is profound hypotension.
- If COPD is a possibility, limit nebulisation to six minutes if using oxygen.

Chapter 12 – Breathing

Table 12.6 Assessing asthma severity.

Mild	Moderate	Severe	Life-threatening
PEF > 75% of best or predicted	PEF > 50–75% of best or predicted	PEF 33–50% of best or predicted	PEF < 33% of best or predicted
$SpO_2 \geq 92\%$	$SpO_2 \geq 92\%$	$SpO_2 \geq 92\%$	$SpO_2 < 92\%$
	Adults: Respiratory rate < 25 breaths/minute Heart rate < 110 beats/minute	**Adults:** Respiratory rate ≥ 25 breaths/minute Heart rate ≥ 110 beats/minute Cannot complete sentence in one breath	**Adults:** Silent chest Poor respiratory effort Exhaustion Altered conscious level Cyanosis Arrhythmia Hypotension
	Children > 5 years Able to talk Respiratory rate ≤ 30 breaths/minute Heart rate ≤ 125 beats/minute	**Children > 5 years** Too breathless to talk Using accessory neck muscles Respiratory rate > 30 breaths/minute Heart rate > 125 beats/minute	**Children > 5 years** Silent chest Poor respiratory effort Agitation Confusion Cyanosis
	Children 2–5 years Able to talk Respiratory rate ≤ 40 breaths/minute Heart rate ≤ 140 beats/minute	**Children 2–5 years** Too breathless to talk Using accessory neck muscles Respiratory rate > 40 breaths/minute Heart rate > 140 beats/minute	**Children 2–5 years** Silent chest Poor respiratory effort Agitation Confusion Cyanosis
	Children < 2 years Audible wheezing Using accessory muscles Still feeding	**Children < 2 years** Cyanosis Marked respiratory distress Too breathless to feed	**Children < 2 years** Apnoea or poor respiratory effort Bradycardia

Note: Only one sign or symptom is required to qualify a patient for a higher severity. For example, an SpO_2 of 91% would place a patient in the life-threatening column, irrespective of other observations.

Side-effects
- Tremor (shaking)
- Tachycardia
- Palpitations
- Headache
- Feeling of tension
- Peripheral vasodilatation
- Muscle cramps
- Rash.

Dosage and administration
- Nebulise with oxygen running at 6–8 l/minute.
- Repeat doses can be administered at an interval of five minutes between doses.
- Six years and above: 5 mg.
- One month to under six years: 2.5 mg.
- Birth: not applicable.

Ipratropium bromide

The indications and contra-indications listed below are taken from the UK Ambulance Services Clinical Practice Guidelines [JRCALC, 2019]. However, you should be familiar with your own service guidelines as restrictions on administration may exist.

Presentation
- Nebules containing ipratropium bromide 250 micrograms in 1 ml or 500 micrograms in 2 ml.

Indications
- Acute severe or life-threatening asthma.
- Acute asthma unresponsive to salbutamol.
- Exacerbation of chronic obstructive pulmonary disease (COPD), unresponsive to salbutamol.

Actions
- Ipratropium bromide is an anti-muscarinic bronchodilator drug. It may provide short-term relief in acute asthma, but beta-2 agonists (such as salbutamol) generally work more quickly.
- Ipratropium is considered of greater benefit in:
  - children suffering from acute asthma
  - adults suffering with COPD.

Contra-indications
- None in the emergency situation.

Cautions
- Ipratropium should be used with care in patients with:
  - glaucoma (protect the eyes from mist)
  - pregnancy and breastfeeding
  - prostatic hyperplasia.
- If COPD is a possibility, limit nebulisation to six minutes.

Side-effects
- Nausea and vomiting.
- Dry mouth (common).
- Tachycardia/arrhythmia.

- Paroxysmal tightness of the chest.
- Allergic reaction.

Dosage and administration
- Nebulise with oxygen running at 6–8 l/minute.
- There is no repeat dose for this drug.
- 12 years and above: 500 mcg.
- 18 months to 11 years: 250 mcg.
- One month to under 18 months: 125–250 mcg.
- Birth: not applicable.

4.2.6 Management

The management of asthma depends on the assessment of severity and the patient's response to treatment (Figure 12.29) [JRCALC, 2019]. In some cases, it may be appropriate to leave patients at home. However, it is vital that the 'red flags' that identify higher-risk patients are considered and those patients are transported to hospital [SIGN/BTS, 2016]. Red flags include:
- still having significant symptoms
- concerns about compliance
- living alone/socially isolated
- psychological problems
- previous near-fatal or brittle asthma
- exacerbation despite adequate dose of steroid tablets already being taken
- presentation at night (due to circadian variation, most common around 04:00)
- pregnancy.

For patients who are safe to be left at home (see Figure 12.29), a short course of steroids has been shown to reduce mortality, relapses, subsequent hospital admission and requirement for beta-2 agonist therapy. This is typically a five-day course of prednisolone [SIGN/BTS, 2016].

Life-threatening asthma
As respiration fails, patients may require assisted ventilation with a bag-valve-mask. Note that increased inflation pressures are likely to be needed to overcome the severe bronchospasm of the lungs. Ideally, these patients need to be intubated by a senior clinician. A critical care paramedic or doctor may also be able to administer additional medications such as IV salbutamol of magnesium sulphate. If the condition is life-threatening call for specialist support early.

Chapter 12 – Breathing

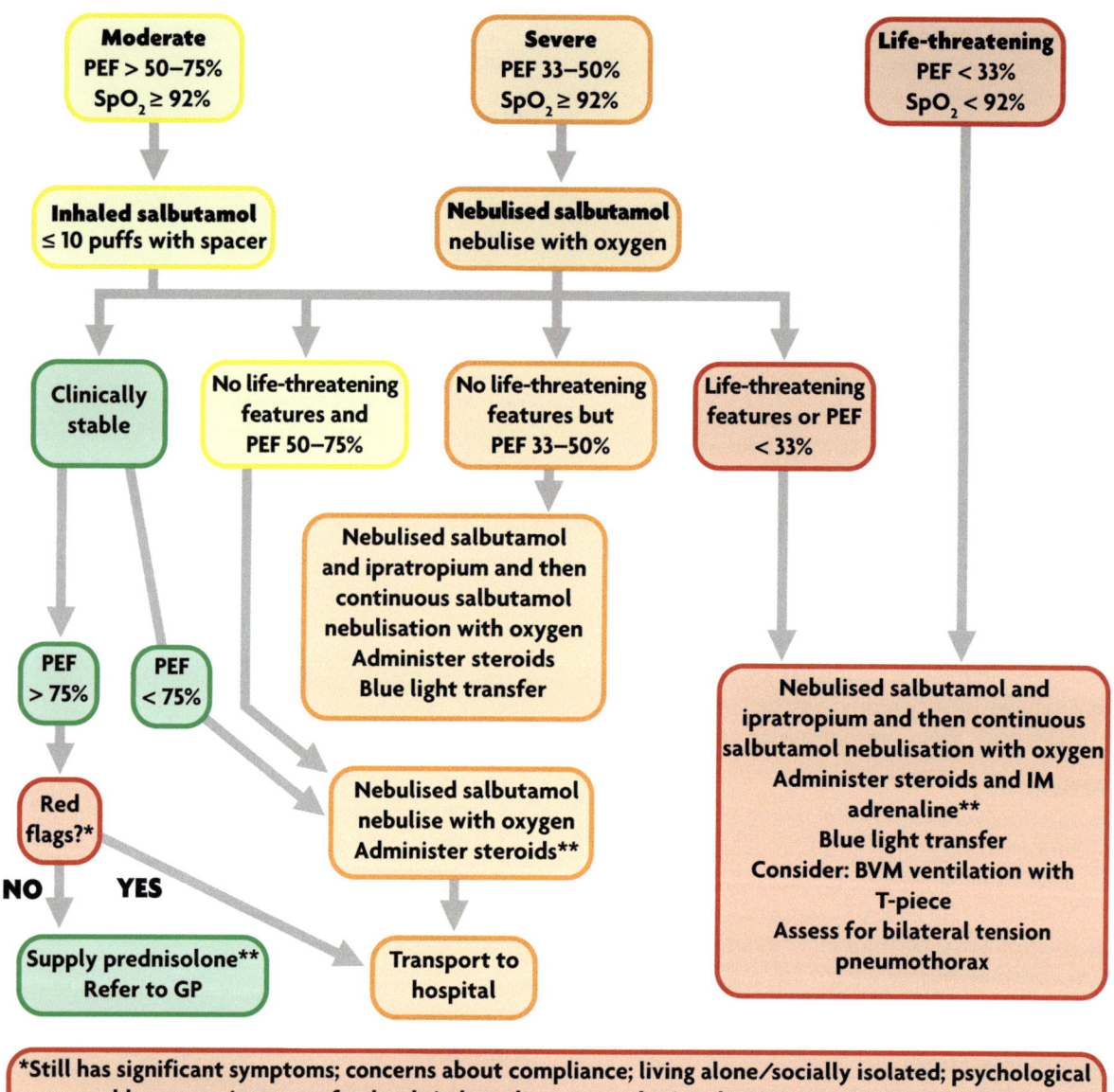

Figure 12.29 Management algorithm for acute asthma.

4.3 Chronic obstructive pulmonary disease

4.3.1 Definitions

Chronic obstructive pulmonary disease (COPD) is an umbrella term for a range of respiratory diseases that result in airflow obstruction. This obstruction is usually progressive and, unlike asthma, is not fully reversible and does not change markedly over several months [NICE, 2018].

The two most important respiratory diseases related to COPD are chronic bronchitis and emphysema. Chronic bronchitis is defined clinically as a persistent cough with sputum production for at least three months of the year for two consecutive years [Hickin, 2015]. Emphysema, on the other hand, is a permanent enlargement of the air spaces below the terminal bronchioles as a result of the destruction of the alveolar walls.

4.3.2 Pathophysiology
COPD
The most important causative factor in chronic bronchitis and emphysema is smoking, although only 15% of smokers develop COPD [Hickin, 2015]. The general effects of smoking in COPD are:
- Inflammation resulting from activation of inflammatory cells which release substances that trigger an immune system response. This activates enzymes that can damage lung tissue, although normally these are kept in check. However, in COPD, so many enzymes are produced that they overwhelm the neutralising mechanism, and lung tissue is digested and destroyed. This is thought to be particularly important in the development of emphysema.
- Inflammation as a direct result of inhaling oxidants in the cigarette smoke (you may have heard of free radicals) which damage the cells directly.

Both of these mechanisms lead to alveolar destruction and production of excess mucus, which is made worse by the impairment of the respiratory cilia, hair-like projections that line the airways and move debris and mucus upwards and out of the respiratory tract [Tortora, 2017].

Chronic bronchitis
Cigarette smoking, occupational exposure and/or recurrent bronchial infections lead to inflammation that narrows the airways and an increase in mucus secretions coupled with inhibition of the cilia. This in turn leads to the accumulation of secretions and bronchoconstriction due to irritant receptor activation, which also causes the chronic productive cough [Hickin, 2015].

Emphysema
In emphysema, the walls of the alveoli are destroyed by enzymes called proteases. These are usually kept under control by another group of enzymes imaginatively called anti-proteases. Once the balance is upset (due to smoking, for example), destruction of the alveoli occurs, leading to a collapse of the airways, resulting in obstruction. In addition, as the walls of the alveoli are destroyed, bullae (small, blister-like air pockets) form on the lung. If these bullae form, air can directly enter the pleural cavity, causing a pneumothorax and collapse of the lung on the affected side [Hickin, 2015].

4.3.3 Oxygen and COPD
Research studies and audits suggest that over-oxygenation increases mortality and morbidity, but careful pre-hospital titration of oxygen administration to patients with COPD can significantly reduce mortality [Austin, 2010]. This is why the oxygen guidelines recommend titrating oxygen administration to patients with COPD between 88–92% [O'Driscoll, 2017].

4.3.4 Signs and symptoms
Patients will usually call for an ambulance during an acute infective exacerbation (sudden worsening) of their COPD.

Features of an acute infective exacerbation of COPD include [JRCALC, 2019]:
- increased dyspnoea
- increased sputum production/purulence (containing pus)
- increased cough
- upper airway symptoms, such as cold and sore throat
- increased wheeze
- reduced exercise tolerance
- fluid retention
- increased fatigue
- acute confusion
- worsening of previously stable condition.

Features that warn of a severe episode of COPD include [JRCALC, 2019]:
- marked dyspnoea
- tachypnoea
- purse-lip breathing
- use of accessory muscles
- acute confusion
- new-onset cyanosis
- new-onset peripheral oedema
- marked reduction in activities of daily living.

Despite the lists above, it is not always clear that the patient with difficulty breathing has COPD. Therefore, you should consider this as a possibility for any patient who meets the following criteria [NICE, 2018]:
- over 35 years of age
- smoker (or ex-smoker)
- have any of the following symptoms:
  - exertional breathlessness
  - chronic cough
  - regular sputum production
  - frequent winter 'bronchitis'
  - wheeze.

4.3.5 Management
The management of the patient with COPD depends on the presence of any time-critical features:
- major ABCD problems
- extreme breathing difficulty (compared to normal)
- cyanosis (although peripheral cyanosis can be normal)
- exhaustion
- hypoxia unresponsive to oxygen (in COPD patients hypoxia is considered to be an SpO_2 below 88%).

These patients require a blue-light transfer to the nearest emergency department and may also require suction, airway management and assisted ventilation. Follow the advice of your senior clinician [JRCALC, 2019].

For patients with no time-critical features, you should ask if they have a treatment plan and follow this, if available. Treatments typically include [JRCALC, 2019]:
- **Oxygen:** Target range of 88–92%. Venturi masks are a good choice for delivering accurate percentages of oxygen, although nasal cannulae may be better tolerated by patients. If you are using a Venturi mask and the patient's respiratory rate is greater than 30 breaths/minute, remember to increase the recommended flow rate by 50%. So if the flow rate should be set at 4 l/minute, then increase this to 6 l/minute.
- **Bronchodilators:** Salbutamol and ipratropium (once only). If the nebuliser is powered by oxygen, nebulisation should be limited to six minutes.
- Patients may need taking to hospital, but depending on how well they respond to treatment, they may be suitable for referral to their GP, respiratory team or advanced paramedic.

4.4 Pneumonia
4.4.1 Definition
Pneumonia is an infection of the terminal bronchioles and alveoli [Hickin, 2015]. It is more common in the elderly and during the winter months [Simon, 2010]. It is often classified in three main ways, although the first is the most commonly used [Dunn, 2005; Osler, 2012]:
- **Setting:** i.e. hospital- or community-acquired pneumonia.
- **Anatomy:** Lobar, if the infection is localised to a lobe of the lung, or bronchopneumonia if the infection is more widespread.
- **Organism:** Bacterial, viral or fungal.

4.4.2 Risk factors for community-acquired pneumonia (CAP)
These are factors that undermine the lung's natural defences and so increase the risk of pneumonia [Hickin, 2015]:
- excessive alcohol
- cigarette smoking
- chronic heart and lung diseases
- bronchial obstruction
- immunosuppression (e.g. due to chemotherapy for cancer)
- drug abuse.

4.4.3 Pathophysiology
This inflammatory process is typically due to a bacterial or viral infection, which has usually entered the lungs having been inhaled from the environment or nasopharynx. Normally, these organisms should be destroyed by the body's lung defences, but infection results if they survive and multiply. This leads to a build-up of fluid and

blood cells (red and white) in the alveoli, known as consolidation [Porth, 2014].

4.4.4 Signs and symptoms

When taking a history, the following symptoms are suggestive of pneumonia [Johnson, 2012]:
- fever with or without rigors
- cough (often productive with green, blood-stained or rusty-coloured sputum)
- pleuritic chest pain
- muscle or joint pain
- when examining a patient you may notice the following signs:
  - high temperature (pyrexia)
  - increased respiratory rate (tachypnoea)
  - increased heart rate (tachycardia)
  - chest sounds such as those shown in Figure 12.30.

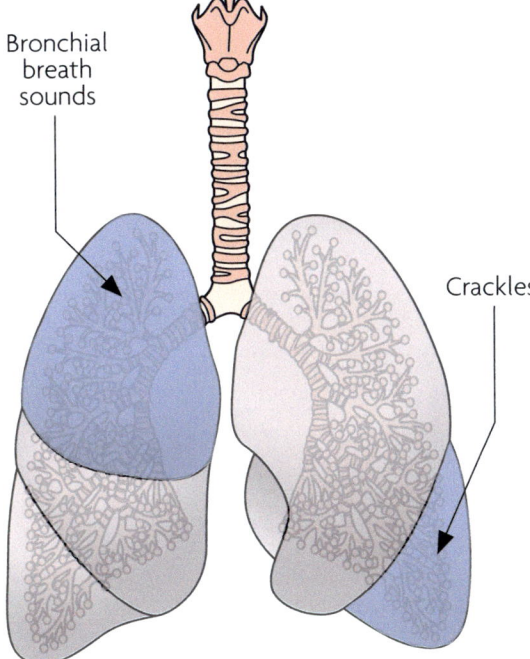

Figure 12.30 Breath sounds in the patient with pneumonia.

4.4.5 Management

Not all patients with pneumonia need to go to hospital. Patients who score a zero on the CRB-65 severity score may be able to be managed at home [BTS, 2010; NICE, 2016a].

CRB-65 severity score
Patients score one point for each of the following:
- confusion
- respiratory rate of 30 breaths/minute or greater
- blood pressure (BP): systolic BP less than 90 mmHg or diastolic BP 60 mmHg or lower
- age: 65 years or older.

You must also consider their social circumstances and home support provision if these patients are to be left at home.

Depending on local arrangements, your senior clinician may refer patients to their own GP or to an advanced practitioner in the ambulance service for further assessment.

Advice
If patients are to remain at home, they should be advised not to smoke, to rest and to drink plenty of fluids. Pleuritic pain can be managed with simple analgesia such as paracetamol.

Transport
Any patient who scores two or more on the CRB-65 severity score should go to hospital. Treatment is supportive and patients should be given oxygen if their SpO_2 is below 94% [JRCALC, 2019].

4.5 Pulmonary embolism

4.5.1 Definition

An embolus is a blood-borne substance (including air) that is transported from one part of the circulation to another, lodging in a vessel that is too small to allow the embolus to pass. When the embolus lodges in the pulmonary vessels, it is termed a pulmonary embolism (PE) [Hickin, 2015]. Deep vein thrombosis (DVT) and pulmonary embolism represent the spectrum of one disease known as venous thromboembolism (VTE) [Tapson, 2008]. Although an embolus can consist of air, fat or amniotic fluid, for example, the most common is a clot from a DVT [Porth, 2014; Konstantinides, 2014].

4.5.2 Risk factors

The risk factors for developing a venous thromboembolism are well known and can

help to identify patients who may have a PE [Konstantinides, 2014]:
- High risk:
  - fracture (hip or leg)
  - major general surgery
  - major trauma
  - spinal cord injury.
- Moderate risk:
  - chronic heart or respiratory failure
  - chemotherapy
  - hormone replacement therapy
  - cancer
  - oral contraceptive therapy
  - paralytic stroke
  - post-partum
  - previous VTE
  - thrombophilia.
- Low risk:
  - bed rest for more than three days
  - immobility due to sitting (e.g. prolonged car or air travel)
  - increasing age
  - obesity
  - pregnancy
  - varicose veins.

4.5.3 Pathophysiology

Thrombi (blood clots) most often form in the deep veins of the calf (hence the name, deep vein thrombosis!) and can grow to lengths of 30–50 cm [Tapson, 2008]. The proximal end of the thrombus can extend into the popliteal vein, where the risk of embolisation is greater. Once the thrombus (or a portion) breaks off, it becomes an embolus, travelling up the femoral vein and into the iliac veins. From there it is free to ascend via the inferior vena cava to the heart. It continues into the right atrium, the ventricle and finally into the lungs via the pulmonary trunk and left and right pulmonary arteries (the only arteries to carry deoxygenated blood), which divide and sub-divide until they form capillaries around the alveoli.

In healthy patients, an obstruction of up to 25% of the pulmonary arterial bed will only cause mild respiratory symptoms, such as shortness of breath. Once this increases to 30–50% there will also be cardiovascular compromise, including cardiac arrest. Patients with pre-existing respiratory and/or cardiovascular disease will be symptomatic at much lower percentages [Konstantinides, 2014].

4.5.4 Signs and symptoms

Common signs and symptoms of PE include difficulty breathing (dyspnoea) and rapid breathing (tachypnoea). Pleuritic chest pain is the most common symptom [JRCALC, 2019].

Other signs and symptoms include:
- Signs:
  - respiratory rate greater than 20 breaths/minute
  - pulse rate greater than 100 beats/minute
  - pulse oximeter reading (SpO_2) less than 92% in air
  - signs of a deep vein thrombosis (DVT), which includes pain, swelling and/or tenderness on only one leg, often in the calf [Simon, 2010].
- Symptoms:
  - difficulty breathing (dyspnoea)
  - pleuritic chest pain
  - substernal chest pain
  - cough
  - haemoptysis (blood from the respiratory tract, usually coughed up)
  - syncope (faint).

4.5.5 Management

Patients with suspected PE need swift transport to hospital. Treatment is mainly supportive of the ABCs (airway, breathing and circulation). Place the patient in a position of comfort (often sitting up, unless they have low blood pressure), provide oxygen if required (to maintain the SpO_2 in the range 94–98%) and be prepared for cardiac arrest [JRCALC, 2019].

Chapter 13 Circulation

1 Cardiovascular system anatomy and physiology

1.1 Learning objectives

By the end of this section, you will be able to:
- state the functions of the cardiovascular system
- describe the anatomy and function of the heart
- state the components of the electrical conduction pathway of the heart
- explain the difference between arteries and veins
- describe the stages of the cardiac cycle.

1.2 Introduction

At the most basic level, the cardiovascular system is composed of blood vessels that transport blood around the body thanks to the work of a pump, the heart. The heart is actually two pumps (the ventricles), each with its own reservoir (the atria), which normally serve two different circulations. The right side of the heart pumps blood to the pulmonary circulation, which travels around the lungs enabling the blood to take up oxygen and give up carbon dioxide. This blood then returns to the left side of the heart, where it is pumped into the systemic circulation to be transported all around the body via the largest artery in the body, the aorta. Both these pumps operate simultaneously and, thanks to valves in the heart, in one direction.

The main functions of the cardiovascular system are [Evans, 2012]:
- transport of nutrients, such as oxygen, glucose (sugar), fatty acids and water
- removal of waste products from metabolic processes, such as carbon dioxide, urea and creatine
- hormonal control, by secreting hormones to their target organs (and secreting some of its own)
- regulation of temperature by controlling heat distribution between the core and skin of the body
- reproduction, by producing penile erection and providing nutrition for the unborn foetus
- host defence, by transporting immune cells and other mediators.

1.3 Heart

The heart is relatively small, considering the work it has to do; it is only about the size of your fist. It sits within the mediastinum, a region in the thoracic cavity that extends from the sternum to the vertebral column, and sits between the lungs. About two-thirds of the heart sits to the left of the body's midline. It is cone-shaped, with the pointed apex orientated anteriorly (to the front), inferiorly (downwards) and to the left, and the flat base directed posteriorly (to the back), superiorly (upwards) and to the right [Tortora, 2017].

1.3.1 Pericardium and heart wall

The pericardium is a fibrous sac that surrounds and protects the heart, keeping it fixed within the mediastinum, but allowing for the vigorous contractions required to move blood around the pulmonary and systemic circulations [Tortora, 2017]. The outer, parietal, layer is fixed to the fibrous pericardium, whereas the inner, visceral, layer (also called the epicardium) forms the outer layer of the heart wall.

The wall of the heart is made up of three layers:
- **Epicardium:** Also known as the visceral layer of the pericardium.
- **Myocardium:** The heart muscle, which makes up most of the bulk of the heart and is responsible for the pumping action that moves blood around the body.
- **Endocardium:** The smooth inner layer, which also covers the valves of the heart and is continuous with the innermost lining (endothelium) of the blood vessels attached to the heart.

Chapter 13 – Circulation

1.3.2 Chambers of the heart

The heart has four chambers. The two superior chambers are called atria and the two inferior chambers are called the ventricles (Figure 13.1) [Tortora, 2017; Evans, 2012].

Right atrium

The right atrium receives deoxygenated blood from the body, via large veins called the superior and inferior vena cava, and from the coronary (heart) circulation via the coronary sinus.

It is separated from the left atrium by a thin partition known as the interatrial septum, and from the right ventricle by the tricuspid valve, so called because it is made up of three cusps. This valve is also sometimes referred to as the right atrioventricular valve.

Right ventricle

The right ventricle makes up most of the anterior surface of the heart and receives blood from the right atrium via the tricuspid valve. To prevent this valve from everting (turning inside out like an umbrella in strong winds) during contraction of the ventricles, the valve is anchored by tendon-like cords known as the chordae tendineae, which connect to papillary muscles. Like the atria, the ventricles are separated by a partition, known as the interventricular septum.

Blood leaves the ventricle via the pulmonary valve, where it enters the pulmonary trunk, which splits into the left and right pulmonary arteries. These arteries are unusual because they transport deoxygenated blood.

Left atrium

The left atrium makes up the majority of the base of the heart. Blood enters the atrium from the lungs via four pulmonary veins and exits through the bicuspid (two cusps) valve. This is also known as the mitral valve (because of the valve's resemblance to a bishop's mitre or hat) and the left atrioventricular valve.

Left ventricle

This forms the apex of the heart and also contains the chordae tendineae and papillary muscle assembly to secure the mitral valve. Blood exits via the aortic valve where it travels up the ascending aorta. Some blood leaves here and enters the coronary arteries to provide oxygen and nutrients to the heart itself. The remaining blood is transported throughout the body.

1.3.3 Electrical conduction pathway

In order to ensure an effective pumping action of the heart, there is a network of specialised autorhythmic (self-excitable) muscle cell fibres that trigger co-ordinated muscle contraction (Figure 13.2), forcing blood around the heart chambers in the direction dictated by the heart valves.

Sinoatrial node

The sinoatrial (SA) node is the main pacemaker of the heart and in textbooks is typically shown as a small area of tissue at the junction of the superior vena cava (SVC) with the right atrium. However, electrophysiology studies have shown that the pacemaker site can spontaneously move down the terminal crest of the right atrium, giving rise

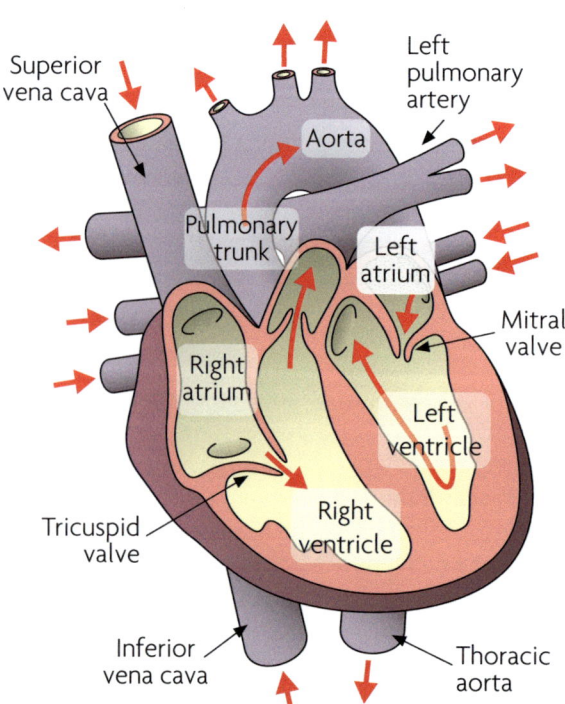

Figure 13.1 Chambers of the heart and related anatomy.

Cardiovascular system anatomy and physiology

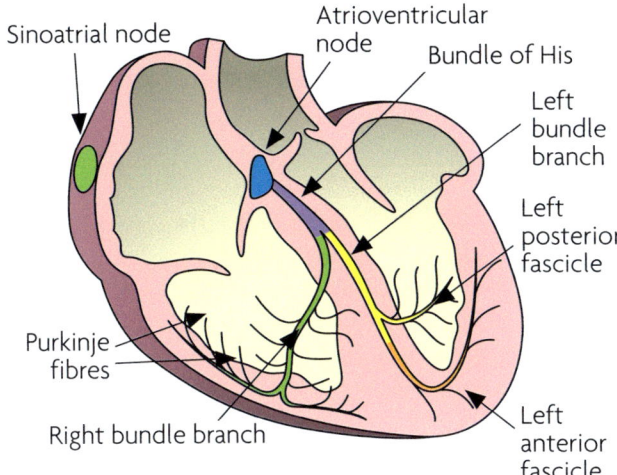

Figure 13.2 The electrical conduction pathway of the heart.

to the phenomenon of the wandering pacemaker and suggesting that there is a much larger area of pacemaker cells [Boyett, 2009].

The SA node is usually supplied by the sinoatrial artery, which branches off the right coronary artery about 50% of the time (it branches off the left circumflex artery the other 50%) [Smithuis, 2008]. Electrical impulses travel from the SA node to the atrioventricular (AV) node and also cross the interatrial septum via a set of specialised cells known as the Bachmann bundle.

Atrioventricular node and bundle of His
The AV node is found in the right atrial wall, close to the opening of the coronary sinus and septal leaflet of the tricuspid valve. Its primary function is to delay the electrical impulse from the SA node long enough for the atria to depolarise, allowing time for atrial muscle contraction to squeeze additional blood into the ventricles (known as the atrial kick). Between the AV node and bundle branches is the bundle of His, which originates in the wall of the right atrium and straddles the interventricular septum. In normal physiology, this is the only way electrical impulses can pass between the atria and ventricles [Garcia, 2015].

Left bundle branch
The left bundle branch starts at the end of the bundle of His, travelling through the interventricular septum, providing fibres that innervate the left ventricle and the left side of the interventricular septum. It splits into two fascicles: anterior and posterior. The left posterior fascicle is a fan-like structure that provides innervation to the posterior and inferior left ventricle via the Purkinje system. Being so widely distributed, it is hard to completely block. The left anterior fascicle, on the other hand, is a single strand, innervating the anterior and superior portions of the left ventricle [Garcia, 2015].

Right bundle branch
The right bundle branch also originates from the bundle of His and sprouts fibres that innervate the right ventricle and right face of the interventricular septum, stimulating the Purkinje fibres. These fibres (named after a Czech physiologist, Jan Purkinje) consist of individual cells located just under the endocardium, and directly innervate myocardial cells causing them to depolarise [Boyett, 2009].

1.3.4 Coronary arteries
The heart requires its own blood supply in order to function properly. There are two main arteries that serve the heart: the right and left coronary arteries, which originate at the base of the ascending aorta (Figure 13.3).

Right coronary artery
The right coronary artery (RCA) runs down the right side of the heart in the coronary sulcus (depression) between the right atrium and ventricle. Most people (around 80%) are right dominant; the RCA gives rise to the posterior descending artery (PDA). In around

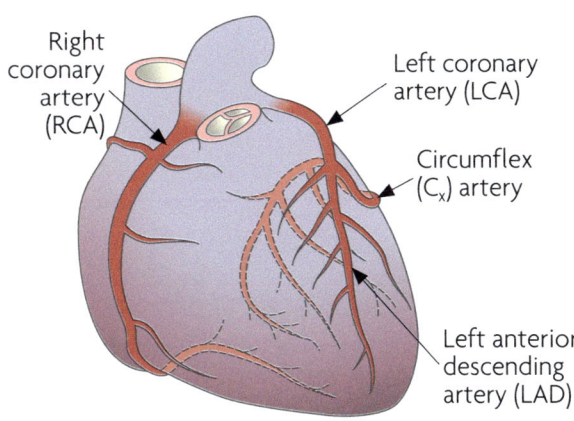

Figure 13.3 Coronary artery anatomy.

8%, this artery arises from the left circumflex (Cx) artery (termed left dominance), with the remainder (12%) being served by both arteries [Goldberg, 2007]. The PDA serves the inferior wall of the left ventricle as well as the inferior part of the septum.

Left coronary artery

The left coronary artery (LCA) passes behind the pulmonary trunk and splits almost immediately into two branches: the anterior interventricular branch (often referred to as the left anterior descending artery, LAD) and the circumflex artery (Cx). The LAD descends obliquely towards the apex of the heart in the anterior interventricular sulcus, supplying the anterior part of the septum and anterior wall of the left ventricle via one or two diagonal branches [Drake, 2015].

1.4 Blood

Blood is a connective tissue consisting of a liquid (plasma) and cells performing a range of essential functions for the body [Tortora, 2017]:
- Plasma makes up around 55% of blood and carries antibodies (an important part of the immune system) and nutrients to the body's tissues, and removes waste products.
- The formed elements make up the remaining 45% and consist of red and white blood cells and platelets.
- Red blood cells (erythrocytes) carry oxygen to the tissues and remove carbon dioxide.
- White blood cells (leukocytes) are an important part of the immune and inflammatory processes.
- Platelets (thrombocytes) along with clotting factors are an essential component of normal blood clotting, particularly in cases of bleeding (haemorrhage).

1.5 Blood vessels

There are five main types of blood vessels in the body. The largest are the elastic **arteries** that leave the heart before subdividing into medium-sized muscular arteries. These further subdivide into even smaller arteries known as **arterioles**. These are important vessels as they control blood flow into the **capillaries**, thin-walled vessels that allow for the exchange of substances between the blood and tissues. The capillaries unite to form small veins, known as **venules**, which subsequently merge to form larger and larger **veins** that return blood to the heart [Tortora, 2017].

1.5.1 Vessel structure

Most blood vessels (except capillaries) are made up of three layers or tunics (Figure 13.4). The internal layer (tunica intima or interna) consists of a smooth inner layer (the endothelium), a basement membrane and, in medium-sized arteries, a layer of elastic tissue that helps to maintain blood pressure. Ordinarily, the endothelial layer is the only one that comes into contact with blood in the lumen of the artery.

The medium-sized veins have one-way valves formed from the endothelial layer. These are designed to prevent blood flow from travelling in the wrong direction (i.e. away from the heart). They resist gravity-induced pooling, particularly in the lower limbs (i.e. the legs).

The next layer is the tunica media. This is made up of smooth muscle and elastic fibres. It is most developed in the medium-sized arteries and least developed in the veins. In the aorta and other large arteries, there is a higher proportion of elastic fibres, making the walls highly compliant and able to stretch easily without tearing when subjected to pressure changes. This is advantageous, because

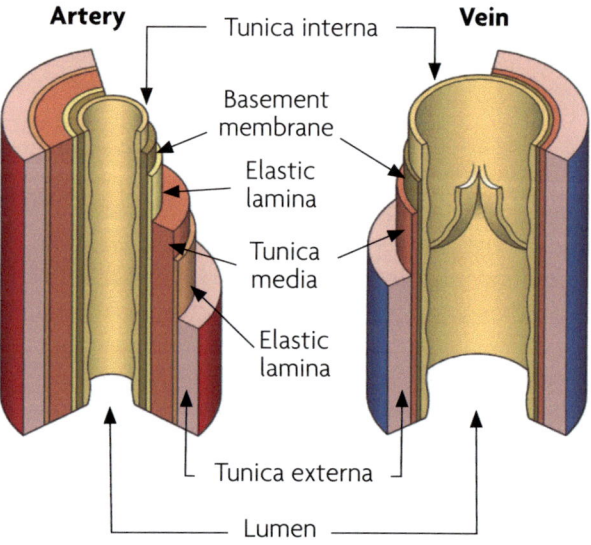

Figure 13.4 The structure of blood vessels.

Cardiovascular system anatomy and physiology

as blood is ejected from the heart, the walls of the aorta stretch, acting as a pressure reservoir that can ensure blood flow continues, even when the ventricles are relaxed [Tortora, 2017].

The final layer is the tunica externa, which is constructed mostly from elastic and collagen fibres, but is also home to the vasa vasorum (the blood supply to the arteries) and nervi vasorum (motor nerves).

1.5.2 Arteries

Figure 13.5 shows the main arteries that branch from the aorta. Don't worry about memorising them all now, you are going to revisit a number in this and other chapters.

1.5.3 Veins

Figure 13.6 shows the main veins that are drained by the superior and inferior vena cavae. It's not necessary to remember them all!

1.6 Cardiac cycle

During a single cardiac cycle, both the atria and ventricles take it in turns to contract and relax, forcing blood from an area of high pressure (due to the contracted muscle) to low pressure. The cycle is short, just 0.8 seconds in a person with an average heart rate of 75 beats/minute [Tortora, 2017; Garcia, 2015].

1.6.1 Atrial systole

This takes about 0.1 seconds. It starts with the sinoatrial (SA) node generating an action potential (electrical signal) when it depolarises (its voltage changes from negative to positive). This in turn causes the depolarisation of the atrial cardiac muscle cells, which contract (atrial systole). Blood is forced out of the atria, through the atrioventricular (AV) valves and into the ventricles, topping them up.

During this period, the electrical impulses from the SA node reach the AV node, pause to allow

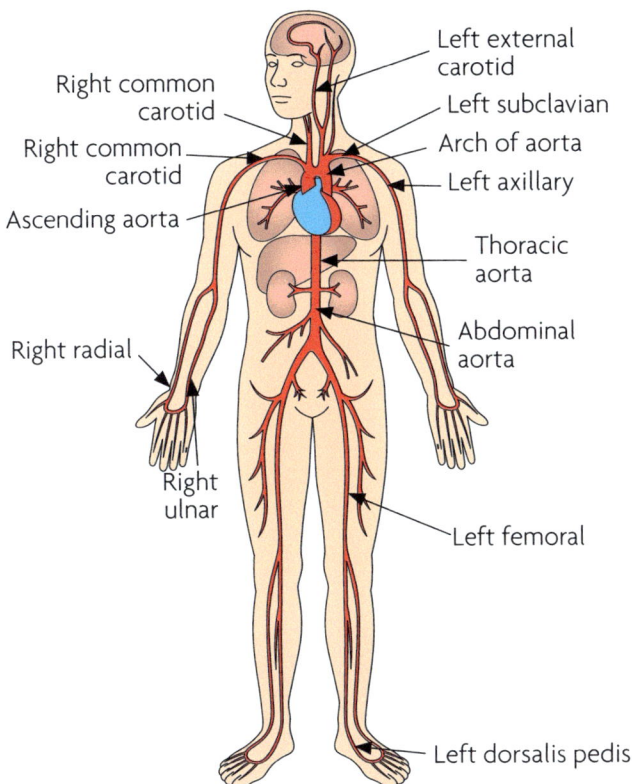

Figure 13.5 The aorta and its branches.

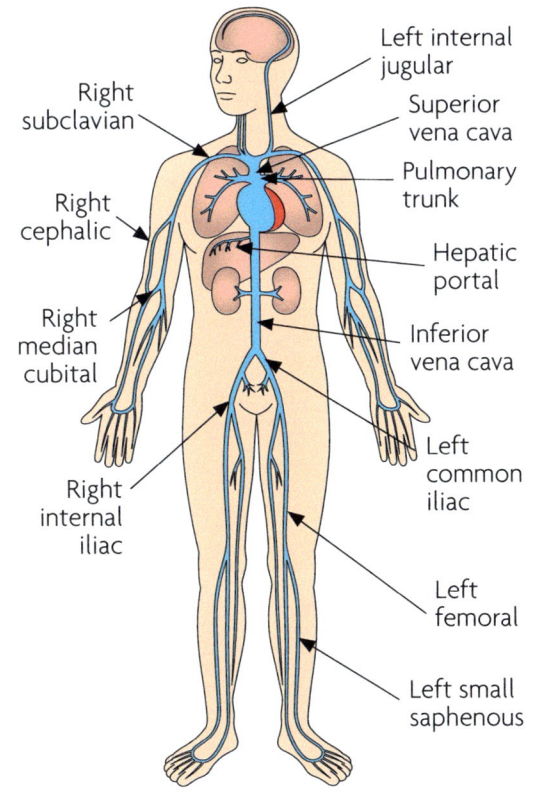

Figure 13.6 Veins of the body.

for atrial muscle contraction and then continue down the bundle of His, the bundle branches and into the Purkinje fibres, leading to ventricular depolarisation.

1.6.2 Ventricular systole

This lasts about 0.3 seconds, and during this time the atrial muscle relaxes (atrial diastole). Ventricular depolarisation causes the ventricular muscles to contract, and as the pressure inside the ventricles increases, the AV valves close and there is a brief period where all four valves of the heart are shut. This is known as isovolumetric contraction and lasts 0.05 seconds.

Contraction of the ventricles continues and eventually overcomes the pressure in the pulmonary and systemic circulations, causing the pulmonary and aortic valves (collectively known as the semilunar valves) to open. Blood is ejected into the pulmonary trunk and ascending aorta.

Meanwhile, the cardiac cells reset their voltage from positive (depolarised) to negative, a process known as repolarisation.

1.6.3 Relaxation period

This is the longest period in a cardiac cycle (around 0.4 seconds) and now both the atria and the ventricles are relaxed. This period is the most shortened when heart rate increases.

Ventricular repolarisation leads to relaxation of the ventricles (ventricular diastole). As the pressure inside the ventricles falls, the semilunar valves close. As with systole, there is a brief period where all four valves are closed (isovolumetric relaxation). The pressure continues to fall, leading to the AV valves reopening and passive filling of the ventricles begins. By the end of diastole, the ventricles will be 75% full, just in time for another action potential from the SA node to start the process all over again.

1.7 Electrocardiograms

The electrical signals that are responsible for the muscle contraction and relaxation during the cardiac cycle can be recorded on an electrocardiogram (ECG) (Figure 13.7). They are useful for determining cardiac rhythm disturbances (arrhythmias) and detecting myocardial injury, such as occurs during a heart attack (myocardial infarction).

As the heart's muscle cells depolarise and repolarise during the cardiac cycle, a potential difference (voltage) is generated, which can be detected on the surface of the body. Each cell generates its own electrical impulse, which has a strength and direction. The sum of all of these vectors is known as the heart's electrical axis and this is recorded on the ECG.

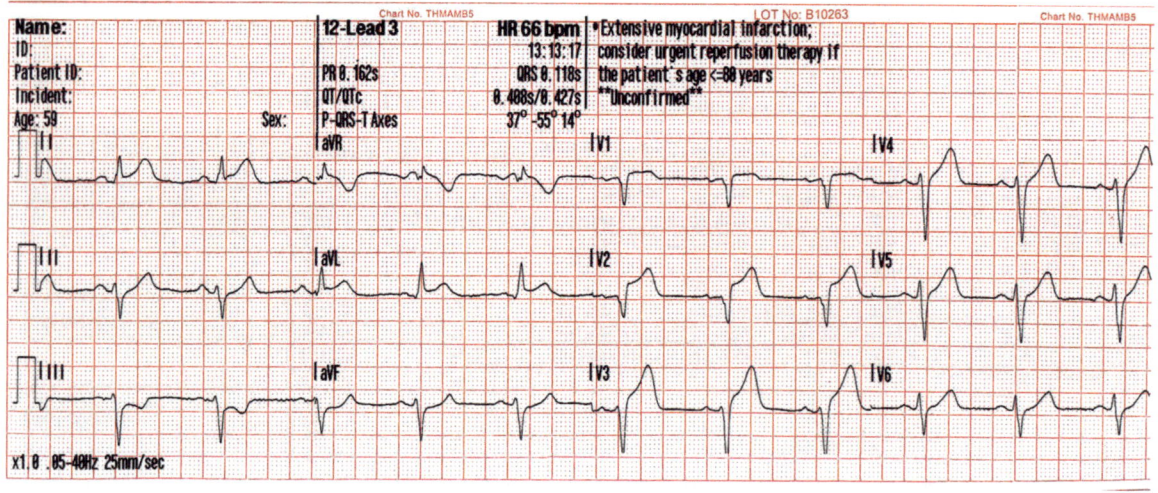

Figure 13.7 An example of a 12-lead ECG.

Recording the ECG is achieved with the use of electrodes that are placed in specific locations on the body to capture the electrical activity of the heart. They are often compared to cameras placed around the heart to build up a three-dimensional picture. In reality, we do not refer to these electrical views as cameras, but as leads, which are not to be confused with the physical leads that the electrodes are attached to. To record a 12-lead ECG, for example, you will only actually place nine or ten physical leads on the patient.

1.7.1 The ECG complex

An ECG complex is made up of a series of waves (a deflection from the baseline), segments and intervals that represent electrical events in the heart (Figure 13.8) [Garcia, 2015]:
- **P wave:** Atrial depolarisation.
- **PR segment:** This is the part of the complex between the end of the P wave and the start of the QRS wave. It should be along the baseline (the line from one TP segment to the next).
- **PR interval:** This is the time period from the start of the P wave to the start of the QRS wave. It should be 0.12–0.20 seconds (three to five small squares).
- **QRS complex:** This represents ventricular depolarisation and is typically made up of a Q, R and S wave. It should be less than 0.12 seconds or three small squares in duration.
- **ST segment:** This is the part of the complex between the end of the QRS wave and the start of the T wave. The point at which the QRS wave ends and the ST segment begins is known as the J point. The ST segment should be on the baseline.
- **T wave:** This wave represents ventricular repolarisation and is the first deflection (positive or negative) that occurs after the ST segment. It should begin in the same direction as the QRS complex.

2 Lymphatic system and immunity

2.1 Learning objectives

By the end of this section you will be able to:
- state the functions of the lymphatic system
- describe the anatomy and physiology of the lymphatic system
- briefly explain immunity and autoimmune disease.

2.2 Introduction

The lymphatic system consists of a network of vessels that transport lymph, essentially interstitial fluid (the extracellular fluid that occupies the microscopic spaces between tissue cells), except that it is inside a lymphatic vessel (Figure 13.9). In addition, there are a number of organs and tissues that play an important role in the creation of lymphocytes: a type of white blood cell that plays an important role in immunity.

The lymphatic system has three key functions [Tortora, 2017]:
- draining excess interstitial fluid (approximately three litres per day)
- transporting fats and fat-soluble vitamins from the gastrointestinal tract
- mounting an immune response to destroy foreign cells and provide protection against diseases.

2.3 Anatomy and physiology

Lymphatic vessels are similar to veins, except that they have thinner walls and more valves to ensure unidirectional flow of lymph. Lymphatic capillaries are larger than blood capillaries and are constructed of overlapping endothelial cells, which

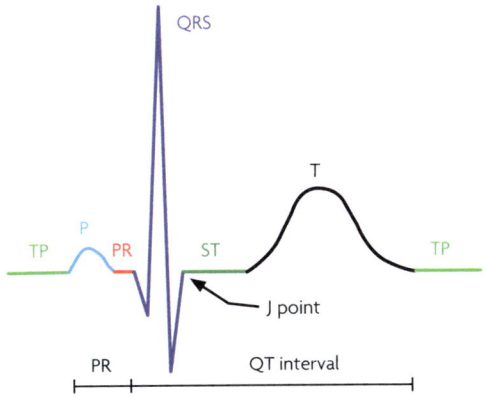

Figure 13.8 Basic components of an ECG complex.

Chapter 13 – Circulation

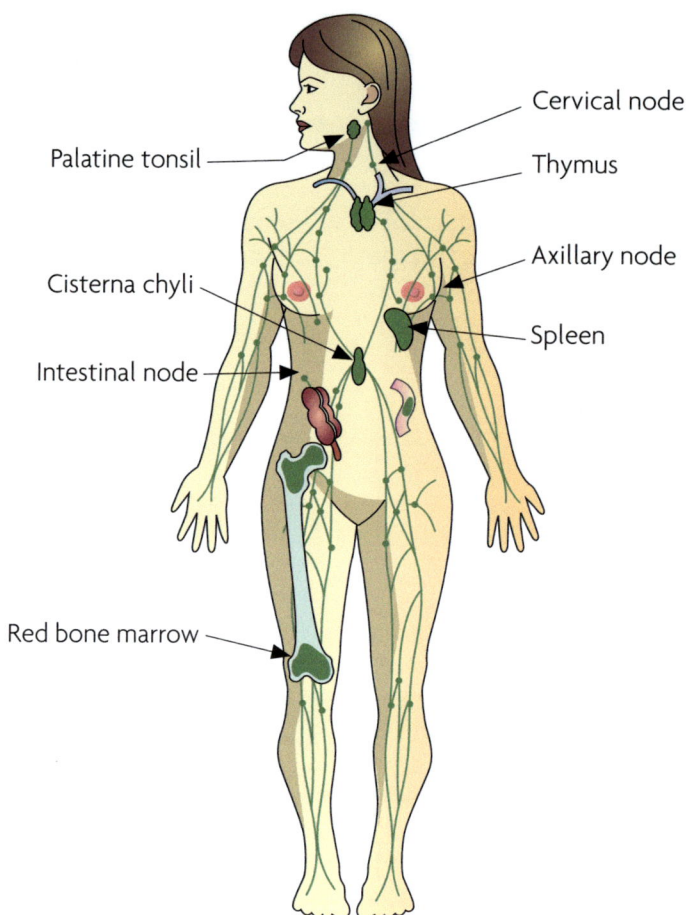

Figure 13.9 The lymphatic system.

separate slightly when interstitial fluid pressure exceeds that of the lymph. This construction also ensures that fluid can enter the lymphatic capillaries, but not leave.

Lymph is moved around the lymphatic vessels and enters the venous circulation at the junction of the internal jugular and subclavian veins. It is 'pushed' around the vessels using the same 'pumps' that move venous blood, i.e. skeletal muscle contraction and changes in intrathoracic pressure that occur during breathing [Tortora, 2017].

2.4 Immunity

In addition to transporting lymph, the lymphatic system is also important in providing immunity, protecting the body from infection. To assist, lymphatic organs and tissues adopt two roles:
- Primary lymphatic organs (red bone marrow and the thymus) create immunocompetent cells (which can mount an immune response to fight infection).
- Secondary lymphatic organs provide a location where most immune responses occur (mainly the lymph nodes and spleen).

2.4.1 Non-specific immunity

Non-specific or innate immunity is a mechanism present from birth to prevent infection. This consists of the skin and mucous membranes as well as internal mechanisms, such as phagocytes (a type of white blood cell) and inflammation.

2.4.2 Specific immunity

Specific or adaptive immunity provides the body with the ability to fight infection caused by specific bacteria, viruses and toxins. When foreign cells and other substances cause an immune response, they are called antigens [Kumar, 2012].

The lymphocytes that play a central role in specific immunity are B-cells and T-cells. B-cells are the main player in the antibody-mediated immune response. Activated B-cells transform into plasma cells, which produce and release proteins called antibodies (also known as immunoglobulins, Ig) that can bind to a specific antigen and disable it. Types of Ig include IgG, the most common type, which provides protection against a range of bacteria and viruses by enhancing phagocytosis and is the only antibody that can cross the placenta from mother to fetus. The least common is IgE, which is responsible for allergic reactions (including anaphylaxis) [Tortora, 2017].

T-cells are either killer T-cells that directly attack antigens (a process known as a cell-mediated immune response) or helper T-cells, which activate killer T-cells and B-cells. When an immune response occurs, a proportion of killer and helper T-cells become memory T-cells. In some cases, these cells can last for decades and ensure that, if subsequent exposure to the same antigen occurs, the response will be much swifter than on first exposure. This 'memory' of antigens is the principle behind vaccination.

2.5 Autoimmune disease

T-cells can only function properly if they can distinguish between foreign cells and substances and the body's own. If this fails, cell- and antibody-mediated immune responses can be mounted against the body. Type 1 diabetes mellitus, for example, involves killer T-cells targeting the beta cells in the pancreas that are responsible for producing insulin. Alternatively, autoantibodies can be created. These attach to self-antigens (i.e. antigens on the body's own cells) and either stimulate or block cell functions. An example of this process leads to Graves' disease, which is caused by an autoantibody mimicking the effect of thyroid-stimulating hormone, which in turn leads to excess production and release of the thyroid hormone [Tortora, 2017].

3 Assessment of circulation

3.1 Learning objectives

By the end of this section you will be able to:
- describe how to accurately measure the following:
  - pulse
  - capillary refill time
  - blood pressure
- explain how to prepare a patient and acquire a 3- and 12-lead ECG
- identify ST-segment elevation myocardial infarction on a 12-lead ECG.

3.2 Introduction

If you are asked to assess a patient's pulse, or obtain a manual blood pressure, you have been given a big responsibility, since only you will know how fast, regular and strong the pulse feels, or when you can hear the Korotkoff sounds in your stethoscope as the blood pressure cuff is deflated.

Treatment decisions are made on the basis of clinical observations, so make sure you record observations accurately.

3.3 Pulse

The alternating expansion and recoil of the elastic arteries after ventricular systole creates a pressure wave, called a pulse, that can be felt in any artery that lies near the surface of the body and which can be compressed against a bone or other firm structure [Tortora, 2017].

Pulses are assessed for two main reasons [Gregory, 2010b]:
- to determine the patient's cardiovascular status
- to provide reassurance and gain a bond with patients who may be anxious.

3.3.1 Pulse locations

Pulses are palpable all over the body, but you should be able to confidently locate the radial, brachial and carotid pulses (Figure 13.10). The other

Chapter 13 – *Circulation*

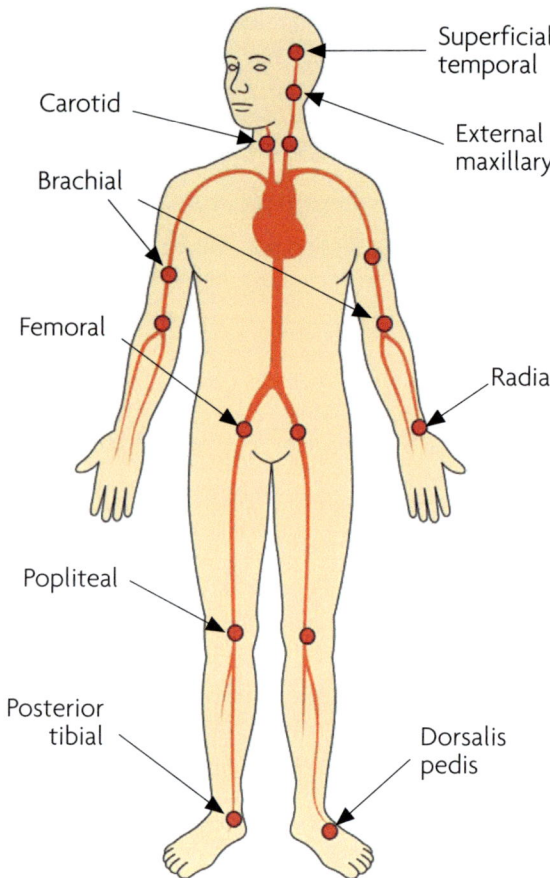

Figure 13.10 The location of common palpable pulses.

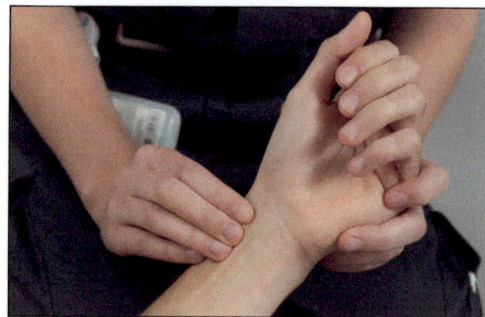

Figure 13.11 Palpating a radial pulse.

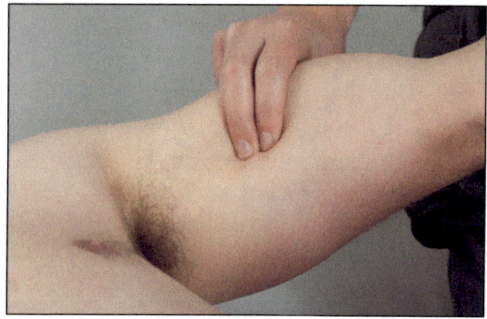

Figure 13.12 Palpating a brachial pulse between the biceps and triceps muscles.

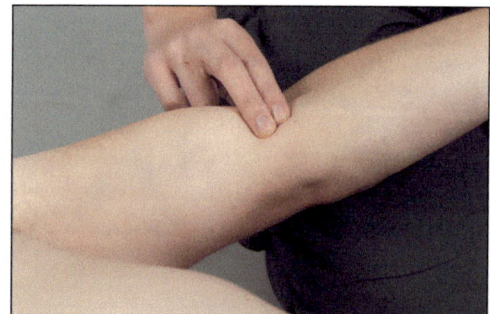

Figure 13.13 Palpating a brachial pulse in the crease of the elbow.

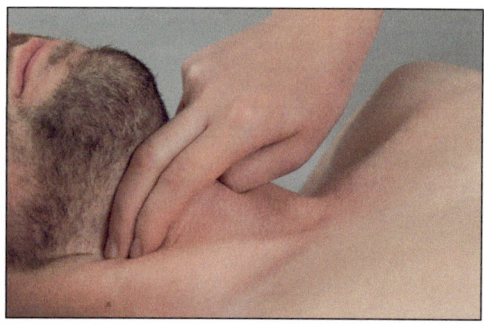

Figure 13.14 Palpating a carotid pulse.

sites are useful for specific conditions, for example, checking that a patient with a leg fracture has a dorsalis pedis pulse.

Radial pulse
The radial artery can be palpated at the wrist, on the radial side (thumb side) of the palmar (inner) aspect of the forearm. It is lateral to the long flexor tendons of the forearm (Figure 13.11) [Allan, 2004].

Brachial pulse
There are two locations for measuring this pulse. The first is in the mid-arm and can be found medially in the cleft between the biceps and triceps muscles (Figure 13.12). However, this is where a blood pressure cuff is usually placed, so in that instance you can also palpate the pulse in the crease of the elbow (antecubital fossa; see Figure 13.13).

The pulse can be palpated just medial to the biceps tendon [Drake, 2015].

Carotid pulse
The carotid artery can be palpated between the larynx and the sternocleidomastoid muscle. Gently press to feel the pulse (Figure 13.14) [Gregory, 2010b].

3.3.2 Assessment
When you assess a patient's pulse, you are looking for four things:
- rate
- rhythm
- volume
- character.

Rate
The normal pulse rate for an adult is 60–100 beats/minute [Allan, 2004]. If the pulse rate is less than 60 beats/minute, this is termed bradycardia; if greater than 100 beats/minute, tachycardia [Talley, 2006].

Causes of bradycardia include:
- sleep
- athletic training
- hypothyroidism
- medications such as beta-blockers
- hypothermia
- some types of arrhythmia (abnormal electrical activity within the heart).

Causes of tachycardia include:
- exercise
- pain
- excitement/anxiety
- hyperthyroidism
- fever
- some types of stimulant drugs such as caffeine and cocaine
- some arrhythmias.

Rhythm
In healthy patients, the rhythm should be regular. However, in certain arrhythmias this regularity can be interrupted. Try to identify whether the irregularity is regular, i.e. seems to occur in a pattern, or the beats are apparently completely random, i.e. irregularly irregular [Gregory, 2010b].

Volume and character
The volume reflects the strength of the pulse. A high volume is typically noted during times when the cardiac output is high, such as during exercise, stress, heat and pregnancy. On the other hand, a low-volume pulse can be due to heart failure or peripheral vascular disease. A weak (also described as 'thready') pulse is most often seen in patients who are suffering from a decreased blood volume (hypovolaemia or shock) [Douglas, 2005].

The character of the pulse is slightly different as you need to picture how the pulse changes during the cardiac cycle. This is tricky to master and will require practice.

3.3.3 Recording a pulse

> **Procedure – To record a pulse**
>
> Take the following steps to record a pulse:
>
> 1. Explain the procedure and obtain consent from the patient.
>
> 2. Place your index, middle and ring fingers along the artery and press gently. Avoid using the thumb as it has its own pulse. Don't push too hard or you will occlude the artery. As a general rule, palpate the radial pulse first in conscious patients and the carotid pulse first in unconscious patients.
>
> 3. In pulses with a regular rhythm, count for 15 seconds and then multiply by four. If the pulse is very fast or slow and/or irregular, then count for a full 60 seconds.
>
> 4. Record the pulse rate on the patient record.

3.4 Capillary refill time
Capillary refill time (CRT) is defined as the time taken for a distal capillary bed to regain its colour after pressure has been applied to cause blanching [Pickard, 2011]. It was introduced during World War II to estimate the degree of shock in battlefield survivors. In 1981, an upper limit of two seconds was arbitrarily chosen as the acceptable upper limit;

this has become the acceptable normal value and is published widely [King, 2014].

This presents a problem, because subsequent research has generally determined that it is not a good indicator of the degree of hypovolaemia in seriously ill and injured adult patients and should not be used [Lewin, 2008].

It does have a place in the assessment of children, although it should not be taken in isolation, i.e. take into account the other aspects of patient assessment that you will undertake, such as pulse rate, respiratory rate, work of breathing, level of consciousness, etc. [King, 2014].

Because the usefulness of CRT is uncertain, you will need to follow your ambulance service guidance about when to use CRT and in which age group.

3.4.1 Assessment

Be aware of the following external factors that can affect the accuracy of capillary refill time (CRT) measurement in children and neonates [King, 2014]:

- **Temperature:** Children in cool environments will have a prolonged CRT, even when they are completely healthy. There is no evidence that CRT is affected by a child's body temperature, such as when they are feverish due to an illness.
- **Ambient light:** Assessing CRT in poor light leads to errors. Ensure you are somewhere well-lit.
- **Site:** CRT is longer in neonates if the heel is used. One study demonstrated that fingertip and sternum CRTs are different in children [Crook, 2013]. Current paediatric guidelines advocate only using the sternum to assess CRT in children [Skellett, 2016].
- **Pressure application:** It is not known how long pressure should be applied prior to assessing CRT, but current paediatric guidelines suggest pressing on the sternum for five seconds [Skellett, 2016].
- **Observer:** When different people (observers) measure CRT at the same time, on the same child, they end up with different results! As a rule of thumb, try to ensure that the same clinician assesses CRT each time.

3.4.2 Recording the capillary refill time

Procedure – To obtain a capillary refill time (CRT)

Follow these steps to obtain a capillary refill time (CRT) [King, 2014]:

1. Ensure the environment is warm and well-lit.
2. Explain the procedure to the parent and to the child if they are able to understand.
3. Apply pressure to the sternum for five seconds to compress blood from the tissues. Apply only enough pressure to cause blanching of the skin.
4. Release the pressure and count how long it takes for the colour of the skin to return to that of the surrounding tissues. This is the CRT.
5. Document your findings.
6. Consider this result in the light of other assessments of the child's cardiovascular status.

3.5 Blood pressure

Blood pressure (BP) is the measurement of the pressure by the blood on the walls of a blood vessel. It is highest in the aorta and large systemic arteries and lowest in the large veins [Tortora, 2017].

The BP that you record consists of two measurements:
- **Systolic blood pressure:** The BP during the systole phase of the cardiac cycle, when the ventricles contract and blood is forced out of the heart. This is the higher reading of blood pressure.
- **Diastolic blood pressure:** The BP during the diastole phase of the cardiac cycle, when the ventricles are relaxed. This is the lower reading of blood pressure.

It is usually measured in millimetres of mercury (mmHg) and recorded as the systolic value over the diastolic, for example 120/80 mmHg.

3.5.1 Assessment

Blood pressure (BP) values

The normal range for adult BP is a systolic value of 120–129 mmHg and/or diastolic of 80–84 mmHg. Hypertension (high BP) is defined as a systolic value of 140 mmHg or higher and/or a diastolic of 90 mmHg or higher [Mancia, 2013].

Hypotension is usually defined as a systolic blood pressure of less than 90 mmHg and this is the threshold for treatment with intravenous fluids in the current UK Ambulance Services Clinical Practice Guidelines [JRCALC, 2019]. However, there is evidence to suggest that, in trauma, a systolic value of 110 mmHg should be the cut-off point for treatment [Eastridge, 2007; Hasler, 2011a; Hasler, 2012]. Even higher values are advocated for the elderly patient [Oyetunji, 2011].

Measurement of BP

Blood pressure can be measured directly, by inserting a sensor into a patient's artery, or indirectly using a cuff, which is applied to a patient's arm. The advantage of direct measurement is that it is accurate and continuous; it is typically used in hospital intensive care units. This method is not practicable outside of hospital and so non-invasive methods are used.

Non-invasive blood pressure (NIBP) measurement

There are two methods of NIBP measurement used by the ambulance service:
- **Auscultatory:** This method uses a stethoscope and an aneroid sphygmomanometer, a device consisting of an inflatable cuff and an aneroid manometer to measure the pressure on a dial (Figure 13.15).
- **Automated:** This consists of an inflatable cuff with a sensor inside that detects the oscillations generated by turbulent blood flow and calculates systolic and diastolic values using an algorithm.

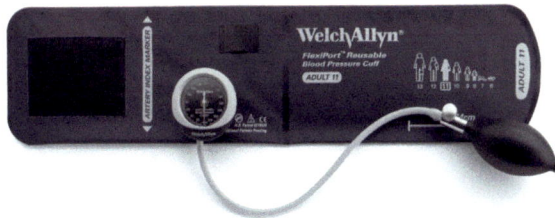

Figure 13.15 An aneroid sphygmomanometer.
Source: Image reproduced by the kind permission of Welch Allyn.

Korotkoff sounds

When using the auscultatory method of measuring BP, you will place a stethoscope over the patient's brachial artery and listen for turbulent blood flow, known as the Korotkoff sounds, after a Russian surgeon, Nikolai Korotkoff, who first described them in 1905 [Talley, 2006].

The sounds are split into five phases [O'Brien, 2003]:
1. The first appearance of faint, repetitive, clear tapping sounds that gradually increase in intensity for at least two consecutive beats is the systolic blood pressure. This corresponds to the restoration of blood flow and is confirmed by the presence of a palpable pulse.
2. A brief period may follow during which the sounds soften and acquire a swishing quality. In some patients, sounds may disappear altogether for a short time.
3. The return of sharper sounds, which become crisper, to match or even exceed the intensity of phase 1 sounds.
4. The distinct abrupt muffling of sounds, which become soft and blowing in quality.
5. The point at which all sounds finally disappear completely is the diastolic pressure.

Note that in some groups of patients, the phase 4 sounds may be heard until the BP measurement reaches 0 mmHg. In these cases, the onset of phase 4 is taken to be the diastolic BP measurement [O'Brien, 2003].

3.5.2 Blood pressure measurement

Procedure – Manual blood pressure measurement

Take the following steps to manually record a blood pressure [Mancia, 2013; Kauffman, 2014; O'Brien, 2003]:

1. Ideally, allow the patient to sit for 3–5 minutes before measuring and obtain consent.
2. Ask about any medical conditions that might prevent a BP being recorded on a particular arm, e.g. mastectomy or arteriovenous shunts in dialysis patients.

Chapter 13 – *Circulation*

Procedure – Manual blood pressure measurement – *cont*

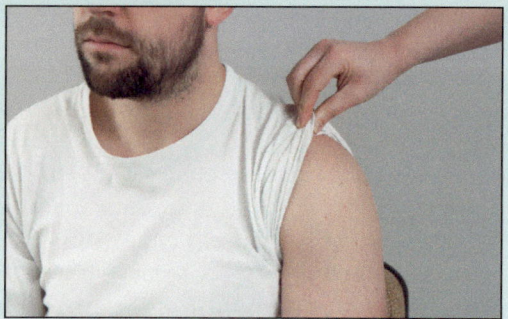

3. Ensure the arm is free of restrictive clothing. Do not apply a cuff over clothes.

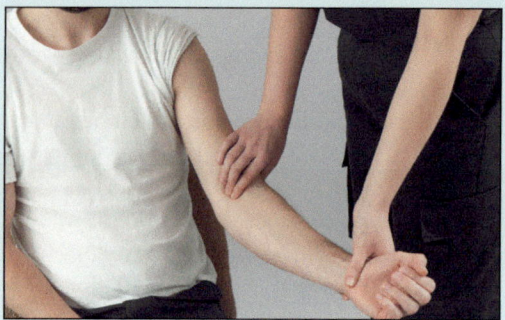

4. Palpate the brachial artery. This can be found by placing the pads of the index and middle fingers of one hand on the biceps tendon and then moving medially and pressing deeply. If you have trouble locating the brachial pulse, ask the patient to extend their arm, which will bring the artery into a more superficial position. Once it is located, ask the patient to relax their arm so that their wrist rests on their thigh.

5. Ask the patient to remain still and not talk during the BP measurement.

6. Select the appropriate cuff size. A standard bladder is 12–13 cm wide and 35 cm long, but ensure you have smaller and larger sizes available.

7. Ensure the cuff is at heart level and wrap snugly around the patient's upper arm and clear of the antecubital fossa, so that the cuff will not touch the stethoscope.

Procedure – Manual blood pressure measurement – *cont*

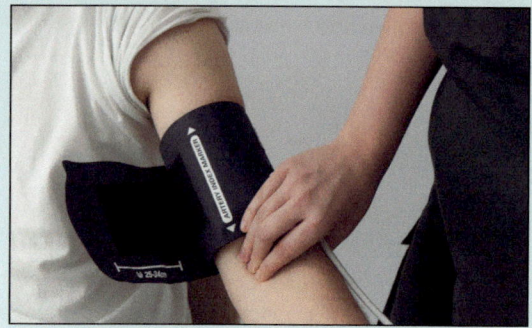

8. Place the artery marker on the cuff over the patient's brachial artery.

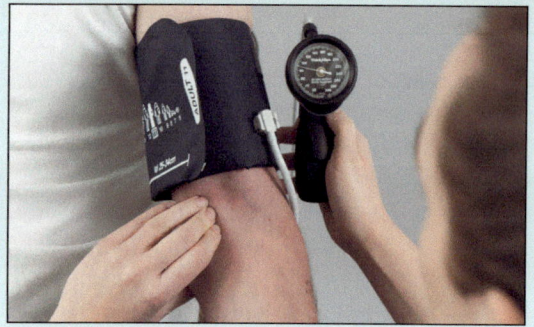

9. Palpate the brachial artery and inflate the cuff until the pulse disappears. Continue to inflate 30 mmHg above this point.

10. Slowly deflate the cuff and note when the pulse returns. This gives an estimation of the systolic blood pressure.

11. Wait 30 seconds and then place the diaphragm of the stethoscope over the brachial artery.

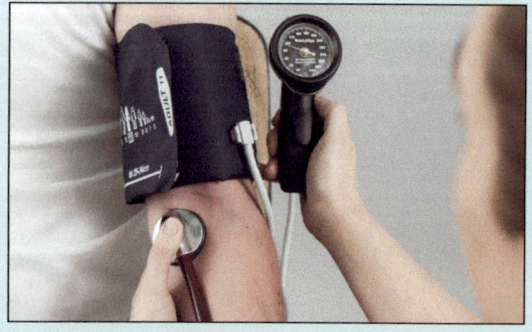

12. Rapidly inflate the cuff 30 mmHg above your estimation of the systolic blood pressure.

Assessment of circulation

Procedure – Manual blood pressure measurement – *cont*

13. Deflate at a rate of 2–3 mmHg per pulse beat.
14. Note the pressure at which you first hear the Korotkoff sounds (systolic BP), the point at which they become muffled (phase 4) and then disappear (phase 5). The disappearance of sounds is usually taken to be the diastolic blood pressure.
15. Document the blood pressure, including which arm the measurement was taken from.

Procedure – Automated blood pressure measurement

Follow the manufacturer's instructions for the measurement of an automated blood pressure. The steps below apply to recording a BP using a LIFEPAK 15 monitor/defibrillator [Physio-Control, 2009]:

1. Press ON.
2. Select the appropriately sized cuff and apply it snugly to the arm in the position described above for manual.
3. Connect the tubing to the cuff and to the NIBP port on the monitor.
4. Change the initial inflation pressure, if necessary.
5. Position the arm in a relaxed and supported position at approximately the same level as the patient's heart. Inform the patient that the cuff will inflate and cause a 'big squeeze' around the arm and that the patient's fingers may tingle.
6. Press NIBP to start the measurement and check that the patient's arm is not moving. When the measurement is complete, the blood pressure measurements are displayed.

Procedure – Manual blood pressure measurement – *cont*

7. Document the blood pressure, including which arm the measurement was taken from.

3.6 Recording an ECG

3.6.1 ECG paper

Electrocardiograms (ECGs) are recorded on standardised graph paper, which is moved past a heated stylus at a standard speed of 25 mm per second. On the vertical axis, the standard calibration amplitude is 10 mm/mV. This is shown by a calibration box, which is printed at the beginning of each line of the ECG (Figure 13.16A) and should be 10 mm tall. It is possible to change both of these settings, so always check your ECG. If standard calibration is used, the horizontal measurement of each large square is 0.2 seconds (Figure 13.16B) and each small square represents 0.04 seconds (Figure 13.16C).

3.6.2 Artefact

The quality of the ECG can be affected by a range of factors. Electrical interference, poor electrode contact, damaged ECG cables, muscle tremors, shivering, hiccups and deep respiration can all lead to artefact or a 'wandering' baseline (Figure 13.17).

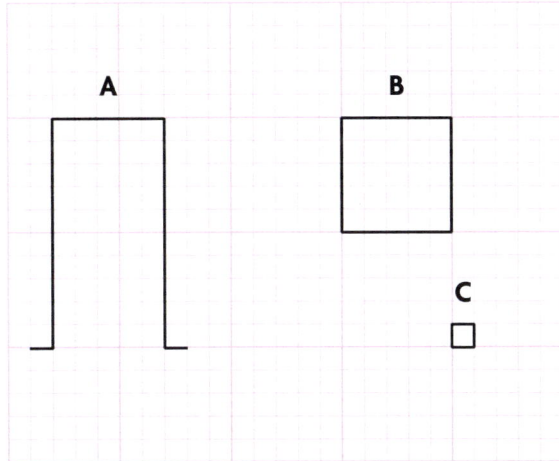

Figure 13.16   Calibration of the ECG and standard square durations.

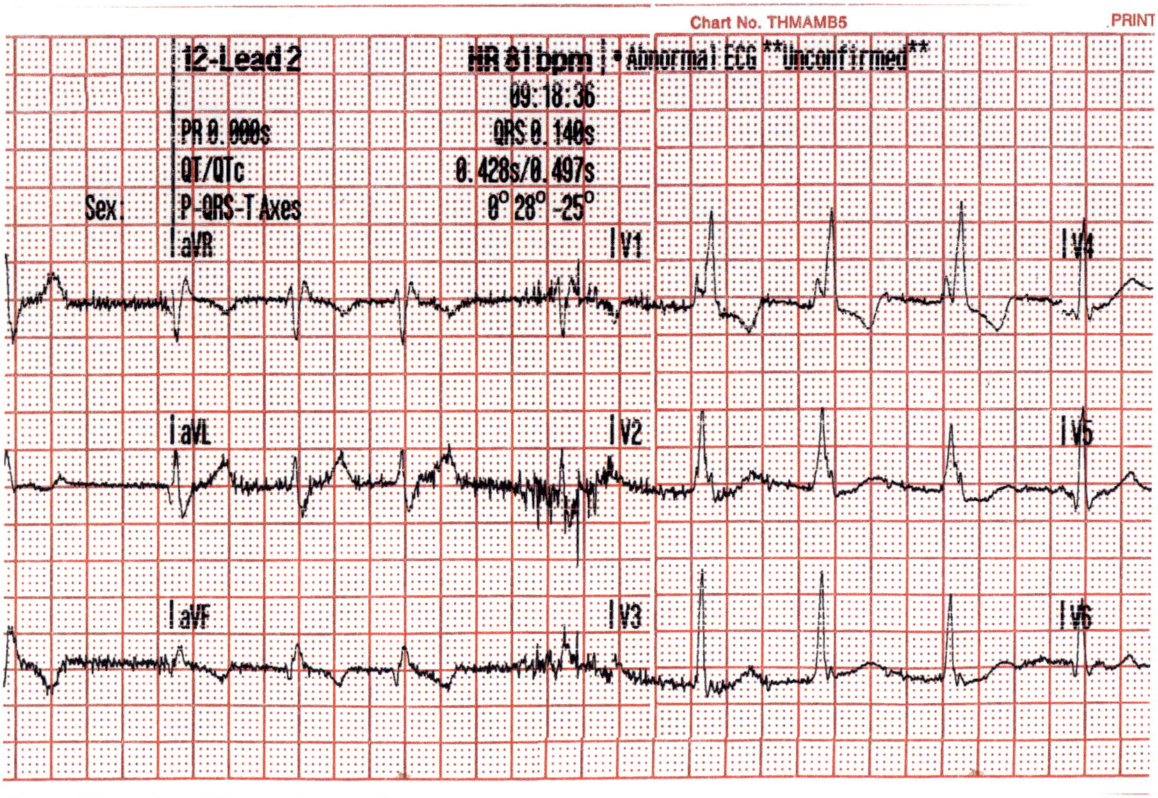

Chapter 13 – Circulation

Figure 13.17 An ECG showing artefact.

3.6.3 Procedure

Procedure – To record a 3- and 12-lead ECG

Take the following steps to record a 3- and 12-lead ECG [Physio-Control, 2009]:

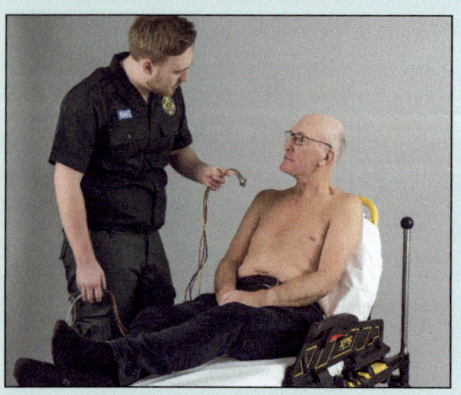

1. Explain the procedure to the patient. Ensure they understand that you are about to remove their top.

Procedure – To record a 3- and 12-lead ECG – *cont*

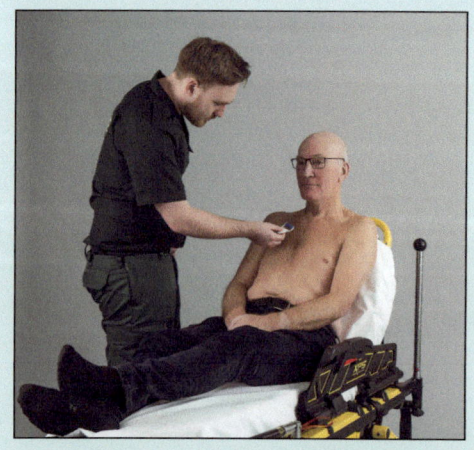

2. Prepare the skin. This will include shaving any hair at the electrode sites, cleaning oily skin with an alcohol wipe, and gently scraping the skin to remove the surface

Procedure – To record a 3- and 12-lead ECG – cont

layer of dead skin cells. Patients who are sweating profusely can be a problem, but an alcohol wipe and/or gauze swabs should help. All of these will improve electrical conduction.

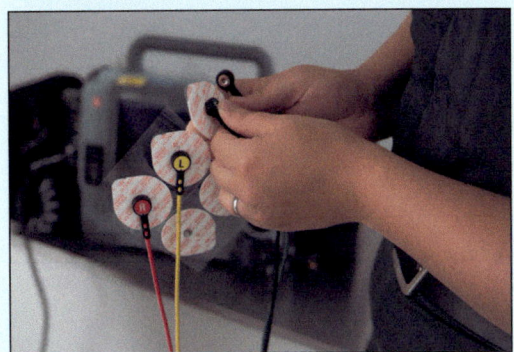

3. Check your electrodes are in date and then attach them to the leads prior to applying them to the patient's skin. When you apply the electrodes flat to the skin, smooth the tape outward and avoid pressing the centre of the electrode. Also, avoid placing electrodes over tendons and major muscle masses.

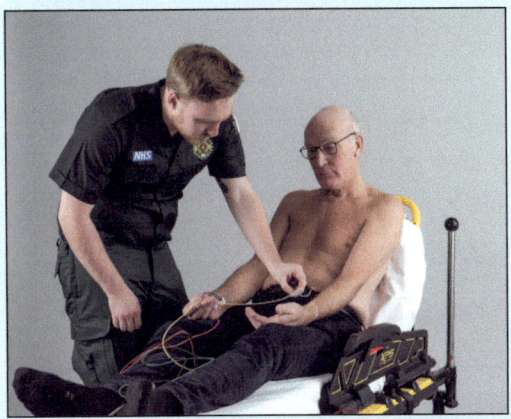

4. Apply the limb leads. Although traditionally placed on the wrists, limb leads can be placed anywhere on the limbs. In cases of either patient and/or vehicular movement, a

Procedure – To record a 3- and 12-lead ECG – cont

more proximal location may reduce artefact [Physio-Control, 2009]. Place the leads as follows:
- **Red:** right wrist/arm
- **Yellow:** left wrist/arm
- **Green:** left ankle/leg
- **Black:** right ankle/leg.

5. Turn on the monitor and record a 3-lead ECG. Label it with the patient's name and date of birth.

12-lead ONLY

The instructions below relate to a 12-lead ECG only.

6. Prepare the chest skin as in step 2 and attach electrodes to the chest leads.

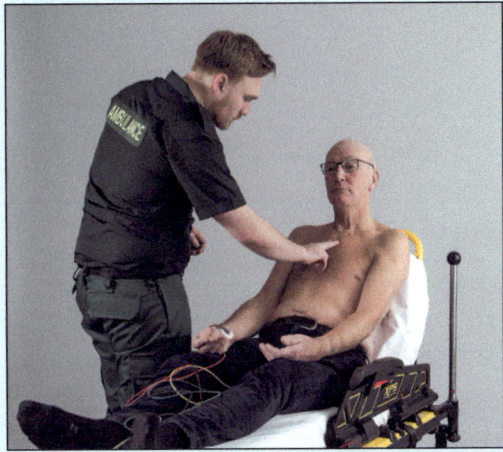

7. Move your finger downwards crossing the manubrium until you feel a small horizontal ridge. This is the sternal angle or angle of Louis, where the manubrium and body of the sternum join.

Chapter 13 – *Circulation*

Procedure – To record a 3- and 12-lead ECG – *cont*

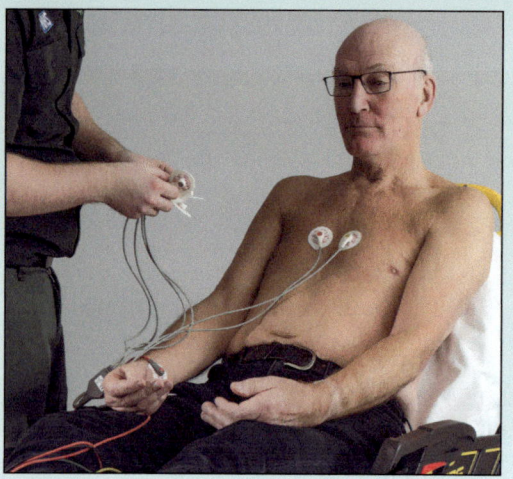

8. Slide your finger laterally and slightly downwards into the second intercostal space and move down two more intercostal spaces to locate the fourth intercostal space. Place lead V1 just to the left (patient's right) of the sternal border, and V2 just to the right (patient's left).

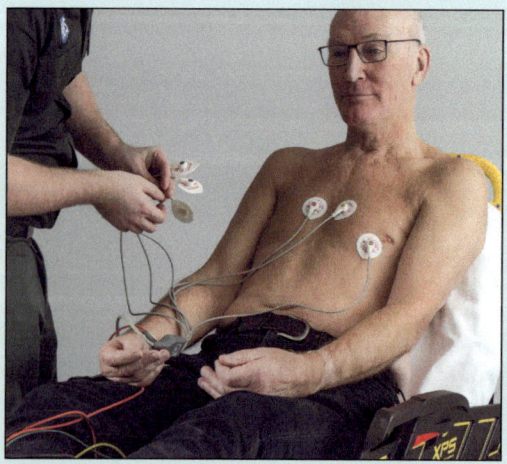

9. Move into the fifth intercostal space and laterally to the mid-clavicular line. This is the location of V4.

Procedure – To record a 3- and 12-lead ECG – *cont*

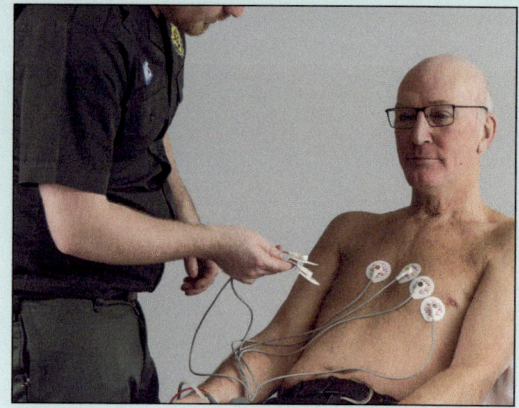

10. Place V3 midway between V2 and V4.

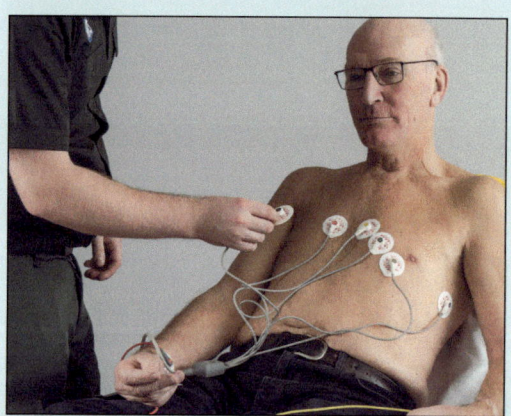

11. Place lead V6 level with V4, and in the mid-axillary line.

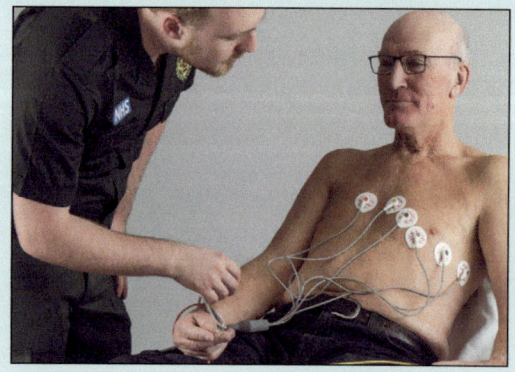

12. Place V5 level with, and midway between, V4 and V6 in the anterior axillary line [Kligfield, 2007].

Procedure – To record a 3- and 12-lead ECG – *cont*

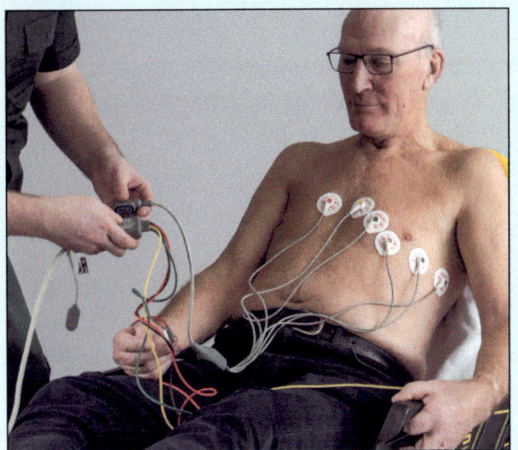

13. Connect the cables to the monitor.

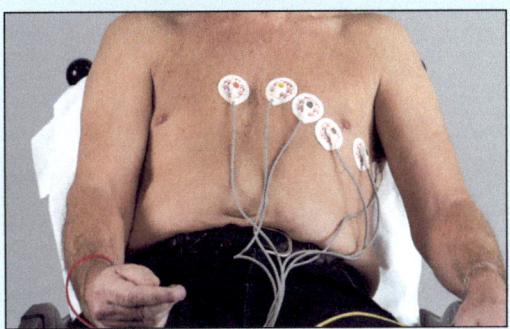

14. Press the 12-lead ECG Analyse button and record a 12-lead ECG. Review the 12-lead ECG to check it is of sufficient quality for diagnostic purposes.

Breasts

Female breasts can make things a bit awkward in terms of placing leads V4–V6. Current guidance provided by two monitor/defibrillator manufacturers states that these leads should be placed under breast tissue. While there is some evidence to suggest that signal reduction by placing electrodes over breast tissue may not be significant, and the procedure has the benefit of ensuring correct anatomical placement of the chest leads, this is not strong enough at present to change the common practice of placing V4–V6 under the breast [BCS, 2017].

3.6.4 12-lead ECG interpretation

Recording a 12-lead ECG is one thing, but interpreting it is quite another. However, in your role, you may not be required to interpret a 12-lead ECG at all. If you are, it is likely to be limited to recognising ST-segment elevation or a left bundle branch block (LBBB) pattern that can suggest an acute coronary syndrome (heart attack) that requires urgent reperfusion. In most cases, this is not actually that difficult. They key is being able to recognise normal and then, having determined that the ECG is not normal, work out what is wrong with it.

The 12-lead ECG is so called because it provides 12 views of the electrical activity of the heart. A standard 12-lead ECG consists of six limb leads (I, II, III, aVR, aVL and aVF from four physical electrodes that you attach to the patient), which look at the electrical activity of the heart in a vertical or coronal plane, and six chest (or precordial) leads that do the same in the transverse plane (Figure 13.18).

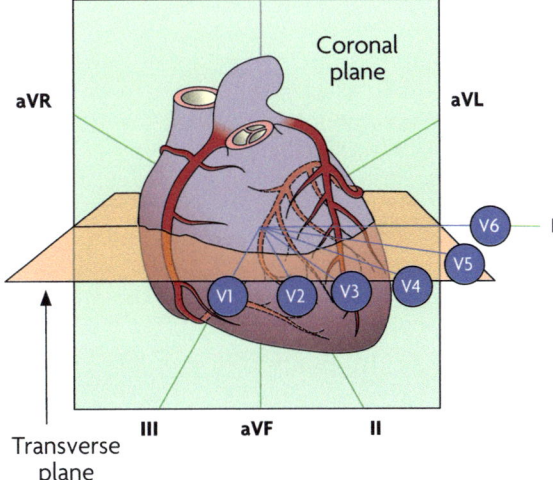

Figure 13.18 The electrical 'views' provided by the limb and chest leads.

Chapter 13 – Circulation

3.6.5 A 'normal' 12-lead ECG

A normal ECG meets the following criteria (Figure 13.19) [Silver, 2003]:

- P waves present and upright in I, II, V2–V6.
- PR interval of 0.12–0.20 seconds (three to five small squares).
- No Q waves > 0.04 seconds in duration in I, II, V2–V6.
- QRS complexes are usually upright in I and II, and less than or equal to 0.12 seconds (three small squares).
- R waves in chest leads should increase in positive voltage from V1 to V4.
- ST segments are isoelectric except in V1 and V2, where some elevation can be normal.
- QRS and T waves should be concordant, i.e. are both positive or negative voltages, in the limb leads.
- T waves should be upright in I, II, V2–V6.
- All waves in aVR should be negative.

If the ECG is not normal, identify the abnormalities that stand out and note any regionalisation of the changes, which are particularly helpful in myocardial injury.

3.6.6 Contiguous leads

Leads that look at the same part of the heart are referred to as being 'contiguous'. Typically, two or more contiguous leads are required when meeting criteria for acute coronary syndromes (Figure 13.20).

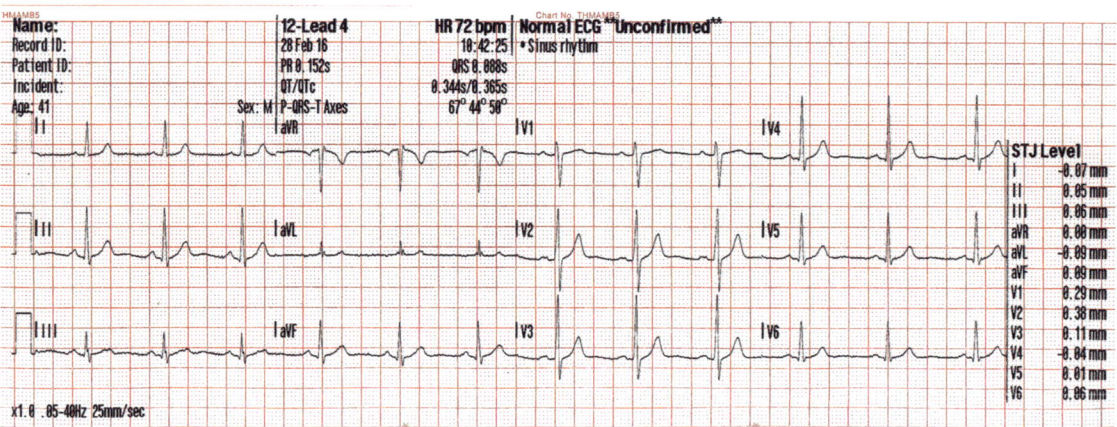

Figure 13.19 A normal 12-lead ECG.

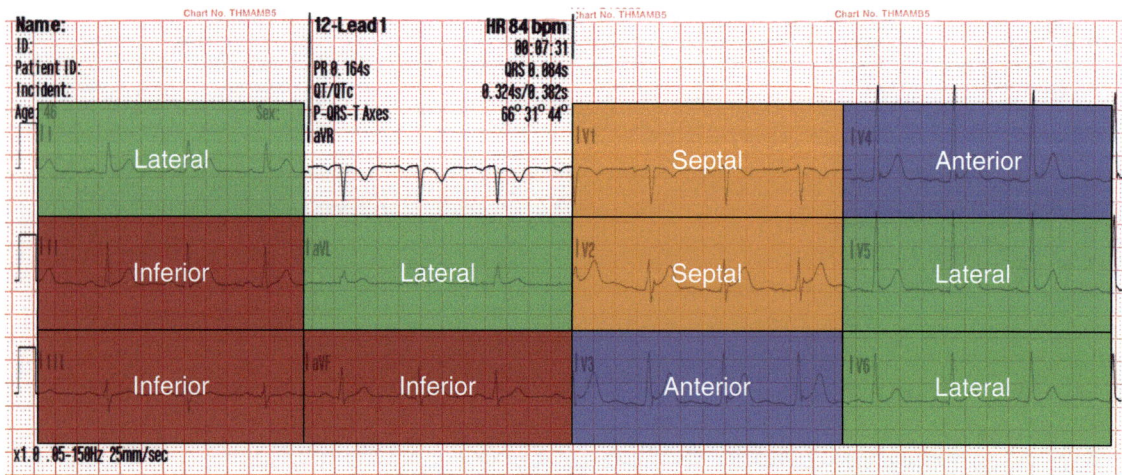

Figure 13.20 Contiguous leads on a 12-lead ECG. Note that chest leads V1–V4 are often grouped together and considered to be anterior leads.

Assessment of circulation

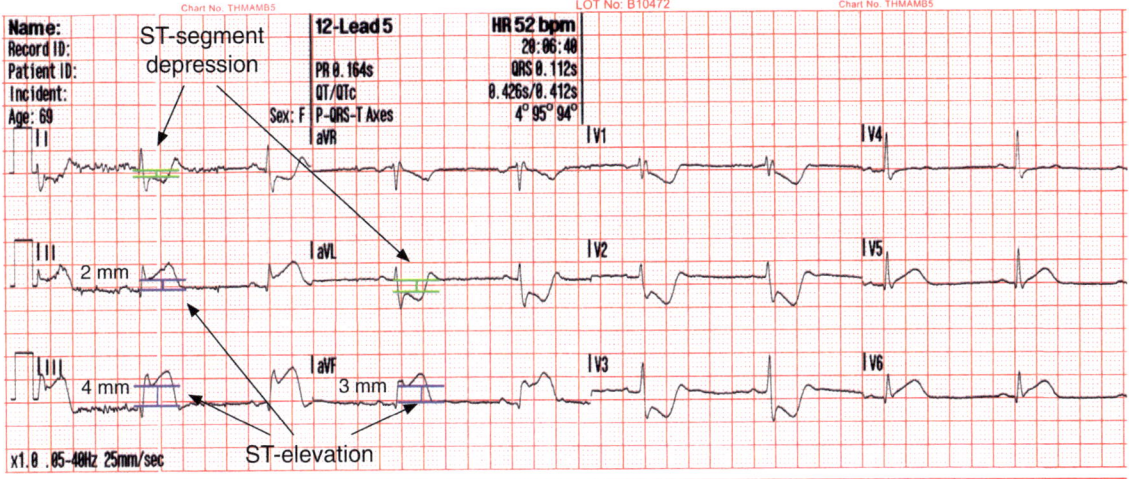

Figure 13.21 An inferior MI. Notice the ST-segment elevation in leads II, III and aVF and the reciprocal ST-segment depression in leads I and aVL. The ST-segment depression in V1–V3 is also a reciprocal change, but this may be due to ischaemia or injury to the posterior wall of the heart. This was caused by a blockage of the patient's right coronary artery.

3.6.7 STEMI (ST-segment elevation myocardial infarction) recognition

ST-segment elevation is present if the J point is raised above the TP segment (taken to be the isoelectric line on an ECG). The UK Ambulance Services Clinical Practice Guidelines suggest that 2 mm or more of ST-segment elevation in two contiguous leads is a criterion for urgent coronary perfusion, but follow local guidance, as some guidelines require only 1 mm of elevation in the limb leads, for example [JRCALC, 2019].

ST-segment depression is also a significant sign, particularly when associated with signs and symptoms of an acute coronary syndrome. It can represent cardiac muscle ischaemia or is a reciprocal change.

Reciprocal changes

The advantage of 12 leads is that you can view the same electrical activity from multiple and, in some cases, opposite views. When there is ST-segment elevation in one lead, you may see ST-segment depression in a lead that is looking at the injury or infarct from the opposite 'side'. On a standard 12-lead ECG, this mainly occurs in the limb leads. So, for example, if you see ST-segment elevation in the inferior leads, II, III and aVF, you might also notice ST-segment depression in the lateral leads of the limbs, I and aVL (Figure 13.21). The septal leads, V1 and V2, may also show ST-segment depression, which if isolated, or associated with ST-segment elevation in the inferior leads, can be a sign that the posterior portion of the heart is ischaemic or injured. There are posterior leads that can be applied, but that is beyond the scope of this book.

Anterior STEMI

A blockage in the left coronary artery or its branches can lead to ST-segment elevation on the anterior and/or lateral leads. Figure 13.22 shows an example of a 12-lead ECG with such changes.

Lateral STEMI

ST-segment elevation can occur in just the lateral leads (I, aVL, V5 and V6), but is often associated with other ST-segment elevation, such as anterior or inferior depending on coronary artery anatomy and which vessels have been affected. Figure 13.23 is an example of anterolateral ST-segment elevation.

3.6.8 Left bundle branch block

Normally, conduction passes through the bundle of His and down the right and left bundle branches. If the left bundle (or both fascicles) become blocked, either

Chapter 13 – *Circulation*

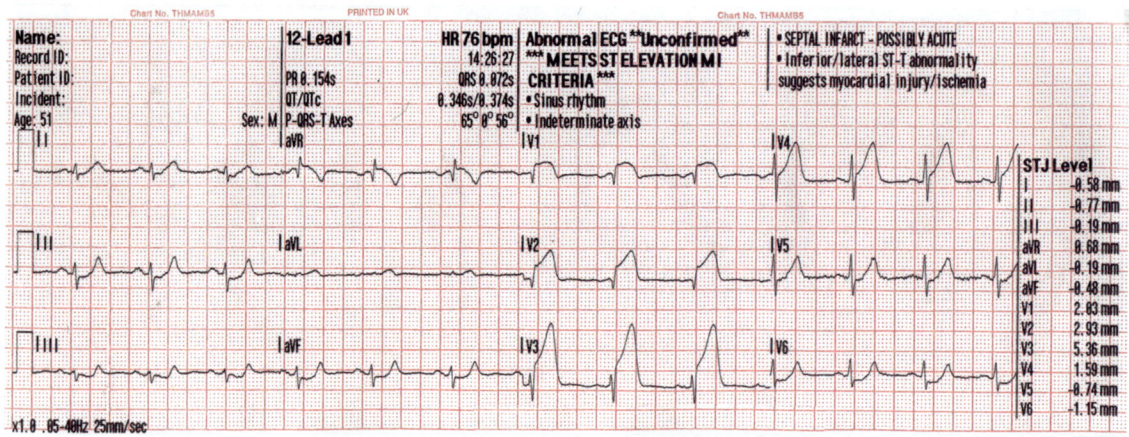

Figure 13.22 An anteroseptal STEMI, i.e. both septal and anterior, often referred to as just 'anterior'. Note the ST-segment elevation in leads V1–V4. The computer interpretation message also indicates that this ECG meets the criteria for STEMI.

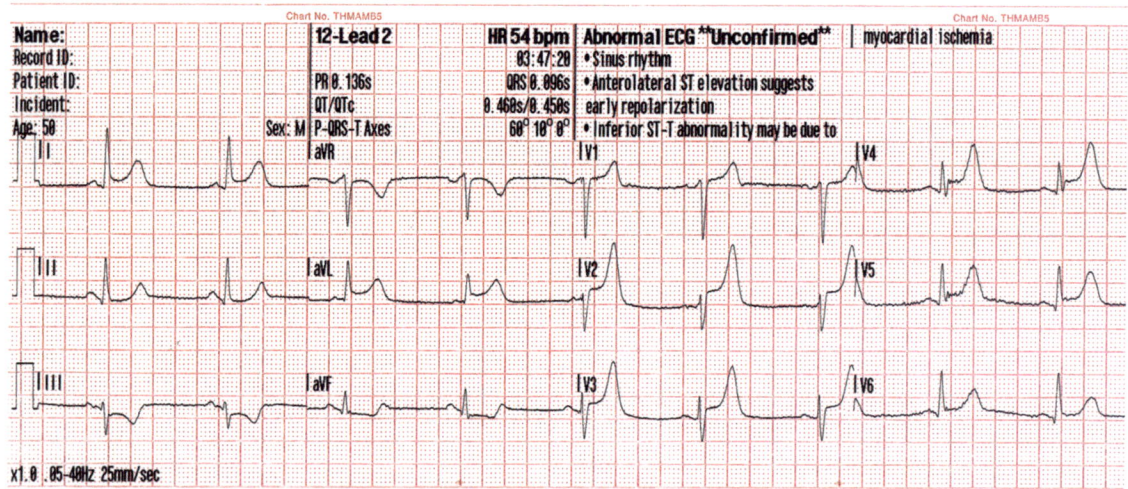

Figure 13.23 An anterolateral STEMI. Note the ST-segment elevation in the lateral leads (I, aVL, V5 and V6) and anterior leads (V2–V4). In this ECG, the computer has not recognised the STEMI yet.

due to cardiac disease, or because of heart muscle injury or infarct, the 12-lead ECG changes dramatically. Due to the block, the right bundle branch conducts electrical impulses as normal, followed by a much slower cell-to-cell depolarisation of the left ventricle. This results in a wide QRS complex.

The three main criteria for diagnosing left bundle branch block (LBBB) on a 12-lead ECG are [Garcia, 2015]:
- QRS duration of ≥ 0.12 seconds
- wide R waves in leads I and V6 with no Q waves
- wide S wave in lead V1 (may have a small R wave).

Figure 13.24 shows a classic LBBB pattern. It is quite characteristic and often described as 'ugly'. If LBBB is assumed to be of new onset (ideally compared with a previous 12-lead ECG) and the patient has signs and symptoms of an acute coronary syndrome, the patient should be considered for urgent reperfusion. Although you are unlikely to have access to a patient's medical records out-of-hospital, it is fairly common for patients who have spent time on a coronary care unit to

Cardiovascular system disorders

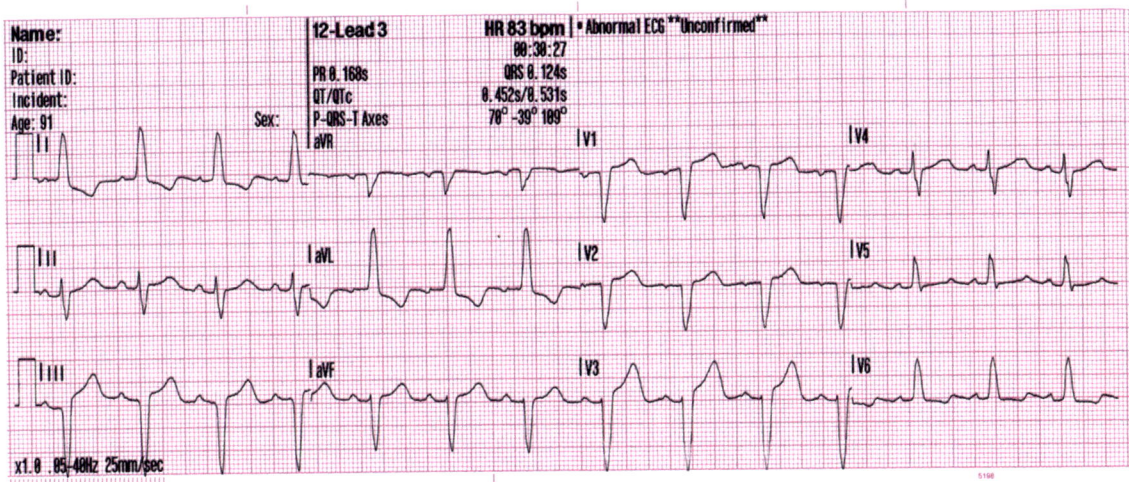

Figure 13.24 LBBB on a 12-lead ECG. Note the QRS duration has been calculated as 0.124 seconds, there are wide R waves in V1 and V6 and a wide S wave in V1.

be sent home with a copy of their discharge ECG, which may prove helpful for comparison.

4 Cardiovascular system disorders

4.1 Learning objectives

By the end of this section you will be able to:
- describe the following conditions of the cardiovascular system and their management:
  - coronary artery disease
  - stable angina
  - acute coronary syndromes
  - heart failure
  - aortic dissection
- explain the types and causes of shock and their management
- briefly outline the pathophysiology of sickle cell disease
- explain the management of a patient in sickle cell crisis.

4.2 Introduction

Many of the cardiovascular conditions you are going to learn about in this section are most commonly caused by the consequences of ischaemic heart disease (IHD), which is the most common cause of death worldwide, with around 1.8 million people dying of it each year in Europe [Ibanez, 2018]. However, this section will also cover some other conditions that affect the cardiovascular system.

4.3 Coronary artery disease

Coronary artery disease (CAD, sometimes called ischaemic heart disease) is almost always caused by atherosclerosis of the coronary arteries. This is a systemic, lipid (fat)-driven immune/inflammatory disease of the medium and large arteries. Over time (usually decades), atherosclerosis causes the formation of plaques: collections of lipids and cholesterol that accumulate in the intimal layer of arteries, some of which attract macrophages (a type of white blood cell). The macrophages secrete protein-dissolving enzymes and engulf the lipids, leaving behind a lipid-rich 'necrotic core' [Falk, 2003].

The interface between the plaque and the lumen of the artery is known as the fibrous cap. If it becomes thickened it can cause narrowing of the artery lumen (stenosis). If significant, this leads to cardiac ischaemia, particularly when myocardial oxygen demand rises, such as when the patient exercises. This can lead to stable or exertional angina. If the plaque ruptures, the artery can become occluded (blocked), leading to an acute coronary syndrome [Aaronson, 2012].

4.4 Stable angina

Angina is a pain or discomfort usually felt across or in the centre of the chest as a tightness or indigestion-like ache. This can radiate to one or both arms, the neck, back or epigastrium (the portion of the abdomen between the diaphragm and umbilicus or belly button). It can be accompanied by belching, which may be wrongly assumed to be due to indigestion [Nolan, 2016].

To be classed as stable it should consist of [Montalescot, 2013]:
- classic chest discomfort as described above
- provoked by exertion or emotional stress
- relieved by rest and/or nitrates (drugs that dilate the vessels) within minutes.

Stable angina is caused by significant stenosis (> 70%) of at least one coronary artery due to coronary artery disease (CAD). This causes narrowing of the artery, which at rest still allows sufficient oxygenated blood to the myocardium. However, during exercise or stress, coronary oxygen demand increases. This demand can be met by increasing blood flow through increasing the diameter of the arteries. However, this is not possible in stenosed vessels and the resulting imbalance of oxygen supply and demand leads to myocardial ischaemia [Aaronson, 2012].

4.4.1 Management

Patients with stable angina are advised to take a dose of glyceryl trinitrate (GTN), wait five minutes and take a second dose. If their pain remains after a further five minutes, they are instructed to call for an ambulance [NICE, 2016b].

If you are the senior clinician on scene and have been called to a patient with stable angina, it is safest to manage patients as if they are suffering from an acute coronary syndrome. If you are working with a paramedic who has recorded a 12-lead ECG and found it to be completely normal, they may manage the patient differently, particularly if the patient's chest pain resolves.

4.5 Acute coronary syndromes

Acute coronary syndromes (ACS) represent a spectrum of three dangerous conditions, all of which constitute medical emergencies and result from a sudden decrease in coronary artery blood flow [Aaronson, 2012]. These three conditions, in order of increasing severity, are:
- unstable angina (UA)
- non-ST-segment elevation myocardial infarction (NSTEMI)
- ST-segment elevation myocardial infarction (STEMI).

Since the treatment of UA and NSTEMI is similar, they are usually considered together. The ST-segment in NSTEMI and STEMI refers to the portion of an ECG complex that may change (STEMI) or not (NSTEMI) during a myocardial infarction (heart attack).

Pathophysiology

The steps that lead to an ACS consist of [Aaronson, 2012]:
1. Rupture of the fibrous cap leads to platelet aggregation (clumping together).
2. Intraplaque thrombus (blood clot) expands the plaque and can occlude the artery if large enough.
3. Intraluminal thrombus resulting in partial or complete occlusion of the artery.
4. Release of vasoconstricting substances associated with platelet aggregation, which makes the vessel constrict and narrow.
5. Endothelial damage promotes further vasoconstriction.

4.5.1 Assessment

The most common presentation of ACS is chest pain felt just under the sternum (substernal) that may be described as heavy, squeezing, crushing or tight, that has lasted for more than 15 minutes and has not been relieved by GTN. The pain radiates to the left arm in about 40% of patients although it can also radiate to the right arm/shoulder or both left and right arms [Body, 2010]. In addition, it can also radiate to the neck, jaw, upper back or epigastrium. The pain can be confused with indigestion and patients may even have tried antacid medication to relieve the discomfort. Pain is not typically altered by deep breathing or coughing. The patient may have other symptoms, such as [JRCALC, 2019]:
- nausea and vomiting
- marked sweating (diaphoresis)

Cardiovascular system disorders

- pale, clammy skin
- shortness of breath
- a feeling of impending doom.

Note that up to 5% of patients do not have chest pain [Valensi, 2011]. These are more likely to be women and have diabetes or a history of heart failure [Canto, 2012].

4.5.2 Aspirin

The indications and contra-indications listed below are taken from the UK Ambulance Services Clinical Practice Guidelines [JRCALC, 2019]. However, you should be familiar with your own service guidelines as restrictions on administration may exist.

Presentation
- 300 milligram aspirin (acetylsalicylic acid) in tablet form (dispersible).

Actions
- Has an anti-platelet action that reduces clot formation.
- Analgesic, anti-pyretic and anti-inflammatory.

Indication
- Adults with clinical or ECG evidence suggestive of myocardial infarction or ischaemia.

Contra-indications
- Known aspirin allergy or sensitivity.
- Children under 16 years.
- Active gastrointestinal bleeding.
- Haemophilia or other known clotting disorders.
- Severe hepatic disease.

Cautions
- As the likely benefits of a single 300 milligram aspirin outweigh the potential risks, aspirin may be given to patients with:
  - asthma
  - pregnancy
  - kidney or liver failure
  - gastric or duodenal ulcer
  - current treatment with anticoagulants.

Side-effects
- Gastric bleeding.
- Wheezing in some asthmatics.

Dosage and administration
- Route: oral – chewed or dissolved in water.
- 300 milligram tablet, no repeat dose.
- In suspected myocardial infarction, a 300 milligram aspirin tablet should be given regardless of any previous aspirin taken.

4.5.3 Glyceryl trinitrate (GTN)

The indications and contra-indications listed below are taken from the UK Ambulance Services Clinical Practice Guidelines [JRCALC, 2019]. However, you should be familiar with your own service guidelines as restrictions on administration may exist.

Presentation
- Metered dose spray containing 400 micrograms glyceryl trinitrate per dose.
- Tablets containing glyceryl trinitrate 2, 3 or 5 milligrams for buccal administration (depends on local ordering).

Actions
- A potent vasodilator drug resulting in:
  - dilatation of coronary arteries/relief of coronary spasm
  - dilatation of systemic veins resulting in lower preload
  - reduced blood pressure.

Indication
- Cardiac chest pain due to angina or myocardial infarction.

Contra-indications
- Hypotension (systolic blood pressure < 90 mmHg).
- Hypovolaemia.
- Head trauma.
- Cerebral haemorrhage.
- Sildenafil (Viagra) and other related drugs – glyceryl trinitrate must not be given to patients who have taken sildenafil or related drugs within the previous 24 hours. Profound hypotension may occur.
- Unconscious patients.

Side-effects
- Hypotension.
- Headache.

Dosage and administration
- Route: sub-lingual for spray and buccal for tablets.
- Sub-lingual spray: 1–2 sprays providing 400–800 micrograms of GTN.
- Buccal: 2, 3 or 5 milligram tablet.
- Repeat every 5–10 minutes.
- No maximum dose, although side-effects may limit repeat dosages.

4.5.4 Management

Patients with ACS require a 12-lead ECG as soon as possible. If this shows a STEMI or equivalent, such as a new-onset left bundle branch block (LBBB), they will receive either mechanical reopening of their arteries, if a receiving hospital capable of performing primary percutaneous coronary intervention (pPCI) can be reached within an appropriate timeframe, or chemical reopening of their arteries (thrombolysis), which can be undertaken by paramedics in some ambulance services. Even if the ECG is completely normal, patients with UA/NSTEMI may still require prompt restoration of coronary blood supply and should be treated as an emergency.

Other treatment will include [JRCALC, 2019]:
- correction of major ABC problems
- administration of aspirin, GTN, clopidogrel as per local and national clinical practice guidelines
- oxygen, if the patient has oxygen saturations of less than 94% on air
- rapid transport to an appropriate hospital.

Note: If patients meet your local ECG criteria for urgent coronary reperfusion, you should follow local guidelines regarding the most appropriate destination for the patient, which may include bypassing the local emergency department for a regional cardiac catheter lab.

4.6 Heart failure

Heart failure is an abnormality of cardiac structure or function, leading to failure of the heart to deliver oxygen at a sufficient rate to meet cell and tissue metabolic needs, despite normal filling pressures [McMurray, 2012].

Patients who have been suffering from heart failure for some time are classed as having chronic heart failure. If their signs and symptoms have not changed in the past month, then it is considered to be stable. On the other hand, if there is an acute deterioration in these patients, they are considered to be suffering from acute decompensated heart failure (often just called acute heart failure, AHF) [Allen, 2007].

Although the most common cause of AHF is sudden worsening of chronic heart failure, about 20–30% of cases are new-onset heart failure, with a small percentage due to malignant hypertensive crisis (blood pressure that is high enough to damage the body's organs) or cardiogenic shock. Up to 25% of cases are caused by an acute coronary syndrome, although these are normally considered separately from 'typical' AHF because of the differing presentation, pathophysiology and treatment [Howlett, 2011].

4.6.1 Anatomy and physiology

Recall from the cardiovascular system anatomy and physiology section that the heart is essentially two pumps in one, with the right side moving deoxygenated blood from the venous to the pulmonary circuit and returning it to the left side, which pumps the oxygenated blood into the arterial circulation. Cardiac output (CO) is the volume of blood ejected from the ventricles every minute and is a product of heart rate and stroke volume. Heart rate is regulated by the autonomic nervous system, and the stroke volume is dependent on three key factors [Tortora, 2017]:
- preload
- contractility
- afterload.

Preload
This is the volume of blood stretching the resting heart muscle at the end of diastole [Porth, 2014], and is largely determined by central venous pressure (CVP) and the compliance of the ventricular walls [Aaronson, 2012].

Contractility
The forcefulness of muscle contraction is known as its contractility; it can be increased by sympathetic nervous system innervation and the

stretching of heart muscle fibres, due to increases in end-diastolic pressures. In a similar way to stretching a rubber band, as heart muscle fibres are stretched by increasing blood volume, they contract with greater force, a characteristic known as the Frank–Starling mechanism [Porth, 2014]. This is an important method the heart utilises to balance left and right ventricular volumes during normal physiological events, such as breathing and change of posture. It also plays an important compensatory role in heart failure [Aaronson, 2012].

Afterload

The final component of stroke volume is afterload. This is the pressure exerted by the systemic circulation that the left ventricle needs to overcome in order to eject blood from the heart [Tortora, 2017].

4.6.2 Pathophysiology

Heart failure usually begins with left ventricular dysfunction caused by myocardial injury (such as myocardial infarction, MI). This causes ventricular enlargement and dilation and impaired contractility. Untreated, this typically gets worse over time and the ventricle becomes less efficient at pumping blood around the systemic circulation. In the long term, this leads to a spiral of increased, but less efficient, cardiac energy expenditure and reduced myocardial perfusion. As a result, the heart becomes increasingly dependent on the sympathetic nervous system to maintain cardiac output [Magner, 2004].

As cardiac reserve (the difference between maximum and resting cardiac output) is consumed by declining heart muscle function, eventually the patient will suffer an episode of acute decompensation. Declining cardiac output on the left side of the heart (left heart failure) causes increased end-diastolic and pulmonary venous pressures as blood backs up into the pulmonary circulation. Fluid begins to accumulate in the lung tissue and this, coupled with the increasing volumes of blood in lung vessels, makes them stiffer and less compliant, causing difficulty in breathing (dyspnoea). In the early stages, this may only occur on lying flat (orthopnoea) and is one of the causes of sudden night-time waking with shortness of breath (paroxysmal nocturnal dyspnoea, PND). Large increases in pulmonary capillary pressure can force fluid into the alveoli, causing pulmonary oedema, severe dyspnoea, decreased gaseous exchange and hypoxaemia [Aaronson, 2012].

Right heart failure has a number of causes, including chronic obstructive pulmonary disease (COPD), pulmonary embolism, heart valve disease and left heart failure. As central venous pressure increases, fluid accumulates in the peripheral tissues, causing pitting oedema in the ankles initially, but rising to the knees and sacrum in severe cases. Other signs of this fluid accumulation can also be seen in the abdomen [Porth, 2014].

4.6.3 Assessment

Heart failure can be difficult to diagnose in the pre-hospital environment, since many of the symptoms are non-specific (Table 13.1), making it difficult to differentiate AHF from other conditions such as pneumonia, chronic obstructive pulmonary disease (COPD) and pulmonary oedema [Williams, 2013]. The more specific symptoms (such as orthopnoea, paroxysmal nocturnal dyspnoea and haemoptysis) are less common [Dobson, 2009].

In AHF, a normal ECG is very unlikely with typical changes including atrial fibrillation and left bundle branch block [Kelder, 2011]. This is unsurprising when you consider that heart failure is unusual in patients without a cause of cardiac injury, such as myocardial infarction [McMurray, 2012].

4.6.4 Management

The management of acute heart failure (AHF) is determined by two key factors in patient presentation: adequate perfusion and signs of congestion [JRCALC, 2019]. Prior to this, however, it is crucial to identify patients with acute coronary syndromes (ACS), particularly ST-segment elevation myocardial infarction (STEMI), as the best treatment for these patients is urgent reperfusion with primary percutaneous coronary intervention (pPCI) or (as a second choice) thrombolysis [McMurray, 2012].

Chapter 13 – Circulation

Table 13.1 History, signs and symptoms of heart failure.

History	Signs	Symptoms
Patient age	Tachypnoea	Shortness of breath
Coronary artery disease	Crackles	Dyspnoea
Hypertension	Dullness to percussion	Orthopnoea
High cholesterol	Reduced SpO$_2$	Fatigue
Valvular disease (e.g. mitra regurgitation or aortic stenosis)	Haemoptysis	Paroxysmal nocturnal dysponea
Known heart failure or myocardial injury	Tachycardia	Reduced exercise tolerance
Loop diuretic use	Peripheral oedema	Ankle swelling
Arrhythmias	Hepatomegaly	
	Ascites	
	Oliguria	

All patients should receive oxygen if their SpO$_2$ is less than 94% on air and a salbutamol nebuliser is acceptable if wheezing is present, in recognition of the potential misdiagnosis of COPD and asthma in this group of patients [JRCALC, 2019]. In patients with signs of inadequate perfusion (reduced level of consciousness, systolic blood pressure less than 90 mmHg and delayed capillary refill time) who do not have signs of congestion (crackles on auscultation, peripheral oedema and distended neck veins), then careful titration of IV fluids is indicated. Follow the guidance of your senior clinician.

Upright positioning, and the administration of GTN and furosemide is advocated for patients without signs of inadequate perfusion and signs of congestion. Evidence for both drugs is lacking, so a decision to administer these drugs (or not) will be taken by a senior clinician, if present.

4.7 Aortic dissection

An aortic dissection occurs when the innermost layer of the aorta is breached, allowing blood to enter the medial layer of the vessel, creating a false lumen [Nienaber, 2012; Thrumurthy, 2012]. Aortic dissection, together with intramural haematoma, penetrating atherosclerotic ulcer and intimal laceration of the aorta due to trauma, form a collection of conditions known as acute aortic syndromes. They all share common clinical characteristics and are difficult to treat [Nienaber, 2012].

Aorta

The largest artery in the body is the aorta. Although a continuous vessel, it is often divided anatomically into the thoracic aorta, above the diaphragm, and the abdominal aorta, below. The thoracic portion of the aorta can be further subdivided into the ascending aorta, which arises from the left ventricle and heads upwards, backwards and to the left, arching over the pulmonary arteries (imaginatively called the arch of the aorta) and becoming the descending aorta, which continues through the thorax and abdomen before finally bifurcating into the common iliac arteries in the pelvis [Drake, 2015].

4.7.1 Pathophysiology

In order for aortic dissection to occur non-traumatically, the medial layer has to degenerate, either due to ageing or genetics.

Cardiovascular system disorders

A thinner and weaker medial layer leads to increased stress on the vessel walls thanks to Laplace's Law, which states that wall stress is directly proportional to the pressure and radius of the vessel and inversely proportional to its thickness. This is compounded by fragmentation of the elastic layers that occurs as part of the ageing process, leading to a reduction in vessel wall compliance. Add hypertension to the mix and the scene is set for aortic dissection [Kumar, 2012].

Aortic dissection occurs when the intima is torn, typically at the sites of greatest wall stress, and is classified according to which part of the aorta is affected (Figure 13.25). In the ascending aorta, the point of greatest wall stress occurs close to the aortic valve on the right lateral wall of the aorta, and in the descending aorta near the ligamentum arteriosum [Ahmad, 2006].

Blood under high pressure is able to split (dissect) the media, forming a false channel, or lumen. Depending on the blood pressure and rate of acceleration of the blood flow, the dissection extends in the direction of blood flow (although can propagate in the opposite direction as well). The blood pressure in the new, false lumen can be high enough to compress and even obstruct the true lumen. Ultimately, the false lumen will either be occluded by thrombus, re-communicate with the true lumen or work its way into other potential spaces, such as the pericardium and pleural or peritoneal cavities [Kumar, 2012; Ahmad, 2006]. As the dissection extends, arteries branching off from the aorta can become affected, leading to cerebral, coronary, mesenteric, renal and limb ischaemia.

4.7.2 Assessment

Patients are more commonly men over 60 years of age [Ranasinghe, 2011]. Pain is the most common presenting symptom of acute aortic dissection, which is typically of sudden onset and very severe [Nienaber, 2012]. However, around 10% of patients will have no pain, particularly if they are diabetic [Thrumurthy, 2012]. Although the textbook description of the pain is tearing or ripping, patients are more likely to describe their pain as sharp [Ramanath, 2009]. Pain location varies depending on the type of dissection. Patients with type II

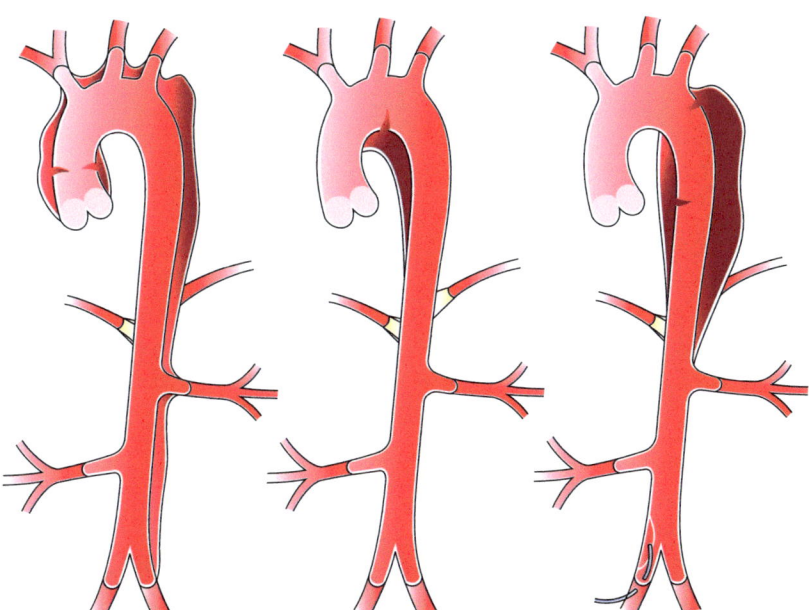

Figure 13.25 DeBakey classification of aortic dissection. (Left) Type I: Originates in ascending aorta; expands to the aortic arch and often beyond into the descending aorta. (Middle) Type II: Originates and is confined to the ascending aorta. (Right) Type III: Originates and is confined to the descending aorta.

dissections (involving the ascending aorta) are more likely to complain of anterior chest pain whereas type III dissections (which do not involve the ascending aorta) are more commonly associated with back and abdominal pain. Pain can radiate into the neck (type II) or interscapular area (type III) and can change as the dissection progresses along the aorta [Thrumurthy, 2012].

Other signs and symptoms to look out for include neurological deficits (for example, loss of consciousness), symptomatic limb ischaemia, pulse deficits between limbs and a systolic blood pressure differential between arms of more than 20 mmHg (Note: not in type III dissections) [Ranasinghe, 2011].

Frustratingly, there are a number of differential diagnoses to consider that not only mimic the signs and symptoms of aortic dissection, but can also be caused by a dissection [Thrumurthy, 2012]:
- acute chest pain
  - myocardial infarction
  - pulmonary embolism
  - spontaneous pneumothorax
- acute abdominal or back pain
  - renal colic
  - perforated viscus
  - mesenteric ischaemia
- pulse deficit
  - non-dissection-related embolic disease
- focal neurological deficit
  - stroke
  - cauda equina syndrome.

4.7.3 Management

Initial treatment common to both types includes strong analgesia (usually opiates, but Entonox is a reasonable alternative if you are not working with a paramedic) to help reduce the sympathetic-mediated release of catecholamines (adrenaline) and trying to calm and reassure your patient while getting them to hospital as quickly as possible, since you are not going to be able to stabilise a patient in the back of your ambulance.

4.8 Shock

Shock is a clinical state in which the delivery of oxygenated blood (and other nutrients such as glucose) to the body's tissues is not adequate to meet metabolic demand [Skellett, 2016]. While the cause of shock may not originate in the cardiovascular system, it will cause an impact, sometimes life-threatening, on the system.

The types of shock vary between textbooks, but five types are included here:
- hypovolaemic shock
- distributive shock
- cardiogenic shock
- obstructive shock
- dissociative shock.

4.8.1 Hypovolaemic shock

This is an acute loss of circulating blood volume either from dehydration (loss of fluids and electrolytes) or from bleeding (haemorrhage) externally or internally. Shock due to blood loss (haemorrhagic shock) has been classified into four classes (stages) [NAEMT, 2020]:
- **Class 1:** The body is able to cope with losses and there are no obvious clinical signs.
- **Class 2:** This is the compensated stage. Blood loss is more significant, but the body has mechanisms to maintain blood pressure despite the reduction in blood volume.
- **Class 3:** This is the decompensated stage. Despite the compensatory mechanisms, blood loss is now too severe to maintain blood pressure. These patients require blood and urgent surgical intervention to stop the bleeding.
- **Class 4:** The irreversible stage. Even if the circulation is restored, the patient is still likely to die.

Note that the original stages of shock described by some trauma courses included blood loss estimates and clinical observations (such as heart and respiratory rate, blood pressure and level of consciousness) that would indicate the stage of shock the patient was experiencing. These have been shown by numerous studies to be inaccurate and so are not included here [Guly, 2010; Mutschler,

2013; Mutschler, 2014]. You will, however, still find them in many textbooks.

Signs of hypovolaemic shock
The classic signs of hypovolaemic shock include [JRCALC, 2019]:
- pallor
- cool peripheries
- anxiety and abnormal behaviour
- increased heart and respiratory rates.

Note that these may not appear until 1,000–1,500 ml of blood has been lost, and even later in some patient groups such as pregnant women, patients on medication such as beta-blockers and fit individuals.

4.8.2 Distributive shock

This type of shock is caused by widespread dilation of the peripheral vascular system because of dilation of the arterioles and/or venules. This in effect creates a larger container for the same blood volume, leading to decreased tissue perfusion. In addition, in causes such as anaphylaxis and sepsis, the vessels become 'leaky', allowing fluid to escape into the tissues and so becoming removed from the general circulation.

Common causes of distributive shock include:
- anaphylaxis
- sepsis
- nervous system-related cause such as spinal cord injury.

4.8.3 Cardiogenic shock

This is due to a primary cardiac problem when the heart is unable to circulate sufficient blood to meet the body's metabolic needs. This is most common following a myocardial infarction, but can also be caused by acute heart failure or arrhythmia.

4.8.4 Obstructive shock

This is an uncommon cause of shock and is due to an obstruction of blood flow to/from the heart. It can be caused by a tension pneumothorax, cardiac tamponade or a massive pulmonary embolism [Evans, 2012].

4.8.5 Dissociative shock

This occurs when the oxygen-carrying capacity of the blood is affected because of inadequate numbers of red blood cells available to carry sufficient oxygen (anaemia) or when competing molecules take up space on the red blood cells that would normally be used to carry oxygen, such as in cases of carbon monoxide poisoning [Skellett, 2016].

4.8.6 Management

Your management of shock will be limited if you do not have a clinician capable of administration of intravenous fluids in the case of hypovolaemic and distributive shock, or who can decompress the chest with needle thoracentesis (or thoracotomy) in cases of tension pneumothorax. However, you can take the following steps, which are still important in preventing further deterioration [JRCALC, 2019; Zideman, 2015]:
- Identify and control sources of external bleeding.
- Administer high levels of supplemental oxygen via a non-rebreathe mask.
- Place patients supine and, if there is no history of trauma, raise their legs. Note that this is only likely to provide transient improvement in vital signs (typically less than seven minutes).
- Promptly transport patients to the nearest emergency department unless there is a local pathway in place for example, for patients with STEMI or major trauma.
- If your service has access to critical care teams that carry blood products, consider contacting them early.

4.9 Sickle cell disease

Sickle cell disease (SCD, or more accurately, homozygous sickle cell anaemia) is the most commonly inherited red blood cell (RBC) disorder and is characterised by haemolysis and vaso-occlusion. It is typically found in people of African, Mediterranean and Asian descent and is associated with a range of symptoms and complications including [Kanter, 2013]:
- acute and chronic pain
- vaso-occlusive crises

- multi-organ injury
- decreased lifespan and quality of life.

4.9.1 Anatomy and physiology

There are in the region of 5.4 million RBCs (erythrocytes) in the adult male, and 4.8 million RBCs in the adult female, per micro-litre of blood. They are biconcave discs with a strong and flexible membrane that tolerates being squeezed, as occurs when they travel around the micro-circulation (e.g. capillaries). They are simple structures, with no nucleus or other organelles, such as mitochondria. As a result, they cannot reproduce or 'repair' themselves, and use anaerobic metabolism to create adenosine triphosphate (ATP, the energy source for the cell), which means that none of the oxygen carried by the cell is metabolised by itself [Tortora, 2017].

Haemoglobin

The lack of organelles in the RBC does make room for haemoglobin (Hb). In fact, each RBC contains approximately 280 million of them. These are the oxygen-carrying proteins that contain a pigment (heme), which is responsible for giving RBCs their characteristic red colour. Normal adult haemoglobin contains four globin chains (alpha-1, alpha-2, beta-1, beta-2), each with a non-protein heme bound to it. At the centre of each heme is an iron ion (Fe_{2+}) that can bind reversibly with one oxygen molecule [Mehta, 2014].

The typical life cycle of an RBC is only 120 days, due to the wear and tear caused by squeezing through capillaries. Over time, the plasma membrane becomes increasingly fragile, making it prone to rupture. Should this occur, fixed phagocytic macrophages in the liver and spleen destroy and remove them from the circulation [Tortora, 2017].

4.9.2 Pathophysiology

SCD arises because of a genetic mutation of the beta-2 subunit of Hb, which leads to the formation of abnormal sickle haemoglobin (HbS). People who inherit two copies of this mutation from their parents will have sickle cell anaemia (HbSS), whereas those who inherit only one HbS become carriers and are said to have a sickle cell trait.

People with sickle cell trait are generally free from symptoms and have some protection from the most common type of malaria. However, since a proportion of their haemoglobin is HbS, they can become symptomatic when hypoxic, e.g. due to severe respiratory illness, anaesthesia, travel in unpressurised aircraft [Longmore, 2014].

When oxygen availability is reduced or demand is high, e.g. hypoxia, stress, acidosis, HbS deforms when giving up its oxygen forming stiff, rod-like structures that bend the RBC into its characteristic sickle (crescent) shape [Tortora, 2017].

These RBCs are fragile, with a reduced lifespan (typically 10–20 days) and due to their shape can occlude the micro-circulation, which leads to ischaemia and infarction, and chronic haemolytic anaemia (a lack of RBCs due to abnormal RBC destruction). This process also leads to inflammation, platelet activation and increased adhesion of RBCs to vascular endothelium, collectively leading to blood vessel damage and blockage [Kanter, 2013].

4.9.3 Signs and symptoms

SCD is a multi-organ disease, leading to a range of symptoms and complications (generally covered by the umbrella term 'sickle cell crisis'), which vary in severity but generally worsen with age. Pain is the most common presenting symptom.

Vaso-occlusive crisis

This is typically due to microvascular occlusion and is triggered by cold, dehydration, infection or hypoxia. In children under three years of age, there may be painful swelling of the hands and feet (sickle cell dactylitis). If the mesenteric circulation is affected, ischaemia can cause abdominal pain, while bone marrow involvement leads to back, pelvic, rib and long bone pain. Vaso-occlusion of the penis can lead to priapism (an unwanted, painful erection). If the central nervous system is affected, the patient can present with stroke or convulsions [Kumar, 2012].

Acute chest syndrome
This can be caused by infection, fat embolism caused by bone marrow necrosis, or pulmonary infarction. This causes a range of signs and symptoms including [Castledine, 2009]:
- shortness of breath
- tachypnoea
- hypoxia
- cough
- fever.

4.9.4 Assessment and management
Follow the standard patient assessment approach and, if you see time-critical signs, promptly transport the patient to hospital and make an alert call. If the patient has a treatment plan, follow it where possible [JRCALC, 2019].

All patients with a sickle cell crisis should receive supplemental oxygen and it is better to over-oxygenate while preparing pulse oximetry measurement than withholding oxygen. Aim for an SpO_2 of 94–98% and administer high concentrations to children. Patients who are wheezing due to bronchoconstriction may benefit from salbutamol [Longmore, 2014].

Perform a 12-lead ECG in patients with chest pain and always offer analgesia. Patients with severe pain ideally require opiate analgesia, but Entonox can be effective, although should not be used for longer than 60 minutes due to the risk of peripheral neuropathy (damage to the peripheral nervous system [Rees, 2003].

Where possible, discourage patients from walking to the ambulance as this can exacerbate the effects of tissue hypoxia [JRCALC, 2019].

Chapter

14 Disability

1 Nervous system anatomy and physiology

1.1 Learning objectives

By the end of this section you will be able to:
- state the functions of the nervous system
- describe the anatomy and physiology of the nervous system.

1.2 Introduction

The nervous system performs three main functions in order to carry out a complex range of tasks including controlling body movements, regulating heart rate, creating memories and producing speech [Tortora, 2017; Briar, 2003]:

- **Sensory function (perception):** Receptors located around the body detect internal stimuli, such as a change in blood pressure, and external stimuli, such as a bad odour, and transmit this via afferent nerves through the cranial and spinal nerves and into the brain and spinal cord.
- **Information transfer and processing:** Nerve cells (neurons) have special projections (axons) that allow the conduction of electrical impulses. These can be delivered to other neurons, and/or modified by or integrated with other impulses to create a complex web that can process sensory information received from afferent neurons.
- **Motor function:** This is the nervous system's response to the processing stage and is communicated via efferent nerves, which carry electrical impulses from the brain via cranial or spinal nerves. This enables the brain to control the body as well as ventilation and circulation.

1.3 Anatomy and physiology

The nervous system (Figure 14.1) consists of the brain and spinal cord (generally referred to as the central nervous system, CNS) and a network of peripheral nerves either originating from the brain (as 12 pairs of cranial nerves) or the spinal cord (as 31 pairs of spinal nerves). Together with small collections of neurons known as ganglia, these form the peripheral nervous system (PNS).

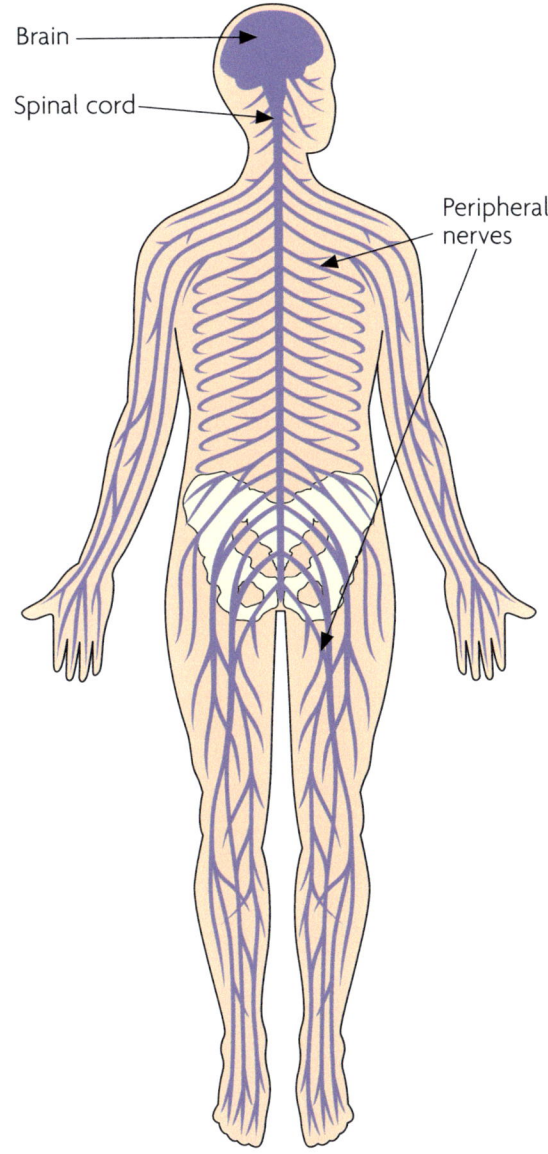

Figure 14.1 The nervous system.

Chapter 14 – Disability

The PNS consists of two divisions. The first is the sensory, or afferent, division, which is composed of large numbers of sensory receptors in the skin. Their nerve impulses are conveyed by somatic sensory fibres, as well as internally around the body (impulses from which are transmitted by visceral sensory fibres), and an extensive network of neurons around the gastrointestinal (GI) tract, collectively known as the enteric plexus, which helps regulate digestion. The other division of the PNS is the motor, or efferent, division. This is split into the somatic nervous system and the autonomic nervous system (ANS) [Marieb, 2013; Tortora, 2017].

1.3.1 Neurons and neuroglia

Neurons are the cells in the nervous system that generate electrochemical impulses enabling the nervous system to function (Figure 14.2). Most consist of [Tortora, 2017]:
- **Cell body:** Where the nucleus and other cellular organelles are found.
- **Dendrites:** The receiving or input portions of a neuron.
- **Axon:** The Long, thin portion of the neuron, which transmits electrical signals from the cell body to the axon terminals. Neurons communicate with each other via chemicals called neurotransmitters, which are released from special axon terminals called synaptic end bulbs.

Neurons vary in size, shape and speed of conduction. For example, neurons that have axons covered with myelin sheaths can conduct electrical impulses much faster than those that do not.

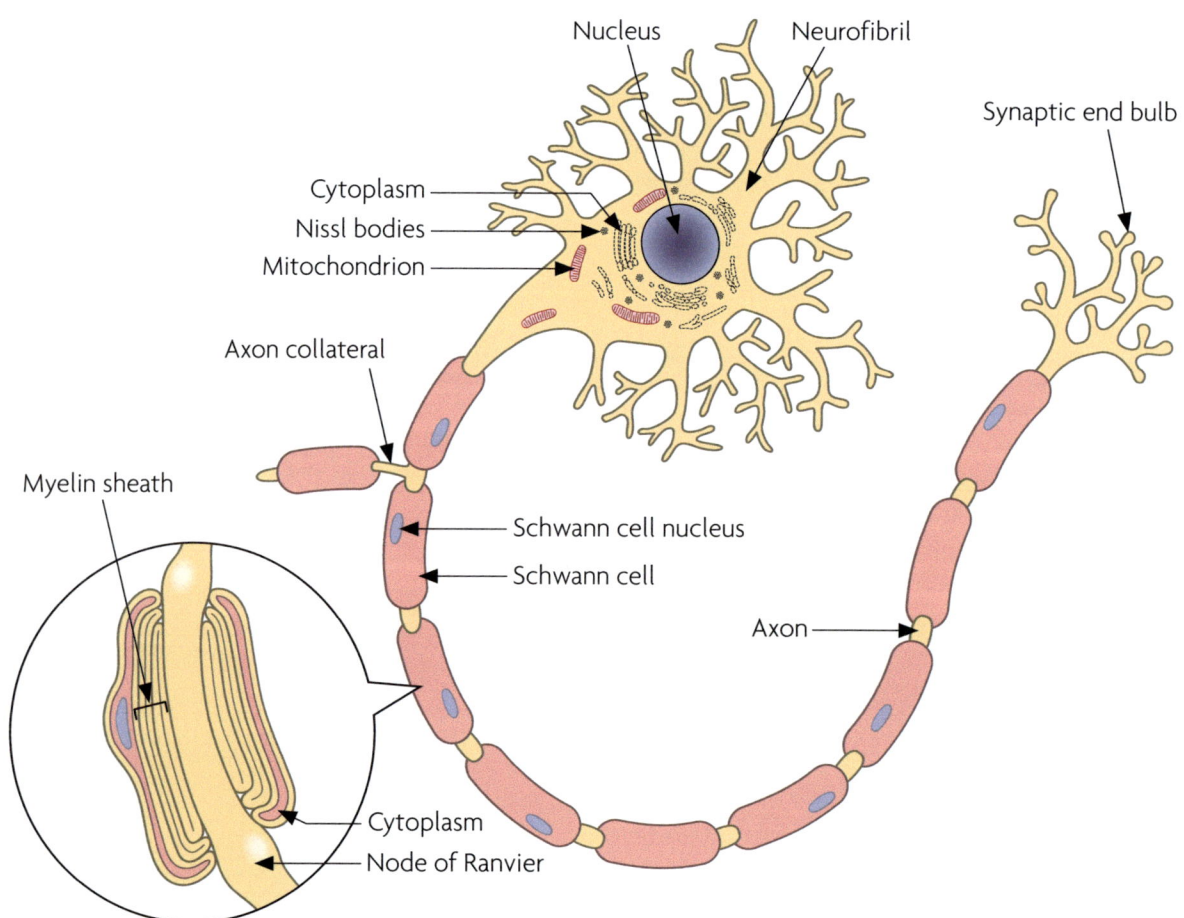

Figure 14.2 A neuron.

Neuroglia are the supporting, non-impulse generating/conducting cells in the nervous system. They have a number of roles including providing structural support for neurons and creating a blood–brain barrier, restricting the movement of substances between the blood and tissue fluids within the CNS. In addition, there are neuroglia that take on the role of a phagocyte, removing debris and damaged tissue [Tortora, 2017].

1.4 Brain

The portion of the central nervous system that is contained within the skull is known as the brain. The brain occupies 80% of the cranial vault, with the remaining 20% made up of cerebral blood (12%) and cerebral spinal fluid (8%). It has a wide range of functions as well as serving as the centre for intellect, emotions, behaviour and memory. The brain is generally divided into four major sections (Figure 14.3) [Tortora, 2017]:
- brain stem
- cerebellum
- diencephalon
- cerebrum.

1.4.1 Brain stem

The brain stem consists of the medulla oblongata, pons and midbrain. Their functions include:
- medulla oblongata
  - relays sensory and motor input between other parts of the brain and spinal cord
  - together with pons and midbrain, controls level of consciousness
  - contains centres to manage heart rate, blood pressure and breathing
  - contains origins of a number of cranial nerves
- pons
  - relays nervous impulses from one side of the cerebellum to the other and between medulla and midbrain
  - contains origins of a number of cranial nerves
  - contains centres to regulate breathing
- midbrain
  - relays motor output from the cerebral cortex and sensory input from the spinal cord to the thalamus
  - controls and co-ordinates movement
  - contains origins of two cranial nerves.

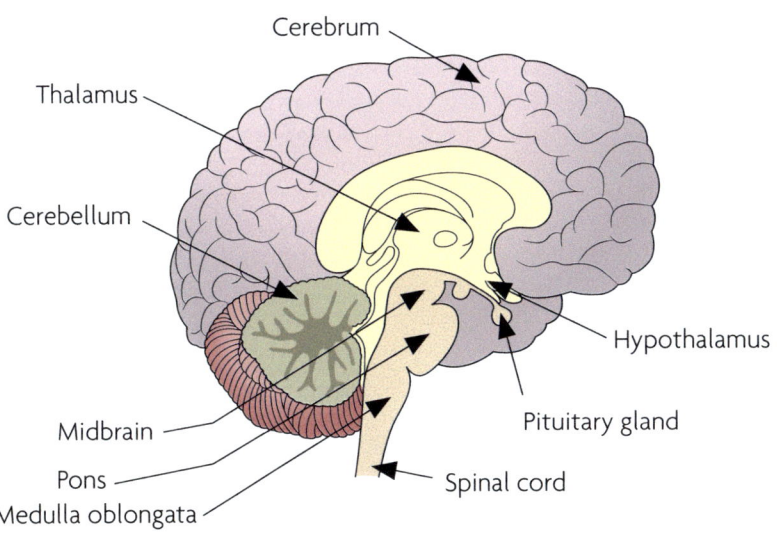

Figure 14.3 The brain.

1.4.2 Cerebellum

This part of the brain is responsible for co-ordinating complex and skilled movements, and regulates posture and balance.

1.4.3 Diencephalon

Located deep within the brain, underneath the cerebrum, the diencephalon is the link between the nervous system and the endocrine system. The diencephalon is comprised of:
- thalamus
  - relays sensory input to the cerebral cortex
  - provides perception of touch, pressure, pain and temperature
- hypothalamus
  - controls and integrates autonomic nervous system activity
  - regulates behavioural patterns and circadian rhythms
  - controls body temperature
  - regulates eating and drinking behaviour.

1.4.4 Cerebrum

The cerebrum allows you to read, write and speak. Various regions are responsible for a range of other functions:
- Sensory areas are involved in perception of sensory information.
- Motor areas control muscular movements.
- Association areas are responsible for complex functions such as memory, personality and intelligence.

The cerebrum is split into two hemispheres and consists of an outer rim of grey matter and an internal region of white matter. The outer rim of grey matter contains the cerebral cortex which, although thin, contains billions of neurons. Each hemisphere can also be further divided into four lobes: frontal, parietal, occipital and temporal.

1.4.5 Meninges

In addition to the skull, the brain is protected by the meninges. There are three of them [Tortora, 2017]:
- **Dura:** Tough outer layer consisting of connective tissue.
- **Arachnoid:** Middle layer. The sub-arachnoid space (between arachnoid and pia layers) is filled with cerebrospinal fluid (CSF).
- **Pia:** Delicate inner layer containing small blood vessels that supply oxygen and nutrients to the brain.

1.4.6 Cerebrospinal fluid

Cerebrospinal fluid (CSF) is a clear, colourless liquid, which protects the brain and spinal cord from physical and chemical injury. It also carries oxygen, glucose and other nutrients that are essential for normal brain function, as well as removing waste products [Tortora, 2017].

1.4.7 Autoregulation

The brain accounts for only 2% of total body weight, yet consumes 25% of the body's glucose. It has no storage mechanism for oxygen or glucose, so needs a continuous supply of blood, which it achieves by the process of autoregulation. This is the intrinsic ability of the brain to constrict or dilate its blood vessels in order to maintain a stable blood flow, which remains constant as long as the mean arterial pressure (MAP) stays between 50 and 150 mmHg [Mittal, 2009].

Mean arterial pressure

The MAP can be calculated from the systolic and diastolic blood pressure values using the following formula:
- Diastolic blood pressure + $\frac{1}{3}$ (systolic blood pressure - diastolic blood pressure)

Fortunately, most automatic blood pressure machines will calculate this value for you. Cerebral blood flow is reliant on the cerebral perfusion pressure (CPP), which is the pressure gradient that causes cerebral blood flow. This must be above 60 mmHg in order to perfuse the brain, and is related to MAP and intracranial pressure (ICP) by the following equation [Marieb, 2013]:
- CPP = MAP − ICP.

1.4.8 Cranial nerves

There are 12 pairs of cranial nerves (CN), which emerge from the skull (cranium, hence their

Nervous system anatomy and physiology

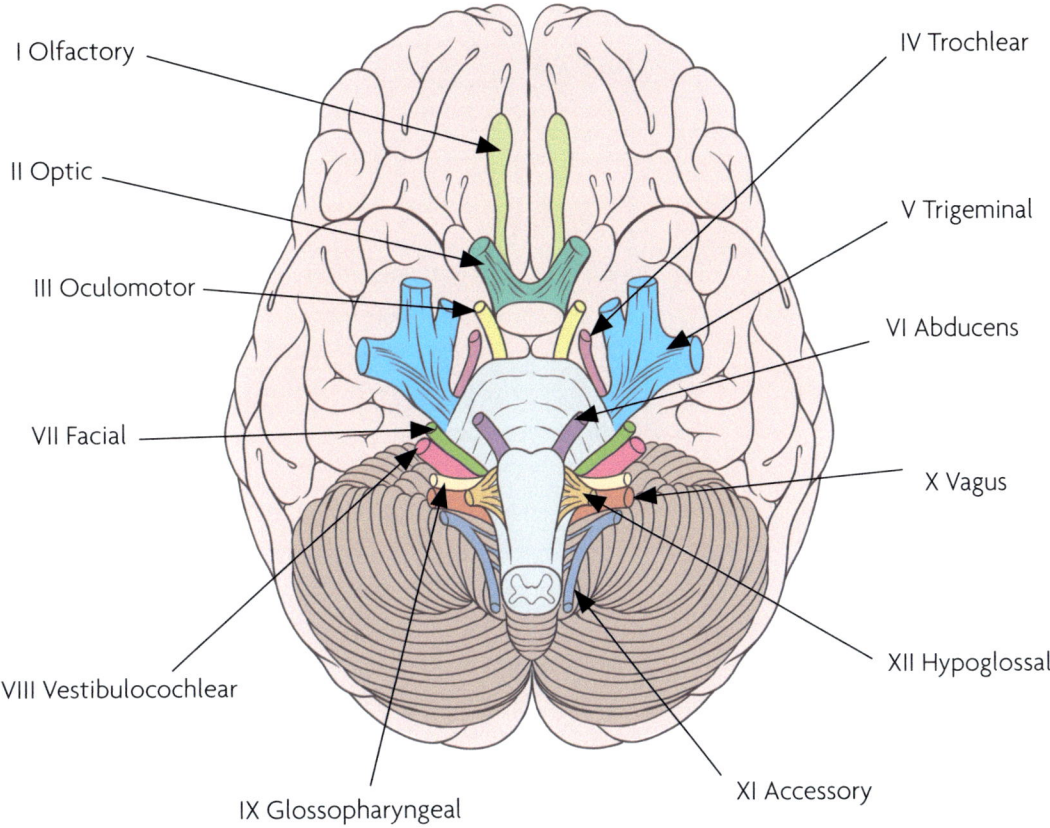

Figure 14.4 Cranial nerves.
Source: Patrick J. Lynch, medical illustrator, derivative work: Beao, derivative work: Dwstultz [CC BY 2.5], via Wikimedia Commons.

name). They are typically labelled using Roman numerals from anterior to posterior (Figure 14.4). All cranial nerves arise from the brain stem and are motor, sensory or motor and sensory nerves [Bickley, 2006]. Table 14.1 provides a summary of the function of the cranial nerves, which be pure motor or sensory nerves, or a mixture of both [Kumar, 2012; Allan, 2004].

1.5 Spinal cord

The vertebral column consists of 33 vertebrae: 7 cervical, 12 thoracic, 5 lumbar, 5 sacral and 4 coccygeal. Part of their function is to provide physical protection for the spinal cord, which the vertebrae encapsulate. Additional protection is provided by vertebral ligaments, meninges and the cerebrospinal fluid (CSF) [Tortora, 2017]. Rather confusingly, there are 31 pairs of spinal nerves: 8 cervical, 12 thoracic, 5 lumbar, 5 sacral and 1 coccygeal (Figure 14.5).

The spinal cord is almost cylindrical in shape, although slightly squashed in the anterior–posterior dimension. Its average diameter is just 12 mm, and in adults it extends from the medulla oblongata to the superior border of the second lumbar vertebra (L2), i.e. it does not extend the full length of the vertebral column. Instead, it tapers to form a cone-like structure called the conus medullaris [Tortora, 2017]. Nerves that originate distal to the conus medullaris form the cauda equina (meaning horse's tail). These nerves have a dorsal root containing afferent fibres, which transmit sensation, and a ventral root containing efferent motor fibres [Gitelman, 2008].

Table 14.1 The cranial nerves and their primary function.

Cranial nerve	Name	Function
I	Olfactory	Sensory nerve conveying sense of smell
II	Optic	Sensory nerve conveying sight
III	Oculomotor	Motor nerve, responsible for eyelid elevation and certain eye movements
IV	Trochlear	Motor nerve responsible for certain eye movements
V	Trigeminal	Sensory nerve responsible for facial and corneal sensation Motor nerve controls muscle used for chewing (mastication)
VI	Abducens	Motor nerve responsible for certain eye movements
VII	Facial	Motor nerve that controls the muscles of facial expression Sensory nerve partially responsible for taste
VIII	Vestibulocochlear	Sensory nerve conveying hearing and assisting with balance
IX	Glossopharyngeal	Sensory nerve partially responsible for taste Motor nerve for pharyngeal muscles
X	Vagus	Motor nerve controlling movements of the larynx, soft palate and pharynx Provides innervation to the heart, lungs and portion of the intestines as part of the parasympathetic nervous system
XI	Accessory	Motor nerve controlling head turning and shoulder shrugging
XII	Hypoglossal	Motor nerve responsible for movement of the tongue

1.6 Somatic nervous system

The somatic nervous system is also sometimes known as the voluntary nervous system, since it allows the person to consciously control their skeletal muscles thanks to somatic nerve fibres that conduct impulses from the central nervous system to the skeletal muscles [Marieb, 2013]. However, the somatic nervous system also includes an involuntary component: reflexes. These are primarily a protective mechanism, for instance removing your hand when you touch something hot [Tortora, 2017].

1.7 Autonomic nervous system

The autonomic nervous system (ANS) is divided into three parts. These are the sympathetic, parasympathetic and enteric nervous systems. They are called autonomic because it was originally believed that they functioned completely independently from the central nervous system (CNS). However, it is now known that the hypothalamus and brain stem regulate ANS activity [Tortora, 2017]. The enteric division is an extensive network of neurons that reside within the walls of the gastrointestinal (GI) tract, pancreas and gall bladder. It has a sensory nervous function enabling the monitoring of the mechanical state of the alimentary canal and the chemical status of the stomach and intestines. In addition, it can output motor signals to modify the motility and secretions of the gut, as well as controlling the diameter of local blood vessels [Briar, 2003].

The sympathetic and parasympathetic divisions of the ANS are often thought of as being at either end of a see-saw. This is true in some organs such as the heart, but in reality this is rather a simplistic view. Some parts of the body receive inputs from

Nervous system anatomy and physiology

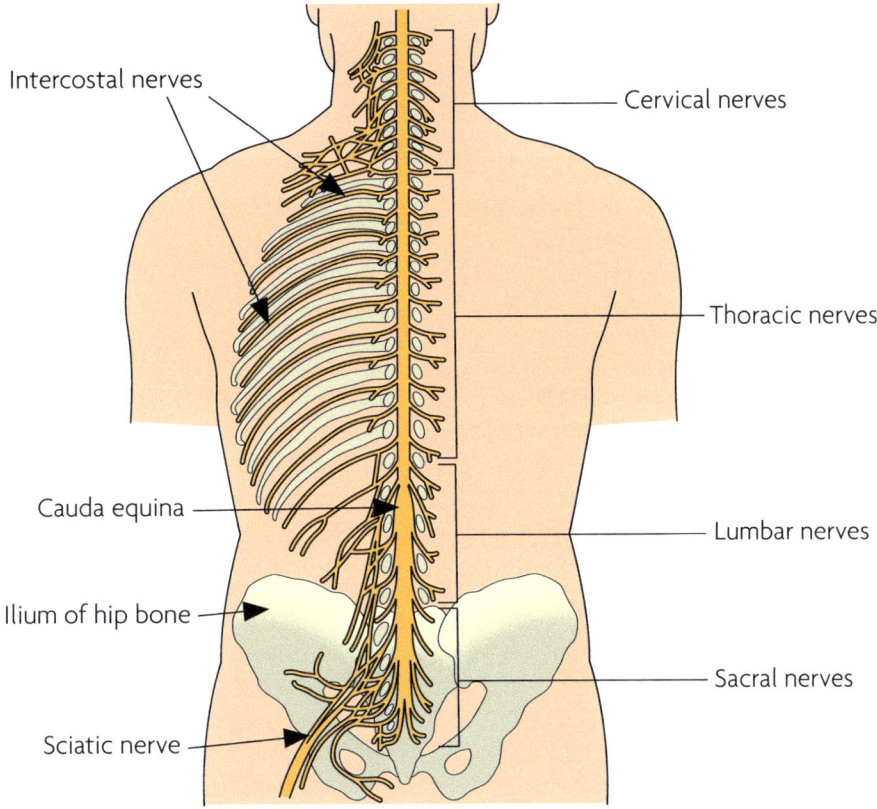

Figure 14.5 Spinal nerves.

only one division, whereas in others the effects of the sympathetic and parasympathetic divisions are similar. However, their actions are carefully controlled and co-ordinated by the hypothalamus.

1.7.1 Sympathetic and parasympathetic divisions

The sympathetic division is often referred to as the fight-or-flight division as its actions prepare the body to respond to stress, facilitating sudden strenuous exercise and increased vigilance. In addition, it helps control blood pressure, thermoregulation, and gut and urogenital function.

The parasympathetic division is often referred to as the rest-and-digest division. Actions of the parasympathetic division include antagonising some effects of the sympathetic division, for example heart rate, gut motility and bronchiole diameter, and controlling many body functions in non-stress states such as GI secretion to aid digestion, micturition and defecation.

Another important difference between the sympathetic and parasympathetic divisions is their structure. Parasympathetic neurons are clustered at either end of the spinal cord, whereas the sympathetic neurons originate from the thoracolumbar section.

1.8 *The eye*

The eye is an asymmetric globe about 2.5 cm in diameter with the anterior boundary surrounded by the eyelid and eyelashes. The eyelids and eyebrows protect the eye, providing shade during sleep, restricting excessive light and foreign objects from causing damage and limiting sweat dripping on to the eyeball. In addition, eyelids spread a film of tears with each blink to prevent the eye from drying out [Tortora, 2017].

The eye itself consists of a layer of photoreceptor cells and associated neurons (the retina), which are encapsulated by a white, tough and rubbery outer coat (the sclera) that is transparent anteriorly (the cornea, Figure 14.6). This is the main refractive component of the eye responsible for focusing light on to the retina. It is assisted in this by the lens, which up until around 50 years of age can change shape to enable focusing on objects closer to the eye [Kapit, 2001].

There are three chambers in the eye: anterior, posterior and vitreous. The anterior chamber is bordered by the cornea anteriorly, and the iris and lens posteriorly, whereas the posterior chamber lies between the iris and the lens. They are filled with aqueous humour, a watery solution full of nutrients to nourish the avascular cornea and lens [Root, 2009].

The vitreous chamber is filled with a different type of fluid: vitreous humour. This is a clear, jelly-like substance that occupies around two-thirds of the eye. It is mostly water, with few cells, but is firmly attached to the peripheral retina and optic disc.

It is also attached, albeit less firmly, to the macula and retinal vessels. Vitreous humour can liquefy and collapse with older age and certain degenerative conditions, a process known as posterior vitreous detachment.

The inner surface of the posterior sclera is lined with a highly pigmented and vascular layer (the choroid), which absorbs and prevents the scattering of light. It thickens anteriorly to become the ciliary body, surrounding the lens. On the anterior portion of the ciliary body sits a thin, pigmented epithelial and fibromuscular layer (the iris), which controls the amount of light entering the eyeball via the pupil. The pupil looks black when you look into it because of the heavily pigmented choroid and retina, but if you shine a light (such as a camera flash) into the pupil, the red of the blood vessels on the surface of the retina is reflected [Tortora, 2017].

The inner coating of the eye (the retina) extends anteriorly to the ora serrata. It is the beginning of the visual pathway and consists of a pigmented layer and the neural layer of the retina. The

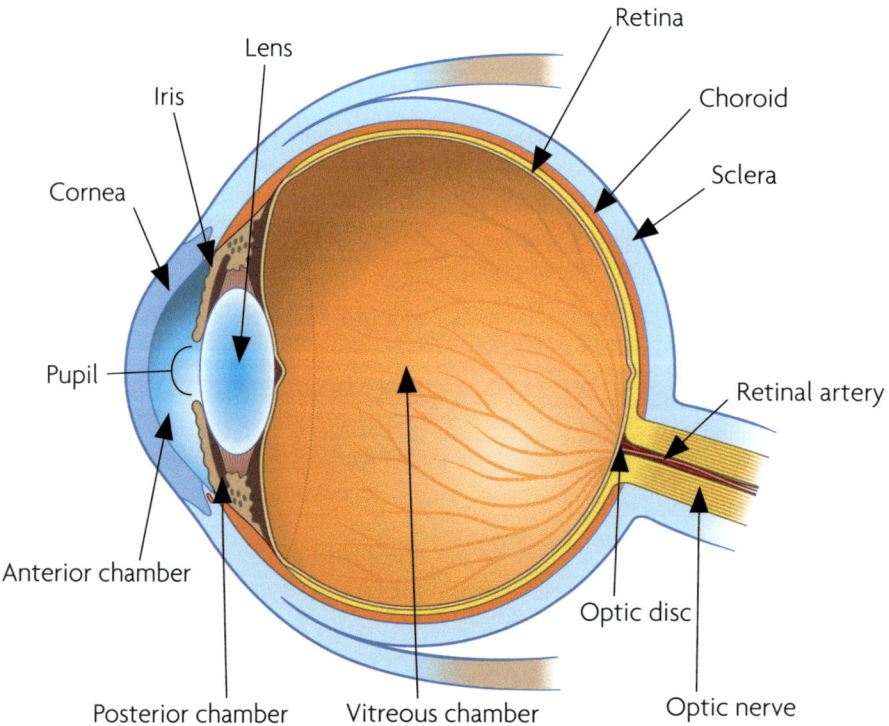

Figure 14.6 Superior view of the transverse section of the eye.

neural (or sensory) layer contains colour- and form-sensitive cone cells and colour-insensitive rod cells, which are connected to optic nerve axons. These extend posteriorly to the optic disc and leave the eye as the optic nerve (CN II). The optic disc is called the blind spot because it contains no rods or cones, but you are usually not aware of this because of your binocular vision.

The macula is the yellow-pigmented area of the retina, responsible for central vision. It contains the fovea centralis, the centre of highest visual acuity in good light, due to the high number of cones present. Rods are more plentiful towards the periphery of the retina, which is why you can see better with your peripheral vision in low light [Root, 2009].

2 Assessment of disability

2.1 Learning objectives

By the end of this section you will be able to:
- describe how to undertake and record the following:
  - Glasgow Coma Scale score
  - pupillary response
  - face, arm, speech test.

2.2 Introduction

A complete assessment of the nervous system is involved and requires a number of tests that are beyond the scope of this book. However, there are several useful and simple tests you can perform that will uncover the presence of serious neurological problems in your patient and help to determine the most appropriate management for them. You have already met one of them, AVPU, in Chapter 10, 'Patient Assessment', and you will learn about a more thorough way to record a patient's level of consciousness using the Glasgow Coma Scale.

2.3 Glasgow Coma Scale

The Glasgow Coma Scale (GCS) was developed in 1974 as a way of objectively testing the level of consciousness in brain-injured patients and to improve communication between healthcare professionals [Teasdale, 1974]. It was originally a 14-point score, but the division of limb flexion into withdrawal and abnormal flexion led to the 15-point score familiar today (Table 14.2) [Teasdale, 2015]. Although designed for in-hospital use, it is now routinely used by the ambulance service and is an important marker for the early management of traumatic brain injury (TBI) [Bazarian, 2003].

The main use for the GCS is to indicate the level of injury or illness, enabling triage and intervention priorities to be established, and then to monitor trends in consciousness over time. In addition, GCS (in theory) provides an objective way of recording and communicating the patient's level of consciousness between healthcare professionals when handing over care [Middleton, 2012].

Scores should ideally be given as their separate components, i.e. eyes, verbal and motor. The motor component, in particular, is of interest to neurosurgeons as it is most predictive of outcome in severe head injuries [Middleton, 2012]. The exact order doesn't matter, although eyes, verbal, motor has been advocated, as the top scores increase incrementally, i.e. eyes = 4, verbal = 5 and motor = 6. This also corresponds to the patient assessment sequence you will follow [Zuercher, 2009].

2.3.1 Recording an accurate GCS

As you approach the patient, and as part of your global assessment (the general impression), take note of local injuries to the eyes, mouth and limbs, the presence of tracheal or tracheostomy tubes, and prior administration of sedative or paralytic drugs, as all of these can affect the accuracy of the GCS. Alcohol consumption does not appear to cause clinically significant reductions in GCS scores in patients with traumatic brain injury (TBI) [Stuke, 2007], even if patients are twice over the legal drink-drive limit [Lange, 2010]. As a result, reductions in GCS scores in the presence of a head injury should not just be attributed to alcohol.

Chapter 14 – Disability

Table 14.2 The Glasgow Coma Scale.

Component	Assessment	Rating	Score
Eye opening	Open before stimulus	Spontaneous	4
	After spoken or shouted request	To sound	3
	After trapezius or fingertip stimulus	To pressure	2
	No opening at any time	None	1
Best verbal response	Correctly gives name, place and date	Orientated	5
	Not orientated, but communicates coherently	Confused	4
	Intelligible single words	Words	3
	Only moans/groans	Sounds	2
	No audible response	None	1
Best motor response	Obeys two-part request	Obeys commands	6
	Brings hand above clavicle to trapezius stimulus	Localising	5
	Bends arm at elbow rapidly, but movement appears normal	Normal flexion	4
	Bends arm at elbow, but clearly abnormal	Abnormal flexion	3
	Extends arm at elbow	Extension	2
	No movement in arms/legs	None	1

Painful stimuli

The aim of a pain stimulus is to assess the level of consciousness and depth of coma, but not to cause long-term pain or damage, which could be considered battery [Waterhouse, 2009]. There are two basic types of pain stimulus to use when assessing GCS: peripheral and central. Use a central pain stimulus first because if the patient opens their eyes and moves their arms in response to this, there is no need to test the peripheral pain response.

The preferred central pain stimulus is the trapezius pinch (Figure 14.7) [Middleton, 2012]. It can be tricky to apply sufficient pressure on the trapezius

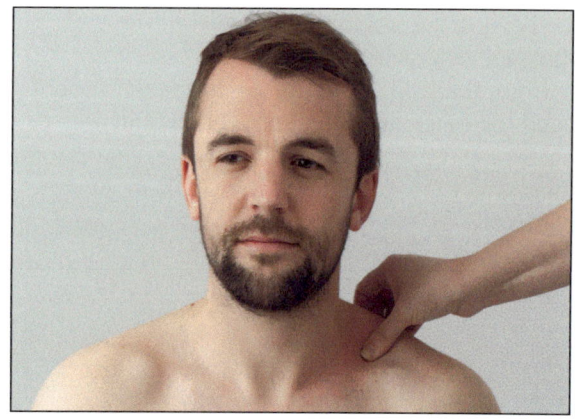

Figure 14.7 Trapezius pinch.

muscle in larger or obese patients and there is some concern about the spinal accessory nerve (which you are stimulating with a trapezius pinch), because it has only a small sensory component compared with its motor function, which increases the risk of a spinal reflex action when you pinch it [Tortora, 2017]. A patient with a spinal injury that affects the arms should not have a trapezius pinch applied.

If a peripheral pain stimulus is required, apply pressure with a pen over the lateral aspect of the distal interphalangeal joint of the index finger. Do not apply direct pressure over the nail bed as this can damage the capillary bed and may result in loss of the nail [Waterhouse, 2009].

2.3.2 Eye opening

If the eyes are open, give the patient a score of 4 and move on to the verbal component. If the patient opens their eyes to spoken or shouted speech (and not necessarily just the command to open their eyes), score a 3. If the patient responds to painful stimuli by opening their eyes, give them a 2, and award a 1 if they fail to respond at all.

2.3.3 Best verbal response

- Orientated patients score 5 and are required to be orientated to person, place, time and the event/situation.
- Confused patients score 4 and can converse, but responses to your questions will reveal disorientation and misunderstanding [Iacono, 2005].
- Inappropriate words score 3 and consist of clear and understandable speech (often swearing or random words). However, it is not possible to hold a conversation with the patient. Repetition of a word or phrase (perseveration) is also awarded a 3.
- Incomprehensible sounds score 2 and consist of moaning and groaning, but no recognisable words. Stroke patients with dysphasia may fall into this category but this is due to a different cause than patients with a moderate or severe TBI who lack sufficient cognition to speak. Make sure you document the difference [Iacono, 2005].
- No verbal response scores a 1 and should be given to patients who make no sound. Follow local guidance about documenting verbal GCS scores for patients who have a tracheal tube in situ (sometimes denoted as NT) or who have been pharmacologically sedated or paralysed [Matis, 2008].

2.3.4 Best motor response

- A patient who obeys commands scores 6. This should be a two-part instruction, such as asking the patient to squeeze and release your fingers or raise and lower their arms [Teasdale, 2014].
- Localisation in response to a stimulus scores a 5 and requires the patient to identify the location of a painful stimulus and attempt to remove it. In the case of a trapezius pinch, you should expect the opposite arm to cross the midline in an attempt to remove the source of the pain (i.e. you!) [Matis, 2008].
- Normal flexion to a stimulus scores 4. This is a normal flexor response where the patient rapidly withdraws their arm and/or abducts the ipsilateral (same side) shoulder [Middleton, 2012]. A peripheral pain stimulus may be required to elicit this accurately.
- Abnormal flexion in response to a stimulus scores 3. This is also sometimes called a decorticate response, and consists of slow adduction and flexion of the arms, flexion of the wrists and fingers, and internal rotation of the legs with plantar flexion of the feet (Figure 14.8).
- Extension to a stimulus (also called a decerebrate response) scores 2. In contrast to abnormal flexion, the arms go into rigid extension alongside the body with pronation of the forearms, and the same leg posture as for abnormal flexion (Figure 14.9) [Iacono, 2005]. Because of the need to record the 'best' score, in the event that there is abnormal flexion on one

Chapter 14 – *Disability*

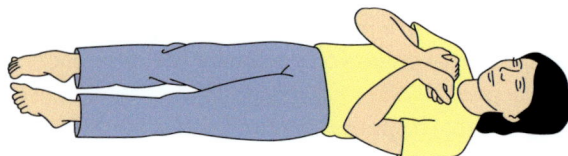

Figure 14.8 Abnormal flexion response.

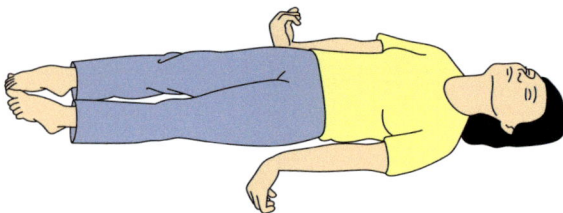

Figure 14.9 Abnormal extension response.

side of the body and extension on the other, the patient should receive a score of 3 not 2.
- No response to pain scores 1. Only score the patient a 1 if they are flaccid and make no movement in response to your painful stimulus.

2.4 Pupillary response

Before switching on your pen torch to check the patient's pupils, have a look at the pupils' relative size to determine whether they are unequal. This is known as anisocoria and is a normal finding in around 20% of the population [Kaeser, 2010]. Look for changes in shape (e.g. oval in acute angle-closure glaucoma, asymmetrical in a penetrating injury).

Pupillary reactions

Test for a direct response to light by shining a light directly on the eye for three seconds [James, 2011]. This should cause a prompt constriction of the pupil. Failure to do so is known as an afferent pupillary defect and indicates severe optic nerve pathology (transected nerve). There will also be failure of the opposite pupil to constrict. If there is no pupillary reaction but the opposite pupil does constrict, consider a traumatic iris paresis. If this test is normal, the patient can be said to have 'pupils equally reacting to light' (PERL).

2.5 *Face, arm, speech test*

With the advent of clot-busting drugs (thrombolytics) for the management of acute stroke, the need for prompt recognition of stroke by ambulance personnel has never been greater. A simple tool that can be used to identify a patient suffering from a stroke is the Newcastle face, arm, speech test (FAST) [NAO, 2010].

The FAST consists of three components [Harbison, 2003]:
- **Facial palsy:** Ask the patient to smile or show their teeth. Look for new lack of symmetry. This is positive if there is an unequal smile, grimace or obvious facial asymmetry.
- **Arm weakness:** Lift the patient's arms together to 90° (45° if they are lying on their back) with the palms uppermost (Figure 14.10). Ask them to hold that position for five seconds. Look for one arm drifting or falling rapidly.
- **Speech impairment:** During the course of a conversation (if the patient can speak), look for new speech disturbance. This may require asking someone who knows the patient. Specifically, look for slurred speech and word-finding difficulties. Ask the patient to identify common objects (such as keys, a cup, a chair and a pen). If the patient has a severe visual disturbance, place the object in the patient's hands and ask them to name it.

The presence of one or more of these signs constitutes a positive FAST (Figure 14.11).

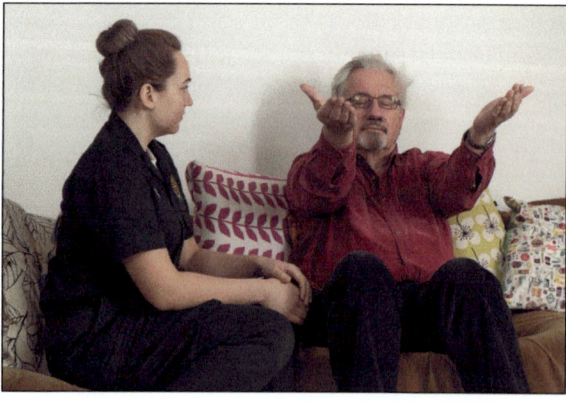

Figure 14.10 A patient performing the FAST.

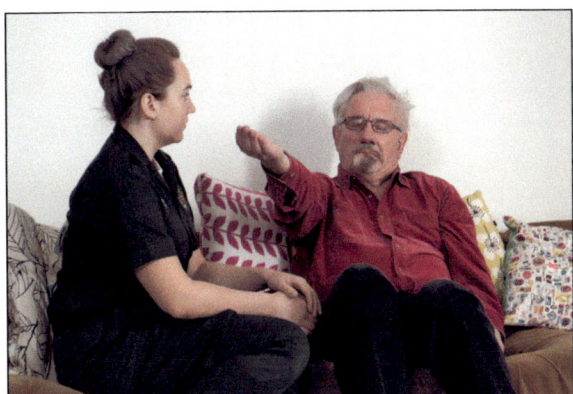

Figure 14.11 A positive FAST, due to a facial palsy and arm weakness.

3 Disorders of the nervous system

3.1 Learning objectives

By the end of this section you will be able to:
- explain the pathophysiology relating to a range of neurological disorders
- describe the management of a range of neurological disorders
- list several causes of coma.

3.2 Introduction

The nervous system is extremely complex and you will learn about only a few of the many disease processes in this section. However, it is important to be able to recognise patients with epilepsy, stroke, meningococcal disease and patients who are unconscious. Timely and appropriate management can result in a better outcome; in some cases, literally the difference between life and death, and/or life-altering disability.

3.3 Convulsions

Epilepsy is not a single condition, but a term used to describe a tendency to have recurrent, unprovoked convulsions (also called seizures and fits). It is the most common of the serious neurological conditions [Smithson, 2012].

Convulsions result from the synchronised and excessive activation of neurons in the cerebral cortex. How this presents clinically depends on where this activity starts and how far and fast it spreads through the brain [Briar, 2003]. Convulsions are divided into two broad categories:

- **Partial (focal) convulsions:** As the name suggests, these originate from a specific area of the cortex, typically the temporal or frontal lobes. They are split into two sub-types [Smithson, 2012; Briar, 2003]:
  - **Simple partial:** Patients remain conscious but may complain of 'butterflies' in their stomach, fear, illusions and hallucinations. These are usually brief.
  - **Complex partial:** This refers to an altered level of consciousness and is characterised by the patient chewing, lip-smacking and fiddling with their hands. These usually resolve within a few minutes.
- **Generalised convulsions:** These convulsions are also divided into two sub-types:
  - **Tonic-clonic:** These convulsions consist of two phases. In the tonic phase, the patient goes stiff (and may cry out), falls (if standing) and bites their tongue as the jaw clenches. This is followed by the clonic phase, characterised by regular jerking movements, which start in the upper limbs. These eventually slow and stop, which may herald the onset of incontinence. Patients typically experience a post-ictal period following a tonic-clonic convulsion, where they may be sleepy and confused. This usually resolves within 20 minutes.
  - **Absence convulsions:** These typically begin in childhood and adolescence and consist of 'day-dreaming', with a few seconds of staring into space, eyelid fluttering, swallowing and head-flopping.

3.3.1 Febrile convulsions

Patients with febrile convulsions are not considered to be epileptic, since the convulsion is provoked by a sudden increase in temperature. The most commonly affected age group is from six months to six years. They are not associated with an increased risk of developing epilepsy in later life [Lissauer, 2007].

3.3.2 Non-epileptic attack disorder

Non-epileptic attack disorder (NEAD, formerly referred to as pseudo-seizures) is a loss of normal function and control of the body by the patient, which resembles an epileptic convulsion, but is thought to have a psychological cause [Dickson, 2017]. This condition can be difficult for specialists to diagnose in the absence of an electroencephalogram (EEG, a bit like an ECG for the brain).

3.3.3 Status epilepticus

Status epilepticus has traditionally been defined as a generalised convulsion lasting for more than 30 minutes, or a series of convulsions, where the patient does not become fully conscious between convulsions, lasting more than 30 minutes [ILAE, 1993]. However, it has been suggested that shortened timescales should be used since most convulsions last fewer than five minutes and those that last more than five minutes generally require therapeutic intervention because they will not stop on their own [Brophy, 2012]. In addition, prolonged convulsions generally become resistant to the drugs typically administered for convulsions, and there is evidence from animal studies that brain injury can occur in under 30 minutes [Meldrum, 1973].

In adults and children, common causes of status epilepticus are withdrawal from or sub-therapeutic doses of anti-epileptic drugs. In children, the most common cause is febrile illness, whereas in adults, stroke is the most common cause. Approximately 16–38% of children diagnosed with status epilepticus are known epileptics. In adults, this figure increases to 42–50% [Chin, 2004; Neligan, 2010].

3.3.4 Post-ictal phase

Patients who suffer a generalised tonic-clonic convulsion, typically enter a post-convulsion (post-ictal) phase that is characterised by a period of unresponsiveness and then a gradual return of consciousness. The patient is likely to be drowsy and disorientated, which can last 15 minutes to an hour (and in some cases, longer). Complaints of a headache are common [Kumar, 2012].

3.3.5 Management of convulsions

As with all patients, start by ensuring they have a patent airway. This can be achieved by a combination of patient positioning (e.g. the recovery position) and airway adjuncts. An oropharyngeal airway can be difficult to insert when patients are convulsing and should not be forced into the patient's mouth. Instead, consider the use of alternatives, such as a nasopharyngeal airway [JRCALC, 2019].

Administer high-concentration oxygen (as close to 100% as possible) via a non-rebreathe mask (or bag-valve-mask) at a flow rate of 15 l/minute. In adults, once a reliable pulse oximetry reading has been obtained, oxygen administration can be titrated to maintain saturations of 94–98%. Children should continue to receive high concentrations of oxygen irrespective of the pulse oximeter reading [JRCALC, 2019].

If patients are still actively convulsing, you can administer the patient's own buccal midazolam if they have been prescribed it. Should they continue fitting for ten minutes after the first dose of midazolam, you should not administer further doses. If a paramedic is available and can obtain intravenous (IV) access, they may elect to administer diazepam IV. If you are on your own, or the paramedic cannot gain IV access, you should transport the patient to hospital as soon as possible.

Don't forget to check for possible causes of the convulsion and manage them appropriately.

Specifically consider:
- hypoglycaemia
- pyrexia due to underlying infection, such as meningococcal septicaemia, for example
- head injury
- alcohol/drug abuse.

Patients who are known epileptics and completely recover from their convulsion may be safe to be left at home. Follow local guidance.

3.3.6 Patient's own buccal midazolam

The indications and contra-indications listed below are taken from the UK Ambulance Services Clinical

Practice Guidelines [JRCALC, 2019]. However, you should be familiar with your own service guidelines as restrictions on administration may exist.

Presentation
- Buccolam oromucosal solution (concentration 5 mg in 1 ml) comes in four pre-filled syringes. The correct dose should be specified in the child's treatment plan or 'epilepsy passport'.

Actions
- Midazolam is a benzodiazepine drug (the same class of drug as diazepam, used by paramedics). The onset of action is typically five minutes depending on the route used to administer the drug. Some 80% of convulsions stop within ten minutes of administration.

Indication
- Generalised convulsion lasting more than five minutes.

Contra-indications
- None.

Side-effects
- Respiratory depression.
- Hypotension.
- Drowsiness.
- Muscle weakness.
- Slurred speech.
- Occasionally agitation, restlessness and disorientation may occur.

Dosage and administration
- Buccal administration with the required dose drawn up and half-administered quickly to each side of the lower buccal cavity (between the cheek and gum).
- Dosage as per patient's individual treatment plan.

3.4 *Stroke*

Stroke is a syndrome consisting of rapidly developing (usually seconds or minutes) symptoms and/or signs of focal central nervous system (CNS) function. The symptoms last more than 24 hours or lead to death. A transient ischaemic attack is essentially the same thing as a stroke, with the exception of the duration of symptoms, which last less than 24 hours and are not caused by a haemorrhage [Ginsberg, 2004]. Stroke is a common cause of death in England with around 30,000 stroke-related deaths each year. Around 57,000 people have a stroke for the first time in England every year, a quarter of them in people under 65 years of age [Public Health England, 2018].

3.4.1 Anatomy and physiology

The brain cannot store oxygen or glucose and so is dependent on a constant supply of blood, which is provided by two pairs of vessels, the vertebral and internal carotid arteries (Figure 14.12). These arteries are interconnected in the cranial cavity to produce an arterial circle (the circle of Willis), which provides an alternative pathway for blood flow should one of the vessels become occluded [Tortora, 2017].

3.4.2 Risk factors

Non-modifiable risk factors for stroke include age, sex, race and family history or previous medical history of stroke, transient ischaemic attacks or myocardial infarction. The chance of having a stroke roughly doubles each decade after the age of 55 years, and although it is more common in men, over half of all stroke deaths occur in women. People of South Asian, African or African-Caribbean origin are more likely to suffer from a stroke [O'Donnell, 2010]. Modifiable risk factors include hypertension, smoking, atrial fibrillation, diabetes, diet, physical activity, alcohol consumption, blood cholesterol and obesity [Rodgers, 2004].

3.4.3 Types of stroke

Strokes can be classified as either ischaemic or haemorrhagic in origin. Ischaemic strokes are the most common and are caused by atherosclerosis or an embolus from the heart, for example. They are responsible for around 85% of all new strokes [ISWP, 2016]. Less common are strokes of vascular origin, caused by haemorrhage. Acute stroke is a medical emergency and the treatment to re-open the arteries is time-dependent, so the sooner

Chapter 14 – *Disability*

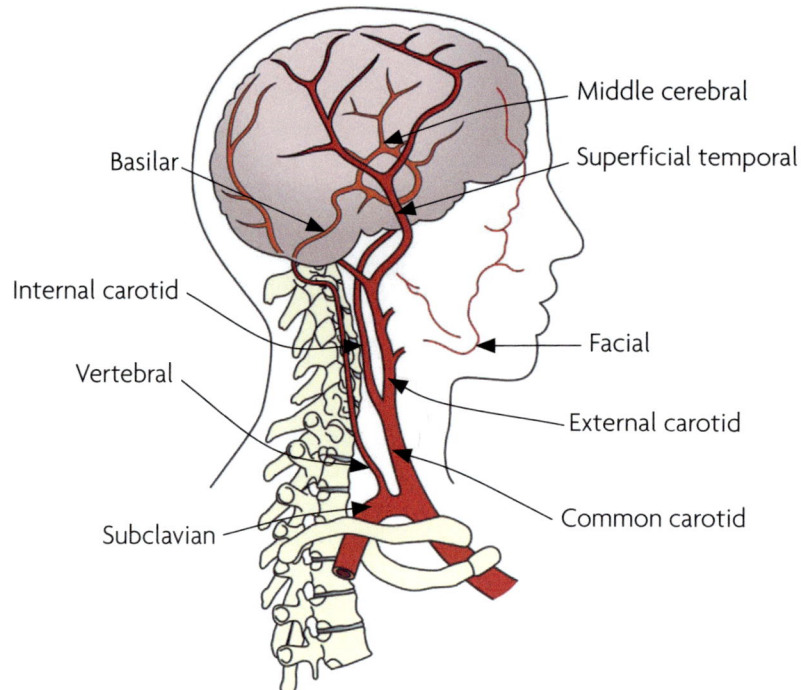

Figure 14.12 Arteries supplying the brain. Note all arteries shown are right-sided except the basilar artery.

patinets are transported to a dedicated stroke centre, the better [JRCALC, 2019].

3.4.4 Assessment and management of stroke

- Assess ABCDE as for all patients.
- Determining the time of onset in stroke is very important for subsequent treatment. Find out when the patient was last free of stroke-like symptoms.
- If the patient has any time-critical A or B problems, then they should be transported to the nearest emergency department. Alert the receiving hospital.
- Oxygen is not recommended unless the patient is hypoxic.
- FAST positive patients with no time-critical A or B problems should be transported to the nearest 'hyperacute' stroke unit. There are likely to be local arrangements in place and eligibility criteria, particularly relating to time since onset of symptoms. Consult local guidelines and don't forget to contact the receiving facility.
- Record a blood sugar; hypoglycaemia is a common stroke mimic.

3.5 *Meningococcal disease*

Meningococcal disease is an umbrella term for a systemic bacterial infection caused by Neisseria meningitidis (meningococcus). It presents as meningitis (inflammation of the meninges), septicaemia or a combination of both [Public Health England, 2019].

Although uncommon, 5% of those affected will die, and up to 36% may have long-term physical, cognitive, and psychological consequences [Public Health England, 2016]. It is most common in infants, followed by children aged 1–4 years of age and a smaller peak in incidence in young adults aged 15–24 years of age [Public Health England, 2018c].

3.5.1 Pathophysiology

Meningococci inhabit the nasopharynx in around 10% of the population, although it is less common in infants (under 5%) and most common in 19-year-olds (over 23%). If the meningococci manage

Disorders of the nervous system

to penetrate the protective mucosa of the nasal passages and enter the bloodstream, they rapidly multiply, doubling in number every 30 minutes.

In some people, meningococci cross the blood–brain barrier, where the bacteria are free to multiply inside the cerebrospinal fluid. This leads to inflammation and swelling in the meninges and brain tissue, raising intracranial pressure, which can result in nervous system damage and even death. Surprisingly, patients with meningococcal meningitis do better than those who go on to develop septicaemia. This is thought to be because the body's immune response has prevented the bacteria from causing an overwhelming sepsis [Ninis, 2010].

3.5.2 Signs and symptoms

A major issue in the recognition of meningococcal disease is the non-specific nature of the signs and symptoms in the initial stages of the disease. These include [NICE, 2015]:
- fever
- nausea/vomiting
- lethargy
- irritable/unsettled
- ill appearance
- refusing food/drink
- headache
- muscle ache/joint pain
- respiratory signs and symptoms.

However, the diagnosis window is short. Many children will have non-specific signs and symptoms in the first 4–6 hours, but can be close to death after 24 hours [Thompson, 2006]. Children who are showing 'classic' signs and symptoms of meningitis or septicaemia are more likely to have the severe disease [NICE, 2015].

3.5.3 Sepsis and shock

The first specific clinical signs to appear are likely to be those of sepsis and shock and include leg pain, abnormal skin colour, cold peripheries and, in older children, thirst. Parents of younger children may also report drowsiness and difficulty in breathing (described as rapid or laboured) [Thompson, 2006]. Don't forget to enquire about how much urine a child has been passing or if they have had a wet nappy recently. Oliguria (low output of urine) is an early sign of shock [Ninis, 2010].

3.5.4 Fever

Many children with septicaemia will become acutely ill with a fever. This can be complicated by a preceding trivial viral illness, but look for a sudden change in the history. Remember that not all children with meningococcal disease have fever, and you should not dismiss a fever responsive to anti-pyretics (such as paracetamol and ibuprofen) as being of viral origin [Ninis, 2010]. Rather counter-intuitively, infants can actually develop hypothermia in sepsis [Wells, 2001].

3.5.5 Rash

The classic sign is a petechial non-blanching rash (Figure 14.13). However, only 10% of children presenting with the rash will have meningococcal disease. The remainder will have a viral infection. On the other hand, febrile and ill children with a purpuric rash (a non-blanching rash of greater than 2 mm in diameter) are very likely to have meningococcal disease [Wells, 2001]. Care needs to be taken with blanching rashes, such as a maculopapular rash, as up to 30% of children may initially present with this, although careful examination will generally yield some non-blanching elements (Figure 14.14) [Hart, 2006].

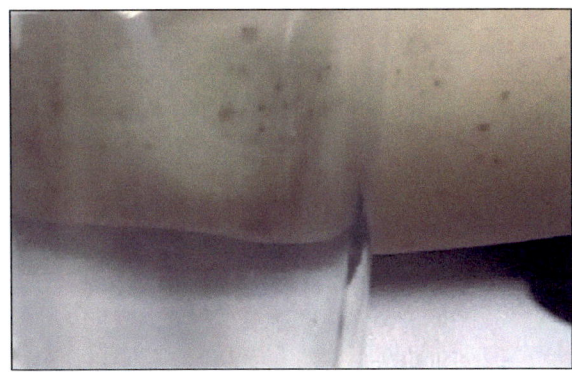

Figure 14.13 Petechial non-blanching rash. Note how this does not blanch under the pressure of a glass.
Source: Courtesy Meningitis Research Foundation www.meningitis.org.

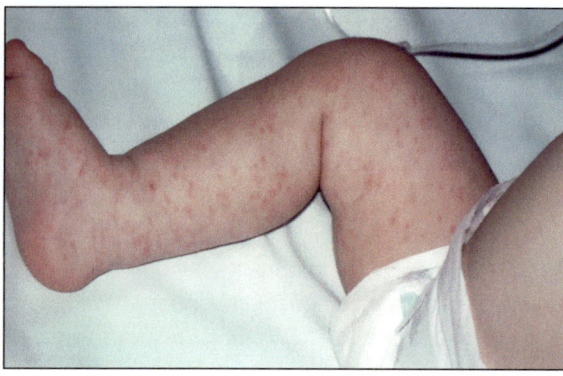

Figure 14.14 Maculopapular rash with scanty petechiae.
Source: Courtesy Meningitis Research Foundation www.meningitis.org.

On dark skin, you may have to check the soles of the feet, palms of the hand, abdomen or conjunctivae and palate. You must fully undress the child and be thorough in your search. Petechial rashes may not be widespread initially and can be easily missed.

3.5.6 Meningism

The signs of meningococcal meningitis can be complicated by concurrent septicaemia in the child, making it difficult to differentiate an altered mental state due to sepsis-induced hypoperfusion from one caused by raised intracranial pressure.

In younger children (particularly those under two years of age), there is less likely to be classic signs of meningism, such as neck stiffness or photophobia. Babies with meningitis sometimes have a full or bulging fontanelle due to raised intracranial pressure and become more distressed when handled than when left alone [Ninis, 2010].

3.5.7 Management

Patients with meningococcal disease are likely to require urgent intravenous antibiotics and fluids. Do not delay on scene and make a time-critical transfer to the nearest emergency department [JRCALC, 2019]. In addition:
- ensure a patent airway
- administer high levels of oxygen to all patients via a non-rebreathe mask
- assist ventilations if necessary
- record a blood glucose and treat hypoglycaemia
- alert the receiving hospital.

3.6 Cauda equina syndrome

Cauda equina syndrome (CES) is a group of signs and symptoms as a result of compression of the cauda equina caused by vertebral disc herniation (most common), low back surgery and spinal tumours (rare).

Although considered uncommon, there were 1,581 cases of CES in England in 2017/18 resulting in 1,175 admissions, 182 as an emergency [NHS Digital, 2018a]. It is a major cause of litigation cases against the NHS, which is unsurprising given that the average age of patients is 53 years (almost half of cases involve patients aged 30–50 years), and that it results in a distressing combination of symptoms including urinary and faecal incontinence as well as loss of sexual function and sensation. It can also leave patients with chronic back and leg pain, as well as requiring them to self-catheterise [Fairbank, 2014].

The Society of British Neurological Surgeons has classified CES into three main types [SBNS, 2009]:
- **Cauda equina syndrome with retention (CESR):** This is characterised by back pain with unilateral or bilateral sciatica, motor weakness of the legs, sensory disturbance in the saddle region, loss of anal tone and established loss of urinary control, i.e. painless retention and overflow.
- **Incomplete cauda equina syndrome (CESI):** This includes the symptoms of CESR, but with altered urinary sensation. This consists of a loss of desire to void, diminished sensation when urinating, a poor stream and the need to strain in order to pass urine. Painful retention may precede painless retention in some cases.
- **Suspected cauda equina syndrome (CESS):** A fence-sitting diagnosis for cases of severe back and leg pains with variable neurological symptoms and signs, and a suggestion of sphincter (urinary and/or anal) disturbance.

3.6.1 Assessment

The most common presentation of CES is back pain and some form of nerve pathology such as weakness, numbness and loss of power/control. Most patients with back pain will not have CES, but you should familiarise yourself with the following red flag symptoms [CESA, 2018]:

- **Back pain/sciatica/leg weakness:** Note that this is not a sensitive indicator as most patients with these symptoms do not have CES. However, note any sudden and severe increase in back pain as this is more indicative of CES [Gitelman, 2008].
- **Bladder disturbance:** Altered urinary sensation is a sign of CESI and includes reduced sensation, poor urinary stream, the need to strain in order to urinate and painful urinary retention. If left untreated, CESI will progress to CESR, at which point loss of urinary control will become established and irreversible, typically resulting in painless urinary retention and overflow [SBNS, 2009].
- **Saddle numbness:** This is an important sign in CES and is characterised by altered sensation around the buttocks, perineum and inner thigh [Kusakabe, 2013]. A good screening question to ask the patient is: 'Can you feel your bottom when you wipe yourself after going to the toilet?' [Fairbank, 2014].
- **Bowel disturbance:** New-onset faecal incontinence, constipation and/or loss of sensation when opening the bowels is suggestive of CES.
- **Sexual problems:** Loss of sensation during sex, erectile dysfunction and loss of clitoral sensation are less common signs of CES, but if present are prognostically a poor sign.

3.6.2 Management

Patients with symptoms of CES should have a magnetic resonance imaging (MRI) scan as soon as possible and, in cases of CESI, undergo surgery within 24 hours of onset. In cases of CESR, surgery can still be effective for up to 48 hours. However, given that nerve generation is a continuous process and not a step-wise one, prompt surgery is probably better [Nater, 2014; Bydon, 2014; Gardner, 2010].

From a pre-hospital perspective, early recognition and expedient transport to an appropriate hospital is the best management, along with the administration of analgesia. Spinal immobilisation is not necessary unless the cause is traumatic or movement of the spine results in worsening of symptoms [NAEMT, 2019].

3.7 *Paralysis*

In medical terminology, paralysis is typically represented by the suffix '-plegia'. This is not to be confused with paresis, which is used to refer to muscle weakness, or incomplete loss of muscle function [Porth, 2014]. Four common terms that you will hear used are [Innes, 2018]:

- **Monoplegia:** Paralysis in a single limb.
- **Hemiplegia:** Paralysis of both limbs on the same side of the body.
- **Paraplegia:** Paralysis of both the lower limbs.
- **Quadriplegia** (also tetraplegia)**:** Paralysis of all four limbs.

3.8 *Coma*

Coma is the absence of consciousness (i.e. unconsciousness) and is often referred to as a loss of consciousness (LOC). This presents as a completely unaware patient unresponsive to external stimuli, with only eye opening to pain and no eye tracking or fixation, and limb withdrawal to a noxious stimulus (usually pain) at best (often with reflex motor movements) [Wijdicks, 2010].

Full consciousness is an awake state in which one is aware of oneself and the environment, including the ability to perceive and interpret stimuli and to interact and communicate with others in the absence of motor deficits [Young, 2019].

Common causes of coma include:
- stroke – ischaemic and haemorrhagic
- cardiac arrest
- alcohol abuse
- substance abuse and overdose
- carbon monoxide poisoning
- sepsis
- bacterial meningitis
- syncope (faint)
- convulsions
- traumatic brain injury
- hyper-/hypoglycaemia.

Chapter 14 – Disability

Uncommon causes of coma include:
- subarachnoid haemorrhage
- brain abscess or tumour
- burns
- hypo-/hyperthermia.

It may not always be possible to determine the cause of coma and the management of the patient may just be supportive. However, for reversible causes, such as hypoglycaemia, convulsions and overdose, it is important to recognise these conditions as the patient can then receive the appropriate treatment out-of-hospital [JRCALC, 2019].

Chapter

15 Exposure

1 Extremes of temperature

1.1 Learning objectives

By the end of this section you will be able to:
- state the normal temperature range for an adult
- explain the terms 'hypothermia' and 'heat-related illness'
- describe the appropriate management for a patient with signs of hypothermia and heat-related illness.

1.2 Introduction

Despite being exposed to a wide range of environmental temperatures, the human body maintains a stable temperature of around 37°C and is maintained in the range 35.8–38.2°C. Normal fluctuations of about 1°C occur over a 24-hour period, with highest temperatures recorded in the afternoon and early evening, and lowest temperatures in the early morning [Marieb, 2013].

Thermoregulation is primarily the job of the hypothalamus, which receives sensory information from peripheral and central thermoreceptors. This is necessary because the different body regions have differing temperatures [Tortora, 2017]:
- Core: Consisting of organs within the skull, thorax and abdomen.
- Shell: The skin.

By controlling the flow of blood to the shell, the hypothalamus can control the amount of heat generated and lost.

1.2.1 Heat-promoting mechanisms

When the external temperature falls, the heat-promoting centre is activated. This maintains core body temperature by [Marieb, 2013]:
- constricting peripheral cutaneous blood vessels
- causing shivering – involuntary contractions of skeletal muscle, which generate heat
- increasing the body's metabolic rate.

In addition, there are a number of behavioural changes that can be promoted:
- putting on warmer clothes
- drinking hot fluids
- increasing physical activity.

1.2.2 Heat-loss mechanisms

Most heat loss occurs via the skin by dilation of cutaneous blood vessels and/or enhanced sweating, allowing for heat loss to occur by [Marieb, 2013]:
- **Radiation:** Infrared waves (thermal energy).
- **Conduction:** Direct contact with cooler objects (such as cold water).
- **Convection:** Since warm air expands and rises, warm air around the body is constantly replaced with cooler air, which absorbs the heat. This process can be enhanced by moving air more rapidly across the body surface, for example by the use of a fan.
- **Evaporation:** As water absorbs heat from the body, it becomes energetic enough to escape the body as a gas, known as water vapour.

1.3 Hypothermia

Hypothermia is defined as a core body temperature of less than 35°C. It is classified into three categories, based on temperature [JRCALC, 2019]:
- mild: 32–35°C
- moderate: 28–32°C
- severe: less than 28°C.

Without a low-reading thermometer, it can be difficult to record accurate core body temperature, so it is important to know the temperature range of the thermometers you use. For example, while consumer tympanic thermometers may have a measurable range of only 34–42.4°C, 'professional' versions can measure down to 20.0°C. Therefore, it is important to suspect that hypothermia might be a factor in the following cases, particularly if

you cannot get a reading from your thermometer [JRCALC, 2019]:
- older patients (over 80 years of age)
- children
- some medical conditions (for example, hypothyroidism and stroke)
- intoxicated patients (alcohol and/or recreational drugs)
- drowning
- patients suffering from exhaustion
- injured and immobile patients
- decreased level of consciousness.

As patients succumb to hypothermia, they move through five stages [Durrer, 2003]:
1. Conscious and shivering.
2. Decreased level of consciousness and not shivering.
3. Unconscious.
4. Not breathing.
5. Death due to irreversible hypothermia.

1.3.1 Management

The mainstay of pre-hospital treatment is to prevent further heat loss. In the mildly hypothermic patient, this is likely to be enough, but severely hypothermic patients will require active rewarming, which realistically can only be performed in hospital [Nolan, 2016]. Adopt the following principles when managing a patient with hypothermia [JRCALC, 2019]:
- Move the patient to a warm environment and remove wet clothes.
- If using a foil blanket, ensure that you wrap the patient in a fabric blanket first.
- Give the patient hot drinks if they are conscious, but not alcohol.
- Do not rub the patient's skin – as with alcohol, this leads to peripheral vasodilation, which worsens hypothermia.
- Avoid rough handling as it can cause arrhythmias and cardiac arrest.
- If intravenous fluids are required, ensure they are warmed prior to administration.
- Patients with a decreased level of consciousness should not be encouraged to walk, but managed horizontally.
- If you have access to a heating blanket, place this over the patient.

1.4 Heat-related illness

Heat-related illnesses can occur as a result of external factors such as the sun, or internal factors such as drugs and exercise. It presents on a continuum, with heat stress the least serious heat-related illness, through to multi-organ dysfunction and even death at the other extreme [JRCALC, 2019]:
- heat stress
- heat exhaustion
- heat stroke
- multi-organ dysfunction.

1.4.1 Heat stress

This is a mild form of heat-related illness and is characterised by [Soar, 2010]:
- normal temperature or mild temperature elevation
- heat oedema: swelling of feet and ankles
- heat syncope: vasodilation causes hypotension
- heat cramps: depletion of salts leads to muscle cramps.

1.4.2 Heat exhaustion

This is a more severe form of heat-related illness, with symptoms mostly as a result of fluid loss and electrolyte imbalances [Soar, 2010]:
- systemic reaction to prolonged heat exposure (hours to days)
- core body temperature over 37°C and less than 40°C
- headache, dizziness, nausea and vomiting, tachycardia, hypotension, sweating, muscle pain, weakness and cramps
- can progress quickly to heat stroke.

1.4.3 Heat stroke

Heat stroke is a systemic inflammatory response to a core body temperature of 40°C or more and is associated with an altered level of consciousness and organ dysfunction [Truhlář, 2015]. It comes in two types: non-exertional heat stroke, which is caused by high external temperatures and/or high humidity, and exertional heat stroke, which is caused by excess heat production. Non-exertional heat stroke tends to occur in the elderly, very young and chronically ill, whereas exertional heat stroke is more typical in active groups such as athletes, manual workers and military recruits [JRCALC, 2019].

Clinical features include [Truhlář, 2015]:
- core body temperature of 40°C or more
- hot dry skin (although sweating is present in around half of all cases)
- extreme fatigue, headache, fainting, facial flushing, vomiting and diarrhoea
- arrhythmias and hypotension
- respiratory distress
- liver and kidney failure.

1.4.4 Management

Heat stress and heat exhaustion

The management of patients with heat-related illness broadly consists of cooling the patient and replacing lost fluid and electrolytes. For patients with signs and symptoms of heat stress, consider the following [Lipman, 2014]:
- remove the patient from the heat source
- passively cool – move the patient into the shade or an air-conditioned ambulance.
- loosen or remove tight-fitting clothing
- provide oral isotonic fluid replacement
- elevate oedematous extremities.

If the patient has developed heat exhaustion, similar management principles apply, except that depending on the patient's level of consciousness, fluid rehydration may have to be intravenous. In addition, cooling should be active, using conductive, evaporative and convective methods. Cold-water immersion is ideal for the ambulant, co-operative patient, but may not be practical otherwise. Alternatives include removing the patient's clothes and spraying or dousing the patient with water. Air movement can be augmented by fanning the patient [Lipman, 2014].

Heat stroke

While supporting the patient's airway, breathing, circulation and disability, begin rapidly cooling the patient while en route to hospital [Truhlář, 2015]. Ice-water immersion is useful, but not practical, so consider the same techniques as for heat exhaustion to cool the patient. Ice packs are useful if they cover the body, not just the neck, axillae and groin, but should not be applied directly to the skin [Lipman, 2014]. Rehydration is safest intravenously as an altered level of consciousness increases the chance of aspiration [Truhlář, 2015].

1.5 Assessment of temperature

There are a range of different thermometers on the market and you may need to use a different type of thermometer depending on the age of the patient, as shown in Table 15.1 [JRCALC, 2022]. Common types include electronic thermometers (Figure 15.1) and tympanic thermometers (Figure 15.2).

Table 15.1 Thermometers according to age.

Infants under four weeks of age	• Electronic thermometer in the axilla
Four weeks and over	• Paediatric infra-red tympanic thermometer
	• Electronic thermometer in axilla

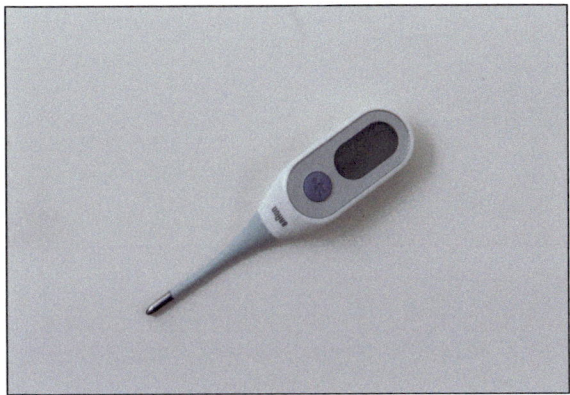

Figure 15.1 Electronic thermometer.

Chapter 15 – *Exposure*

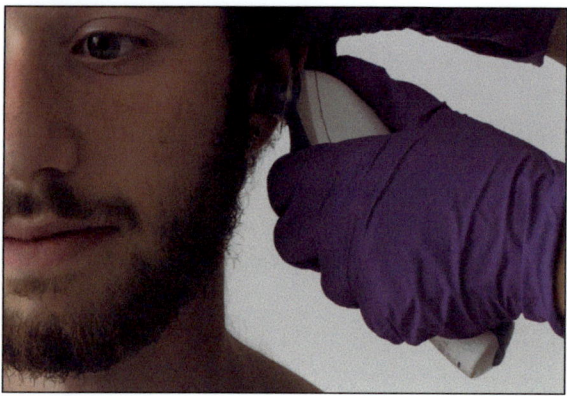

Figure 15.2 Tympanic thermometer.

Out-of-hospital, a peripheral temperature is gained to provide an estimation of what the temperature is in the core of the patient.

Temperature readings are broadly accurate, but they can be impacted by factors including:
- build-up of ear wax
- patient lying on one side for a prolonged period
- wearing of ear defenders or muffs prior to temperature being taken
- having stood outside for a prolonged period
- water or snow in the ear.

When taking a series of temperature measurements, always use the same site and procedure to try and improve accuracy. For example, if you are using the tympanic thermometer and you take the first reading from the right ear, you should use the right ear for all further temperature assessments

1.5.1 Procedure

Procedure – Electronic thermometer in axilla
Take the following steps to record a temperature:
1. Turn on the thermometer, check it is clean and functional and apply a fresh cover to the probe. Once you have turned it on, the thermometer will be able to perform any self-checks.

Procedure – Electronic thermometer in axilla – *cont*

2. Place the tip of the thermometer high in the axilla, in the fold where the arm meets the chest. Get the patient to bring their arm down to the side so the thermometer is covered.
3. Leave in place until the thermometer has finished measuring. Usually there will be a visual or audible indication that this has happened.
4. Remove and read the temperature.

Procedure – Infra-red tympanic thermometer
This is a general description on how to use an infra-red tympanic thermometer. You may need to vary this procedure based on different models available.

1. Turn on the thermometer, check it is clean and functional and apply a fresh cover to the probe. Once you have turned it on, the thermometer will be able to perform any self-checks.
2. The thermometer works by taking an infra-red reading of temperature directly from the tympanic membrane. As the ear canals are not straight, you should first try to straighten the canal slightly.
   a. For children under one, gently pull the pinna of the ear directly backwards.
   b. For children over one and adults, pull the ear gently upwards and backwards.
3. Place the probe into the ear. It should be placed straight down in the canal so the tip of the device is facing the tympanic membrane. At this point, some devices will 'pre-warm' the tip of the measuring probe to help ensure the results are accurate. They will emit a beep and the screen display will change when they are ready to use.
4. Push the button that measures temperature and hold the probe still until it has completed; this can take a few seconds.
5. Remove from the ear and read the temperature.

2 Drowning

2.1 Learning objective

By the end of this section, you will be able to:
- explain the pathophysiology and management of drowning.

2.2 Introduction

The definition of drowning has been complicated in the past and so in 2002 (at the World Congress on Drowning, held in Amsterdam) a single definition was agreed. As a result, drowning is now defined as a process resulting in primary respiratory impairment from submersion/immersion in a liquid [Idris, 2003]. Whether the victim lives or dies after this process is not important, they have still drowned. If they do not survive, then they have fatally drowned [Szpilman, 2012].

2.3 Pathophysiology

When a drowning victim is unable to keep water (the most common liquid in drowning incidents) from their mouth, it is spat out or swallowed. If still conscious, victims will then attempt to hold their breath, but this is likely to continue for less than a minute, depending on levels of panic and the temperature of the water. Once the inspiratory drive is too high to resist, the victim will take a breath and water will be aspirated into the airways [Szpilman, 2012]. Laryngospasm may occur, but this is rapidly terminated by cerebral hypoxia, and active ventilation, with aspiration of water, will resume. It was once thought that laryngospasm might be responsible for drowning victims who were found not to have aspirated (so called dry-drowning). The theory was that the victim died due to hypoxic cardiac arrest because of laryngospasm or breath holding [Layon, 2009]. However, autopsy studies have concluded that this is unlikely, as water does not passively seep into the lungs [Modell, 1999; Piette, 2006]. To drown therefore requires active ventilation while the victim is submerged (i.e. under the water and still alive).

Whether due to laryngospasm or breath holding, with no gas exchange the victim becomes increasingly hypoxaemic, hypercarbic and acidotic.

Unless they are rescued, the victim will succumb to hypoxaemia, leading to loss of consciousness and apnoea [Layon, 2009]. The cardiac rhythm deteriorates, usually following a sequence of tachyarrhythmias, bradyarrhythmias, pulseless electrical activity (PEA) and asystole [Szpilman, 2012].

Immersion in cold water (10°C or less) produces large and rapid reductions in skin temperature, which in turn leads to cold shock. This term refers to a collection of physiological responses including an inspiratory gasp (which can result in drowning if the victim's airway is submerged), hyperventilation, hypocapnia, tachycardia, peripheral vasoconstriction and hypertension [Datta, 2006]. Cold shock is thought to be caused by stimulation of cutaneous cold thermoreceptors, which results in an excessive sympathetic nervous system response. The magnitude of the cold shock response is reduced by the victim's clothing, their habituation to cold (regular winter swimming in just your Speedos, for example) and orientation on immersion [Shattock, 2012].

If the victim is fully submerged in cold water, the diving response may be activated. This is caused by cooling of the cold thermoreceptors on the face, which are innervated by the trigeminal nerve. This results in a profound sinus bradycardia due to parasympathetic nervous system stimulation of the heart, an expiratory apnoea due to inhibition of central respiratory neurons, and sympathetic nervous system-mediated vasoconstriction of the trunk and limbs. A similar response is also possible by stimulation of vagal receptors in the pharynx and larynx [Angell-James, 1975].

It has been suggested that this simultaneous stimulation of both sympathetic and parasympathetic pathways of the autonomic nervous system results in an 'autonomic conflict', leading to life-threatening arrhythmias that may result in death in susceptible individuals (Figure 15.3) [Shattock, 2012].

Although the tonicity of the water (for example, sea water versus fresh water) was once thought to be important, the effect on the lungs is ultimately

Chapter 15 – *Exposure*

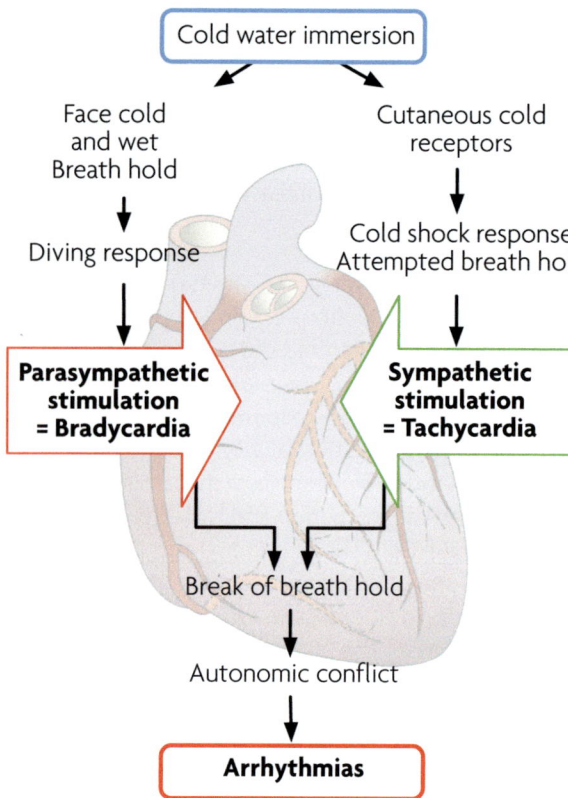

Figure 15.3 Autonomic conflict.

the same, although with a different osmotic gradient. The fragile alveolar-capillary membranes are disrupted, leading to increased permeability and movement of fluid, plasma and electrolytes [Orlowski, 1989]. Clinically, this leads to significant amounts of blood-stained pulmonary oedema and decreasing gaseous exchange of oxygen and carbon dioxide. Following drowning, the presence of additional fluid in the lungs and the loss of surfactant lead to increasing areas of the lungs becoming regions of low, or no, ventilation and perfusion (pulmonary shunting), and there is widespread atelectasis (collapse of a portion of lung) and bronchospasm [Layon, 2009]. Similarly, the haemodynamic and cardiovascular effects seen in drowning are not related to tonicity either, but primarily are a consequence of anoxia [Orlowski, 1989].

2.4 Management

Try to avoid getting wet. You should only go into the water to rescue a drowning victim as a last resort and only if you are adequately trained and equipped. Many victims who are drowning can help themselves with firm coaching or will have already been rescued by bystanders or professional rescuers, who can have a dramatic impact on the victim's outcome. On beaches with a lifeguard, for example, only around 0.8% will require cardiopulmonary resuscitation (CPR) [RNLI, 2017]. This is in stark contrast to the 30% of victims requiring CPR when rescued by untrained bystanders [Venema, 2010].

If you need to rescue the victim, remember to 'call, reach, throw, wade and row'. As previously mentioned, encourage victims to self-rescue first. Next, try to reach them with an object such as a pole, tree branch or even items of clothing. Consider throwing something that is buoyant, ideally a rescue ring with a lifeline attached. Wading into the water is the next possibility as long as someone on the shore has hold of you, the water is shallow enough to stand in and the victim is within reach. Alternatively, use a boat, if available.

Get the victim out of the water as soon as possible and place them supine (on their back), with head and torso at the same level, and check for breathing. If they are breathing but unconscious, provide high-flow oxygen via non-rebreathe mask as per clinical guidelines and place them in the recovery position. They are at high risk of gastric regurgitation, so ensure that you have suction available [JRCALC, 2019].

Victims of prolonged immersion in water (typically 30 minutes or more, but less as water temperature decreases) may also suffer the added complication of circum-rescue collapse [Golden, 1997]. This is due to the increased hydrostatic pressure from the water on the victim's legs and torso increasing venous return and cardiac output. Central baroreceptors mistake this for hypervolaemia resulting in increased diuresis (production and excretion of urine). In addition, peripheral vasoconstriction will occur as the water is cold relative to the body, which magnifies this response [Lord, 2005]. Once the victim is removed from the water, the hydrostatic pressure is lost, exacerbating the hypovolaemia. This can also be compounded by hypothermia and physical effort (if the victim attempts to remove him- or herself from the water, for example). The sudden drop in venous return can reduce coronary perfusion enough to induce cardiac arrest. For this reason, it is advised to remove victims horizontally from the water if possible [Szpilman, 2012].

Hypothermia is likely to occur so wet clothes should be cut off, but minimise movement. Hypothermic patients are at risk of cardiac arrhythmias, including ventricular fibrillation, even with minor movement [Althaus, 1982]. Get the patient covered with blankets and in a warm ambulance as soon as possible.

Chapter

16 Medical and Surgical Emergencies

1 Anaphylaxis

1.1 Learning objectives

By the end of this section you will be able to:
- explain the term anaphylaxis and its common causes
- describe signs and symptoms that a patient with anaphylaxis may present with
- state the management of anaphylaxis including the administration of adrenaline using the patient's own auto-injector.

1.2 Introduction

Anaphylaxis is a serious allergic reaction that is rapid in onset and is life-threatening [Muraro, 2014]. Its hallmark is rapidly developing life-threatening airway/breathing/circulation (or any combination of the three) problem(s) and it is usually associated with skin and mucosal changes [Soar, 2008]. The incidence of anaphylaxis is not known, but it is estimated that 0.3% of the European population will have an anaphylactic reaction at some point in their lives [Panesar, 2013]. In England, for example, 4,836 patients were admitted with a primary diagnosis of anaphylaxis in 2017/18 [NHS Digital, 2018a].

The most common causes (triggers) are food, medication and insect stings [Panesar, 2013]. In children, food is the most common cause of allergy, whereas in adults, it is medication [Capps, 2010]. Death is unlikely more than six hours after exposure to a trigger, but cardiac arrest can occur in minutes, particularly if the trigger is medication that has been administered intravenously. Envenomation typically causes cardiac arrest within 15 minutes; food takes a little longer on average, at around 30 minutes [Pumphrey, 2000].

1.2.1 Pathophysiology

Two types of cells are instrumental in the chain of events that can lead to anaphylaxis: basophils and mast cells. Basophils are granular leukocytes (a type of white blood cell) that migrate to sites of inflammation, leaving the capillaries and entering the tissues where they release heparin, histamine and serotonin, intensifying the inflammatory reaction [Tortora, 2017]. Mast cells are connective tissue cells found in high numbers near tissues that are exposed to the outside world. Examples include the skin, oral mucosa (which includes the lips and tongue), conjunctiva, the lungs and digestive tract [Prussin, 2006].

Most triggers lead to anaphylaxis due to the production of the immunoglobulin E (IgE) antibody, which cross-links with an antigen to activate high-affinity IgE receptors (FcεRI) on basophils and mast cells. This process is essentially irreversible and initiates a series of cellular events, leading to activation of an enzyme, tyrosine kinase, and an influx of calcium into basophils and mast cells. The result is a rapid release of preformed mediators such as histamines, prostaglandins, leukotrienes and platelet-activating factor (there are over 100 in total) [Paiva, 2010]. The actions of several mediators are summarised in Table 16.1.

Table 16.1 Actions of specific mediators.

Mediator	Actions
Histamine	Vasodilation Increased vascular permeability Increased heart rate and contraction Increased glandular secretion
Prostaglandin D_2	Bronchoconstriction Pulmonary and coronary vasoconstriction Peripheral vascular dilation
Leukotrienes	Bronchoconstriction Increased vascular permeability
Platelet-activating factor (PAF)	Increased vascular permeability

Chapter 16 – Medical and Surgical Emergencies

Of particular concern in fatal cases of anaphylaxis is the activation of human heart mast cells. These are located between myocardial muscle and around blood vessels. Low doses of preformed mediators can cause coronary artery spasm, myocardial injury and arrhythmias [Simons, 2007].

1.3 Signs and symptoms

Anaphylaxis is likely when all of the following criteria are met [Nolan, 2016]:

1. Sudden onset and rapid progression of symptoms, particularly after exposure to a known trigger (allergen).
2. Life-threatening airway and/or breathing and/or circulatory problems.
3. Skin and/or mucosal changes (e.g. generalised urticaria, pruritus or flushing, and swollen lips/tongue/uvula, also known as angioedema).

Note: Up to 20% of anaphylaxis cases do not have skin and/or mucosal changes, particularly reactions that occur intra-operatively in adults and food-/insect sting-induced reactions in children. Patients with severe anaphylaxis resulting in significant hypotension may not exhibit any cutaneous symptoms until their blood pressure is restored

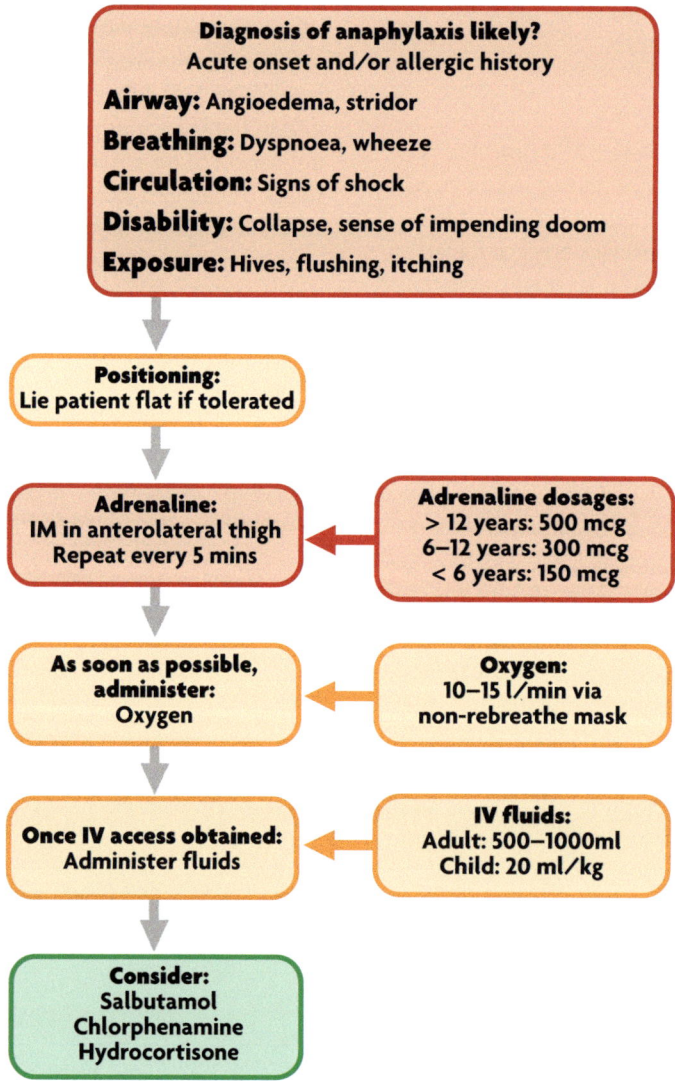

Figure 16.1 Emergency management of anaphylaxis.

[Lee, 2011]. Exposure to a known allergen can help with the diagnosis.

1.4 Management

Conduct a standard <C>ABCDE assessment to determine whether your patient is likely to be suffering from anaphylaxis. Try to identify the trigger and remove it if possible (e.g. stop any drug infusions, remove bee stings). However, if this is not possible, then do not delay treatment. If you suspect food-induced anaphylaxis, encouraging the patient to vomit is not recommended [Soar, 2008].

Lie the patient flat where possible with or without legs raised. Note that patients with A or B problems are likely to be more comfortable sitting up, but do not allow patients to sit or stand if they feel faint as this can cause cardiac arrest.

Give intramuscular (IM) adrenaline immediately to prevent cardiorespiratory arrest [JRCALC, 2019]. Where possible, administer adrenaline into the anterolateral thigh as there is a greater margin of safety, it is quick to administer and the peak plasma concentration is higher when adrenaline is administered in the thigh compared to the deltoid [Simons, 2001]. In the event of a cardiac arrest, however, the patient should receive their adrenaline IV [Truhlář, 2015]. Doses of adrenaline can be repeated every five minutes depending on patient condition.

Administer high-flow oxygen at 10–15 litres per minute initially. If local guidelines allow, consider administering nebulised salbutamol (Figure 16.1) [Truhlář, 2015; JRCALC, 2019].

If you are working with a suitably qualified clinician, they are likely to obtain IV access and administer fluid and second line treatments, such as antihistamines and hydrocortisone. In addition, you may be asked to set up a nebuliser to administer bronchodilators such as salbutamol and ipratropium [JRCALC, 2019].

Note: Adrenaline is also known as epinephrine, particularly in American texts.

1.4.1 Auto-injectors

Patients who are known to have anaphylactic reactions may have been provided with their own adrenaline auto-injector. Common systems in the UK include Jext® and Epipen® and are typically available as 300 microgram adult and 150 microgram child doses.

1.4.2 Procedure

Procedure – for Jext® auto-injector

Take the following steps to administer adrenaline with a Jext® auto-injector [ALK-Abello, 2018]:

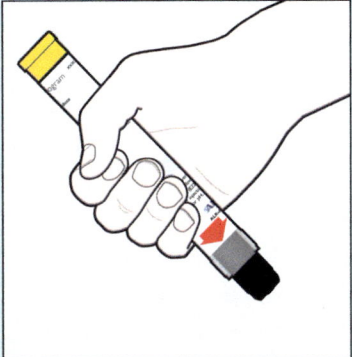

1. Grasp the Jext® injector in your dominant hand (the one you use to write with) with your thumb closest to the yellow cap.

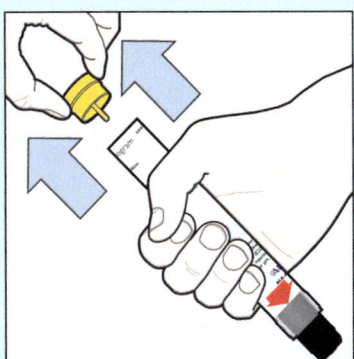

2. Pull off the yellow cap with your other hand.

Chapter 16 – *Medical and Surgical Emergencies*

Procedure – for Jext® auto-injector – *cont*

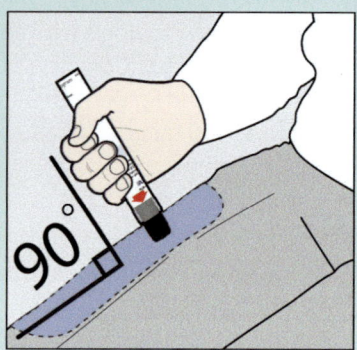

3. Place the black injector tip against the patient's outer thigh, holding the injector at a right angle (approximately 90°) to the thigh.

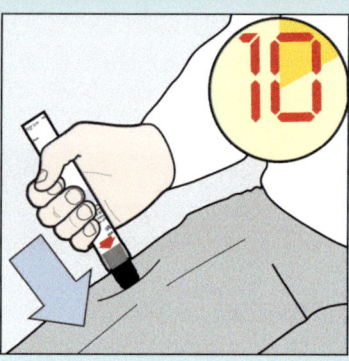

4. Push the black tip firmly into the outer thigh until you hear a 'click' confirming the injection has started, then keep it pushed in. Hold the injector firmly in place against the thigh for ten seconds (a slow count to ten) then remove. The black tip will extend automatically and hide the needle.

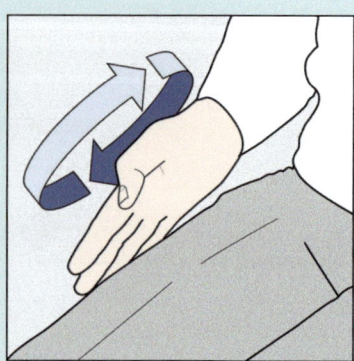

5. Massage the injection area for ten seconds.

2 Sepsis

2.1 Learning objectives

By the end of this section you will be able to:
- explain what sepsis and septic shock are and how they occur
- state how you would recognise a patient with sepsis or red flag sepsis
- describe the out-of-hospital management of sepsis.

2.2 Introduction

Sepsis is a life-threatening condition that arises when the body's response to an infection injures its own tissues and organs. It leads to shock, multiple organ failure and death if not recognised early and treated promptly [Czura, 2011]. Sepsis is estimated to cause 46,000–67,000 deaths a year and is responsible for more deaths than lung, bowel and breast cancer combined [UKST, 2017]. Around 90% of patients with sepsis arrive at hospital by ambulance, most commonly presenting with a respiratory tract infection [Gray, 2013; Daniels, 2011].

Septic shock is a subset of sepsis that has a higher risk of mortality than sepsis alone [Singer, 2016]. Septic shock causes particularly profound circulatory, cellular, and metabolic abnormalities. Since determining the presence of septic shock can be difficult out-of-hospital, a pragmatic alternative is to treat any patient who is hypotensive despite fluid resuscitation as if they have septic shock. These patients are high risk, as are others with any of the 'red flag' signs/symptoms shown in Figure 16.2. To ensure that these patients receive urgent attention, it is important that the receiving hospital is alerted that the 'patient has suspected sepsis' [JRCALC, 2019].

2.3 Risk factors for sepsis

Certain groups of patients are at higher risk of developing sepsis [JRCALC, 2019]:
- infants and older people (over 75 years or very frail)
- patients with impaired immune systems, for example:
  - cancer patients receiving chemotherapy
  - diabetic patients

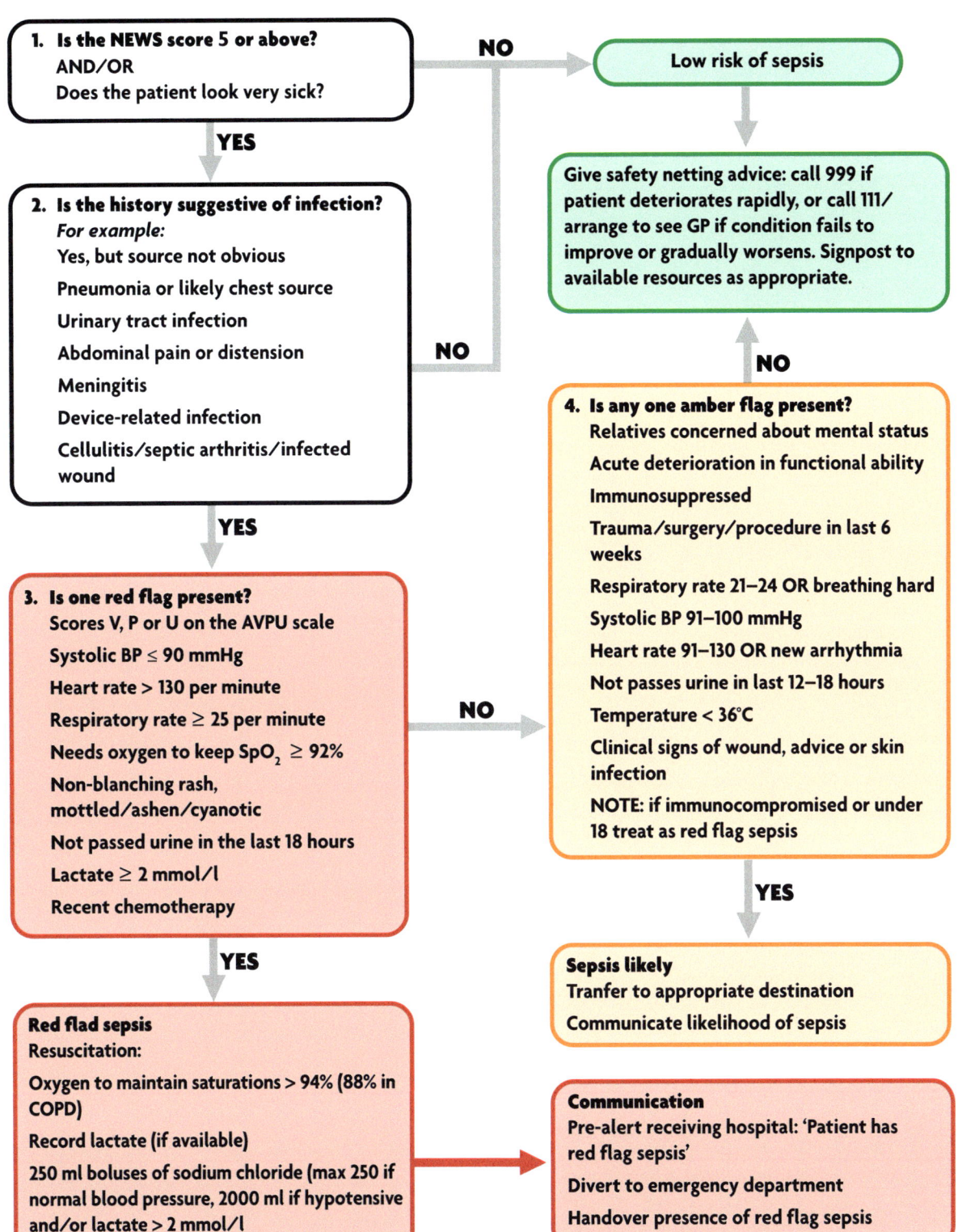

Figure 16.2 Pre-hospital sepsis screening tool.

Chapter 16 – *Medical and Surgical Emergencies*

- patients without a spleen (due to splenectomy)
- patients with sickle cell disease
- patients taking long-term steroid drugs or immunosuppressant drugs for conditions such as rheumatoid arthritis
- patients who have had recent surgery (in the previous six weeks)
- intravenous drug users
- pregnant women.

2.4 Recognition

To simplify the identification of sepsis (particularly red flag sepsis), a screening tool has been developed for pre-hospital use (Figure 16.2) [JRCALC, 2019]. You should suspect sepsis in any patient who presents with fever and/or feeling unwell, and who has a National Early Warning Score (NEWS2) of five or more and/or looks unwell with a history of infection. A history of infection might be indicated by the presence of [UKST, 2017]:

- pneumonia
- urinary tract infection
- abdominal pain/distension
- cellulitis/septic arthritis/infected wound
- device-related infection
- meningitis.

Next, look for the presence of any red-flag signs/symptoms that may indicate the presence of red-flag sepsis (Figure 16.2). Patients who do not meet the criteria for red-flag sepsis but have sepsis still require further assessment and appropriate management to prevent their clinical condition deteriorating. Identifying sepsis before arrival at the ED and, even more importantly, ambulance crews stating that they suspect the patient has sepsis reduces patients' time to receive antibiotics and the sepsis care bundle in the ED [Studnek, 2012; Band, 2011].

2.5 Management

All patients with suspected sepsis should be given oxygen to achieve a target saturation of 94–98%, or 88–92% for patients with chronic obstructive pulmonary disease (COPD). Patients who are hypotensive (systolic blood pressure <90 mmHg or a mean arterial pressure of <65 mmHg) should be given intravenous (IV) fluids, typically in bolus doses of 500 ml over 15 minutes. You may be required to assist your senior clinician with obtaining IV access and setting up an IV infusion [JRCALC, 2019].

3 Endocrine system disorders

3.1 Learning objectives

By the end of this section you will be able to:
- describe the relevant anatomy and physiology of the endocrine system
- describe the types and causes of diabetes
- describe two diabetic emergencies
- explain how to record a blood sugar measurement
- briefly outline the pathophysiology of Addison's disease
- explain how to manage a patient suffering from an Addisonian crisis.

3.2 Introduction

The endocrine system consists of a collection of glands located throughout the body (Figure 16.3)

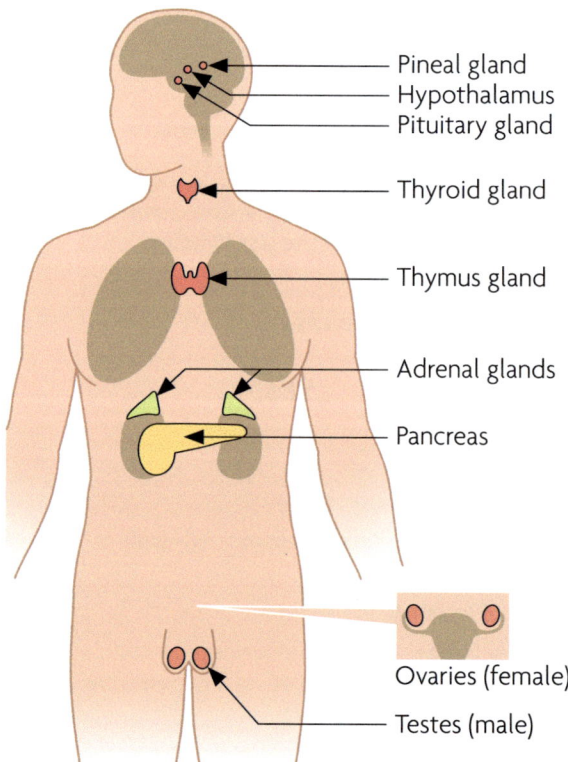

Figure 16.3 The endocrine system.

that are responsible for the secretion of hormones: molecules that are released from endocrine glands and regulate the activity of cells in other parts of the body. The endocrine system works alongside the nervous system to help co-ordinate the function of all of the body's systems [Tortora, 2017].

The endocrine system consists of the pineal, pituitary, thyroid, parathyroid and adrenal glands. In addition, there are a number of organs and tissues that are not strictly endocrine glands, but do secrete hormones. These include the pancreas, ovaries, testes, liver and heart.

3.3 Anatomy and physiology of the pancreas

The pancreas is a mixed endocrine (secretes chemical substances into the blood stream) and exocrine (secretes chemical substances into ducts) gland, situated posterior to the stomach, and extends across the posterior abdominal wall from the duodenum on the right to the spleen on the left (Figure 16.4). It is retroperitoneal, apart from its tail [Tortora, 2017].

Around 99% of the cells in the pancreas are involved in the production of pancreatic enzymes. The cells are organised into clusters called acini. Among the acini are collections of endocrine tissue called pancreatic islets, or islets of Langerhans after the German scientist Paul Langerhans, who first described them [Jolles, 2002].

There are five types of cells in the pancreatic islets, which have a range of functions, including regulation of blood glucose (Table 16.2).

3.3.1 Blood sugar regulation

Falling blood glucose levels normally activate a series of glucose counter-regulatory processes to prevent, or quickly correct, hypoglycaemia. This is crucial, given that the brain's demand for glucose is fairly constant and the intake of (exogenous) glucose from eating is intermittent. This is accomplished by the dynamic control of endogenous production of glucose by the liver (and, to a lesser extent, the kidneys) and reduction of glucose consumption by non-neural tissue, such as muscle [Briscoe, 2006].

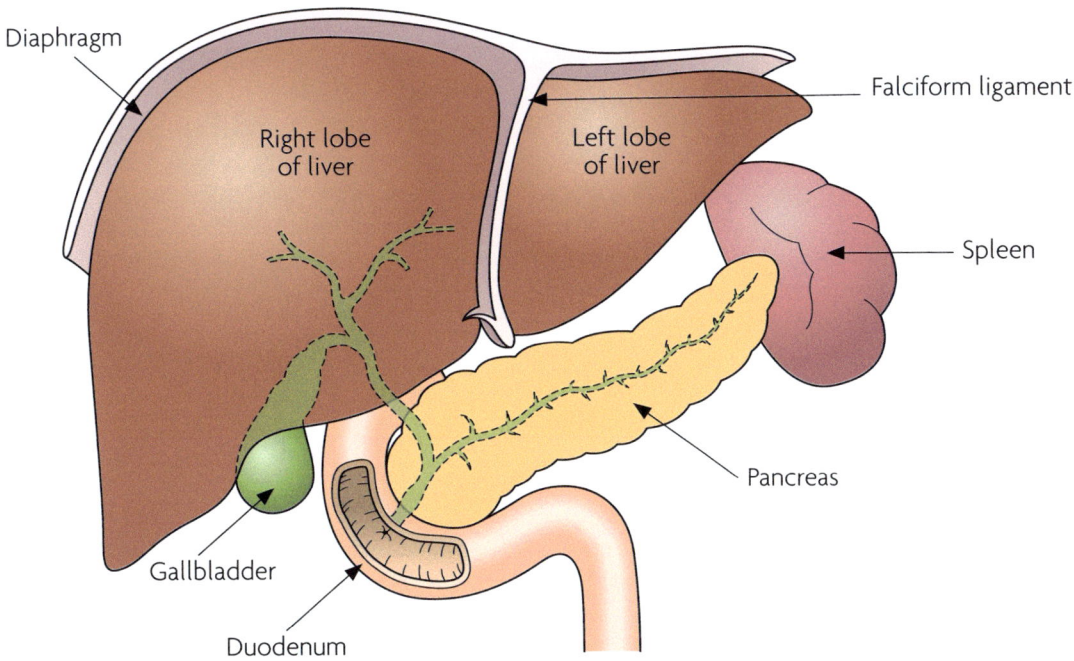

Figure 16.4 The pancreas and other selected abdominal organs.

Table 16.2 Cells of the pancreatic islets.

Cell	Hormone	Action
Alpha	Glucagon	Increases blood glucose
Beta	Insulin, amylin	Insulin: reduces blood glucose Amylin: delays gastric emptying, inhibits insulin
Delta	Somatostatin	Inhibits glucagon and insulin release
PP (or F)	Pancreatic polypeptide	Inhibits somatostatin secretion, gallbladder contraction and secretion of pancreatic digestive enzymes
Epsilon	Ghrelin	Stimulates hunger

Hormonal control of blood glucose is largely dependent on the endocrine pancreas via the hormones insulin and glucagon. Insulin increases transport of glucose across cell membranes and is released by the beta cells. It targets the muscle, fat and liver cells causing gluconeogenesis (a process that creates glucose) and synthesis of triglycerides, fatty acids and proteins [Tortora, 2017].

Glucagon targets the liver, promoting the conversion of glycogen into glucose and the creation of glucose from lactic and amino acids. This results in increased glucose release by the liver into the blood. Glucagon release is inhibited by insulin and increased by falling blood glucose levels.

Defence against hypoglycaemia (also called glucose counter-regulation) can be broadly classified into physiological and behavioural responses [Briscoe, 2006]. As blood glucose falls (although still within 'normal' limits), insulin secretion from the beta cells is reduced, leading to increased glucose production by the liver and virtual cessation of glucose use by tissue sensitive to insulin.

When blood glucose falls below 4 mmol/l, glucagon release is increased from the alpha cells, further increasing glucose production and decreasing insulin release. In addition, adrenaline release from the adrenal medulla is increased by the sympathetic nervous system. Adrenaline has similar effects on the liver as glucagon, but can also stimulate renal production of glucose and plays a role in reducing insulin-stimulated glucose uptake [Elliott, 2011].

If blood glucose continues to fall, a more intense sympathetic-mediated adrenaline release causes a behavioural response in the form of hunger, as well as other autonomic symptoms, such as palpitations, sweating and pallor [Graveling, 2009].

3.4 Anatomy and physiology of the adrenal glands

The adrenal (or suprarenal) glands are situated in the retroperitoneum, within the renal fascia and on the superior and medical aspects on each kidney (i.e. on top and towards the middle; see Figure 16.5). They are shaped like a flattened pyramid, and in adults are around 3–5 cm tall, 2–3 cm wide and 1 cm deep. When viewed in cross-section, it is clear that they are, in fact, two glands in one, with a smaller, inner medulla, responsible for secreting the catecholamines adrenaline and noradrenaline, and an outer cortex, which makes up over 80% of the gland.

The adrenal cortex is subdivided into three zones (Figure 16.5):
- An outer zona glomerulosa, which secretes mineralocorticoids, the most important being aldosterone. This helps regulate levels of sodium (Na^+) and potassium (K^+), by increasing reabsorption of sodium from the distal

Endocrine system disorders

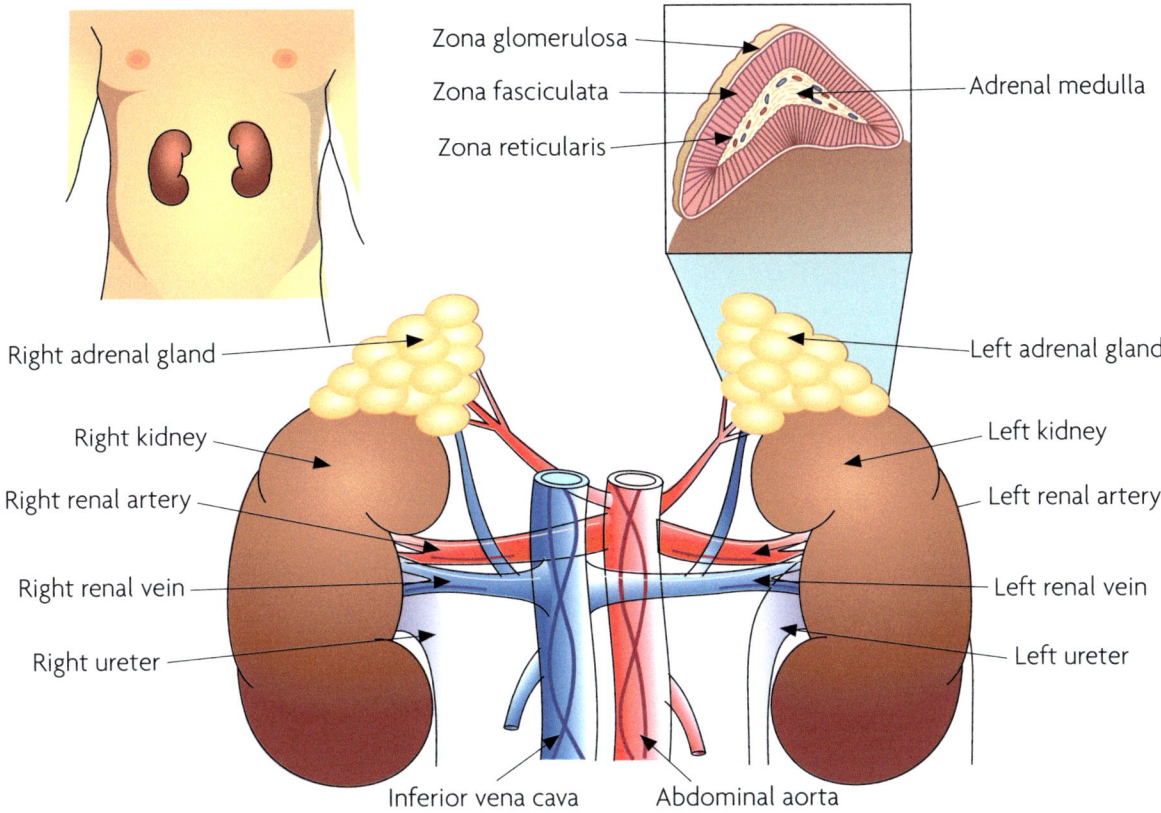

Figure 16.5 The kidneys and adrenal glands.

tubules of the kidneys, the sweat glands and the gastrointestinal (GI) tract. It also increases excretion of potassium. Finally, aldosterone helps to regulate blood pressure.
- A middle zona fasciculata, which secretes glucocorticoids, mainly cortisol (also known as hydrocortisone). Cortisol has a number of functions including glucose formation, the breakdown of proteins and triglycerides, reducing numbers of white blood cells involved in inflammatory processes and depressing the immune system response. It is also a permissive hormone, allowing other hormones to exert their effects.
- An inner zona reticularis, which secretes sex steroids such as oestrogen, progesterone and androgen. These are not crucial in acute emergencies, but can have a significant impact on the lifestyle of patients with Addison's disease [Arlt, 2002].

3.4.1 Glucocorticoids

Cortisol (the chief glucocorticoid and 'stress' hormone) release is controlled by a small area of the brain, located just under the thalamus – the hypothalamus. This area receives input from a number of different areas of the brain including the limbic system, cerebral cortex, thalamus, reticular activation system and external sensory signals from internal organs and even the retina. It forms the major interface between the nervous and endocrine systems.

In response to some form of stress, e.g. cold, fasting/starvation, hypotension, haemorrhage, surgery, infection, pain from wounds and fractures, severe exercise and even emotional trauma, neurosecretory cells in the hypothalamus release corticotropin-releasing hormone (CRH). This hormone travels to the anterior pituitary gland where it is stimulated to release adrenocorticotrophic hormone (ACTH). ACTH travels through the blood stream until it reaches the adrenal glands and stimulates the zona fasciculata to synthesise and release cortisol.

Once blood levels of cortisol are high enough, levels of ACTH reduce thanks to a negative feedback mechanism acting on both the hypothalamus (inhibiting the release of CRH) and the anterior pituitary.

3.5 Diabetes

Diabetes mellitus is a common metabolic disorder typified by chronic high blood sugar (hyperglycaemia). It is a major cause of morbidity and premature death due to long-term complications such as heart attack, stroke, kidney failure and blindness [Holt, 2010].

There are two types of diabetes [WHO, 1999]:
- **Type 1:** Previously referred to as insulin-dependent diabetes (IDDM). Patients with type 1 diabetes are unable to produce any insulin, usually due to autoimmune disease that destroys the insulin-producing beta cells in the pancreas [Holt, 2010]. Insulin is a hormone that increases transport of glucose across cell membranes and is released by the beta cells. It targets the muscle, fat and liver cells to promote the creation of glucose [Tortora, 2017].
- **Type 2:** Previously referred to as non-insulin dependent diabetes (NIDDM). Patients with type 2 diabetes have a relative insulin deficiency due to varying degrees of insulin resistance. This is by far the most common type of diabetes, accounting for around 90% of all people with diabetes in the UK.

3.5.1 Causes/risk of diabetes

Underlying causes of diabetes generally fall into four categories [Holt, 2010]:
- **Genetic:** A family history of type 1 diabetes or other autoimmune disease is linked to a higher risk of developing type 1 diabetes in the family. Likewise, type 2 diabetes also has a familial component, although this connection is rather more complicated.
- **Obesity:** This increases the risk of developing type 2 diabetes, particularly in people with a body mass index over 25 kg/m^2 or large waist circumference.
- **Age:** People are living longer and beta cell function declines with age, leading to a chance of developing diabetes in old age.
- **Ethnicity:** Some ethnic groups are at higher risk of developing diabetes, particularly those of South Asian and Afro-Caribbean origin.

3.6 Diabetic emergencies

Blood sugar is typically maintained within a narrow range of 3.0 to 5.6 mmol/l [JRCALC, 2019]. Diabetic patients are generally encouraged to keep their blood sugar at 4.0 or higher, with a target range of 4.0–7.0 mmol/l for children [NICE, 2016c] and the same target of 4.0–7.0 mmol/l for adults (except on waking, when a target of 5–7 mmol/l is advised for adults) [NICE, 2016d].

There are two main types of diabetic emergency that you will encounter on an ambulance:
- hypoglycaemia
- severe hyperglycaemia, which can be further divided into diabetic ketoacidosis (DKA) and hyperosmolar hyperglycaemic state (HHS).

3.7 Hypoglycaemia

Hypoglycaemia in diabetics commonly occurs due to a relative excess of insulin in the blood and a compromised physiological and behavioural response to falling blood glucose levels. Since injected insulin and hypoglycaemic drugs such as sulphonylureas are not perfect pharmacokinetically, there are typically periods where there is an excess of insulin in the blood and falling blood glucose levels. The performance of the counter-regulatory defences is crucial in determining whether the patient will develop significant hypoglycaemia.

3.7.1 Pathophysiology

If the beta cells do not release insulin, such as occurs in type 1 and end-stage type 2 diabetes, glucagon release is usually impaired and the physiological defence relies completely on the nervous system response to falling blood glucose

Endocrine system disorders

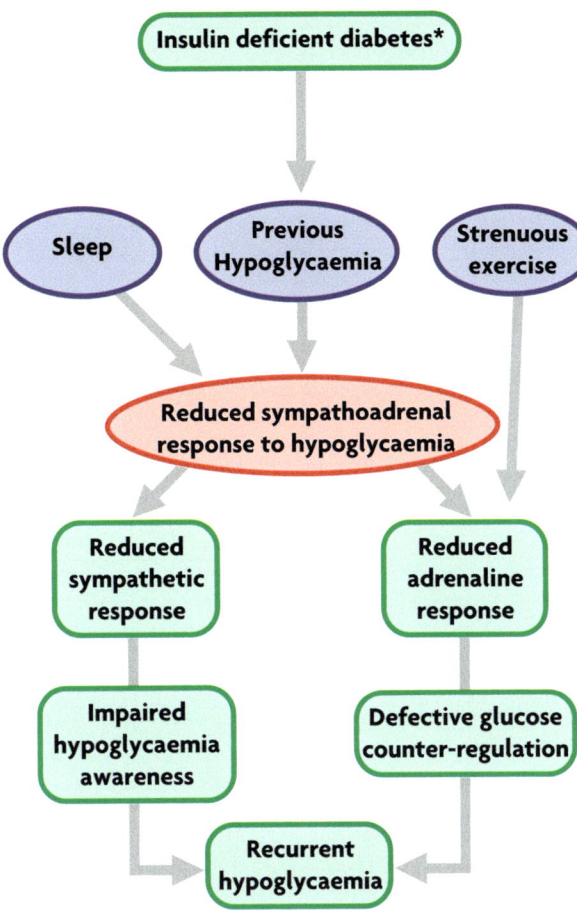

*i.e. there is no insulin decrease or glucagon increase, when blood glucose levels fall due to exogenous insulin administration.

Figure 16.6 Hypoglycaemia-associated autonomic failure.

levels [Cryer, 2008]. However, there are a number of factors that can dampen this response and cause a hypoglycaemia-associated autonomic failure (Figure 16.6).

The three main causes of hypoglycaemia-associated autonomic failure are previous episodes of hypoglycaemia, strenuous exercise and sleep. The mechanisms are not well understood, but repeated episodes of hypoglycaemia impair increases in adrenaline release and hypoglycaemic symptoms in both diabetics and non-diabetics in subsequent falls in blood glucose [Elliott, 2011]. Strenuous exercise causes a late hypoglycaemic response 15 hours after the event and often at night. Sleep further dampens the nervous and adrenal responses to falling blood glucose and patients have reduced arousal from sleep [Cryer, 2008]. Thus, not only is the physiological defence potentially overcome, but the behavioural defence is also affected by an impaired awareness of hypoglycaemia. This is compounded by old age, patients with long-standing diabetes, the consumption of alcohol and very tight glycaemic control [Elliott, 2011].

3.7.2 Signs and symptoms

Although diabetic patients are generally encouraged to keep their blood sugar at 4.0 mmol/l or higher, some will experience symptoms of hypoglycaemia at blood sugar levels higher than this, making recognition important. Some signs and symptoms of hypoglycaemia include [Deary, 1993]:
- sweating
- palpitations
- shaking
- hunger
- confusion
- drowsiness
- odd/aggressive behaviour
- speech problems
- headache
- nausea.

3.7.3 Management

If the patient is still conscious and able to take oral glucose, then administer 10–20 g of glucose. You can find 10 g of glucose in:
- 225 ml Lucozade Energy Original
- 100 ml Coca-Cola
- 3 teaspoons of sugar (actually, 12 g).

In addition, commercial preparations of glucose are available including Glucogel, Dextrogel and Hypo-Fit. Administration of oral glucose can be repeated after 10–15 minutes, if required.

If the patient is unable to take oral glucose due to impaired consciousness, is uncooperative or there is a risk of aspiration, then either IM glucagon or IV glucose should be administered. This decision will be a judgement call by the senior clinician (if present) and will depend on whether IV access can be obtained.

Chapter 16 – Medical and Surgical Emergencies

The most common presentation of IV glucose for ambulance staff is a 500 ml bag containing 10% glucose. This replaced earlier pre-filled syringes of 50% glucose as it was found to be just as effective and possibly more beneficial to the patient, since lower doses are required, resulting in lower post-treatment glucose levels [Moore, 2005].

Higher concentrations are available, including 20% and 50%, although 50% glucose is not recommended due to the risk of extravasation injury and difficulty in administration.

All glucose infusions should be administered via a wide-bore cannula having first ensured correct placement with a 10–20 ml flush. A dose of 10 g of glucose equates to 100 ml of the 10% solutions, which is administered over 15 minutes. [JRCALC, 2019]. This can be repeated after 10 minutes following the first administration.

Where it is not possible to administer oral or IV glucose, then glucagon can be administered IM once only. The adult dose is 1 mg. This may not be effective in patients with inadequate stores of glycogen such as those who are intoxicated, alcoholic or anorexic. If IV access is not possible, then it is preferable to smear oral glucose around the patient's mouth [Moore, 2005].

Diabetic patients who suffer an episode of severe hypoglycaemia will often fully recover and can be discharged at the scene safely as long as their blood sugar is above 5 mmol/l, they consume 20–40 g of carbohydrates and meet any local criteria for discharge at the scene. It is recommended that patients are referred to a diabetes specialist, as their treatment regimen may need to change [Walker, 2006; Roberts, 2003a].

However, patients should be encouraged to attend hospital in the following circumstances and as directed by local guidance [JRCALC, 2019]:
- elderly (although no specific age range is cited in the literature)
- low BMI
- live alone
- not diagnosed as diabetic
- taking oral hypoglycaemic agents (mainly sulphonylureas such as glibenclamide or gliclazide
- blood glucose <5 mmol/l after treatment
- treated with glucagon
- co-morbidity (for example, renal failure/dialysis, chest pain, arrhythmias, alcohol consumption, dyspnoea, convulsions or focal neurological signs)
- signs of illness/infection.

3.8 Severe hyperglycaemia

Severe hyperglycaemia (sometimes referred to as hyperglycaemic crisis) manifests as two conditions: diabetic ketoacidosis (DKA) and hyperosmolar hyperglycaemic state or syndrome (HHS, previously known as hyperosmolar non-ketotic coma, HONK) [Van Ness-Otunnu, 2013].

3.8.1 Diabetic ketoacidosis

DKA is a complex metabolic state characterised by:
- hyperglycaemia
- acidosis
- ketonaemia.

It is a common and potentially life-threatening complication of type 1 diabetes mellitus (T1DM) mainly, compared to HHS, which typically affects only patients with type 2 diabetes mellitus (T2DM).

3.8.2 Hyperosmolar hyperglycaemic state

HHS does not have a universally agreed definition, but it is generally accepted that the following must be present for the patient to be diagnosed with HHS [Scott, 2015]:
- hypovolaemia (secondary to severe dehydration)
- blood sugar >30 mmol/l without signs of hyperketonaemia or acidosis
- blood osmolality >320 mOsmol/kg (not measured out-of-hospital).

3.8.3 Pathophysiology

Diabetic ketoacidosis
DKA and HHS share the complications of severe hyperglycaemia, but early mechanisms are different. In DKA, insulin production is absent or severely

reduced. This, coupled with increased levels of insulin counter-regulatory hormones (e.g. cortisol, glucagon, growth hormone and catecholamines), enhances hepatic gluconeogenesis (glucose creation) and glycogenolysis (breakdown of stored glucose in the form of glucagon). This leads to severe hyperglycaemia that is exacerbated by simultaneous reduction in glucose take-up by the peripheral tissue because of the lack of insulin.

Although blood glucose is high, there is a glucose famine inside the cells, so body fat (adipose tissue) is used to create energy by increasing lipolysis and decreasing lipogenesis. Circulating free fatty acids (FFAs) are metabolised and converted into ketone bodies by the liver [Lupsa, 2014]. At a normal blood pH (sometimes called physiological pH, typically a pH of 7.35–7.45), ketones dissociate and the excess hydrogen ions bind to the circulating bicarbonate. Since the ketones are now missing a hydrogen ion, they become negatively charged (anions), leading to the metabolic acidosis of DKA.

Hyperosmolar hyperglycaemic state
Although HHS is also caused by a decrease in insulin and increase in counter-regulatory hormones, the fundamental difference between HHS and DKA is that there is still sufficient insulin production to prevent significant ketosis (and the associated severe metabolic acidosis) but not the severe hyperglycaemia that is a key feature of the condition. As before, hyperglycaemia is caused by increased gluconeogenesis, accelerated conversion of glycogen to glucose and inadequate utilisation of glucose by the peripheral tissues, particularly muscle.

As blood glucose concentration and osmolality (a measure of the body's fluid–electrolyte balance) of extracellular fluid increase, an osmolar gradient is created, which draws water out of cells [Pasquel, 2014]. In the initial stages, glomerular filtration rate (GFR) is increased, leading to glucosuria and osmotic diuresis, which in turn causes dehydration, hyperosmolality and electrolyte loss. While the GFR is maintained, severe hyperglycaemia does not occur. However, once kidney function is adversely affected and hypovolaemia occurs due to excessive fluid losses, GFR declines and severe hyperglycaemia results.

Deaths from severe hyperglycaemia are thankfully rare, with cerebral oedema the most common cause of death in DKA; children and adolescents are most vulnerable to this. Other serious complications include hyperkalaemia and (ironically) hypoglycaemia following corrective treatment [Savage, 2011]. Cerebral oedema is also a cause of death in HHS, along with prolonged convulsions and central pontine myelinolysis (damage to the myelin sheaths of neurons in the pons), the leading cause of which is suspected to be rushed correction of osmolality by medical staff [Scott, 2015].

3.8.4 Signs and symptoms
DKA and HHS typically present in different groups of patients and over differing time periods. DKA most commonly occurs in T1DM (although advanced/severe T2DM patients are also at risk). HHS on the other hand is almost exclusively seen in T2DM and is more common in the elderly [Lupsa, 2014], although its incidence in teenagers and young adults is on the rise [Scott, 2015]. DKA typically presents within hours to days of onset whereas HHS does not occur for many days to weeks, which explains why the metabolic derangement and dehydration in HHS are so much more severe than in DKA [Savage, 2011].

Typical signs and symptoms of severe hyperglycaemia are common to both DKA and HHS (except where highlighted in the list below) [Lupsa, 2014; Corwell, 2014]:
- polyuria
- polydipsia
- blurred vision
- fatigue
- weakness
- weight loss
- vomiting and abdominal pain (DKA) (probably due to delayed gastric emptying and ileus because of electrolyte abnormalities and/or acidosis)
- fruity breath odour (DKA)
- Kussmaul breathing (DKA)

- focal neurological signs such as hemiparesis (HHS)
- altered mental state, although this can range from confusion to coma
- signs of dehydration such as dry mucous membranes, poor skin turgor, long furrows on tongue.

3.8.5 Management

Out-of-hospital management of a hyperglycaemic crisis is limited. Your focus should be on prompt recognition and transport of the patient to definitive care while managing <C>ABCDE [JRCALC, 2019; Skellett, 2016]:

- Ensure airway patency, with patient positioning, suction and adjuncts, as required, particularly in patients with a reduced level of consciousness.
- Adults need supplemental oxygen if the patient's SpO_2 is <94%. Children should receive high-flow oxygen titrated to a target range of 94–98%. Patients can expire CO_2 with spontaneous breathing far more effectively than with artificial ventilation, so avoid assisting/interfering unless the patient is in respiratory failure or arrest.
- Your senior clinician may commence rehydration en route to hospital, since fluid deficits of patients with DKA are typically 100 ml/kg; in HHS, they can range from 100–220 ml/kg, i.e. up to 16.5 l in a 75 kg patient.
- The UK Ambulance Services Clinical Practice Guidelines advocate 250 ml bolus doses of 0.9% saline up to a maximum of 2 l. However, in children, fluid is restricted to a single dose of 10 ml/kg due to the risk of cerebral oedema [JRCALC, 2019].
- Assess level of consciousness and watch for the patient's general trend (e.g. decreasing Glasgow Coma Scale (GCS) score). In children, watch for signs of rising intracranial pressure (posturing in response to pain, reducing GCS score, rising blood pressure with decreasing heart rate). Don't forget to record the patient's blood glucose, but be wary of results that do not fit the clinical picture (e.g. a low blood sugar reading in a patient with 'classic' signs of hyperglycaemia).

3.9 Blood sugar measurement

You will obtain blood glucose measurements as part of your clinical assessment. As with all diagnostic tests, they are not perfect and are prone to error if the correct technique is not used. Common causes of error include [Lunt, 2010]:

- Incorrect calibration chip used to read the test strips.
- Contamination of the test finger with glucose-rich foods or dilutional error due to inadequate hand drying or the patient licking their finger clean.
- Expired strips or strips stored in adverse environmental conditions such as heat, humidity or extreme cold.
- Patient conditions such as extremes of haematocrit (e.g. anaemia) and hypoxia. Shocked patients may have a reduced capillary blood glucose reading compared to a venous blood sample. Consider taking venous blood in these patients (particularly as you are likely to be cannulating them anyway).
- Aspirin, paracetamol and vitamin C can all raise blood glucose, although this may not be clinically significant.

3.9.1 Procedure

Take the following steps to record a blood sugar measurement with an Accu-Chek® Aviva blood glucose meter:

Procedure – To record a blood sugar measurement with an Accu-Chek® Aviva blood glucose meter

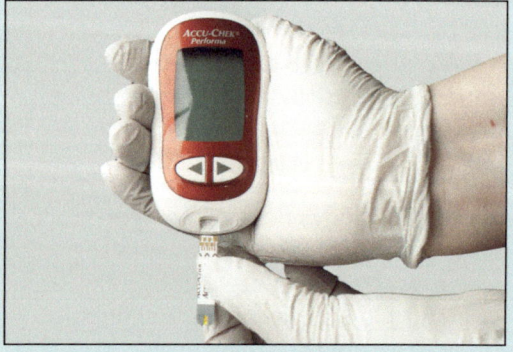

1. Wash and dry your hands or use alcohol gel and put on gloves. Select an appropriate site, which is typically the side of a finger in an adult or older child (non-dominant hand, if possible) and the heel of the foot

Endocrine system disorders

Procedure – To record a blood sugar measurement with an Accu-Chek® Aviva blood glucose meter – *cont*

in a younger child or infant. Clean the area with water or water-soaked gauze and dry thoroughly. Insert the test strip into the meter and check that the meter turns on automatically. Alcohol swabs do not remove traces of glucose as effectively as water so should not be used. Hand-washing is preferable, but if that is not possible, simple cleansing wipes are almost as effective.

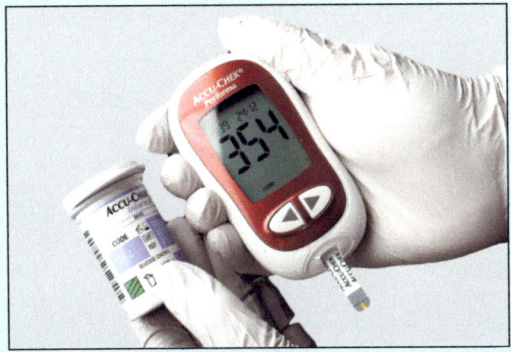

2. Ensure that the code number of the display matches the code number on the test strip container.

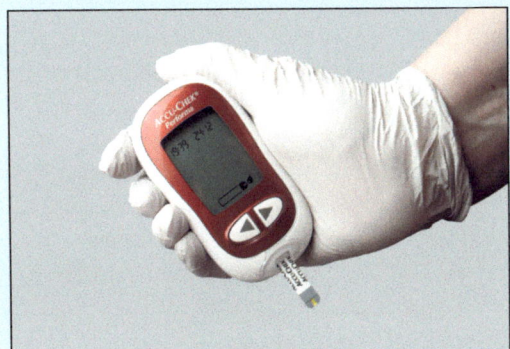

3. On the screen, an icon showing the test strip and a flashing blood drop will appear. Ask the patient to dangle their arm down at their side to encourage blood flow to their fingertips.

Procedure – To record a blood sugar measurement with an Accu-Chek® Aviva blood glucose meter – *cont*

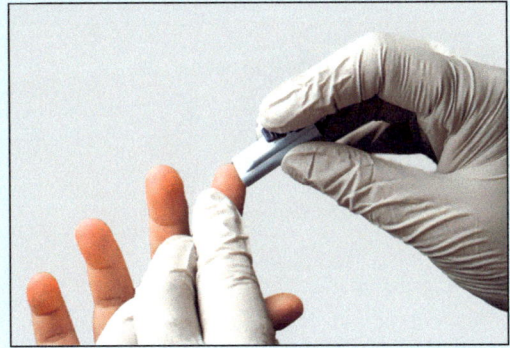

4. Prick the target area with a lancet, disposing of it in a sharps bin after use.

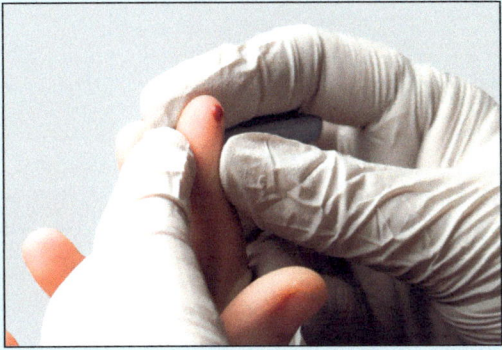

5. With the patient's hand facing downwards, gently squeeze their finger to assist the flow of blood.

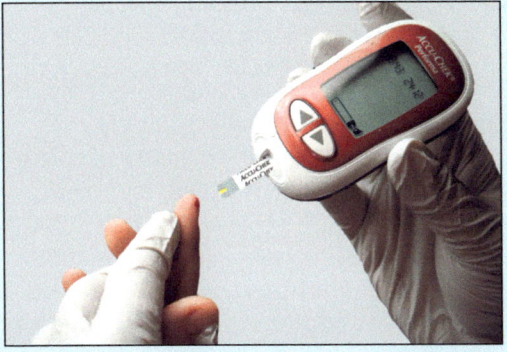

6. Touch the blood drop to the front edge of the yellow window of the test strip. When you have enough blood, you will see an egg timer icon flash.

Procedure – To record a blood sugar measurement with an Accu-Chek® Aviva blood glucose meter – *cont*

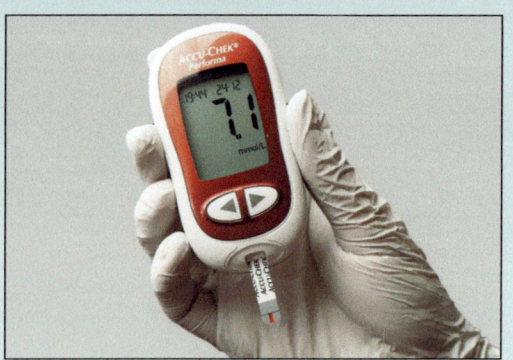

7. The blood sugar result will appear on the display. Note this value on the patient's clinical record.

3.10 Addison's disease

Addison's disease falls under the umbrella term of primary adrenal insufficiency. This is a clinical syndrome caused by a number of diseases that all have decreased secretion of cortisol (the 'stress' hormone) and aldosterone by the adrenal glands in common [Husebye, 2009].

There are numerous causes of Addison's disease. Pre-existing diseases are more commonly seen in patients with Addison's disease, particularly other autoimmune-related diseases such as Graves' disease, type 1 diabetes, premature ovarian failure and coeliac disease [Hellesen, 2018].

The majority of patients with Addison's disease in developed countries have the autoimmune form of the disease, whereby the adrenal cortex is progressively destroyed by the body's own immune system. There are approximately 9,000 people in the UK who have autoimmune Addison's disease [ADSHG, 2016a]. It typically affects young and middle-aged people and is more common in women than men [Husebye, 2009].

3.10.1 Adrenal crisis

A number of factors can lead to a patient with Addison's disease (and other causes of primary

Table 16.3 Common precipitating factors for adrenal crisis.

Cause	Incidence (%)
Vomiting	33
Diarrhoea	23
Flu-like illness	11
Major infection	6
Surgery	6
Blackout/LOC	6
Injury/severe pain	4
Shock	4
Other	3
Severe fatigue/inadequate medication	2
Unknown	1
Anxiety/psychological upset/stress	1

adrenal insufficiency) going into 'crisis'. The most common cause is vomiting and/or diarrhoea [White, 2010], but other precipitating factors are given in Table 16.3 [White, 2010]. Around 8% of patients with Addison's disease will have at least one adrenal crisis requiring administration of hydrocortisone. The vast majority of these patients rely on a healthcare professional to administer a hydrocortisone injection. In one study, only 12% were able to administer it themselves, with a further 17% having the drug administered by a partner, relative or friend [White, 2010].

3.10.2 Signs and symptoms

The most obvious signs of Addison's disease are cachexia and overpigmentation of the skin, which occurs due to loss of the negative feedback mechanism that controls melanocyte-stimulating hormone from the anterior pituitary gland [Innes, 2018]. The patient may look tanned, although this sign is sometimes subtle. Check for pigmentation of the palmar creases, and muddy brown patches in the mucous membranes of the lips and mouth. Enquire specifically about salt-craving, which can occur in hyponatraemia. Symptoms can be remembered by using the ADDISONS mnemonic [ADSHG, 2016b]:

A	Always tired
D	Dizzy when standing
D	Drop in blood pressure on standing
I	Inexplicable weight loss
S	Skin colour changes
O	Only eating sparingly/anorexia
N	No strength in handgrip or limbs
S	Sick or nauseous.

Patients in adrenal crisis typically present with severe hypotension or shock, acute abdominal pain, vomiting and pyrexia [Charmandari, 2014].

Other clues that may indicate your patient has Addison's disease include a MedicAlert bracelet and glucocorticoid and mineralocorticoid replacement medication, most commonly hydrocortisone and fludrocortisone [Baker, 2009]. In patients with type 1 diabetes, there may be a history of deteriorating blood sugar control, with recurrent hypoglycaemic episodes [Charmandari, 2014].

3.10.3 Management of adrenal crisis

This is a life-threatening emergency. Patients are usually told to double or even treble their oral dose of hydrocortisone when unwell or injured, but they may not be able to manage medication orally if they are vomiting [Baker, 2009]. It is essential therefore that they receive intravenous (IV) hydrocortisone (or intramuscular, IM) as soon as possible. Follow local guidance, but you may be able to administer the patient's own hydrocortisone via the IM route. If there is doubt, it is better to administer it than to withhold it.

Patients may become hypotensive and hypoglycaemic, both of which are best treated with IV fluids and glucose, respectively. However, do not delay on scene if a paramedic is not available. Oral glucose or IM glucagon can be administered, if required. Frequently re-check blood glucose as these patients are at risk of recurring hypoglycaemia. Alert the receiving hospital and make sure you pass on that the patient has Addison's disease to the staff, as the patient will require repeated doses of hydrocortisone every 6–8 hours.

4 Poisoning

Poisoning is the exposure by ingestion, inhalation, absorption or infection to a quantity of a substance or substances that may result in illness or death. Over 70% of emergency department (ED) admissions involving poisoning are deliberate, with paracetamol the most common drug involved [Baker, 2014].

4.1 *Toxidromes*

A toxidrome is a collection of signs and symptoms associated with a particular class of toxins. Drugs are grouped together based on these signs and symptoms, which provides some indication as to which drugs have been taken and helps guide management of the poisoning. It is not perfect, as not all signs and symptoms will be present in your patient, and overdoses of multiple types of drug are common, leading to variable signs and symptoms [Boyle, 2009]. Common toxidromes are summarised in Table 16.4. These include [JRCALC, 2019; QAS, 2018a; NPIS, 2019]:

- sympathomimetic
- anticholinergic
- cholinergic
- opioid
- sedative-hypnotic
- serotonin syndrome.

4.2 *Assessment and management*

Acute poisoning is a dynamic medical illness and patients can quickly deteriorate. Altered level of consciousness (LOC), decreased airway reflexes and hypotension are common problems. To properly assess and manage the poisoned patient, the following approach has been advocated,

Table 16.4 Common toxidromes.

Toxidrome	Signs/symptoms	Example causes
Sympathomimetic	Tachycardia, hypertension, Mydriasis (dilated pupils), Diaphoresis (sweating), Piloerection ('goose bumps') Hyperthermia, seizures	Caffeine, cocaine, amphetamines, Ritalin, LSD, theophylline, MDMA (ecstasy) Novel psychoactive substances: synthetic cannabinoids such as 'Spice' or 'Mamba' and synthetic cathinones such as mephedrone (can also cause serotonin syndrome) Alcohol/drug withdrawal
Anticholinergic	Confusion Mydriasis, near-vision blurred Decreased salivation, dry mouth, intense thirst and difficulty swallowing Marked flushing of face and chest, although not related to cholinergic blockade Elevated body temperature, blockade of sweat glands Urinary retention Absent bowel sounds **NOTE:** Children especially at risk due to receptor sensitivity, particularly children with Down's syndrome	Anticholinergics, e.g. atropine Antihistamines, e.g. chlorphenamine, hydroxyzine, diphenhydramine Antipsychotics, e.g. chlorpromazine, olanzapine, thioridazine Antispasmodics, e.g. clidinium, hyoscyamine, oxybutynin
Cholinergic	Sweating Lacrimation (crying) Miosis (pinpoint pupils) Rhinorrhoea (runny nose) Frothing at mouth due to salivation and bronchorrhoea Vomiting Bradycardia Urinary incontinence Diarrhoea	Nicotine Nerve agents, e.g. sarin Organophosphates
Opioid	Miosis, altered level of consciousness, decreased bowel sounds and respiratory depression (rate and depth) Nausea and vomiting can occur **NOTE:** Opioid: compounds related to opium Opiates: drugs derived from opium Endogenous opioids: naturally occurring ligands for opioid receptors	Morphine, codeine, tramadol, heroin, fentanyl, methadone, oxycodone, hydrocodone

Toxidrome	Signs/symptoms	Example causes
Sedative-hypnotic	Altered level of consciousness Slurred speech Ataxia Amnesia Cardiovascular and respiratory depression Decreased bowel sounds	Barbiturates, e.g. thiopental, phenobarbitol Benzodiazepines, e.g. diazepam, lorazepam Z-drugs, e.g. zopiclone, zolpidem Drugs of abuse, e.g. GHB
Serotonin syndrome	Delirium Mydriasis Sweating Tachycardia Clonus, myoclonus, hyperreflexia, increased limb tone Increased bowel sounds Nausea	Drugs abuse, e.g. MDMA, amphetamines Antidepressants, e.g. tricyclics, citalopram, fluoxetine, sertraline Monoamine oxidase inhibitors Novel psychoactive substances: synthetic cathinones such as mephedrone
Alcohol	Vomiting Slurred speech Confusion Convulsions Unconsciousness Change in rational thinking Hypoglycaemia	Alcohol containing product or a mixture of alcohol containing products

which you might find easier to remember with the mnemonic Resus–RSI–DEAD [Murray, 2015]:

- **Resus**citation
  - airway
  - breathing
  - circulation
  - detect and correct
    - hypoglycaemia
    - convulsions
    - hyper-/hypothermia
  - emergency antidote administration
- **R**isk assessment
  - drug
  - dose
  - time since ingestion
  - clinical features and course
  - patient factors
- **S**upportive care and monitoring
- **I**nvestigations
  - screening
    - 12-lead ECG
    - paracetamol levels
  - specific
    - **d**econtamination
    - **e**nhanced elimination
    - **a**ntidotes
    - **d**isposition.

4.2.1 Resuscitation

As for all life-threatening emergencies, you should address the ABCs. Note that in some types of poisoning, standard resuscitation algorithms may not be effective. Detect and correct hypoglycaemia. Drugs such as insulin, sulphonylureas, beta-blockers, quinine and salicylates (aspirin) can cause hypoglycaemia. Convulsions are typically generalised in poisoning, so look for another cause if your patient presents with partial convulsions. IV benzodiazepines are the first-line treatment. Profound hypothermia can mimic or cause cardiac arrest and prolonged CPR is usually required (not dead until warm and dead). Hyperthermia is also associated with significant morbidity and death. Closely monitor any patient with a temperature greater than 38.5°C; if over 39.5°C, rapid in-hospital intervention is required if multi-organ failure and neurological injury is to be avoided [Murray, 2015].

There are a number of antidotes to poisoning that are carried by the ambulance service, including naloxone for opioid overdose and atropine for organophosphorus agent intoxication. There are a number of others, but these are generally only available in hospital; in the case of anti-venom for snake bites, for example, only specialist centres will keep a stock [Baker, 2014].

4.2.2 Risk assessment

Making a risk assessment is a key element in poisonings and guides subsequent treatment. Consider the difference between an adult patient who takes an accidental overdose of their Adcal calcium supplements, which has a low toxicity (constipation in large doses), versus a 75 kg patient who has taken 10 g paracetamol in the last hour (more than the toxic dose of 75 mg/kg) because they wanted to end their life [NPIS, 2019].

Assuming that patients are alert and orientated, they may be able to tell you what they have taken. In addition, check for discarded packets of medication and try to determine how many are missing. Prescribed medication will have a dispensed date, which may help, although if planning is involved, then patients may have been hoarding medication prior to the attempt. The drug, dose and time since ingestion should fit with the patient's current presentation. If it does not, revise your risk assessment.

Since poisoning is a dynamic process, time-points when a patient is at particular risk can be identified. For example, life-threatening events in tricyclic antidepressant overdoses occur within six hours; if the ingestion is well beyond that, then the patient is less likely to be at risk [NPIS, 2019]. However, some sustained-release medications may require 24 hours or longer of observations in hospital. In order to determine the most appropriate action, it is important to understand whether the drug/poison is toxic in the quantity that the patient has been exposed to. In the UK, TOXBASE is the most commonly used online database, but it is possible to contact the National Poisons Information Service (NPIS) by telephone, although this is typically undertaken via your clinical hub in the emergency operations centre (EOC) or at the local emergency department (ED) than by ambulance staff on scene.

Psychosocial assessments are important, but, from an ambulance service perspective, all deliberate overdoses should be assessed in hospital [Baker, 2014].

4.2.3 Supportive care and monitoring

Morbidity and death from poisoning typically arise from the targeting of the respiratory, cardiovascular and/or central nervous system by the poison. Therefore, a period of observation is usually appropriate in the local ED, and some patients will need critical care interventions, resulting in a stay in the hospital's intensive care unit. This is most likely to occur in patients who require intubation and ventilation, prolonged or invasive haemodynamic monitoring or support and haemodialysis [Murray, 2015].

4.2.4 Investigations

All unconscious patients should have a serum paracetamol level checked, which cannot at present be conducted by ambulance staff. Figure 16.7 shows some of the signs that can help differentiate between the various toxidromes to help guide treatment. In addition, you should record a 12-lead ECG, as many drugs taken in overdose can lead to significant ECG changes.

4.2.5 Decontamination

Activated charcoal is recommended by the National Institute for Health and Care Excellence (NICE) when a person who has self-poisoned presents to the ambulance service within one hour of ingestion, is

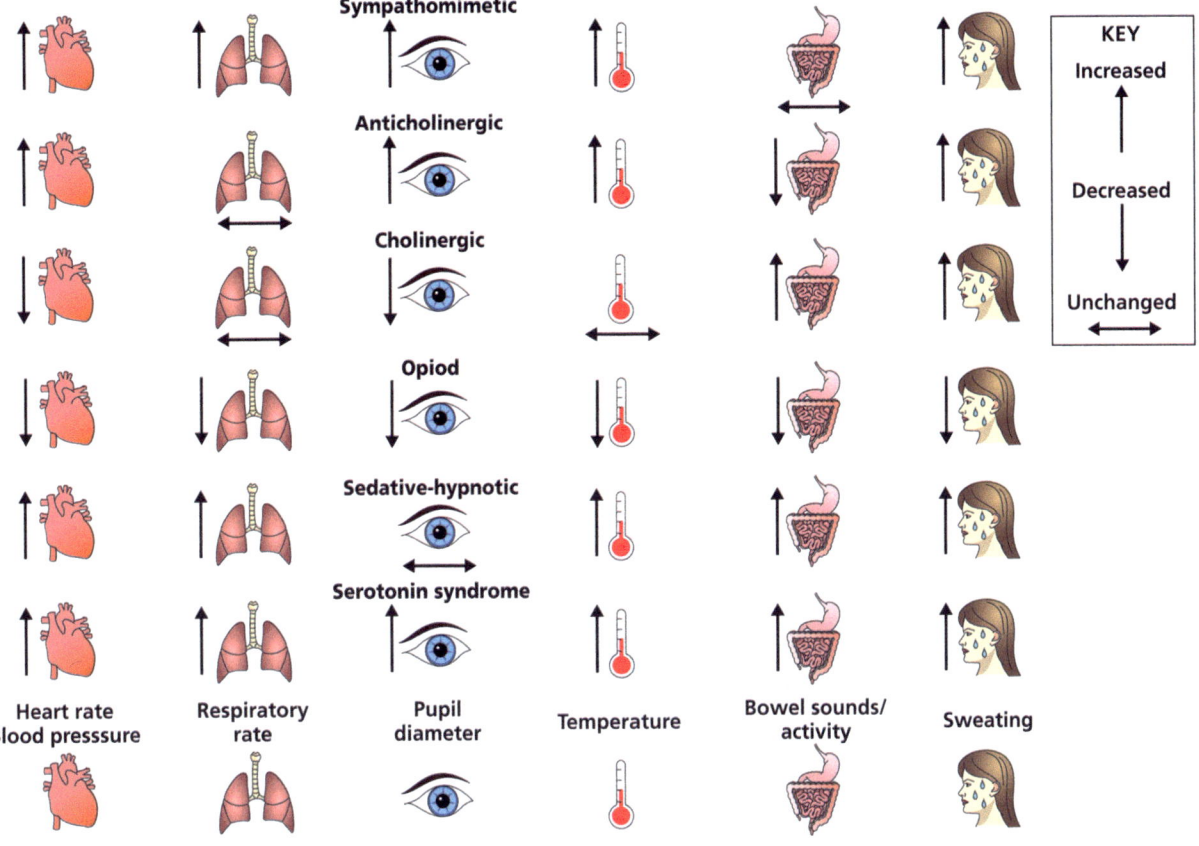

Figure 16.7 Toxidrome signs.

fully conscious and able to protect their own airway. However, this should be offered only when the substance(s) ingested is/are likely to be adsorbed by activated charcoal and when the person is considered to be at risk of significant harm [NICE, 2004].

Note that vomiting occurs in 30% of patients given activated charcoal within an hour. It is ineffective if the poisons are hydrocarbons, alcohols, metals or corrosives [Murray, 2015].

4.2.6 Enhanced elimination

This will not be conducted in the ambulance, but may include multiple doses of activated charcoal as well as more advanced procedures.

4.2.7 Antidotes

Some drugs do have an antidote and there are antivenoms available for some snake and other bites available in the UK. However, most antidotes also have their own contra-indications and adverse side-effects, and should only be given when appropriate.

4.2.8 Disposition

It may be suitable to leave patients with non-intentional exposures at home if they meet the following criteria (and your local non-conveyance guidelines) [JRCALC, 2019]:
- The substance is verified by TOXBASE or the NPIS as being harmless.
- A responsible adult is present.
- Advice is provided to the patient to seek medical advice if they become unwell.
- The patient's health visitor or GP is informed.

However, as previously mentioned, all intentional overdoses should have a mental health assessment.

Table 16.5 Out-of-hospital treatment options for overdose.

Toxidrome	Initial treatment
Alcohol	Acute alcohol poisoning is usually transient. However, patients will need monitoring and supportive treatment whilst they recover. In some situations, it can be serious and lead to other secondary complications including hypothermia and hypoglycaemia. Always measure the blood glucose of any confused patient or any patient you believe may have consumed a significant quantity of alcohol. You should be aware that alcohol can significantly enhance the effects of other drugs such as opioids or benzodiazepines, if taken simultaneously.
Opiates	The main concern with opiates is respiratory depression so your management should primarily focus around establishing a patent airway and ventilating the patient, if required, to maintain oxygenation and an appropriate $ETCO_2$. Depending on your local service, you may be able to administer IM naloxone; you will be trained in this procedure locally if appropriate.
Caustic irritant	Encourage the patient to drink a cup of milk if they are able to do so safely. Do not induce vomiting.
Paracetamol or paracetamol-containing products	Even small amounts of paracetamol taken in overdose can be dangerous. Any patient thought to have taken a paracetamol overdose will require urgent blood measurements. In some circumstances, it may be possible to give the patient activated charcoal to reduce the amount of paracetamol being absorbed into the body.

At the opposite end of the spectrum, some patients will require transfer to a specialist centre for definitive care.

Table 16.5 outlines out-of-hospital treatment options for overdose on some of the commonest forms of toxidromes. As an AAP, you may not be able to provide all of these treatments, but it is important you are aware of them [JRCALC, 2019].

5 The acute abdomen

5.1 Learning objectives

By the end of this section you will be able to:
- describe the anatomy and physiology of the digestive system
- list a number of causes of an 'acute abdomen' and describe their signs and symptoms
- explain the management of a patient with an 'acute abdomen'.

5.2 Introduction

The term 'acute abdomen' refers to abdominal conditions that are characterised by a rapid onset of severe symptoms, which require prompt admission to hospital and may require surgical intervention. Because of the number of organs and structures within the abdominal cavity, it can be difficult to make a diagnosis, but this does not matter out-of-hospital, as long as serious red-flag symptoms have been recognised and acted on.

5.3 The abdominal cavity

The abdominal cavity extends from the diaphragm to the pelvic cavity, although it is continuous with this and some abdominal organs descend into the pelvic cavity. The arched dome shape of the diaphragm extends well above the costal margin, allowing the ribs to provide protection for the liver, spleen, upper poles of the kidneys and the adrenal (suprarenal) glands. The spine provides additional protection, although the anterior and lateral aspects of the abdomen are more exposed, since the abdominal muscles provide only modest protection. Organs are either suspended by double folds of the peritoneum (a membrane that lines the abdominal cavity), known as mesenteries, or bound to the posterior abdominal wall. In addition, some organs are located posterior to the peritoneum and are termed retroperitoneal, including the kidneys, adrenal glands and ureters [Tortora, 2017].

Organs contained within the abdominal cavity include [Drake, 2015]:
- major elements of the digestive system (Figure 16.8)
- posterior end of oesophagus, stomach, small and large intestines, liver, pancreas and gallbladder

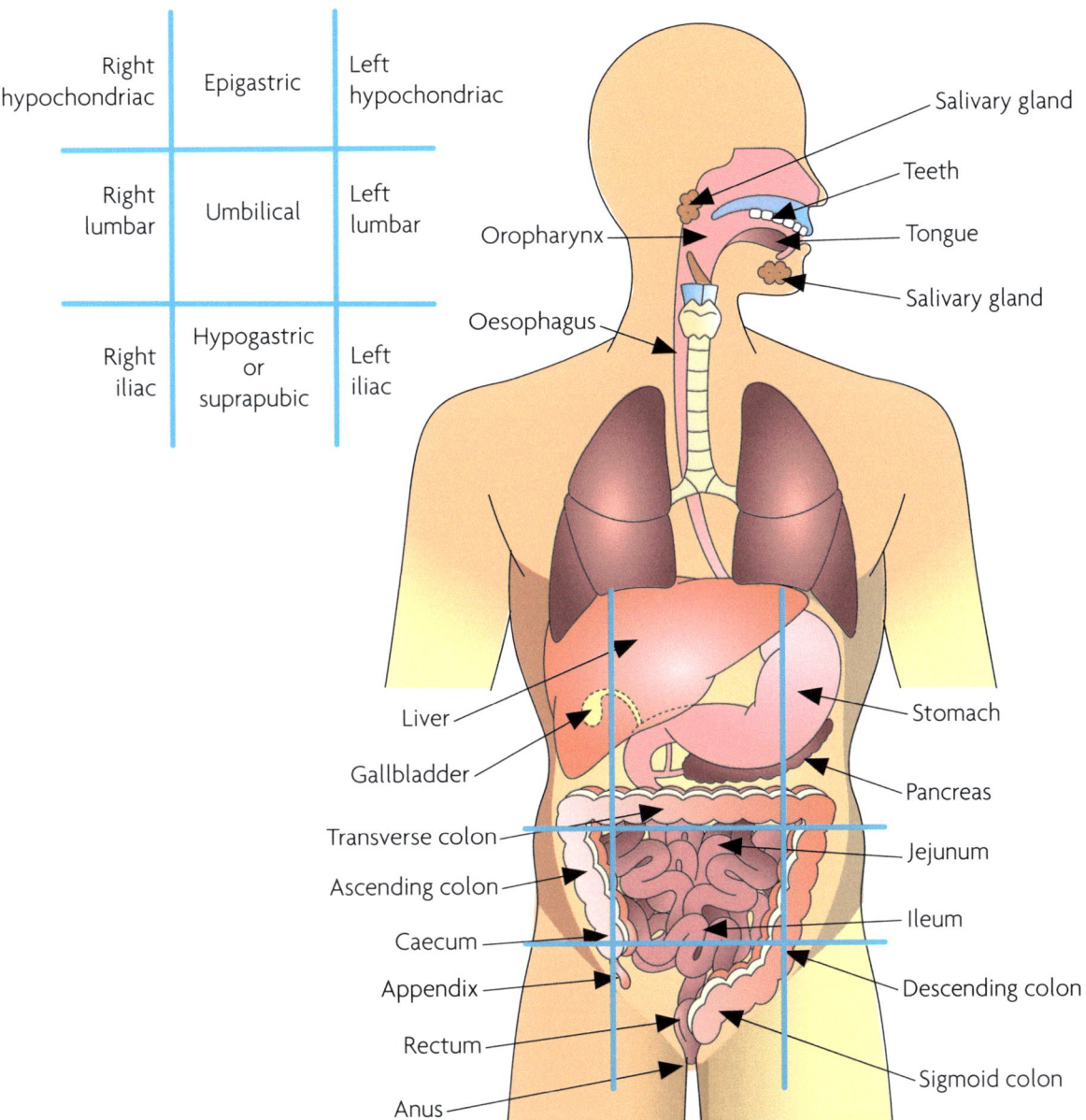

Figure 16.8 Overview of the digestive system.

Chapter 16 – Medical and Surgical Emergencies

- components of the urinary system (kidneys and ureters)
- major neurovascular structures (e.g. abdominal aorta, inferior vena cava).

5.4 Locating abdominal organs

To make it easier to relate surface anatomy to the underlying organs, the abdomen is often divided into nine (Figure 16.8) or four (Figure 16.9) regions. Dividing the abdomen into nine is achieved by drawing two mid-clavicular lines extending to the mid-inguinal point vertically, and two horizontal lines, one in the transpyloric plane, midway between the pubic symphysis and jugular notch, and the second running between the tubercles of the iliac crests [Drake, 2015].

5.5 The digestive system

The digestive or gastrointestinal (GI) system performs six main functions [Tortora, 2017]:
- ingestion
- secretion
- mixing and propulsion
- digestion
- absorption
- defaecation.

It consists of an alimentary canal (the GI tract) and associated accessory organs, forming a continuous tube that runs from mouth to anus. Starting at the oral cavity, the teeth pulverise, and saliva softens and partly digests the food that is in the mouth. The tongue assists with mechanical manipulation of the food and flips what's left into the pharynx during swallowing.

Boluses of food move down the oesophagus due to regular peristaltic contractions and enter the stomach, where the food is treated to mechanical and chemical digestion, resulting in the formation of a semi-fluid mass known as chyme. This enters the small intestine for further digestion, aided by bile from the gallbladder, which passes down the bile duct and into the duodenum and helps digest fat and neutralise stomach acid. In addition, digestive enzymes from the exocrine pancreas also enter the duodenum. Molecular-sized nutrients are extracted from the small intestine and transferred by blood and lymph capillaries to the liver for processing.

Finally, the proximal half of the large intestine absorbs minerals and water, while the remaining portion acts as a storage unit for undigested and unabsorbed material, which continues to the rectum ready for discharge via the anus.

5.6 Abdominal pain

Abdominal pain is a common presentation to emergency and urgent care services. As has already been discussed, diagnosing abdominal pain can be very challenging due not only to the sheer number of things that can go wrong with the abdomen, but also because of the arrangement of organs within, which makes it very difficult to pinpoint the exact issue.

It is likely that you will transport any significant abdominal pain to hospital for further assessment, but in the initial phases, you should consider the following as part of your examination [Kumar, 2012]:
- the site, intensity, character, duration and frequency of the pain

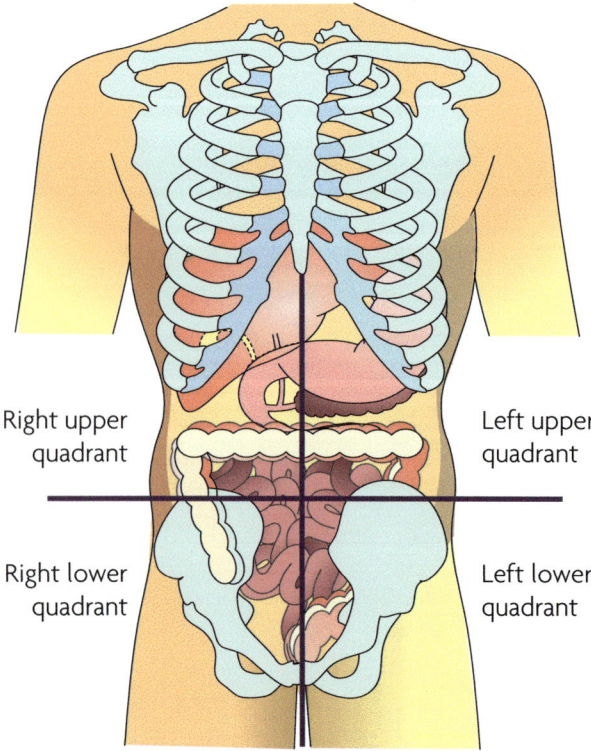

Figure 16.9 Abdominal quadrants.

The acute abdomen

- the aggravating and relieving factors
- associated symptoms, including non-gastrointestinal symptoms.

You should be particularly concerned when abdominal pain presents with altered vital signs (tachycardia, hypotension, etc.) [Leath, 2017]. Table 16.6 provides examples of conditions that cause abdominal pain [JRCALC, 2019].

5.7 Management of abdominal pain

The focus of management for abdominal pain patients will be to stabilise and transport them to the ED. If you suspect that the patient has any of the conditions in Table 16.6 or has any life-threatening ABC problems, consider requesting support from a senior clinician and/or transport the patient to hospital as an emergency.

Table 16.6 Conditions that cause abdominal pain.

Condition	Characteristics of pain	Associated symptoms
Leaking or ruptured abdominal aortic aneurysm (AAA) Consider AAA in patients over 50 years old who present with the symptoms listed. Most deaths occur in the elderly	Sudden severe abdominal pain or backache Renal colic-type pain: a new diagnosis of renal colic in a patient over 50 years old raises the concern of AAA even in the absence of a palpable mass **Note:** Given that <25% of all AAA patients present with classic signs and symptoms there is a risk of misdiagnosis	Collapse Hypotension with bilateral lower limb ischaemia History of smoking Hypertension and hypercholesterolaemia
Appendicitis Frequently misdiagnosed. Approximately one-third of women of childbearing age with appendicitis are considered as having pelvic inflammatory disease or UTI	A constant pain, increasing in intensity often starting in the periumbilical area Pain may settle in the right lower quadrant, but the location may vary in the early stages Older patients may present with generalised pain, distension and decreased bowel sounds	
Acute cholecystitis Accounts for approximately 30% of patients attending the ED for acute abdominal pain	A sharp pain in the right upper quadrant of the abdomen May experience right shoulder-tip pain The pain is worse when breathing deeply and on palpation of the right upper quadrant	Nausea and vomiting Increased temperature >38°C History of fat intolerance
Intestinal obstruction A partial or complete obstruction of the small or large intestine	Abdominal pain that is cramping in nature	Abdominal distension Nausea and vomiting Absolute constipation (late stage)

continued

Chapter 16 – Medical and Surgical Emergencies

Table 16.6 Conditions that cause abdominal pain. *continued*

Condition	Characteristics of pain	Associated symptoms
Peptic ulcer An erosion of the lining of the stomach or small intestine forming an ulcer	Central burning abdominal discomfort Back pain Perforation may lead to abrupt-onset epigastric pain	Nausea and vomiting Haematemesis Fatigue Weight loss
Acute pancreatitis Inflammation of the pancreas	Constant pain in the upper left quadrant or middle of the abdomen The pain may radiate to the patient's back	Abdominal tenderness Hypotension Nausea and vomiting Dehydration Shock History of alcohol abuse or gallstones
Diverticular disease Inflammation of the diverticula in the large intestine	Abdominal pain in the lower left quadrant	Nausea and vomiting Altered bowel habits Bloating Increased temperature >38°C
Ectopic pregnancy Pregnancy is not implanted in the uterus. This affects around 1 in 80 people and accounts for 13% of all pregnancy-related deaths	Pain in the lower abdomen, pelvic area or back NB Patients may present atypically, but pain is almost always present	Nausea Missed last menstrual period (though can occur before this) History of pelvic inflammatory disease Previous ectopic pregnancy If the pregnancy ruptures, patients may report: – severe lower abdominal pain – shoulder-tip pain – feeling faint/collapse

Other treatment will include:
- Gather and frequently reassess vital signs – record these on your documentation.
- Place the patient in the position of most comfort.
- Administer adequate pain relief – consider if further pain relief than what you are able to administer is required; if so, request appropriate backup.
- Be prepared for the patient to deteriorate and to initiate resuscitation if necessary.

6 Urinary system disorders

6.1 *Learning objectives*

By the end of this section you will be able to:
- describe the anatomy and physiology of the urinary system
- explain the assessment and management of a patient with a urinary tract infection (UTI)
- describe the nature and purpose of renal dialysis

- explain the management of a patient on renal dialysis.

6.2 Introduction

The urinary system carries out a number of important functions, including [Tortora, 2017]:
- regulation of blood volume and composition
- regulation of blood pressure
- glucose synthesis
- excretion of waste products in urine.

All of these functions are carried out by the kidneys. The other organs and tissues that make up the urinary system provide transport for the storage and excretion of urine.

6.3 Anatomy and physiology

The urinary system is made up of two kidneys, two ureters, a bladder and urethra (Figure 16.10).

6.3.1 Kidneys

The kidneys are red-brown kidney bean-shaped organs that are located just above the waist and lie between the peritoneum and posterior wall of the abdomen. The right kidney is lower than the left to accommodate the liver above. Due to the important functions of the kidney, they receive around 25% of resting cardiac output, about 1,200 ml per minute, via the renal arteries [Tortora, 2017]. As with other blood vessels, these subdivide into smaller and smaller vessels, before reaching the glomerular capillaries in the nephrons (Figure 16.11).

The functional unit of the kidney is the nephron (Figure 16.12). This consists of a renal corpuscle (itself made up of the glomerulus and Bowman's capsule) and the renal tubule, which is split into three sections: proximal convoluted (tightly coiled) tubule (PCT), loop of Henle and distal convoluted tubule (DCT).

Blood enters the renal corpuscle from the afferent arteriole. Due to the high pressures, water and most solutes leave the glomerulus and enter the Bowman's capsule before flowing into the PCT. The total sum of all filtered fluid that leaves the Bowman's capsule every minute is known as the glomerular filtration rate.

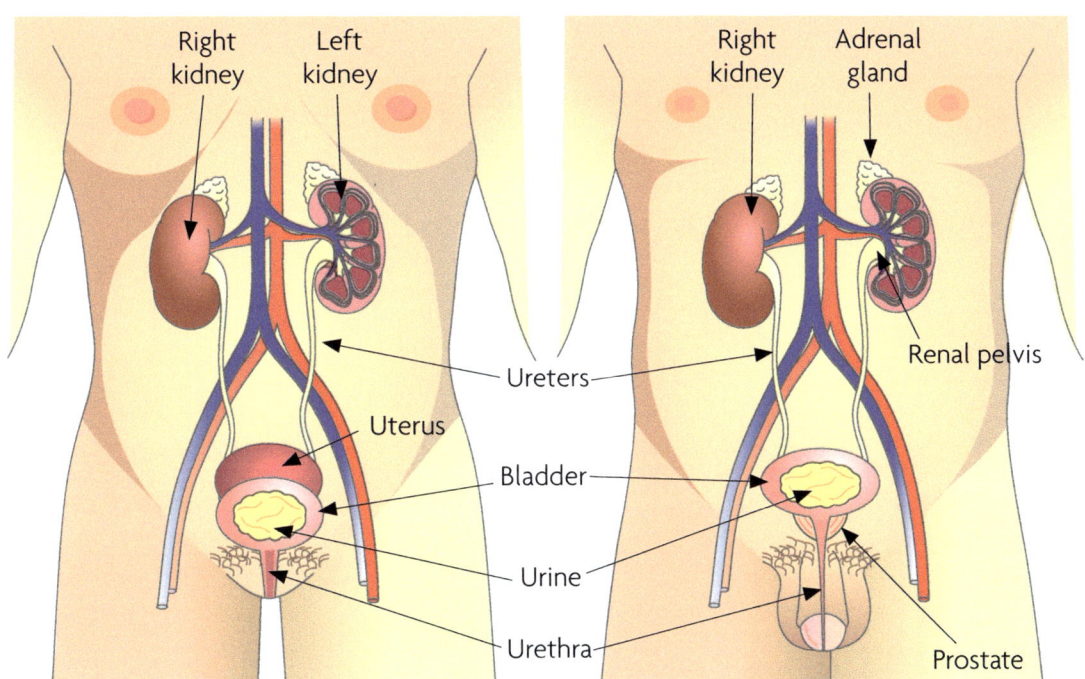

Figure 16.10 The urinary system in females (left) and males (right).

Chapter 16 – Medical and Surgical Emergencies

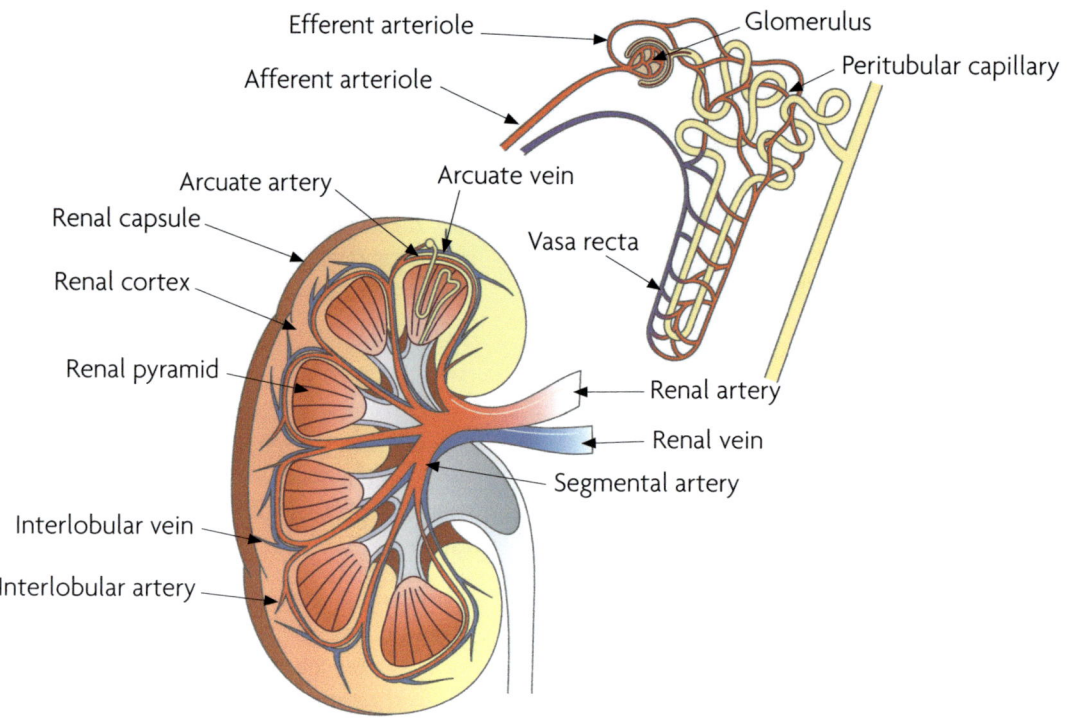

Figure 16.11 Blood supply to the kidneys.

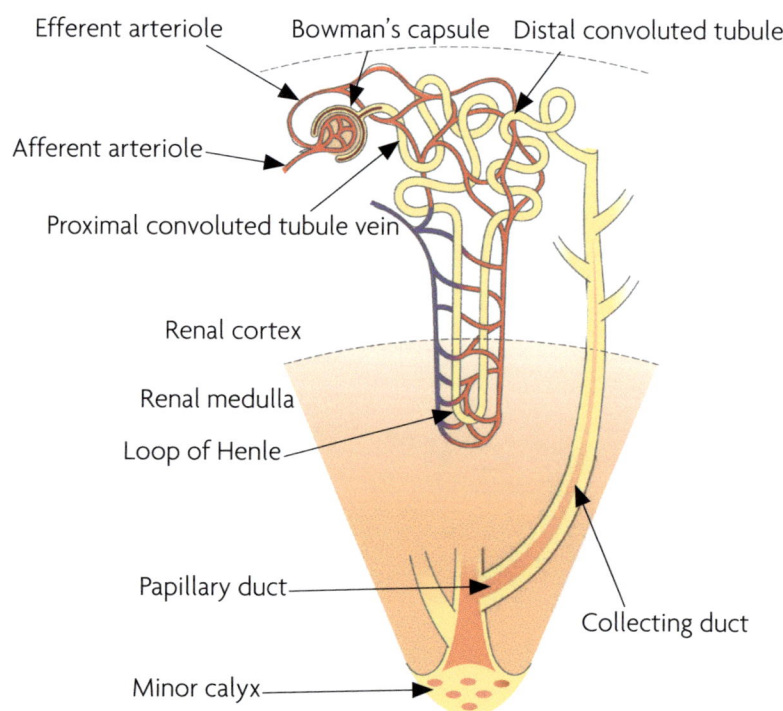

Figure 16.12 A cortical nephron. These make up around 80% of nephrons. The remainder are juxtamedullary nephrons, which have much longer loops of Henle, enabling them to produce very diluted or concentrated urine.

As the filtered fluid passes through the PCT, around 65% of the water and virtually all of the glucose, amino and lactic acids as well as water-soluble vitamins are reabsorbed back into the blood. The remainder travels into the loop of Henle, where a further 15% of water together with quantities of solutes such as potassium, sodium, calcium, bicarbonate and chloride are reabsorbed. Finally, in the DCT further reabsorption of water, sodium and calcium occurs. By the time the filtered fluid reaches the end of the DCT, up to 95% of filtered water and solutes have been reabsorbed back into the blood [Tortora, 2017].

6.3.2 Ureters, bladder and urethra

The remaining fluid and solutes that leave the collecting duct are now urine. This drains out of the minor calyx into the major calyx and into the renal pelvis. From here it drains into the ureters and moves into the bladder by a combination of rhythmic contractions of its muscular walls (peristalsis), pressure and gravity.

The urinary bladder is sited in the pelvic cavity just posterior to the pubic symphysis. It is a hollow and expansible organ that has a maximum capacity in the region of 700–800 ml. The last stage is the urethra, which allows urine to be excreted from the body.

6.4 Urinary tract infections

A urinary tract infection (UTI) occurs when there is microbial infiltration of the normally sterile urinary tract.

UTIs can affect the urethra (urethritis) and urinary bladder (cystitis), collectively termed lower UTIs, and/or ascend to the kidneys (pyelonephritis) where, unsurprisingly, it is termed an upper UTI. One other important anatomical level is the systemic circulation, infection of which results in sepsis.

UTIs are typically classed as mild or severe, which is defined by the number of symptoms the patient reports (more on this later). Three or more symptoms are classed as severe, and this has implications for treatment. UTIs can also be classed as complicated or uncomplicated. In an otherwise healthy adult female, acute cystitis or pyelonephritis would be considered uncomplicated; in 70–95% of cases, it is caused by *Escherichia coli* (E. coli). If the patient is male and/or has a structural or functional abnormality of the urinary tract, or suffers from kidney disease and certain other diseases, such as diabetes, then typically the UTI would be considered to be complicated.

6.4.1 Signs and symptoms

The classic symptoms of a UTI include [Nickerson, 2007]:
- **Dysuria:** Pain or a burning sensation when urinating.
- **Frequency:** Urinating more often.
- **Nocturia:** Having to get up in the night to urinate.
- **Urgency:** A reduction in the time between feeling the need to urinate and actually having to pass urine. If the patient cannot hold on until they reach a toilet, urge incontinence results.

Haematuria (blood in the urine) does sometimes occur (more common in upper UTIs) and the urine can also be offensive-smelling. Elderly patients may have minimal urinary symptoms, but consider this as a differential diagnosis if there is a history of new-onset confusion or incontinence.

Infants and children
In newborns and infants, the presentation of a UTI can be vague, so should be considered when there is a history of fever, irritability (the infant, not the parents) and vomiting. As children get older, they will present more typically, with symptoms such as dysuria, for example [Lissauer, 2017].

Pyelonephritis
Upper UTIs classically present with loin to groin pain on the affected side, although some patients may just complain of back pain. The pain is often colicky and sharp in nature, with

patients struggling to get comfortable and so are restless. Costovertebral angle (formed by the 12th rib and spine) tenderness may be detected on physical examination. Haematuria is more common as are signs and symptoms of systemic illness, such as fever, rigors and profuse sweating [Nickerson, 2007].

6.4.2 Management
Not all UTIs need anti-microbial drugs or a trip to the emergency department. Even acute pyelonephritis can be treated in the community unless the patient has nausea or vomiting or other signs of systemic illness. Follow local guidelines on possible referral pathways.

Children
All children under the age of three months with a suspected UTI should be taken to hospital for review. All children under the age of three years should have a urine sample sent for culture, which probably means a trip to the hospital, unless you have an alternative arrangement in place locally. For children over three years of age, a positive urine dipstick result is likely to indicate a UTI and can be treated with antibiotics. However, even in children over three years of age, if there are signs that they have a systemic illness, pyelonephritis, a history of recurrent UTIs or have had no response to treatment within 24–48 hours, then they too require a trip to the ED [RCGP, 2018b].

6.5 Renal dialysis
Most of the patients you meet who are undergoing renal dialysis (also called renal replacement therapy) are likely to have chronic kidney disease. This is defined as abnormal kidney function or structure for more than three months that has implications for health [NICE, 2015d].

There are two main types of renal dialysis:
- peritoneal dialysis
- haemodialysis.

6.5.1 Peritoneal dialysis
Peritoneal dialysis involves placing a tube into the patient's peritoneal cavity through the abdomen through which a special fluid, called dialysate, is passed. The fluid enters the peritoneal space where waste products usually removed by the kidneys, such as urea, travel down their concentration gradients from the body into the dialysate. The dialysate is then replaced and the process repeated. Modifications to this process include [Kumar, 2012]:
- **Continuous ambulatory peritoneal dialysis:** Dialysate resides in the peritoneal space continuously, except when it is exchanged. The exchanges need to be performed 3–5 times a day and involve 1.5–3.0 litre bags of dialysate. An exchange takes about 20–40 minutes depending on the volume to be exchanged.
- **Automated peritoneal dialysis:** Also known as nightly intermittent peritoneal dialysis; as the name implies, this uses an automated device to manage the exchange overnight while the patient sleeps, which can be more convenient for the patient.

6.5.2 Haemodialysis
Haemodialysis works by pumping blood out of the patient through an array of semipermeable membranes (the dialyser) that brings the blood into close contact with dialysate, which is pumped into the dialyser in the opposite direction to the blood (Figure 16.13). This allows for the removal of waste products, but requires high flow rates, typically 200–300 ml/minute of blood and 500 ml/minute of dialysate. In order to facilitate this, the patient requires a surgical procedure to connect either a radial or brachial artery to the cephalic vein. Approximately 6–8 weeks after this procedure, the vein distends and thickens, making it suitable for the large-bore needles that are required for haemodialysis [Mahon, 2013]. Due to the greater efficiency of haemodialysis over peritoneal dialysis,

Urinary system disorders

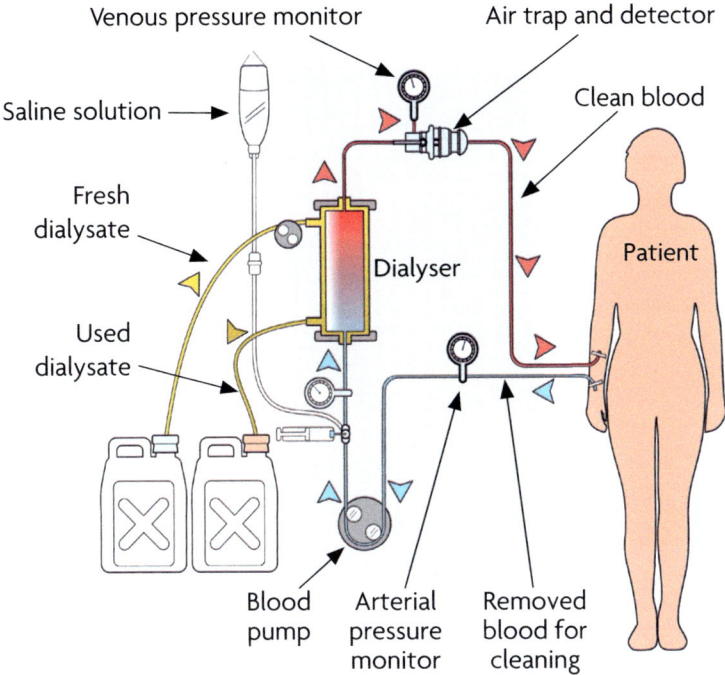

Figure 16.13 A haemodialysis circuit.
Source: YassineMrabetTalk (Own work from Image: Hemodialysis schematic.gif.) [CC BY-SA 3.0], via Wikimedia Commons.

patients need to have dialysis 'only' three times a week, for around 4–5 hours.

6.5.3 Complications

Bacterial peritonitis (inflammation of the peritoneum) is the most serious complication of peritoneal dialysis. However, other complications include fluid leaks, hernias, pain and rectal and vaginal prolapse.

Patients on haemodialysis can have a number of complications too (intradialytic complications) [Mahon, 2013]:
- fever and chills
- headache
- chest pain
- cardiac arrest
- air embolism
- hypotension
- nausea and vomiting.

6.5.4 Management

If you are called to a patient on dialysis at home, either follow their instruction or that of a carer. Remember, they are experts in the management of their condition and will have been taught how to disconnect themselves from their dialysis equipment or device. If this is not possible, you will have to disconnect them.

Chapter 16 – *Medical and Surgical Emergencies*

Procedure for peritoneal dialysis

Take the following steps to remove a patient from peritoneal dialysis [QAS, 2018a]:

1. Put on gloves and ensure an aseptic technique.
2. Turn equipment off at the machine ON/OFF switch (if it is an automated system).
3. Turn tubing flow off from the machine or hanging bag via clamp or roller lock and repeat for the drainage bag.
4. If necessary (where it cannot be identified how to stop the solution flow), clamp catheter tubing at either side of connector port using available clamps already in situ (if available), or umbilical cord clamps (in the maternity pack).
5. Disconnect patient from device and place a cap on the catheter end.

Procedure for haemodialysis

Take the following steps to remove a patient from their haemodialysis machine [QAS, 2018a]:

1. Put on gloves and ensure an aseptic technique.
2. Turn equipment off at the machine ON/OFF switch (if automated system).
3. Clamp catheter tubing using available clamps already in situ, or umbilical cord clamps (in the maternity pack).
4. Disconnect patient from device and leave the cannula in situ with or without extension tubing attached (depending on type of set).
5. Connect a cap to the cannula or extension tubing where necessary to maintain sterility.
6. In the case of severe bleeding during the procedure from the therapy site, apply pressure and bandage as required maintaining pressure (for up to 20 minutes).

Chapter

17 Trauma

1 Major trauma services

1.1 Learning objectives

By the end of this section you will be able to:
- define trauma and major trauma
- state the costs of traumatic injuries to the economy
- outline the inclusive trauma system that has been implemented in England
- explain the role of regional trauma networks including major trauma centres and trauma units.

1.2 Introduction

Trauma is the acute physiological and structural change (injury) that occurs in a patient's body when an external source of energy transfers to the body faster than the body's ability to sustain and dissipate it. Major trauma describes serious and often multiple injuries where there is a strong possibility of death or disability [NAO, 2010]. It is also often defined using the injury severity score (ISS), with a score of over 15 classed as 'major' [Kehoe, 2015].

Major trauma is the leading cause of death in people under 45 years of age, with road traffic collisions the most common cause [McCullough, 2014]. Prior to the introduction of major trauma networks, costs to the NHS were estimated to be around £300–400 million per year to manage major trauma and lost economic output was estimated to be in the region of £3.3–3.7 billion [NAO, 2010].

Since the 1960s, successive reports into the management of major trauma have criticised its ad hoc and unstructured management, as well as highlighting avoidable deaths. However, it was not until the National Confidential Enquiry into Patient Outcome and Death [Findlay, 2007] that there was a significant political shift towards the introduction of regional trauma services, which are present today. Evidence suggests that this approach is working, with an increase of nearly one-fifth in the odds of surviving major trauma, resulting in over 1,600 lives saved between the introduction of the networks in 2012 to early 2018 [Crawford, 2018].

1.3 Inclusive trauma systems

An inclusive trauma system is a model for trauma care where there is collaboration between ambulance services, hospital trusts, commissioners, public health representatives and others to plan and manage patients injured due to major trauma [NHSCAG, 2010].

This has led to the creation of a trauma care pathway that highlights the location and capability of hospitals within the region, when and which patients should be transferred to specialised units, and provides ambulance services with guidelines on appropriate destinations for major trauma, which is often not the closest emergency department. In addition, their acute care and rehabilitation once in hospital is also an integral part of the pathway.

1.3.1 Trauma networks

Regional organisation of major trauma services is managed by trauma networks: a collaboration of providers within a geographical area. At the core of this network is the major trauma centre (MTC), a multi-speciality hospital that can manage all types of injuries and provide senior doctor (consultant) level of care.

Other hospitals within the trauma network are either designated as trauma units (TUs), or local emergency hospitals. The role of a trauma unit will depend on its capabilities. Those with limited facilities are expected to stabilise and transfer serious cases but admit those with less serious injuries. More capable hospitals may be able to manage most injured patients, particularly if they do not have multiple injuries, from acute care through to rehabilitation and recovery [NICE, 2016e].

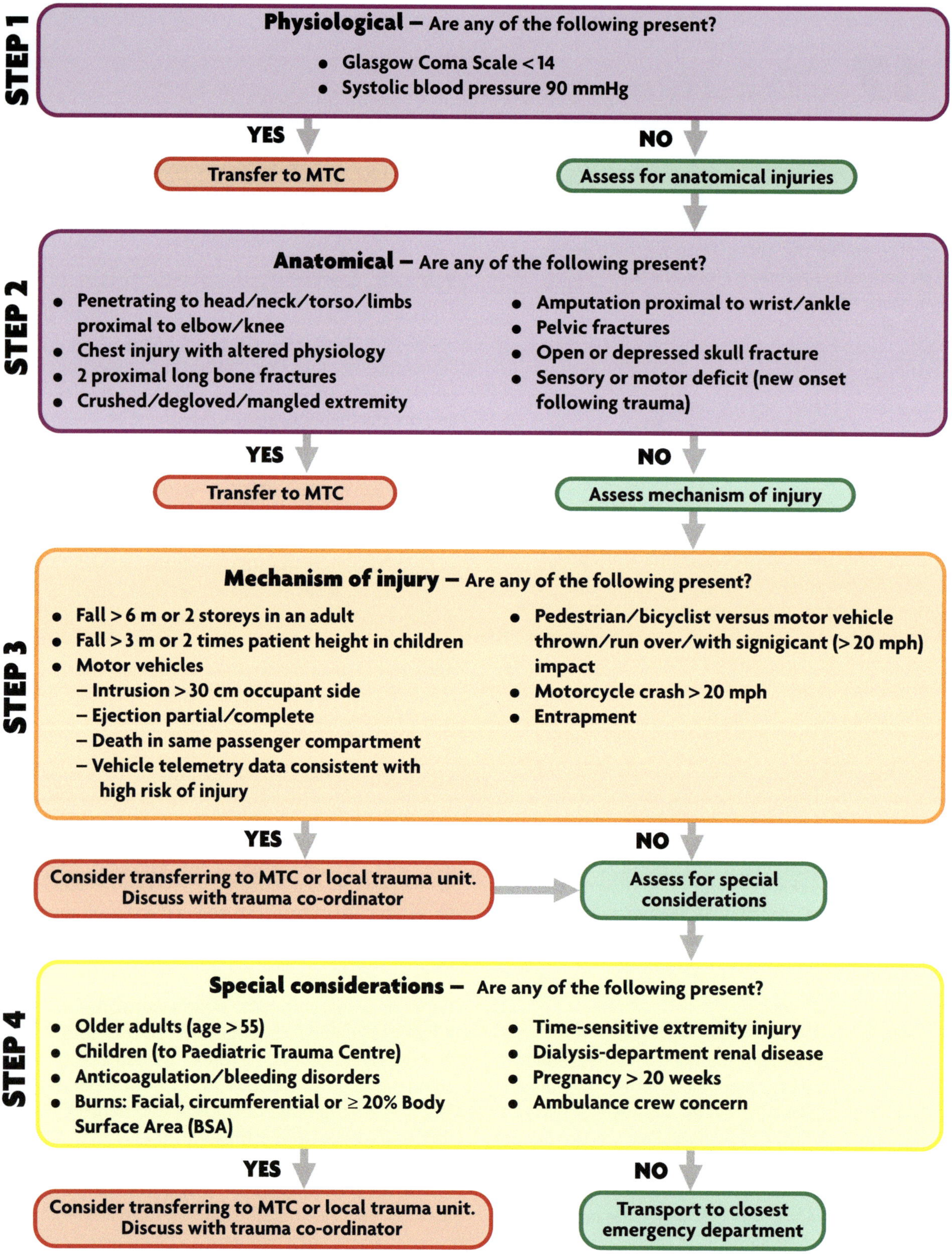

Chapter 17 – *Trauma*

STEP 1

Physiological — Are any of the following present?
- Glasgow Coma Scale < 14
- Systolic blood pressure 90 mmHg

YES → Transfer to MTC

NO → Assess for anatomical injuries

STEP 2

Anatomical — Are any of the following present?
- Penetrating to head/neck/torso/limbs proximal to elbow/knee
- Chest injury with altered physiology
- 2 proximal long bone fractures
- Crushed/degloved/mangled extremity
- Amputation proximal to wrist/ankle
- Pelvic fractures
- Open or depressed skull fracture
- Sensory or motor deficit (new onset following trauma)

YES → Transfer to MTC

NO → Assess mechanism of injury

STEP 3

Mechanism of injury — Are any of the following present?
- Fall > 6 m or 2 storeys in an adult
- Fall > 3 m or 2 times patient height in children
- Motor vehicles
  - Intrusion > 30 cm occupant side
  - Ejection partial/complete
  - Death in same passenger compartment
  - Vehicle telemetry data consistent with high risk of injury
- Pedestrian/bicyclist versus motor vehicle thrown/run over/with signigicant (> 20 mph) impact
- Motorcycle crash > 20 mph
- Entrapment

YES → Consider transferring to MTC or local trauma unit. Discuss with trauma co-ordinator

NO → Assess for special considerations

STEP 4

Special considerations — Are any of the following present?
- Older adults (age > 55)
- Children (to Paediatric Trauma Centre)
- Anticoagulation/bleeding disorders
- Burns: Facial, circumferential or ≥ 20% Body Surface Area (BSA)
- Time-sensitive extremity injury
- Dialysis-department renal disease
- Pregnancy > 20 weeks
- Ambulance crew concern

YES → Consider transferring to MTC or local trauma unit. Discuss with trauma co-ordinator

NO → Transport to closest emergency department

Figure 17.1 Major trauma triage tool.

Emergency hospitals do not routinely receive acute trauma (except minor injuries), but are expected to promptly transfer those patients to trauma units or the MTC.

1.4 Major trauma triage tool

In order to assist ambulance service staff with making decisions about the most appropriate destination for their patients, a pre-hospital major trauma triage tool should be used (Figure 17.1). The tool will be based on an assessment of anatomical injuries and physiological parameters to determine whether a patient should be conveyed to an MTC or TU [NICE, 2016f]. Note that there is some local variation in assessment criteria (for example, rather than a Glasgow Coma Scale (GCS) score < 14, some services use a motor component score of < 4). In addition, there is variability in the transportation time allowed to take patients to an MTC, bypassing local hospitals. When the trauma networks started, this was set to 45 minutes, but has now been extended to 60 minutes.

2 Mechanism of injury

2.1 Learning objectives

By the end of this section you will be able to:
- define mechanism of injury and outline the different types
- explain the kinetics associated with trauma
- describe the mechanisms that can cause injury to the head, spine, chest, abdomen and pelvis.

2.2 Introduction

The mechanism of injury (MOI) can be defined as the sum of all physical forces that result in the patient's injury, and is primarily concerned with the transfer of energy. Since human tissue, organs and systems can only withstand a limited range of physical, environmental and physiological stress, injury occurs when the energy delivery to the body exceeds these limits. The tolerance to external energy delivery is dependent on which type of tissue(s) have been targeted; the age and physical health of the patient; and the type, magnitude and duration of the energy that has been transferred [Greaves, 2008].

There is evidence that a good review of the mechanism of injury can help to predict injury patterns, the need to be treated at a trauma centre and likelihood of death [Haider, 2009; Lerner, 2011].

2.2.1 Types of trauma

Trauma is generally divided into two types [NAEMT, 2020]:
- **Blunt:** Injuries that do not cause penetration of the skin by an external object. Typical mechanisms of blunt trauma include road traffic collisions (RTCs) involving vehicles, pedestrians, motorcyclists, etc.; fall from a height; serious sports injuries; and blast injuries (although this mechanism often also causes penetrating trauma). Blunt trauma is the most common type of trauma in the UK [Kehoe, 2015].
- **Penetrating:** Injuries caused by projectiles penetrating the skin. Examples include stab and gunshot wounds and blast injuries involving shrapnel and secondary projectiles. In the UK the most common form of penetrating trauma is knife injuries.

2.3 Kinetics

Kinetics is the study of the relationship between motion and its forces.

In a road traffic collision, there are three collisions. The first occurs when the vehicle a person is travelling in collides with another object. Newton's first law of motion states that a physical body will remain at a steady speed and direction (i.e. velocity) or at rest until an external force acts upon it. In the case of a person driving their car, this force may be due to a collision with another vehicle or other object, such as a tree. During a head-on collision with a tree, for example, the vehicle stops abruptly, but the occupant inside will still be moving at the same velocity as they were prior to the collision until they come into contact with the inside of the vehicle (the second collision). The third collision occurs when the person's internal organs and tissues make contact with the body's hard surfaces, such as the skull or chest wall [NAEMT, 2020].

Newton's second law states that the force an object exerts is equal to its mass multiplied by its acceleration, or in the case of a collision, mass multiplied by the deceleration. Thus, rapid decelerations, such as a car hitting an immovable object or striking another vehicle travelling in the opposite direction at speed, for example, lead to large forces being exerted.

Newton's third law states that for every force, there is an equal and opposite force, meaning that the force applied to the tree in our head-on collision example is exerted on the vehicle too, leading to damage to the vehicle and, potentially, the occupants.

2.4 Energy

Energy is a measure of an object's ability to do work, or transfer energy to another object. The law of conservation states that energy cannot be destroyed, only transformed.

Energy comes in at least five forms [Greaves, 2008]:
- **Kinetic:** Related to motion, and the most common type of injury-causing energy.
- **Thermal:** Kinetic energy of molecular motion, measured as temperature; the cause of burns.
- **Electrical:** The flow of electrical charge. This type of energy mainly causes damage through conversion to thermal energy.
- **Chemical:** Energy created or consumed during the alteration of electrical charge in chemical reactions. Explosions are often due to chemical reactions.
- **Nuclear:** Energy released as a result of nuclear fission (the splitting of an atom into smaller parts, with associated energy release).

In trauma, it is usually kinetic energy that is of interest and this can be represented by the formula [Greaves, 2019]:
- kinetic energy $= \frac{1}{2}mv^2$

where m is the mass of the object and v its velocity. From this, it is clear that it is the velocity of the object that makes the greatest difference to the amount of kinetic energy available to be transformed. Human tolerance to kinetic energy is influenced by the magnitude of the energy (the force applied) and the duration of the exposure, specifically the change in velocity. This is typically deceleration, for example a person's feet hitting the floor after a fall from a height, or when a car strikes a large tree at speed. However, excessive acceleration can also cause injury, for example when a pilot is ejected from a jet aircraft [Greaves, 2008].

2.4.1 Energy transfer

The energy exchanged during trauma is the same, whether it is blunt or penetrating. Cavitation, the formation of a cavity or hollow, occurs during trauma as tissues in the body move away from the point of impact and their usual position. Thanks to the elastic properties of tissues, the body shape of the torso usually returns to its usual position, i.e. the cavitation is temporary. However, this can hide serious internal injury to organs and tissues that have had the kinetic energy of the impact transferred to them. Other denser tissues, such as bone, may remain deformed, giving clues to the presence of injury [Greaves, 2008].

In penetrating trauma, temporary cavitation occurs, but there is also a permanent cavity that remains once the temporary cavity has collapsed due to the elasticity of the tissues. In low-energy penetrating trauma, such as a stab wound, temporary cavitation may be minimal, but with higher energies, such as those in a gunshot, the temporary cavity can become significant in terms of injury to surrounding tissues [Kuhajda, 2014] and by generating a sub-atmospheric pressure within, causing external debris and dirt to be 'sucked in' to the wound [NAEMT, 2020].

The mechanical damage that remains after trauma does not necessarily correlate to the severity of injury. For example, a screwdriver plunged through the chest that damages the heart may leave only a small external injury, but is likely to be more serious than a gunshot wound to the patient's knee (Figure 17.2).

Penetrating projectiles do not always follow a straight path and can ricochet off internal organs and bone as the projectile decelerates. Although entrance and exit wounds are sometimes visible, determining which is which is not clinically

Mechanism of injury

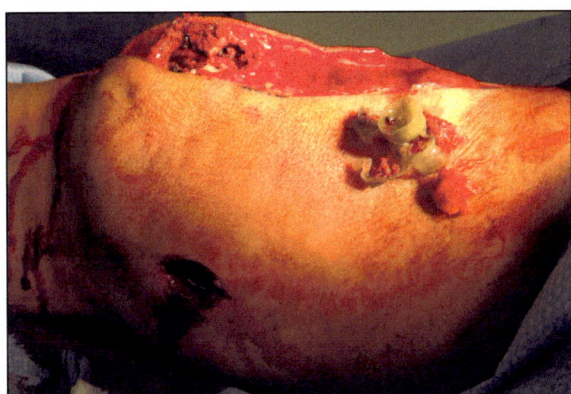

Figure 17.2 A close-range gunshot wound to the right knee, with a shotgun. Note the smaller entrance wound towards the bottom of the picture and the much larger exit wound.
Source: DiverDave (Own work) [CC-BY-SA-3.0 or GFDL], via Wikimedia Commons.

important. Note that the absence of an exit wound means that all of the projectile's kinetic energy has been transferred to the body [Stefanopoulos, 2014].

2.4.2 Elderly patients and pre-existing disease

The Trauma Audit Research Network (TARN) collects data on patients experiencing major trauma in the UK. A recent review of this data showed that over the last few decades the demographic of people experiencing major trauma and the causes of it are rapidly changing. In 1990, the mean age of patients was 36.1 years and the most common cause of major trauma was an RTC. By 2013, this had changed with the mean age rising to 53.8 years and the most common cause of major trauma being a fall from fewer than two metres [Kehoe, 2015].

Older adults are suffering more major trauma, so the age of the patient should be a consideration when assessing the severity of traumatic injuries. For example, it is unlikely that a fall from standing height will be fatal to a young healthy person, whereas for an elderly patient who may have a pre-existing disease, such as osteoporosis, such a fall has a far greater chance of causing fatal injury [TARN, 2017]. This recognition of major trauma in older people is now the focus of a lot of work

and you may hear the phrase 'silver trauma' when referring to trauma in the elderly [RCEM, 2018].

2.5 Mechanisms that cause injury

There are many mechanisms that can result in a host of both isolated and multiple injuries to the human body. Some of the more common mechanisms and the injuries they cause to the head, spine, thorax, abdomen and pelvis are covered in this section.

2.5.1 Head

If the head is travelling ahead of the body, such as during a headfirst fall, it is the first structure to receive the force of the impact and energy transference. The continued movement of the rest of the body results in compression, which can damage the scalp and skull. If the skull fractures, bony fractures can end up damaging the brain. The same damage can also be caused by the application of an external force, such as occurs as a result of a blow to the head during an assault [NAEMT, 2020].

The brain is soft and compressible and can move following the application of external forces. This can lead to shearing of brain tissue as well as rupture of the blood vessels surrounding the brain, leading to intracranial haemorrhage.

If a projectile penetrates the skull, the damage can be very severe as the kinetic energy is distributed within the confines of the skull. Small calibre bullets, for example, may not have enough energy to exit the skull, but instead contour around it, leading to extensive damage [NAEMT, 2020].

2.5.2 Spine

The main mechanisms that cause spinal injury can be divided into abnormal flexion, extension, rotation and compression. Extension or flexion with rotation are the main causes of injury to the cervical spine [Lencean, 2003; Greaves, 2019; NAEMT, 2020].

Flexion
Hyperflexion injuries are typically caused by RTCs where lap-belts (rather than three-point belts)

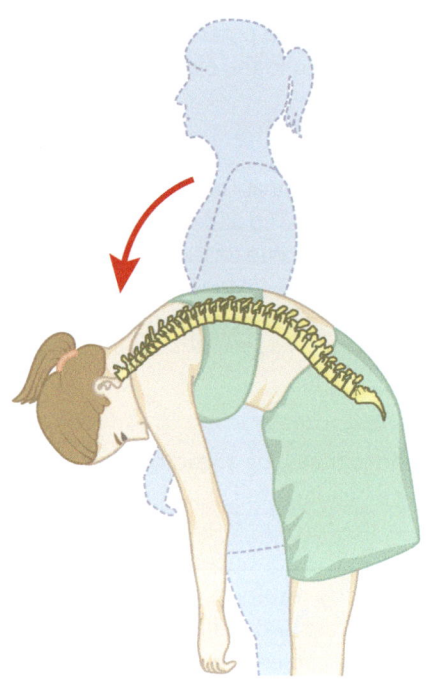

Figure 17.3 Flexion.

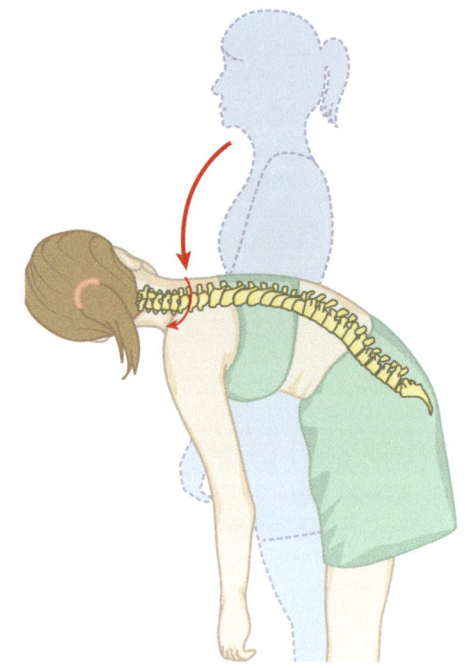

Figure 17.4 Flexion with rotation.

are used, direct blows to the occiput and rapid deceleration in flexed positions such as diving and contact sports like rugby. Hyperflexion on its own is uncommon in the cervical spine, since the chin abutting the chest limits flexion (Figure 17.3).

Flexion with rotation

The design of the first two cervical vertebrae allows for significant rotation. Injuries due to this mechanism are considered unstable as there is little in the way of bony or soft-tissue support. Not surprisingly, this mechanism is much more likely to produce significant cervical injury and is often caused by lateral-impact RTCs or direct trauma. Note that rotation rarely occurs in isolation (Figure 17.4).

Extension

These injuries are generally only found in cervical and lumbar regions and can be caused by hanging, striking the chin on a steering wheel during a collision or a rear impact collision where the headrest is improperly positioned (Figure 17.5).

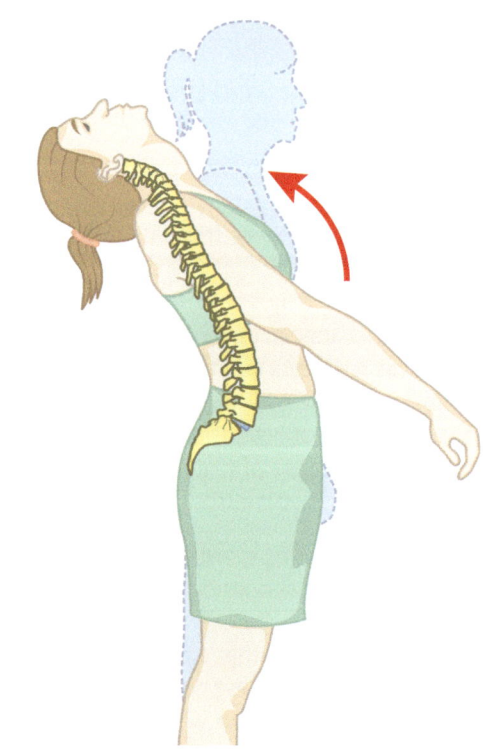

Figure 17.5 Extension.

Mechanism of injury

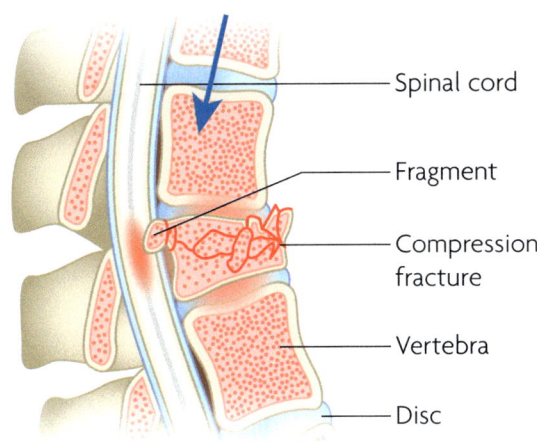

Figure 17.6 Compression.

Compression
Wedge fractures are the most common type of compression fracture of the lumbar and thoracic spine, but if a weight falls on the head or if the patient lands on their head after a fall, then the cervical vertebrae can be fractured and/or ligaments ruptured. Most fractures caused by compression are stable, but spinal cord injury can occur if the vertebral body is shattered and fragments of bone become embedded in the cord (Figure 17.6).

Combination
A combination of two or more of the above mechanisms can occur depending on the nature, direction and duration of force applied to the patient. Carefully considering the mechanism will help you to predict which type of force(s) may have been applied. For example, if a person dives from a pool side and hits their head on the bottom of the pool then the most likely form of injury is compression with potentially some flexion or extension.

2.5.3 Thorax

Severe blunt thoracic trauma most commonly occurs as a result of RTCs (about 70–80%) where high speeds are involved, leading to rapid deceleration. This causes shearing forces that can rupture large blood vessels, tear the bronchial airways and damage the lungs, causing a pneumothorax, for example. Even with lower velocity mechanisms, such as direct blows to the chest, fractures of the rib cage and sternum, as well as bruising to the underlying structures including the heart and lungs, can occur [NAEMT, 2020]. It is common for elderly patients to receive significant chest wall injuries from a fall from standing height.

In penetrating trauma, the most serious consequences arise as a result of rupture of the major blood vessels, which can lead to serious haemorrhage. In the UK, knife crime is the most common form of penetrating chest trauma [Greaves, 2019]. Projectiles penetrating the chest wall can also cause an open pneumothorax.

2.5.4 Abdomen

Abdominal injury is most commonly caused by blunt trauma, usually due to RTCs, and often as part of a multi-system pattern of injuries. If the abdomen comes into contact with the steering wheel during rapid deceleration, crush injuries can occur. Compression of the abdominal organs increases the intra-abdominal pressure, which in turn can rupture the hollow organs and/or the diaphragm. Penetrating trauma is less common, and in the UK is more likely to be as a result of a stab wound than gunshot. Fortunately, less than half of all stab wounds actually penetrate the peritoneum (the lining of the abdominal cavity) [Greaves, 2008].

2.5.5 Pelvis

As with any trauma patient, you should consider the MOI to provide an indication as to possible underlying injuries. Pelvic ring fractures usually require high forces, so it is no surprise that the most common cause is RTCs. Front-seat passengers in head-on collisions, and those on the side of impact in T-bone-type collisions in cars, are most common. These are closely followed by motorcyclists, pedestrians and falls from heights [Gabbe, 2011; Papadopoulos, 2006]. However, a significant subgroup are the elderly, who will typically fall from standing and may have osteoporosis [Garlapati, 2012].

Figure 17.7 shows the three main types of pelvic ring fracture (there is an additional type, which is just a combination of the other three) and the direction of forces required to cause them [Burgess, 1990].

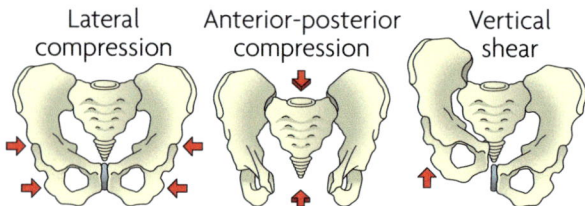

Figure 17.7 Types of pelvic fracture. The red arrows indicate the direction of force.

Lateral compression (LC) fractures
These are the most common type of pelvic ring fracture and are caused by internal rotation of the pelvic ring due to a direct force applied to the iliac crests, or indirectly via the femoral head [Garlapati, 2012]. These forces typically result in pubic rami fractures on one or both sides anteriorly, which places severe strain on the sacroiliac joints. If these become displaced, the pelvis will be unstable. The typical mechanism of injury is a side-impact RTC or fall from a height.

Anterior–posterior compression (APC) fractures
These are most commonly caused by a frontal collision between a pedestrian and a vehicle, front-seat passengers in a frontal RTC and crush injury [NAEMT, 2020]. With these mechanisms, either the pubic rami are fractured or the symphysis pubis is disrupted, resulting in the pelvic bones springing apart and externally rotating. This is often called an 'open book' injury. Posteriorly, the sacroiliac ligaments can be torn and/or the posterior aspect of the pelvic bones fractured [McCormack, 2010].

Vertical shear (VS) fractures
These are the least common type of injury but are the most likely to kill your patient [NAEMT, 2020]. These fractures occur when one of the pelvic bones is displaced vertically, leading to a fracture of the pubic rami and disruption of the sacroiliac joint on the same side. These are typically caused by falls from heights, with the patient landing on one leg first. Because of this, blood vessels are often torn, leading to severe retroperitoneal haemorrhage (which can easily accommodate the body's entire blood volume [Leenen, 2010]) and severe damage to soft tissues.

Combined mechanical (CM) fractures
These are a combination of the other types of fractures, typically caused by a multitude of forces applied in different directions, for example during a rollover RTC.

2.5.6 Blast injury

Blasts (or explosions) cause complex multi-system injury due to the significant transfer of kinetic, heat and other energies. Injuries are generally classified into the five types shown in Table 17.1 [NAEMT, 2020; Jorolemon, 2018; Scott, 2017].

2.5.7 Suspension trauma

The use of the word 'trauma' in suspension trauma is a bit of a misnomer, as there is often no physical injury. Instead, it is really a form of syncope that occurs when the body is held motionless in a vertical position for a period of time (5–30 minutes) [Lee, 2007c]. This position causes venous pooling in the legs, which can result in a 20% reduction in circulating volume. The reduction in venous return leads to a reduced venous return to the heart, which reduces cardiac output and arterial blood pressure and leads to syncope (fainting). Ordinarily, a patient would collapse and assume a horizontal position, which would reverse this process. However, in suspension trauma, the victim is kept upright, typically due to being suspended in a harness from a rope, for example, and death can occur, although this appears to be uncommon [Thomassen, 2009].

Table 17.1 Blast injury categories.

Category	Cause	Possible injuries
Primary	Injuries caused by patient contact with blast shock wave (Figure 17.8)	Gas-containing organs may be damaged, including lungs and gastrointestinal tract
Secondary	Injuries due to flying fragments and debris striking the patient	Entire body can be affected, leading to lacerations and fractures
Tertiary	Blast wave propels patient against objects. Crush injuries secondary to structural damage and building collapse	Penetrating injuries
Quaternary	Other explosion-related injuries and illnesses	Blunt and crush injuries
Quinary	Injuries resulting from additives, for example bacteria and radiation ('dirty bombs')	Burns

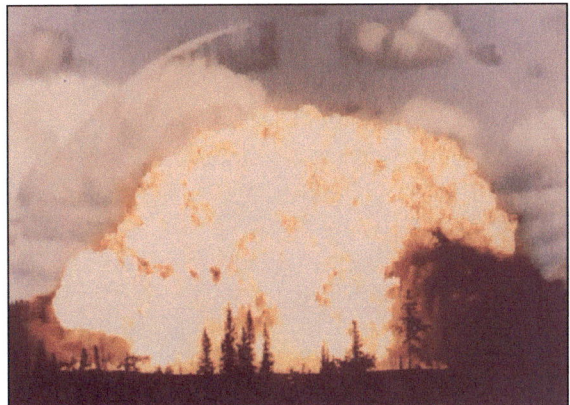

Figure 17.8 An explosion with visible blast wave.

3 Integumentary system anatomy and physiology

3.1 Learning objective

By the end of this section you will be able to:
- describe the anatomy and physiology of the integumentary system.

3.2 Introduction

The integumentary system (or skin) is the largest organ of the human body, in terms of both surface area and weight. In adults, skin has a surface area of 2 m^2 and weighs 5 kg [Tortora, 2017]. It is composed

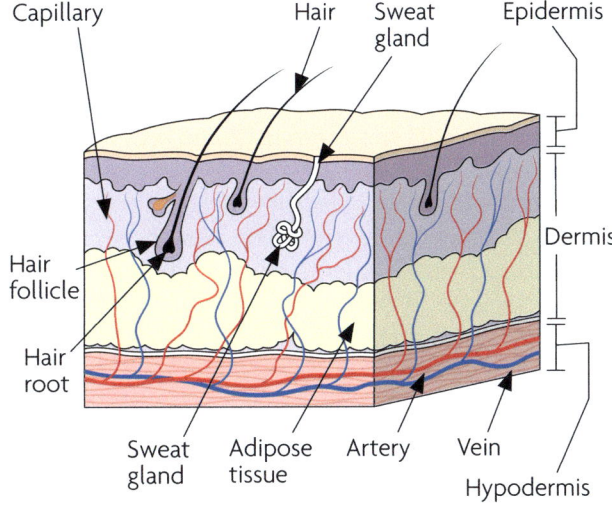

Figure 17.9 Cross-section of the skin.

of two main layers: the epidermis and dermis. Under the skin is a supportive subcutaneous layer, known as the hypodermis or superficial fascia (Figure 17.9) [Dykes, 2002].

3.3 Epidermis

This is the outermost layer and consists of five sublayers. Most of the cells (90%) are keratinocytes, which produce a tough, fibrous protein (keratin). This helps to protect the skin and tissues from heat and microbes. Keratinocytes also produce lamellar granules which decrease water entry and loss, and prevent entry of foreign material. Around 8% of the cells are melanocytes, which produce melanin. This is taken up by keratinocytes, protecting the cell's nucleus from the harmful effects of ultraviolet (UV) light. Keratin is either a yellow-red or brown-black pigment and contributes to skin colour. The remaining cells consist of Langerhans cells, which help in the body's immune response, and Merkel cells, which are involved in touch perception [Tortora, 2017].

It takes around 2–3 weeks for a cell starting at the lowest layer of the epidermis to become a keratinocyte and migrate up to the top layer (stratum corneum) and slough off [AAOS, 2011].

3.4 Dermis

This deeper layer of skin mostly consists of connective tissue, elastin and an extracellular matrix, which provides strength and pliability. However, it also contains blood and lymphatic vessels, nerve fibres, hair follicles and sebaceous and sweat glands. The dermis is divided into two regions: the papillary and the reticular. The papillary region comprises connective tissue that anchors the epidermis and a dense network of capillaries and small blood vessels, in nipple-like projections called dermal papillae. These play an important part in temperature regulation. In addition, the dermal papillae also contain free nerve endings, which act as pain and fine touch receptors (Meissner corpuscles) [Tortora, 2017].

The reticular region makes up 80% of the dermis and consists of dense, irregular connective tissue. Interlocking collagen fibres run in various planes, forming 'lines of cleavage'. Surgeons try to make incisions parallel to these lines, since the skin does not gape as much, resulting in less scarring [Thompson, 2008].

3.5 Hypodermis

Also known as the superficial fascia, this layer contains subcutaneous fat, connective tissue, sweat glands, muscle and bone. It helps to insulate the body, absorbs shocks to the skeletal system and enables the skin to move easily over underlying structures [AAOS, 2011].

3.6 Physiology

The skin provides a range of functions, which any damage can impair [Tortora, 2017; Thompson, 2008]:
- Protection against infection by forming a physical barrier to microbes and foreign material.
- Sensory perception of pain, pressure, heat and cold.
- Thermoregulation using nerves, blood vessels and sweat glands to control body temperature.
- Excretion of trace amounts of water and body waste, while helping to prevent dehydration.
- Maintenance of mineralisation of bones and teeth and synthesis of vitamin D.
- Absorption of lipid-soluble substances such as fat-soluble vitamins and drugs through the skin.

4 Wounds and bleeding

4.1 Learning objectives

By the end of this section you will be able to:
- describe the types of bleeding
- explain how to appropriately assess and manage bleeding
- explain how to detect concealed bleeding
- describe various types of wounds and how to manage them
- discuss the implications of foreign objects in wounds
- explain complications associated with bleeding and wounds.

4.2 Introduction

Wounds and bleeding are a common reason for an ambulance to be requested. Even in the emergency ambulance service, these calls will vary in their severity, from injuries that require basic first aid only, through to life-threatening wounds and bleeding that require prompt and more advanced intervention in order to prevent death.

4.3 Bleeding

Bleeding is the loss of blood from a damaged blood vessel. You will often hear the term 'haemorrhage' used, which is usually reserved for severe bleeding

Wounds and bleeding

in medical circles. Bleeding is often classified by the type of vessel involved (i.e. artery, vein or capillary) or whether it is external or internal [SJA, SAA, BRC, 2016].

4.3.1 Assessment

Sources of bleeding

Bleeding can be defined by whether it is visible on the outside of the body and/or which type of vessel is responsible [Gregory, 2010a; SJA, SAA, BRC, 2016]:

- **Internal:** This bleeding is concealed within the body and can be hard to detect. The thorax, abdomen, pelvis and long bones provide good hiding places for significant volumes of blood. The mechanism of injury and the presence of shock without signs of external haemorrhage can help with diagnosis. These patients need to be in hospital to stop the bleeding.
- **External:** This bleeding is visible and should be detected during your primary and/or secondary survey. This bleeding can usually be controlled.
- **Arterial:** Blood inside the arteries is under relatively high pressure and so bleeding can lead to significant blood loss. It is characterised by bright red (oxygenated) blood, spurting in time with the heartbeat.
- **Venous:** Since veins carry blood back to the heart, they typically carry deoxygenated blood and so bleeding is a darker red. Since the pressure is lower, blood does not spurt but flows freely. However, blood loss can still be severe, particularly from veins in the neck and legs.
- **Capillary:** These are the smallest blood vessels in the body and carry a mixture of oxygenated and deoxygenated blood, so the colour of bleeding will vary. Blood loss tends to be small as blood oozes from wounds.

Estimating blood loss

Estimating blood loss accurately is very difficult and ambulance staff (and doctors/nurses/ midwives) generally do not do this well [Frank, 2010; Bose, 2006; Ashburn, 2012]. Table 17.2 provides examples of what various volumes of blood loss look like (this was originally designed for estimating obstetric blood loss) [JRCALC 2019; Bose, 2006]. Fractures can cause significant blood loss, depending on the bone(s) affected and whether the fracture is open or closed (Table 17.3) [NAEMT, 2020]. Remember to check for signs and symptoms of shock (this was covered in the common cardiovascular conditions section in Chapter 13, 'Circulation').

Table 17.2 Visual guide to estimating blood loss.

Blood loss (ml)	
60	
500	

Table 17.3 Approximate internal blood loss due to fractures.

Fracture	Blood loss (ml)
Rib	125
Radius or ulna	250–500
Humerus	500–750
Tibia	500–1,000
Femur	1,000–2,000
Pelvis	1,000–entire circulating volume; in adults that can be 5,000–6,000 ml

4.3.2 Management

In light of learning from military experience in previous conflicts [Hodgetts, 2006], the old assessment mnemonic of ABC has been changed to <C>ABC [JRCALC, 2019]. This is to highlight the important of recognising and managing catastrophic bleeding immediately in the primary survey, even before airway management if the two cannot be managed simultaneously [Nutbeam, 2013]. Once the scene assessment has been completed, you need to check for, and manage, any actual or potential catastrophic haemorrhage. Only once this has been completed can you continue with the remainder of the primary survey.

During the assessment of circulation (the second C), any interventions to manage catastrophic haemorrhage must be reassessed to ensure that bleeding is being controlled appropriately. Don't forget the bleeding you cannot see. 'Blood on the floor plus four more' is a good way to remember the areas where significant blood loss can accumulate, i.e. the thorax, abdomen, pelvis and long bones [Greaves, 2010].

Most external haemorrhages can be controlled with simple first-aid measures such as direct pressure and elevation of the bleeding extremity. In some cases, additional interventions are required, but these should be introduced in an incremental fashion, as shown in the haemostasis escalator (Figure 17.10) [Lee, 2007b; Moorhouse, 2007].

Catastrophic haemorrhage management
If you suspect the bleeding is likely to cause death in minutes (i.e. is a catastrophic haemorrhage), you are likely to ascend the haemostasis escalator rather faster than for non-catastrophic haemorrhage. If the haemorrhage involves a limb, then an arterial tourniquet should be immediately applied. Should the first tourniquet not adequately control the bleeding, then a second tourniquet should be applied above the first. If bleeding continues, pack the wound with a haemostatic gauze and apply a fresh dressing. Apply firm direct pressure [JRCALC, 2019].

In other body areas, such as the head, neck and torso, it will not be possible to use a tourniquet. In this instance, you should apply a wound dressing to the site of bleeding and apply firm pressure directly over the wound. Elevation is unlikely to be appropriate with these types of bleeds. If direct pressure fails to stem the bleeding, then wound packing should be undertaken and may be supplemented with haemostatic agents. Where haemostatic agents are used, they should be placed as close to the bleeding point as possible and then direct pressure should be applied for at least three minutes. After this, a dressing should be applied over the top that keeps the haemostatic dressing in place and applies pressure to the bleeding site.

Assess limb positioning and consider whether the use of splinting may help to reduce bleeding. Straightening angulated fractures and applying a pelvic binder may help to reduce blood loss [NICE, 2016f].

Non-catastrophic haemorrhage
For other, non-catastrophic external haemorrhage, you can move up the haemostasis escalator. Start by applying direct pressure, with or without a dressing and, if the injury is below the knee or elbow, consider elevating the affected limb above the level of the heart, if practicable. If this does not control the bleeding, consider applying further dressing while continuing to apply firm direct pressure [JRCALC, 2019].

If bleeding continues, you should treat the haemorrhage as a potential catastrophic bleeding event. For limbs, this means applying a tourniquet; in the case of head, neck or torso wounds, packing with haemostatic dressing. As with catastrophic haemorrhage, consider whether the use of splinting of a limb or applying a pelvic binder would help reduce blood loss.

Tourniquet

Limb positioning, traction and splints

Wound packing ± haemostatic agents

Direct pressure ± elevation of limb

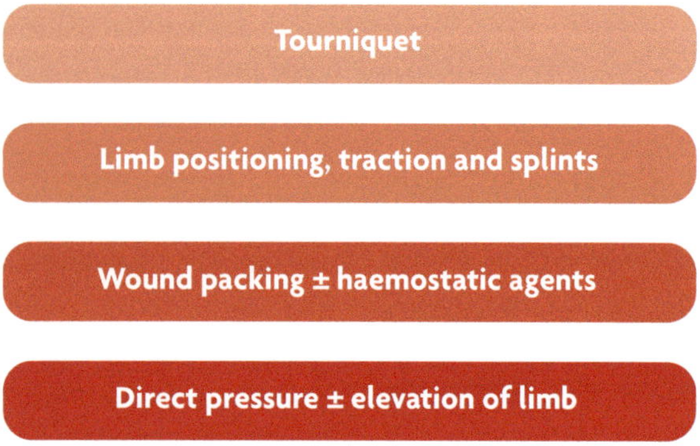

Figure 17.10 The haemostasis escalator.

Wounds and bleeding

4.3.3 Tourniquets

The use of tourniquets (Figure 17.11) has caused controversy, but they do have a place in civilian ambulance services for use in specific circumstances [Lee, 2007b]:

- Extreme life-threatening limb haemorrhage, or limb amputation/mangled limb with multiple bleeding points, to allow immediate management of airway and breathing problems. Following treatment of any airway or breathing problems, the need for a tourniquet can be reassessed in the circulatory assessment and may be converted to a simple method of haemorrhage control.
- Life-threatening limb haemorrhage not controlled by simple methods.
- Point of significant haemorrhage from limb is not peripherally accessible due to entrapment (and therefore it is not possible to initiate simple methods of haemorrhage control such as direct pressure).
- Major incident or multiple casualties with extremity haemorrhage and lack of resources to maintain simple methods of haemorrhage control.

However, incorrectly applied tourniquets can actually increase blood loss if venous, but not arterial, vessels are occluded [FPHC, 2017]. Even correctly applied tourniquets can cause local tissue injury from direct contact with the tourniquet and, when left in place for more than two hours, can lead to muscle and skin damage [Walters, 2005]. In addition, tourniquets cause severe pain and patients must receive adequate analgesia.

4.3.4 Procedure

Procedure – Application of CAT tourniquet

The following steps are a suggested method for applying a CAT tourniquet [NAR, 2019; FPHC, 2017]:

1. Identify the need for a tourniquet during the primary survey, assessing for catastrophic haemorrhage. Once identified, apply as quickly as possible. Warn the patient it may hurt.

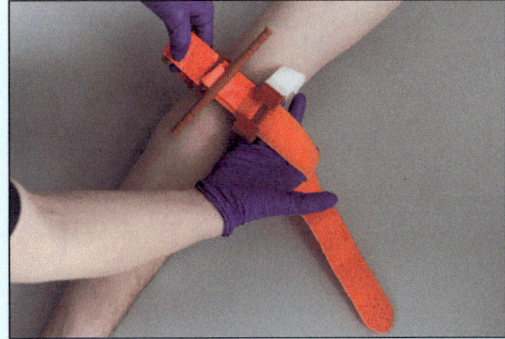

2. Apply the tourniquet 2–3 inches above the bleeding site directly to the skin.

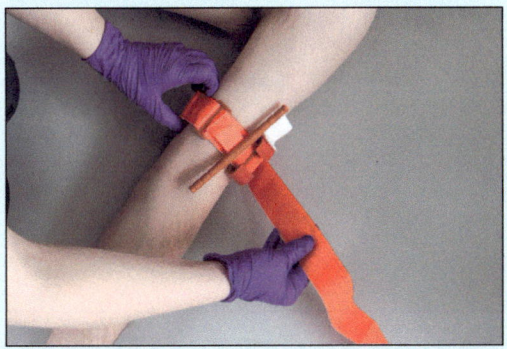

3. Take the slack out of the tourniquet by pulling the strap tight and secure the strap by sticking down the hook and loop material (velcro).

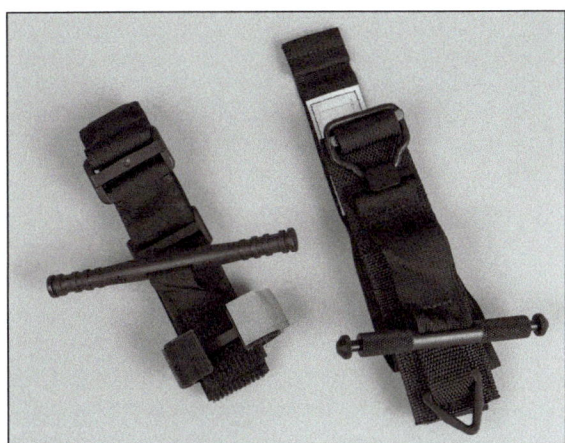

Figure 17.11 Two tourniquets: a CAT tourniquet on the left and a SOFTT-W on the right.

Chapter 17 – Trauma

Procedure – Application of CAT tourniquet – *cont*

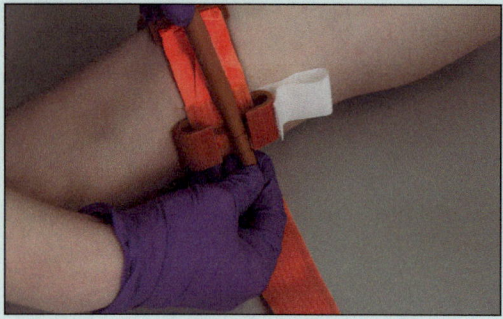

4. Turn the tourniquet windlass until the catastrophic bleeding stops. Secure windlass by continuing to turn until it can sit into the holder.

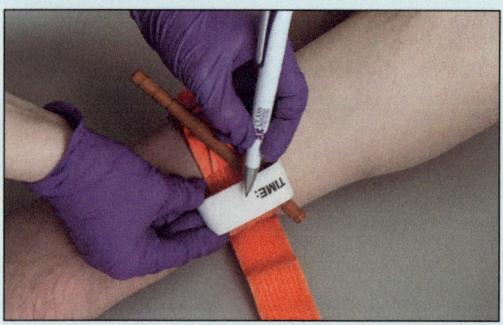

5. Record the time of tourniquet application.
6. Reassess during the assessment of circulation. If bleeding continues, apply a second tourniquet proximal to the first.
7. Frequently reassess and tighten tourniquet as required. Provide analgesia.

4.3.5 Procedure

Procedure – Application of SOFTT-W tourniquet

The following steps are a suggested method for applying a SOFTT-W tourniquet [FPHC, 2017]:

1. Identify the need for a tourniquet during the primary survey, assessing for catastrophic haemorrhage. Once identified, apply as quickly as possible. Warn the patient it may hurt.

Procedure – Application of SOFTT-W tourniquet – *cont*

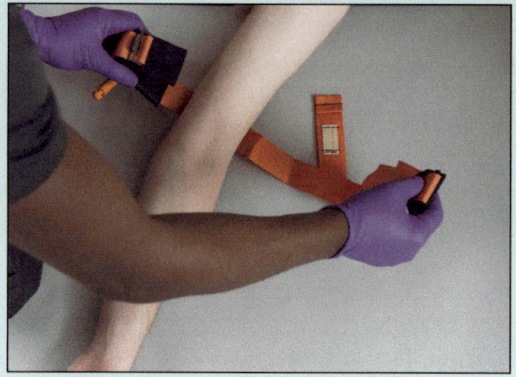

2. Apply the tourniquet 2–3 inches above the bleeding site directly to the skin.

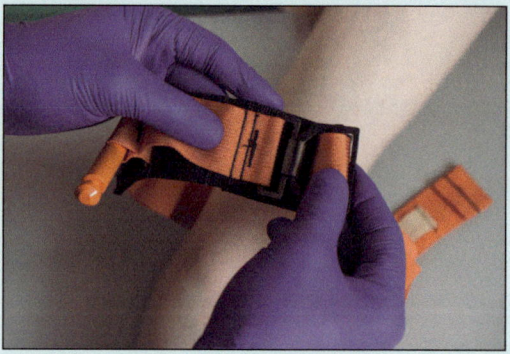

3. Clip the buckle on the strap to the receiver on the body of the tourniquet.

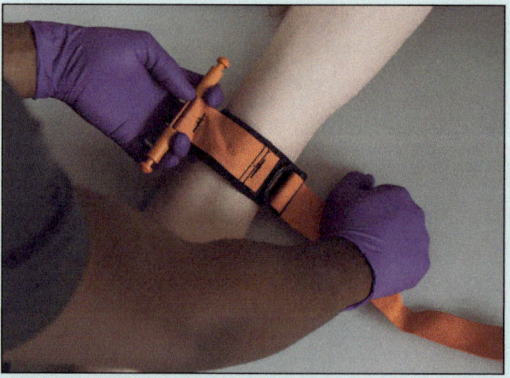

4. Pull the strap until the slack has been removed and the tourniquet is tight to the skin.

Wounds and bleeding

Procedure – Application of SOFTT-W tourniquet – *cont*

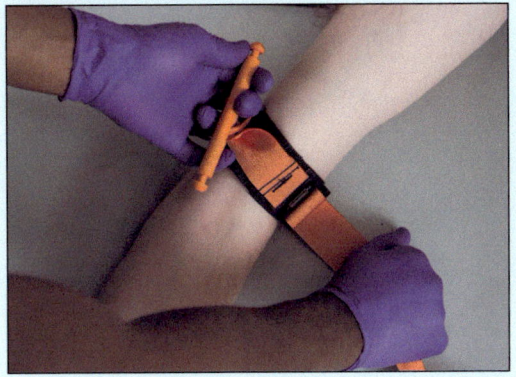

5. Turn the windlass until catastrophic bleeding stops.

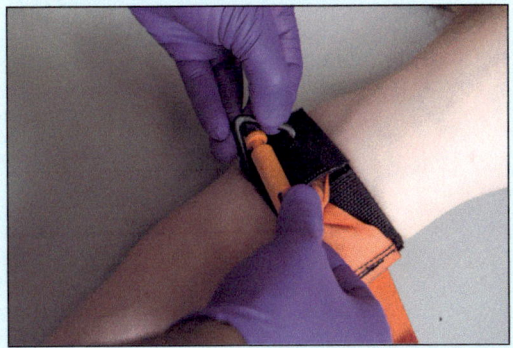

6. Continue to tighten until the windlass can be hooked into the holder.

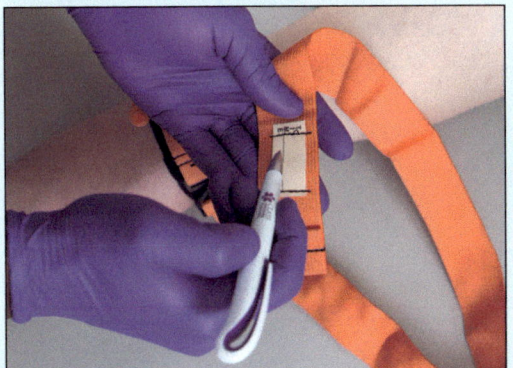

7. Record the time of application; this might be on the space provided on the tourniquet, but more likely will either be on the patient or the clinical record.

Procedure – Application of SOFTT-W tourniquet – *cont*

8. Reassess during the assessment of circulation. If bleeding continues, apply a second tourniquet proximal to the first.

9. Frequently reassess and tighten tourniquet as required. Provide analgesia.

4.3.6 Haemostatic agents

Where direct pressure and wound packing are ineffective, and in areas such as the groin, neck and axilla, where tourniquet application is not possible, haemostatic agents can be used to control haemorrhage [JRCALC, 2019; Boulton, 2018]. Modern haemostatic agents usually come as dressings, into which the active ingredients have been impregnated. They work by either concentrating clotting factors, acting as a precursor to coagulation, or are mucoadhesive [Boulton, 2018] (Figure 17.12).

4.4 *Wounds*

A wound is an injury to living tissue, breaking its continuity. There are seven basic categories [Purcell, 2016; Gregory, 2010b]:

- **Contusion (bruises):** Caused by bleeding from damaged blood vessels under the skin. They cause a bluish/purple discolouration beneath the skin and are typically caused by blunt trauma.
- **Abrasion (grazes):** Injuries caused by friction shearing the skin away. These usually involve the superficial layers of the skin but can go much

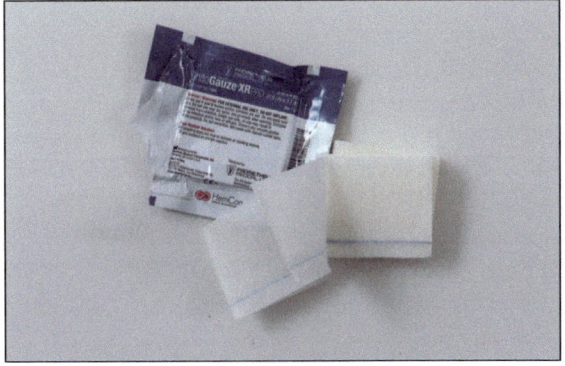

Figure 17.12   Haemostatic dressings.

deeper. They can be very painful and are often dirty, with embedded grit and mud.
- **Laceration (tear):** Tearing or splitting of the skin due to blunt trauma. These cause a ragged wound, which can extend through the skin surface to the underlying structures.
- **Incision (cut):** A break in the continuity of the skin by a sharp implement, such as broken glass or a knife. These are usually clean wounds (unless the implement is dirty) with neat edges.
- **Puncture (stab):** A penetrating wound caused by an object that is pointed and narrow, such as a nail or knife. Although these wounds are typically small, they can be deep, causing serious damage to vessels and other body structures below the skin.
- **Burn:** An injury caused by energy transfer to the body's tissues, causing necrosis and an associated inflammatory reaction (covered in section 7, 'Burns' later in this chapter).
- **Gunshot:** A complicated wound caused by a projectile moving at speed. The wound consists of an entry point, with varying amounts of tissue destruction and cavitation underneath the skin, and, if there is sufficient energy left, an exit wound.

There are a range of external and internal factors that can lead to wound formation [Thompson, 2008]:
- **External:** Mechanical (friction), chemical, electrical, temperature extremes, radiation and microorganisms.
- **Internal:** Circulatory system failure, endocrine (e.g. diabetes), neuropathy, haematological, malignancy (cancer).

4.4.1 Management

Wound management will be determined by the size and nature of the wound and the presence of complicating factors. The main initial problems are bleeding, pain and the risk of infection [Purcell, 2016]. Always enquire about tetanus immunisation in any patient who has a wound with a higher risk of infection, such as a dirty wound, or a wound caused by a bite (human or animal) or involving a puncture by a dirty object [SJA, SAA, BRC, 2016]. In addition, consider whether there has been damage to other structures such as blood vessels, nerves, tendons and ligaments, which can have life-changing consequences if not managed appropriately. For example, consider a pianist who damages their hand causing damage to ligaments. Although the external wound may be minor, without prompt management of the ligamentous injury, their fingers may not function properly in the future.

If the wound is small and bleeding easily controlled, clean the wound:
- Use a wet gauze to clean the edges of open wounds, wiping away from the wound to avoid contaminating it further. Continue until all visible dirt and blood has been removed.
- Irrigate wounds with tap water as rubbing or scrubbing can cause tissue damage, and swabs or cotton wool can leave fibres in the wound.

Once cleaning is complete, cover with a sterile, non-adherent dressing.

If there is a foreign object in the wound, it may be possible to remove it if it's small (e.g. grit) by irrigating the wound with water or using tweezers. However, larger objects or those that appear firmly embedded should not be removed, but left in place and a sterile, non-adherent dressing applied. These objects do need to be removed as they may lead to infection, so follow local guidance and your clinician as to the next step in the patient's management [Purcell, 2016].

Larger wounds are going to require closure by someone trained in wound care. This may be in hospital, but it might also be possible for a specialist paramedic or minor injuries unit to manage the closure, helping to avoid the need to take the patient to the emergency department. Follow your local guidelines when selecting the most appropriate pathway.

5 Assessment and management of the trauma patient

5.1 Learning objectives

By the end of this section you will be able to:
- explain the assessment and management of patients with a range of traumatic injuries
- describe the complications associated with a range of traumatic injuries.

5.2 Introduction

The approach to the trauma patient is similar to that of all patients, with an initial scene assessment, followed by a primary and secondary survey. However, there are some aspects of this process that are specific to trauma. In addition, there are a range of complications that can arise as a result of traumatic injury to specific regions and a number of these are going to be covered in this section, specifically injuries to the head, spine, thorax, abdomen and pelvis.

5.3 Scene assessment

The SCENE mnemonic can be used to ensure that you cover all aspects of an initial trauma scene assessment [JRCALC, 2019]:

- **S:** Safety. A dynamic risk assessment should highlight current as well as potential dangers. If you are not equipped in terms of kit and expertise to deal with the scene, withdraw and request specialist help, for example from the hazardous area response team (HART). Remember to continually reassess safety as the situation can change quickly. Make sure you are wearing appropriate personal protective equipment (PPE).
- **C:** Cause, including mechanism of injury (MOI). Finding out what happened is important in order to appreciate likely injuries and energy transfer. However, ensure that the scene matches the story you are being told, as you may have come across a crime scene or case of abuse.
- **E:** Environment. Consider whether there are any environmental factors that need to be taken into account. These may complicate your extrication by affecting access to and from the scene and/or increase the risk of harm to the patient, due to increased risk of hypothermia, for example.
- **N:** Number of patients. Determine the number of patients early on in your assessment to help you determine whether you can manage the scene on your own. It may also help to identify patients who have either wandered off from the scene or who have been ejected from a vehicle, for example, and are currently hidden from view.
- **E:** Extra resources needed. Depending on the number of patients, the severity of their injuries and the nature of the incident, you may need additional help from other emergency services, such as the police, to keep a scene safe, or additional ambulances, including the air ambulance, for patient transport. You should also consider advanced care providers including critical care teams and BASICS who might be available and request them early.

5.4 Primary survey

The aim of the primary survey is to identify threats to life promptly and intervene as soon as they are found. The steps of the primary survey should be undertaken sequentially, unless there are enough personnel to allow for simultaneous assessment and treatment [Halliwell, 2011].

5.4.1 Procedure

Procedure – Primary survey

Take the following steps to undertake a primary survey in the trauma patient [JRCALC, 2019; NAEMT, 2020; Nutbeam, 2013; Greaves, 2019]:

1. **General impression:** As you approach the patient, perform a global assessment. Are they sitting up and watching you approach, with well-perfused skin and a normal effort of breathing, or are they lying unresponsive, pale and clammy and gasping for breath with an expanding pool of blood leaking from a wound?

2. **Catastrophic haemorrhage:** This is bleeding that is likely to cause death within minutes, so cannot wait until airway and breathing have been addressed. Typically, bleeding can be controlled with direct pressure and elevation of the bleeding site, but catastrophic bleeding is likely to require the use of haemostatic dressings or tourniquets (see section 4, 'Wounds and bleeding', earlier in this chapter).

3. **Airway with cervical spine consideration:** If a patient has suffered significant blunt trauma or the MOI suggests that the cervical spine may have been damaged, provide

Procedure – Primary survey – *cont*

prompt manual in-line stabilisation (MILS). This should be applied as soon as there are sufficient personnel at scene to do so, but should not commit a member of the team if more important treatments are required. Assess the airway by looking for obvious obstruction, listening for noisy airflow (snoring or gurgling) and feeling for air movement.

4. Manage the airway using appropriate airway manoeuvres, such as:
   - jaw thrust
   - suction
   - naso- and oropharyngeal airways.
5. **Breathing:** Administer high-flow oxygen to patients to obtain a target saturation of 94–98%, even if they have COPD.
6. Examine the neck for:
   - tracheal deviation
   - wounds and swellings
   - emphysema (surgical/subcutaneous)
   - laryngeal crepitus
   - veins.
7. Look for obvious chest injuries, wounds, bruising, flail segments, and equal rise and fall on both sides of the chest. Assess the rate, depth and quality of respiration:
   - Ventilate with a BVM if respirations absent or fewer than 10 breaths/minute.
   - If respirations are greater than 30 breaths/minute, it may also be clinically appropriate to ventilate the patient. Follow the advice of the senior clinician at scene.
   - Monitor closely if respirations are in the range 10–30 breaths/minute.
8. Listen (auscultate) over both axillae for air entry. If bilateral air entry is not heard, the clinician may use percussion to indicate the underlying problem.
9. Feel for equality of chest movement and note any instability or crepitus.

Procedure – Primary survey – *cont*

Note: This assessment should include examination of the back of the chest, although it may not be appropriate to log roll the patient to do this. If the patient is supine, feel as much of the back as you can without excessively moving the patient.

10. Manage breathing problems as you find them. This may include:
    - applying an appropriate dressing to sucking chest wounds
    - a clinician inserting a cannula into the chest to decompress a tension pneumothorax
    - positioning to support a patient with a flail segment (not possible if the patient has a suspected spinal injury).
11. **Circulation:** If a catastrophic haemorrhage was encountered at the start of the primary survey, reassess this now.
12. Assess both central and distal pulses (carotid and radial, typically), noting rate, rhythm and volume. Note the skin colour, temperature and the presence of clamminess. If additional personnel are available, the blood pressure can also be measured.
13. Assess for signs of blood loss, remembering the phrase 'blood on the floor plus four more':
    - Externally: Don't forget to consider bleeding into clothing, splints and dressings.
    - Chest: Completed during assessment of breathing.
    - Abdomen: Look for bruising or external marks and feel for rigidity and to elicit tenderness.
    - Pelvis: Examine the pelvis for obvious deformity or bruising. The pelvis should not be manipulated or 'sprung' to assess for instability. A suggestive MOI is often sufficient to immobilise the pelvis, especially if it is accompanied with haemodynamic instability.

Procedure – Primary survey – *cont*

- Long bones: Assess long bones, particularly the femurs, but do not be distracted by fractures that are more peripheral and not likely to cause sufficient bleeding to endanger life at this stage of the primary survey.

14. Manage bleeding appropriately (see section 4, 'Wounds and bleeding', earlier in this chapter). Splint pelvic fractures prior to moving the patient. Limb fractures can wait until you are en route if the patient is critically injured unless they are major long bone fractures such as a femur.

15. The clinician may wish to gain intravenous access now if fluids and/or tranexamic acid are required.

16. To minimise clot disruption, patient movement should be kept to a minimum. Use an orthopaedic (scoop) stretcher where possible.

17. **Disability:** Calculate the Glasgow Coma Scale (GCS) score for the pre-hospital major trauma triage tool. Assess pupil size, equality and reaction to light. Don't forget to check the blood glucose.

18. **Exposure/environment:** To identify all injuries, it is necessary to remove the patient's clothing. In cases of severe injury or suspected spinal injury, clothes should be cut off the patient to minimise movement. Take care to prevent hypothermia as this can dramatically increase their chances of dying (up to three times higher if core body temperature drops below 35°C [Balvers, 2016]). It may be more appropriate to remove patients to a heated ambulance before completing this step.

5.5 *Secondary survey*

The secondary survey should only commence once all life-threatening injuries identified in the primary survey have been addressed and, in the case of severely injured patients, once they are on the way to hospital [NAEMT, 2020; JRCALC, 2019; Greaves, 2019].

5.5.1 Procedure

Procedure – Secondary survey

Take the following steps to perform a secondary survey in the trauma patient:

1. **Vital signs and history:** Obtain a full set of observations, a history of the injury-inducing event and a brief medical history (e.g. SAMPLE).

2. **Head**
   - Reassess the airway to ensure patency and check the mouth for bleeding, lacerations and loose teeth.
   - Look at and feel the entire head and face to identify lacerations, bruising, fractures and burns.
   - Re-check the pupils and GCS score.
   - Inspect the nose and ears for the presence of blood and cerebrospinal fluid (CSF) leakage as this may suggest a basal skull fracture. Other signs, such as bilateral bruising around the eyes or behind the ears, can take 12–36 hours to appear.

3. **Neck:** The clinician may choose to examine the neck. To do this, they will feel the back of the neck and then, depending on the situation and local guidelines, may ask the patient to move their neck. Until the senior clinician decides otherwise, the neck should be held still, using manual in-line stabilisation (MILS). If the clinician decides that a cervical spine collar is required, then it should be applied at this stage.

Procedure – Secondary survey – *cont*

4. Reassess for signs of life-threatening injury, indicated by:
   - tracheal deviation
   - wounds and swellings
   - emphysema (surgical/subcutaneous)
   - laryngeal crepitus
   - veins.
5. **Chest:** Repeat the assessment carried out in the primary survey. Look for obvious chest injuries, wounds, bruising or flail segments. Note the presence of seat-belt marks.
6. Assess the rate, depth and quality of respiration:
   - Ventilate with a BVM if respirations absent or fewer than 10 breaths/minute.
   - If respirations greater than 30 breaths/minute, it may also be clinically appropriate to ventilate the patient. Follow the advice of the clinician.
   - Monitor closely if respirations are in the range of 10–30 breaths/minute.
7. Listen (auscultate) over as much of the chest (front and back) as possible. If bilateral air entry is not heard, the clinician may use percussion to indicate the underlying problem.
8. Feel for equality of chest movement and note any instability.
9. **Abdomen:**
   - Look for open wounds, bruising and seat-belt marks. Try to view as much of the front and back as possible.
   - Feel the whole abdomen for tenderness, guarding and rigidity.
10. **Pelvis:**
    - Check for blood loss from the urethra or vagina.
    - Note the presence of bruising around the perineum and scrotum (in males).
    - Discourage urination.

Procedure – Secondary survey – *cont*

11. **Extremities:** Thoroughly examine the lower and then upper limbs. Look for wounds and fractures. Check motor, sensory and circulatory (MSC) function in all four limbs:
    - Motor: Ask the patient to move the limb.
    - Sensory: Apply light touch to evaluate sensation.
    - Circulation: Assess a distal pulse and skin temperature.

5.6 Head injuries

Common causes of traumatic brain injury (TBI) include road traffic collisions, falls, assault and direct blows to the head [Shivaji, 2014]. The worst outcomes are associated with [Moppett, 2007]:
- penetrating injuries
- non-accidental injury in children aged under five years
- pedestrians and pedal cyclists
- ejection from a vehicle.

Other clues at the scene include a 'bulls-eye' pattern on a vehicle windscreen and significant damage to protective helmets, if a patient was wearing one at the time of the injury [JRCALC, 2019].

Once a primary brain injury has occurred, it cannot be undone. Fortunately, good pre-hospital management can help to minimise the impact of secondary brain injury. This can be broken down into three areas:
- Recognise the injury that will indicate that a traumatic brain injury may be present.
- Understand the pathophysiology relating to traumatic brain injury.
- Manage the patient appropriately.

5.6.1 Recognition

Suggestive signs and symptoms of TBI include [Pante, 2010]:
- lacerations, contusions or haematomas to the scalp
- boggy areas when palpating the scalp

- visible fractures or deformity of the skull
- Battle's sign or 'panda eyes' (not apparent for several hours)
- cerebrospinal fluid and/or blood leaking from the nose or ears
- Cushing's triad: rising blood pressure, reducing heart rate and irregular respirations
- dizziness
- nausea and vomiting
- abnormal pupils and/or pupil reaction
- visual disturbances (double or blurred vision, seeing 'stars')
- severe headache
- altered level of consciousness
- perseveration (repeatedly asking the same questions)
- amnesia
- paraesthesia/paralysis of the extremities
- convulsions
- posturing
- abnormal respirations.

5.6.2 Pathophysiology

In the traumatically injured brain, autoregulation starts to fail and blood flow in affected areas of the brain changes, relying on higher than normal mean arterial pressures to maintain perfusion.

If a cerebral oedema or haematoma develops, CSF is displaced and the quantity of venous blood in the cranium is reduced. In the early stages of rising intracranial pressure (ICP), blood pressure will be fairly stable. However, in the later stages when the cardiovascular centre in the medulla becomes ischaemic, the Cushing reflex is triggered, resulting in peripheral vasoconstriction and a rise in blood pressure. This in turn leads to a reflex bradycardia. Respiration is also affected, leading to irregular respirations (hence the term 'Cushing's triad') [Moppett, 2007].

5.6.3 Management

The mainstay of management for patients with TBI is preventing hypoxia, treating hypotension and transporting patients quickly to definitive care. There is a link between head injury and injury of the cervical spine [NICE, 2014], so an assumption of spinal injury should be made, unless your clinician is confident at clearing the patient's cervical spine on scene. Cervical collars have been shown to raise intra-cranial pressure (ICP) [Maissan, 2018]; due to this, your senior clinician may choose not to apply a collar, but to instead rely on MILS [Connor, 2013].

Airway compromise is common after severe TBI and needs to be managed early to prevent hypoxia. Even brief episodes of hypoxia can cause secondary injury, which can be disastrous for head injury patients [Yan, 2014]. Provide 100% oxygen via a non-rebreathe mask and aim for oxygen saturations of 94–98% [JRCALC, 2019]. Continuous monitoring of oxygen saturations is important. Assess adequacy of ventilation and provide assistance if required. If you are able to monitor $EtCO_2$, aim for normocapnia, as both hypocapnia and hypercapnia have been shown to increase mortality [Hammell, 2009].

As with oxygen saturations, a single drop of systolic blood pressure to less than 90 mmHg doubles the patient's risk of death [Moppett, 2007]. Make sure you keep your clinician informed if you notice the blood pressure close to this value.

When transporting, it can be helpful if the patient's head is kept slightly up to help prevent a rising intra-cranial pressure [Greaves, 2019], but this can be challenging when immobilised.

Many of these patients may benefit from additional treatments that are available from pre-hospital critical care teams, especially if their level of consciousness is reduced, which may include an emergency pre-hospital anaesthetic. Consider asking for assistance early if your head injured patient is agitated or has a low GCS.

5.7 *Maxillofacial injuries*

Maxillofacial injury (i.e. involving the maxilla and/or face, but referred to as just facial injury in this chapter) is common, with an estimated 500,000 facial injuries occurring each year in the UK, 180,000 of them serious (requiring specialist treatment or hospital admission) [Jalo, 2009]. Causes include road traffic accidents, assault, falls and sport-related injuries [Patel, 2016]. Alcohol is a common factor, especially in relation to injuries from assault.

5.7.1 Facial structures and injuries

Orbit

A blow to the eye can cause the orbit to 'blow out' and fracture. The most common location for this to occur is the inferior portion (floor). This injury may not necessarily lead to any external tenderness, but signs and symptoms of a blowout fracture include [Purcell, 2016; NAEMT, 2020]:
- Enophthalmos: The eyeball retracts into its socket.
- Double vision (diplopia) and/or loss of upward vision.
- Pupils at a different horizontal level to each other.
- Loss of sensation above eyebrow and over cheek.

Zygoma

Fractures of the zygoma, typically caused by assault and RTCs, lead to a depression of the cheek. They are commonly associated with orbital fractures, ocular injury and epistaxis [Purcell, 2016]. Paraesthesia may be present as in orbit injury. It is worth noting that fractures to the orbitozygomatic complex are the most commonly missed eye injury [Greaves, 2008].

Maxilla

The maxilla is most commonly fractured by RTCs, but other blunt injury causes include assault and sport injuries. Maxilla fractures are often associated with injuries to other middle facial structures. Fractures form three classic patterns of separation from the skull, which were first described by a French physician, René Le Fort (Figure 17.13) [Le Fort, 1901; NAEMT, 2020]:
- **Le Fort I:** Horizontal detachment of the maxillae from the nasal floor. The passage of air through the nares may be affected and the oropharynx can be compromised by blood clots and/or oedema in the soft palate.
- **Le Fort II:** This is a pyramidal fracture, including both maxillae, the medial aspect of the floor of the orbit and the nasal bones. Since the sinuses are well vascularised, this can lead to severe bleeding
- **Le Fort III:** Complete craniofacial disruption allowing movement of the whole of the middle

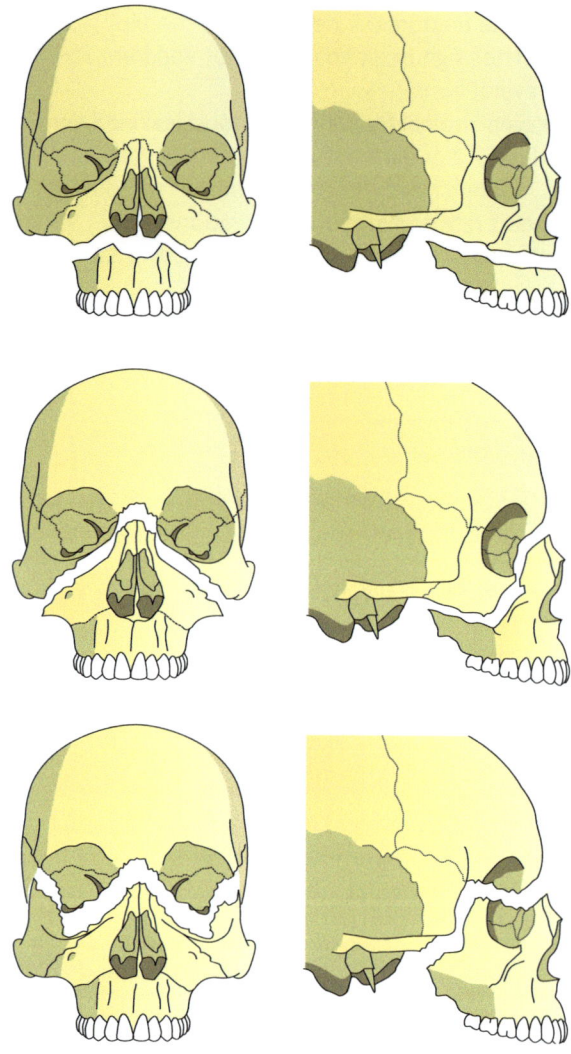

Figure 17.13 Le Fort I (top), Le Fort II (middle), Le Fort III (bottom)

third of the face, which can cause airway compromise and is associated with traumatic brain injury.

Since the base of the skull is sloping, the bones forming the middle third of the face have a tendency to slide backwards and downwards, obstructing the airway and causing an anterior open bite, which splints the front teeth open [Greaves, 2008].

Mandible

The mandible and its associated structures form the lower third of the face. The necks of the mandibular condyles are a point of weakness and are often fractured following blunt trauma to the chin. The combination of bilateral condylar and midline (symphyseal) mandibular fractures is sometimes referred to as a guardsman's fracture.

Teeth
Teeth are frequently avulsed (knocked out) as a result of facial trauma and can be inhaled if the patient is unconscious. In addition, avulsed teeth can displace into the soft tissues, including the lips. A fracture to the crown of a tooth is extremely painful and may prove to be the patient's main complaint.

Soft tissue
The facial tissues have an abundant blood supply, which can lead to dramatic-looking wounds and bleeding. However, it is uncommon for these to result in hypovolaemia (except in children) and other causes should be assumed to be responsible, particularly in the initial stages of your assessment. Large lacerations on the face often gape due to muscle pull and those in the middle third of the face can swell rapidly, masking underlying fractures. If swelling involves the eyelids, this can prevent examination of the globe of the eye, potentially hiding damage to the patient's vision [NAEMT, 2020].

5.7.2 Management: General

The management of facial injuries follows the same principles as for any trauma patient, but the airway is likely to occupy a significant portion of your time. Follow the standard <C>ABC approach, although note that catastrophic haemorrhage in isolated facial trauma is rare, but may require critical care teams who carry facial packing kit not normally available on ambulances.

Generally, patients with facial injuries are best managed sitting up and leaning forward, to allow for drainage of blood and debris from the mouth and reduce venous return. Cervical spine injury needs to be considered, but use assessment guidelines such as the NEXUS or Canadian c-spine rules to stratify the risk. Arguably, any conscious patient who asks to sit up should be allowed to do so on the basis of the following [Perry, 2008]:

- A talking patient has intact airway reflexes and will be able to protect their airway if sitting forward.
- To be able to sit up, the patient requires sufficient muscle tone that will provide spinal stability.
- Persistent/repeated requests to sit up are an indication of either impending airway compromise or the desire to vomit, requests that can be misinterpreted as the patient being 'difficult' due to alcohol or brain injury.
- Spinal immobilisation is only appropriate for co-operative or unconscious patients. Agitated patients or those who actively resist your attempts to immobilise them should be left to adopt a position they choose. Forcible restraint against active movement increases forces applied to a potentially unstable spine.

5.7.3 Management: Airway

Unconscious patients
Clear any debris from the mouth, (e.g. broken teeth) using suction or forceps if you are trained to do so. Although cervical spine injury needs to be considered, the lack of a patent airway will kill the patient first. If neck movement is required, this is acceptable, although it is reasonable to try and keep this to a minimum [Austin, 2014]. Even a jaw thrust results in some cervical spine movement, albeit less than a head tilt–chin lift manoeuvre [Prasarn, 2014]. However, these can be difficult to perform in patients who have faces covered in blood.

If the patient has a Le Fort fracture that has resulted in the maxilla moving posteriorly, reduce it by holding the upper jaw and pulling forward firmly. If the mandible has become displaced due to bilateral condylar fractures, this too should be reduced as the tongue is likely to end up resting on the posterior wall of the oropharynx, increasing the risk of airway occlusion. This can be achieved by pulling forward on the mandible and, if necessary, taking hold of the tongue with some gauze, although this position will have to be maintained and a suture or surgical towel clip is more convenient, although neither of these is standard ambulance equipment [Greaves, 2008]!

If, despite these manoeuvres, the airway cannot be cleared, then the senior clinician may have to perform other manoeuvres to ensure the airway is clear.

Oropharyngeal airways (OPAs) are not always helpful in facial injuries as they can easily dislodge, particularly with the alterations in airway anatomy that occur with facial fractures. In addition, they are not suitable for responsive patients. Nasopharyngeal airways (NPAs) are generally better tolerated, but should be used with caution in patients with fractures to the middle third of the face, as these are associated with fractures to the base of the skull. The use of a bag-valve-mask can also be challenging with fractures of the mid-face as the application of the mask to the face can displace the fractures and further occlude the airway. However, in serious facial injuries the real enemy is bleeding, and neither an OPA nor an NPA will prevent aspiration and both can block with clots and other debris. Intubation and facial packing is ideal, but will require a critical care team.

Conscious patients
In awake supine patients, facial bleeding may not be obvious if the patient is able to swallow the blood. This is problematic as it increases the risk of the patient vomiting. Conversely, patients with mandibular fractures may actually have trouble swallowing efficiently, leading to difficulty in keeping the airway clear. Be wary of patients on anticoagulants, as significant airway-threatening swelling can occur, even in the absence of fractures. Retropharyngeal swelling is important to note as it is also a marker for cervical spine injury [Perry, 2008].

Watch for repeated requests/attempts to sit up. This may be a sign that your patient is going to vomit. If they are immobilised and you are on your own (in the back of an ambulance en route to hospital), the most practical method to clear the airway is to tilt the patient's head down and suction at high pressures, rather than attempt to log roll the patient.

5.7.4 Management: Breathing
This should be managed as for other traumatic injuries, although facial injuries sustained as a result of a road traffic collision are often accompanied by chest and abdominal injuries, including diaphragmatic rupture.

5.7.5 Management: Circulation
With the exception of significant middle third fractures, bleeding from the facial injuries is unlikely to lead to hypovolaemic shock, so look for an alternative cause. Mid-face fractures can be tricky as this portion of the face has an extensive collateral supply from the internal and external carotid arteries. Reducing maxilla fractures may assist in staunching haemorrhage, which can be otherwise difficult to control. Asking the patient to bite on gauze may help, but nasal bleeding needs to be controlled with anterior and posterior nasal packing, if available.

5.7.6 Management: Disability
Many patients with facial injuries are going to be under the influence of alcohol, but don't assume that the abnormal neurology they display is due to this (and don't forget the blood sugar measurement, either). If in doubt, treat agitation unresponsiveness and cyanosis as sign of inadequate oxygenation and ventilation.

Pupil signs can be misleading if the patient has cranio-orbital trauma, as mydriasis (pupil dilation) can occur even in the absence of raised intracranial pressure. Soft tissue swelling of the eyelids can prevent the eye being seen at all. In this case, holding a pen torch against the swollen eyelid can at least assist in the detection of blindness.

Speech is often poor and/or slurred, secondary to either alcohol, facial fractures, tongue swelling and/or dental malocclusion, so don't rush in deciding that your patient is FAST positive.

5.7.7 Specific management: Eye injuries
Eye injuries can be categorised into four types [Purcell, 2016]:
- chemical burns
- corneal abrasions
- blunt trauma
- foreign bodies.

Chemicals splashed into the eye should generally be considered to be an emergency as they can lead to severe corneal injury and blindness [Purcell, 2016]. Ensure that you do not get contaminated by wearing appropriate PPE, and then irrigate the eye with copious amounts of water for 20 minutes [FPHC, 2018], ensuring that you do not contaminate the unaffected eye. Don't waste time identifying the chemical at the expense of starting irrigation and transporting the patient. In some work settings, specific antidotes may be available and can be used in place of water [Zideman, 2015].

A corneal abrasion is a superficial injury to the surface of the cornea. It can be caused by a foreign body, leaves or branches, fingernails and contact lenses, for example. This is not normally a serious injury, but is often very painful. Patients will require an ophthalmic assessment, but this may be able to be performed by a local minor injuries unit or advanced practitioners within your service. Similar injuries can be caused by flash burns. These are a form of radiation burn caused by sun lamps or a welder's flash, for example. However, the onset of pain and other symptoms can take several hours to develop [Purcell, 2016].

Blunt trauma to the eye is typically caused by mechanisms such as a blow from a fist or a small ball (for example, a squash ball). It's important to assess visual acuity. This is typically undertaken with a Snellen chart, a chart containing letters of reducing size. This can be approximated, by asking the patient to read text from a book or newspaper, for example. Even if their vision appears unaffected, they still require a thorough eye examination. Follow local guidance for a suitable destination or referral.

Foreign bodies such as grit or a loose eyelash can safely be rinsed out of the eye. If the object is in the upper eyelid, instruct the patient to grasp the eyelashes of their upper eyelid and gently pull it over the lower lid [SJA, SAA, BRC, 2016]. Any foreign bodies that are embedded in the cornea or are intra-ocular should not be removed and the patient should be taken to hospital.

5.7.8 Specific management: Nosebleed

A nosebleed, or epistaxis, is a common occurrence with multiple causes, including [NHS, 2017c]:
- direct trauma to the nose
- nose-picking
- blowing the nose too hard
- bleeding disorders such as haemophilia
- anti-coagulant and anti-platelet drugs such as warfarin and aspirin
- the inside of the nose being too dry (because of a change in air temperature).

The source of bleeding in children and young adults is usually from the anterior portion of the nasal septum (called Little's area), whereas bleeding in older adults can occur anteriorly and posteriorly, which is more difficult to access [Purcell, 2016].

Assessment
Obtain a good history. This will provide clues as to whether this is a one-off occurrence due to aggressive nose-picking, for example, or due to the patient having high blood pressure and poorly controlled anti-coagulant drug therapy.

Management
Take the following steps to control a nosebleed [Purcell, 2016; NHS, 2017c]:
- Instruct the patient to sit down and lean forward to reduce the likelihood of blood entering the oropharynx and being swallowed.
- Ask the patient to squeeze the soft part of their nose for ten minutes. They must not release the pressure before this time. Alternatively, you may have nose clips available that can be used instead of the patient applying pressure.
- Advise patients to breathe through their mouth and gently spit blood out of their mouth, rather than swallow it, as this can lead to vomiting.
- Once ten minutes are up, instruct the patient to release the pressure and see if the bleeding has stopped. If bleeding continues, reapply pressure for a further ten minutes and reassess. If bleeding still continues, reapply pressure for a further ten minutes.
- If bleeding continues for more than 30 minutes, appears to be from a posterior bleeding point, or the patient is on anti-coagulant medication,

transport the patient to hospital unless you have access to advanced practitioners who can pack the nose.

5.8 Spinal injuries

Spinal injuries, or more specifically spinal cord injuries (SCIs), are rare, with around 12–16 per million of population a year in the UK [NHS England, 2013c]. In adult major trauma, approximately 10% of patients will sustain a spinal fracture/dislocation, but fewer than 2% will sustain an SCI. The most common cause is a fall (46%), although, significantly, a third of these are falls of fewer than 2 m in height. Falls are closely followed by road traffic collisions (40%), whereas the other causes, such as sports injuries (under 3%), stabbings (1%) and shootings (0.6%), are much rarer. SCIs most commonly occur at the cervical level (45%), followed by thoracic (29%), lumbar (24%) and multi-level injuries (2%) [Hasler, 2011b].

Risk factors for SCI include [Hasler, 2011b]:
- male sex
- under 45 years of age
- reduced Glasgow Coma Scale score
- accompanying chest injury
- dangerous mechanism (falls greater than 2 m in height, sports injury, RTC, shooting).

5.8.1 Recognition

The signs and symptoms also depend on the completeness of the SCI. The classic picture in complete SCI is vasodilation, relaxed muscles and loss of sensation below the injury, as well as loss of temperature regulation mechanisms such as vasodilation and sweating. This can lead to a poikilothermic state, where the body adopts the temperature of the surrounding environment (whether hot or cold). Depending on how high the SCI injury is, the blood pressure can dramatically fall, for example to 80 mmHg systolic in high cervical injuries, but there is no compensatory tachycardia, since the sympathetic signals to the heart are blocked. In fact, parasympathetic division dominance leads to bradycardia, further reducing cardiac output. In an incomplete SCI, there is a mixed picture of paralysis and paraesthesia, but not profound hypotension or bradycardia, making the absence of these signs unreliable in excluding SCI in unconscious patients [Harrison, 2007].

5.8.2 Pathophysiology

Key to the maintenance of homeostasis within the autonomic nervous system (ANS) are the cerebral cortex and hypothalamus, which provide appropriate excitatory and inhibitory inputs to various areas in the medulla, which plays a crucial role in cardiovascular control. This relies on feedback from afferent sensory impulses from central and peripheral baroreceptors. Thus, it is not difficult to see that SCI, depending on the level and completeness of the injury and cord interruption, can dramatically affect the body's ability to keep control of the ANS [Krassioukov, 2012].

Despite the common use of words like 'transection', 'cutting' and 'severing' of the spinal cord after a traumatic injury, in reality a spinal cord lesion (abnormality or damage) is primarily caused by ischaemic necrosis. Traumatic injury mechanisms include displacement of one or more vertebral bodies, causing compression and/or stretching of the cord, which may result in no visible injury, but leads to oedema and vascular disruption. However, not all SCI is due to trauma. Other causes include spinal tumours, vascular thrombosis or haemorrhage, and infection and abscesses caused by tuberculosis or meningitis [Gupta, 2009].

The space within the vertebral canal is very limited and an oedematous spinal cord is soon compressed. This disrupts blood and oxygen flow, resulting in ischaemic tissue and, ultimately, necrosis. The rapid cessation of signal transmission that this process causes leads to a range of signs and symptoms that are termed 'spinal shock' [Harrison, 2007].

Nerves originating from T1–T5 are responsible for most heart and vascular control, and injuries below this level typically do not have such a dramatic effect on the ANS. However, an injury at T6 or above can lead to interruption of sympathetic division control from the brain. Parasympathetic innervation of the heart arises from the brain and so is typically unaffected, making the parasympathetic division dominant.

5.8.3 Management

All patients who are suspected of having a spinal injury should be immobilised as soon as possible. Remember that the whole spine must be immobilised. The techniques and equipment involved in order to perform this safely are described in the skeletal immobilisation section.

Remember that spinal immobilisation is not a risk-free procedure. Potential complications of spinal immobilisation include [JRCALC, 2019]:
- airway problems (including increased risk of aspiration)
- increased intracranial pressure
- restricted respiration
- dysphagia
- skin ulceration/pressure sores
- pain.

Patients with isolated penetrating trauma to the head or limbs do not require immobilisation, but if, in torso or neck trauma, it is possible that the projectile could have passed near or through the spinal cord and there are signs of spinal cord injury, then immobilisation may be appropriate.

In blunt trauma, there are guidelines that allow clinicians to discontinue immobilisation, so you may on occasion be asked to stop immobilising a patient once a thorough assessment has been completed [JRCALC, 2019].

5.9 Thoracic injuries

Thoracic trauma accounts directly for 25% of all trauma deaths and is a contributing factor to around another 50% [Greaves, 2019]. Major causes are road traffic collisions, industrial accidents and domestic and sporting injuries [Greaves, 2008]. The most common problem associated with severe thoracic injury is hypoxia [JRCALC, 2019]. This can occur due to respiratory and/or cardiovascular causes, which are summarised in Table 17.4 [Greaves, 2008].

5.9.1 Pneumothorax

The lungs are surrounded by a pleural membrane. The outer layer (parietal pleura) lines the chest wall and the inner layer (visceral pleura) covers the lungs. Between them is the pleural space, which is lubricated to ensure that the surfaces glide smoothly over one another as well as creating a surface tension that results in the surfaces 'sticking together'.

Table 17.4 Causes of hypoxia from thoracic injury.

Respiratory	Cardiovascular
Open pneumothorax	Large haemorrhage
Tension pneumothorax	Tension pneumothorax
Massive haemothorax	Pericardial tamponade
Ventilatory failure (e.g. flail chest)	Rupture of major blood vessels
Pulmonary contusion	Myocardial contusion

Pneumothorax, or air in the pleural space, is generally classified as being spontaneous if there is no obvious causal factor, or traumatic if there is an external cause [Noppen, 2010]. In the event that air within the alveoli can escape into the pleural space, or there is an external breach of the thoracic cavity allowing atmospheric air to enter the pleural space, the normal physiology of ventilation is disrupted and the lung collapses [Yarmus, 2019]. Spontaneous pneumothorax is regarded as common and normally benign so long as it does not progress to a tension pneumothorax [Yoon, 2013].

A traumatic pneumothorax is caused by penetrating trauma, such as stab and gunshot wounds or impalements; blunt trauma that leads to rib fractures and increased intrathoracic pressure; and bronchial rupture and barotrauma, where changes in pressure of the air delivered to the lungs lead to expansion. This phenomenon has been reported in air crew and scuba divers [Sharma, 2008].

Open pneumothorax
In an open pneumothorax, air enters the pleural space thanks to a communication between atmospheric air and the pleural space, for example as a result of penetrating trauma (Figure 17.14). As the chest expands during inspiration, air enters the

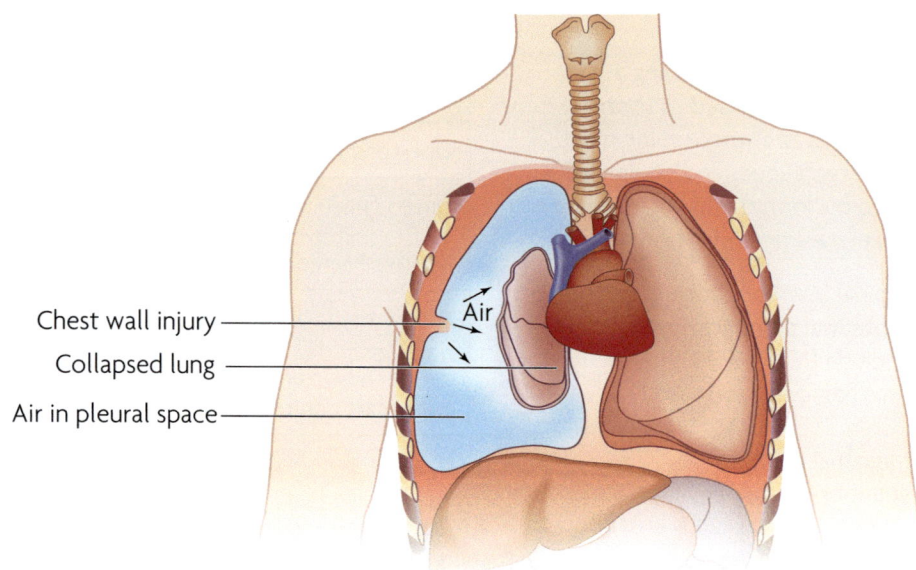

Figure 17.14 An open pneumothorax. A penetrating chest injury has resulted in an opening between the outside and inside of the chest wall.

pleural space. If the wound is large enough, there may be free movement of air into and out of the affected lung during respiration. If the wound is similar in size to the glottic opening to the lower airway, then atmospheric air preferentially enters via the wound, leading to ineffective ventilation of the alveoli. The sound heard as air moves into and out of the wound has led to these types of injury being referred to as 'sucking chest wounds' [NAEMT, 2020; Greaves, 2008].

Tension pneumothorax

Tension pneumothorax is an uncommon, but life-threatening, condition that can prove rapidly fatal to patients, particularly those who are being ventilated with positive pressure [Leigh-Smith, 2005]. It most often occurs in [MacDuff, 2010]:

- ventilated patients in intensive care
- trauma
- cardiac arrest
- acute exacerbations of asthma and COPD
- blocked or clamped chest drains
- non-invasive ventilation.

As with other types of pneumothorax, air enters the pleural space on inspiration, but cannot escape during expiration due to the presence of a one-way valve formed by a pleural defect. This leads to increasing intra-pleural pressure on the affected side of the chest, worsening the lung collapse and causing diaphragmatic depression (see Figure 17.15). In severe cases, and dependent on mediastinal distensibility, this can compress the contralateral lung.

It's worth noting that a tension pneumothorax typically develops far more slowly in spontaneously breathing awake patients, compared to ventilated and sedated patients who can experience hypotension and a rapid decline in oxygen saturations in just a few minutes, hastened by the administration of positive-pressure ventilation [Leigh-Smith, 2005; MacDuff, 2010].

Assessment

Arguably, the most important type of pneumothorax to be recognised is one under tension. However, the clinical course of a tension pneumothorax is not the same for all patients, with the progression of clinical deterioration for an awake, spontaneously breathing patient likely to be considerably longer than for those who are being ventilated with positive-pressure ventilation [Leigh-Smith, 2005].

Assessment and management of the trauma patient

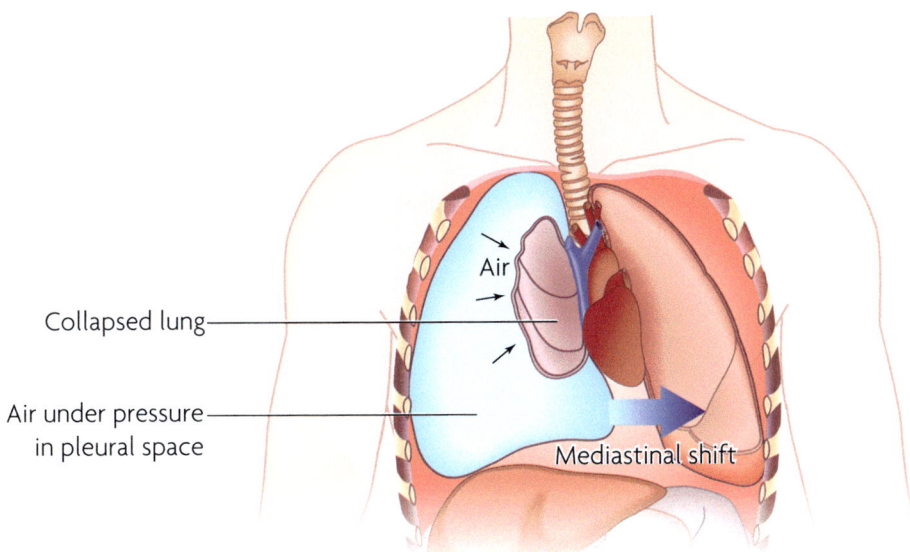

Figure 17.15 A tension pneumothorax including mediastinal shift.

Signs and symptoms of a tension pneumothorax in awake patients include:
- pleuritic chest pain (sharp pain, worse on breathing in and out)
- air hunger
- respiratory distress
- tachypnoea (rapid breathing rate)
- tachycardia (rapid heart rate)
- falling oxygen saturations (SpO_2)
- agitation
- on the same side as the injury:
  - hyperexpansion
  - hypomobility
  - decreased breath sounds
- pre-terminal (near death):
  - decreasing respiratory rate
  - hypotension
  - decreasing level of consciousness.

Do not rely on tracheal deviation or distended neck veins as these can be difficult to determine [Spiteri, 1988].

In ventilated patients, the clinical deterioration is likely to be far more alarming. In addition, ventilated patients are more likely to suffer a cardiac arrest, whereas awake patients tend to suffer from respiratory arrest initially [Leigh-Smith, 2005].

Management
Patients with a simple pneumothorax with no signs of cardiovascular compromise, suggesting tension, should be closely monitored en route to hospital, but are typically managed conservatively [Lee, 2007a]. All patients with a pneumothorax should receive oxygen at the appropriate target range (usually 94–98%, except for patients with COPD, who should be managed at either 88–92% or their usual range [JRCALC, 2019]). If the patient maintains saturations of 94–98% without oxygen, it may not be required.

If there is an open pneumothorax, then the clinician may choose to cover it with a commercial chest seal [Lee, 2007a]. However, these can block, so closely monitor the patient and remove the dressing if the patient shows signs of tension pneumothorax [Yoon, 2013]. Patients with signs of a tension pneumothorax require prompt decompression by needle thoracentesis, which involves inserting a large-bore cannula into the patient's chest and should only be performed by a paramedic or other senior clinician.

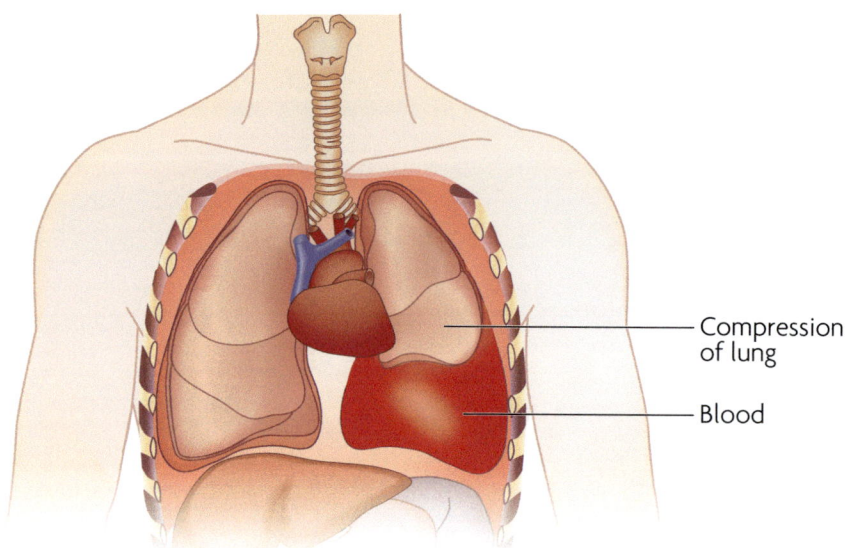

Figure 17.16   A haemothorax.

5.9.2 Haemothorax

Haemothorax, or blood in the thoracic cavity, usually occurs as a result of penetrating trauma (Figure 17.16). Life-threatening haemorrhage can occur in cases of severe lacerations of the lung, large vessels in the mediastinum and the heart. Each hemithorax (literally, half of the chest) can easily accommodate half of the patient's circulating blood volume before the physical signs are obvious [Greaves, 2008].

However, this amount of bleeding will lead to the signs and symptoms of shock. Since blood occupies space usually reserved for the lung, lung collapse occurs, leading to absent or decreased lung sounds, reduced chest wall expansion on the injured side and dullness on percussion [Leech, 2016].

There are few treatment options available outside of hospital; usually, expedient transport to the nearest major trauma centre is indicated.

5.9.3 Flail chest

Blunt chest trauma can lead to multiple rib and sternal fractures. In the event that two or more ribs are broken in two or more places, the chest wall will lose the rigid structure that usually supports the chest. A flail segment will start to move paradoxically, that is, it will move inwards during inspiration and outwards on expiration (Figure 17.17) [Athanassiadi, 2010]. If this area is large enough, it results in compromised ventilation. However, it is usually bruising of the underlying lung that leads to hypoxia and there can also be significant blood loss, with each rib fracture causing around 100 ml of blood loss [Greaves, 2008].

The flail segment is not always obvious as muscular spasm can support the segment until the muscles are exhausted. However, these injuries are painful and your clinician is likely to want to provide intravenous analgesia [JRCALC, 2019]. Do not attempt to splint the flail segment as this is likely to further impair ventilation [NAEMT, 2020].

5.10 *Abdominal injuries*

The abdominal cavity extends from the diaphragm to the pelvic bones and from the vertebral column to the muscles of the abdomen and flanks (Figure 17.18). Organs are classed as peritoneal if they are covered by a lining called the peritoneum. These include the spleen, liver, stomach, gallbladder, parts of the large intestine and most of the small intestine, and

Assessment and management of the trauma patient

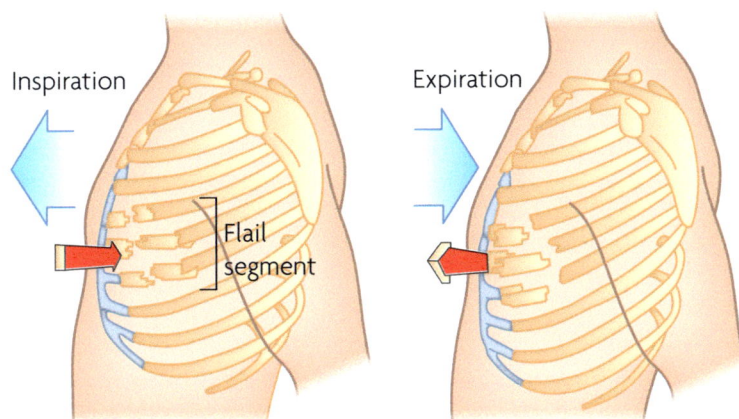

Figure 17.17   Flail chest.

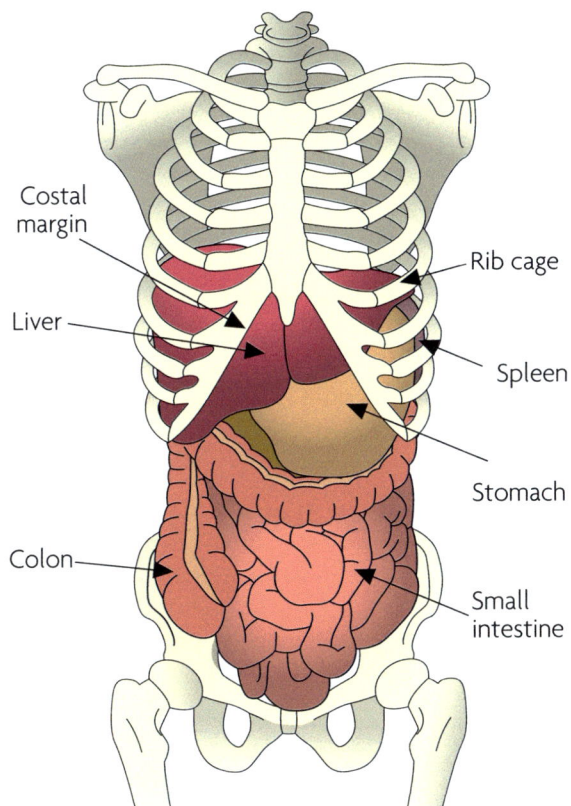

Figure 17.18   The abdominal cavity.

In blunt trauma, the spleen, liver and structures that are firmly fixed, such as the retroperitoneal organs, are most commonly injured due to shearing forces associated with rapid deceleration. Penetrating trauma can also cause serious damage and severe bleeding. Depending on the angle at which the penetrating object enters, thoracic injury is also possible, particularly in upper abdominal stab injuries [NAEMT, 2020].

Patients suffering from abdominal trauma may not exhibit many symptoms initially, although you should suspect internal injury in any shocked patient with a suggestive mechanism of injury. Look at the abdomen for signs of injury, such as bruising, abrasions and seat-belt marks. Gently feel the abdomen for signs of tenderness, but don't be reassured by a normal examination [JRCALC, 2019].

There is no specific management of blunt abdominal trauma, but in penetrating trauma, if the injury has caused the bowel to protrude (evisceration) out of the abdomen, you should not push it back in. Instead, cover it with a dressing soaked in warm saline [NAEMT, 2020].

If the penetrating object is still in place in the patient's abdomen, do not attempt to remove it. Instead, secure it appropriately, although if it is pulsating, allow some movement of the object, but not its removal [JRCALC, 2019].

the female reproductive organs [Tortora, 2017]. The retroperitoneal space is the area behind the peritoneum. This area contains the kidneys, ureters, pancreas, parts of the small and large intestine, and the aorta and vena cava [JRCALC, 2019].

5.11 Pelvic injuries

Fractures of the pelvic ring are uncommon, with around for 20–37 per 100,000 people suffering a fracture, about 2–8% of all skeletal injuries [Garlapati, 2012; McCormack, 2010]. However, pelvic fractures are found in up to 20% of injuries involving a significant mechanism of injury resulting in multiple injuries. The major cause in the younger population is road traffic collisions (RTCs), with around 44–64% of pelvic ring fractures due to the patient being involved in an RTC. Vehicle speed and compartmental intrusion are important factors [Adams, 2002]. The overall mortality rate is around 12%, although it can be as high as 50% for open pelvic fractures [Lee, 2007c]. There is some evidence that recent advances in trauma care including the more prolific use of pelvic binders and increasing availability of major trauma care systems is helping to reduce the number of fatalities due to pelvic fracture [Siada, 2017].

All pelvic fractures cause some bleeding, although the source can vary. Bleeding from cancellous bone that has been fractured is common, but bleeding can also occur from lacerations to retroperitoneal veins and the internal iliac arteries. Arterial bleeding accounts for up to 25% of haemodynamically unstable pelvic ring fractures [McCormack, 2010], but most bleeding is actually low-pressure bleeding (i.e. not arterial) and usually responds well to appropriate stabilisation (such as with a pelvic binder or external fixator) and tamponade [Abrassart, 2013].

5.11.1 Associated abdominal injuries

As well as the potential vascular damage that pelvic ring fractures can cause, the soft tissues are also vulnerable, and injuries to the anorectum, vagina, urethra and nerves can occur. The most common is bladder injury, typically caused by compression or tearing of the bladder wall. Urethral and anorectal injuries are more common with straddle injuries, for example when a motorcyclist straddles the fuel tank during an RTC, resulting in the separation of the two pelvic bones and severe tearing of the pelvic floor [Leenen, 2010].

5.11.2 Pelvic binders

If you elect to apply a pelvic binder, make sure it is positioned correctly. Generally, the binder should be placed over the greater trochanters, but it is commonly placed too high. In a 2018 study at a UK trauma centre, 40% of binders applied in the pre-hospital setting were found to be too high on arrival to hospital [Naseem, 2018]. Placing binders too high can actually worsen pelvic injury. Pelvic binders should be placed directly against the patient's skin. As with cervical collars, pelvic binders are not risk-free, so consider whether their application is appropriate. Indications for the application of a pelvic binder are shown in Figure 17.19, but follow local guidance [Scott, 2013].

5.12 Suspension trauma

Patients who are suspended at height need rescuing as soon as possible, particularly if they are unconscious or have pre-syncopal symptoms such as [HSE, 2009b]:
- light-headedness
- breathlessness
- numbness of the arms or legs
- visual disturbance
- sweating
- pallor
- nausea
- dizziness.

Do not attempt rescue if you are not trained to do so. The hazardous area response team (HART) may be required if other on-site support is not available. If the patient cannot be immediately rescued, elevating the legs of the patient into a horizontal position may increase the time that suspension will be tolerated.

Once the patient has been rescued, assess and treat the patient's airway, breathing and circulation as normal, including placing the patient in a supine position [HSE, 2009b]. There is no evidence that leaving patients in a seated or semi-recumbent position is beneficial [Thomassen, 2009].

5.13 Musculoskeletal injuries

Musculoskeletal injuries are very common, and you are likely to see the whole spectrum of injuries from

Assessment and management of the trauma patient

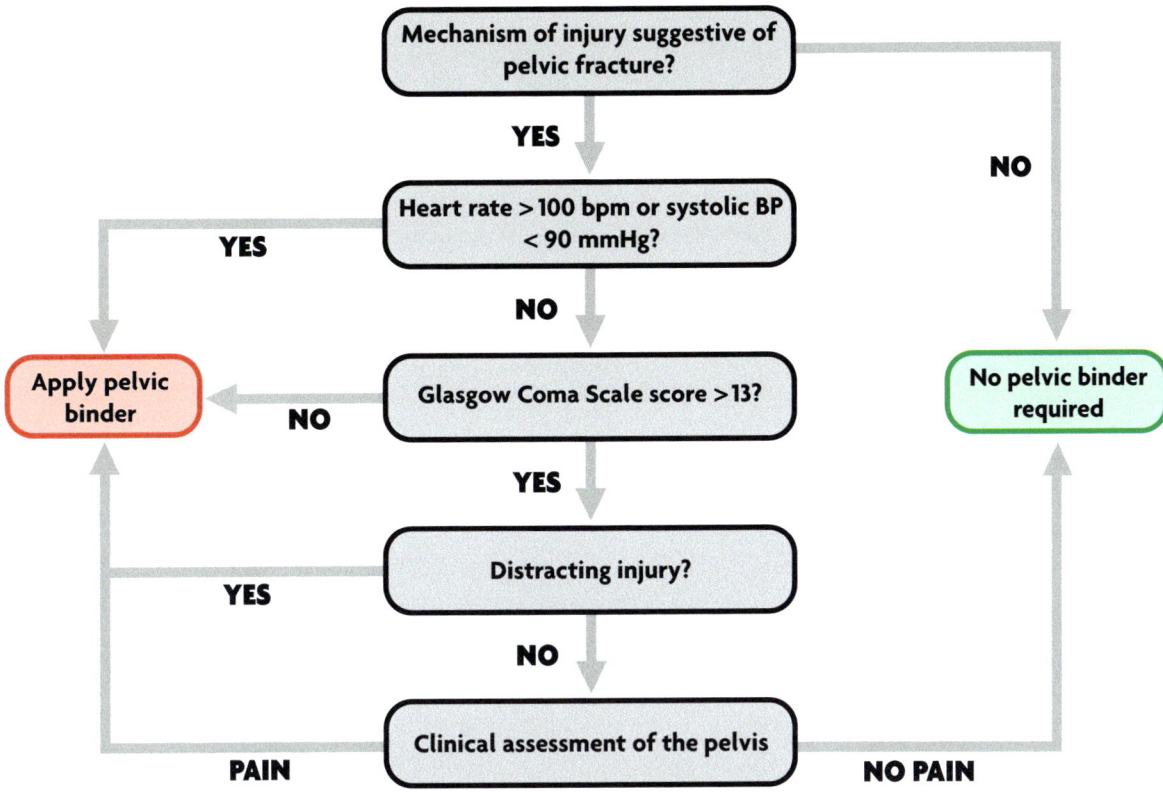

Figure 17.19 Indications for the application of a pelvic binder.

sprains to fractures. Joint injuries can be particularly debilitating, so it is important that you have a low threshold for referring or transporting patients to ensure that they can receive a thorough assessment and appropriate management. Although the principles here mainly apply to limb injuries, they can be applied to other musculoskeletal injuries.

Adopt a methodical assessment and always obtain a good history before you start examining the patient:
- history
  - mechanism of injury (MOI)
  - symptoms and any change over time
  - previous injuries/past medical history
- examination
  - joint above/below
  - look
  - feel
  - move
  - nerves and vessels.

5.13.1 History

It is important that you determine the exact mechanism of injury. A good way to do this is to produce a mental image of the direction, magnitude and duration of the force that was applied to the injured limb or joint. For example, in ankle injuries, it can be useful for the patient to show you the position of the ankle at the time of injury (although do get them to use the uninjured ankle to do this!) [Wardrope, 2008]. In lower limb injuries, check whether the patient could weight bear immediately after injury occurred and be alert for any repeated 'giving way' of knee or ankle joints and past injuries.

Ask about symptoms and their progress over time. For example, swelling that developed within minutes of the injury is more likely to be due to bleeding in the joint space (i.e. a haemarthrosis). In patients with knee injuries, make sure you enquire about weight-bearing immediately following the injury, as a complete loss of function (e.g. being stretchered off the field) following injury is not a good sign. Common symptoms of knee injuries are generally pain, swelling and loss of function, but ask about paraesthesia (pins and needles) and additional injuries.

Finally, enquire about the patient's past medical history, and note joint conditions, such as arthritis, as patients such as haemophiliacs and those taking anti-coagulant medication are at an increased risk of bleeding.

5.13.2 Examination

In lower limb injuries, observe the patient walking and standing, if they are able. In knee injuries, for example, patients who cannot straighten their injured knee might walk on the ball of their foot. In upper limb injuries, patients may be cradling an injured arm or, in the case of a dislocated shoulder, dangling the affected limb and holding it to the body with their uninjured arm [Purcell, 2016].

Joint above/below
Depending on the mechanism, forces can be transmitted along limbs, resulting in injuries elsewhere, for example a knee or hip injury following a fall, or a proximal humerus injury when falling on an outstretched hand.

Look
Check for swelling, erythema (redness), bruising and/or deformity. If the injury is to a limb, compare with the uninjured side. Limbs that are clearly abnormally angled are almost certainly broken (fractured). Do not attempt to realign the bones, but splint in the position you find them. If the bone is protruding through an open wound (an open fracture), cover with a sterile dressing to prevent further contamination.

Feel
Gently palpate the area surrounding the injury in a systematic fashion. It is not necessary to directly palpate the most tender area of an injury, but instead note its location.

Move
If the injured area or limb is not obviously fractured, ask the patient if they can slowly move it. Note whether the range of movement of a joint is reduced by comparing it with the other limb. Instruct the patient to stop the movement if it is painful and splint the joint to prevent further movement.

Nerves and vessels
Check sensation below the injury and compare it with the other side. Note reduced or absent sensation and paraesthesia (pins and needles). In limbs, check for a pulse below the level of an injury. In the case of an obvious deformity of a limb, an absent pulse below the level of an injury should be treated as an emergency.

Special tests
A number of special tests exist to help determine whether or not an x-ray is required. Two such examples are the Ottawa Ankle and Ottawa Knee rules. Based on a series of criteria, it is possible for a clinician to determine whether or not an x-ray of the potential injury is required. It is beyond the scope of this text to cover these tests in detail here, but you should be aware of them for when you see your clinical colleagues using them in practice.

5.13.3 Fractures and dislocations

A fracture is a break (or breaks) in a bone. There are a number of types [Tortora, 2017] (Figure 17.20):
- **Transverse:** A single horizontal break through the bone, splitting it into two parts.
- **Comminuted:** A fracture that results in the bone being split into more than two parts.
- **Oblique:** The bone is broken diagonally along its shaft.
- **Spiral:** Caused by a twisting force.
- **Open:** Sometimes called a compound fracture. A fracture with a wound at the site of the injury caused by bone pushing through the skin.
- **Closed:** Sometimes called a simple fracture. A fracture where no puncturing of the skin has occurred.
- **Greenstick:** An incomplete fracture where only one side of the periosteum fractures. This fracture is common in children because their bones are soft and porous.

A dislocation is an abnormal separation of joint surfaces. They can occur in isolation or be associated

Assessment and management of the trauma patient

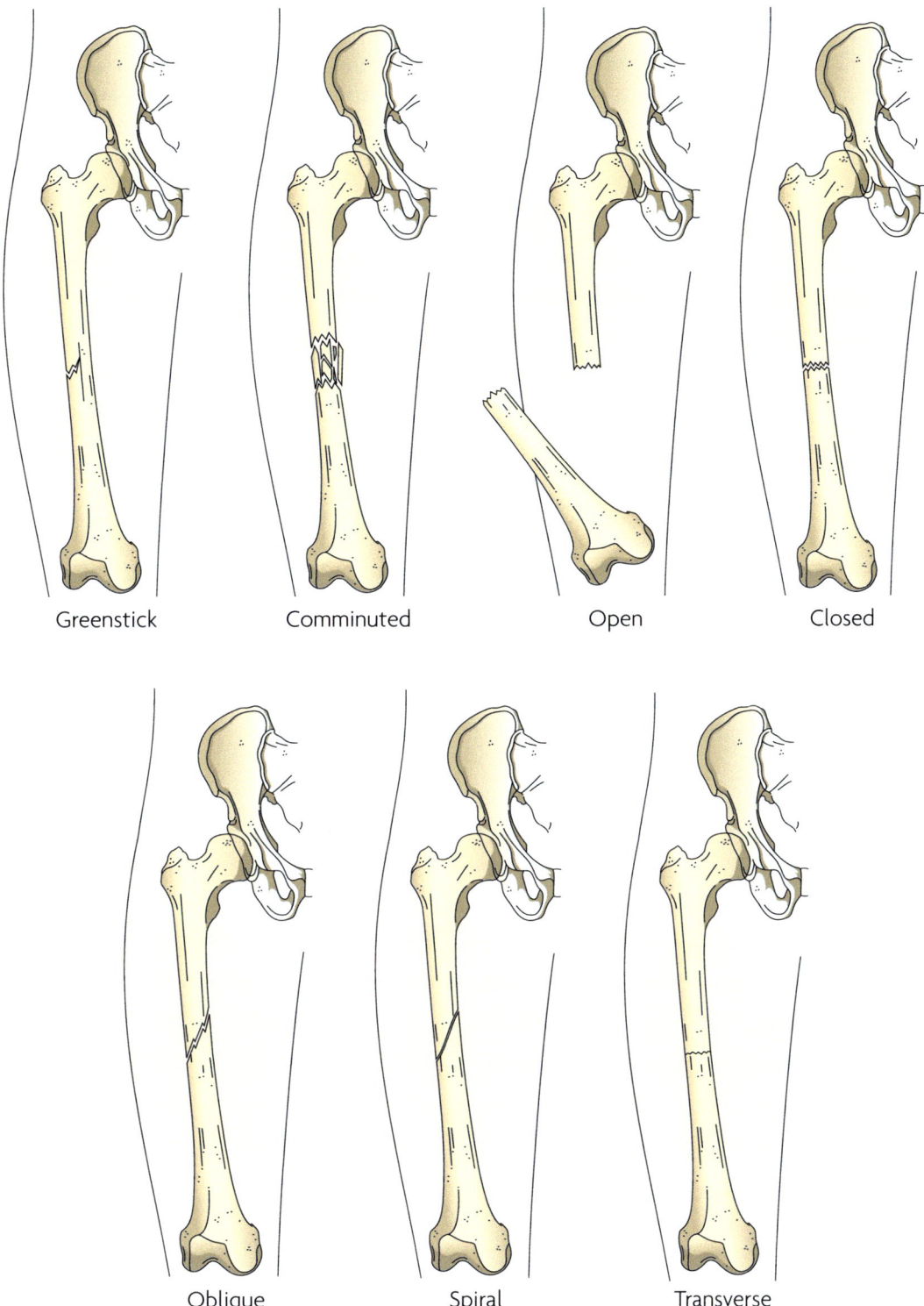

Figure 17.20 Types of fracture.

with a fracture (or fractures). Since joints are kept in place by soft tissues such as ligaments, these will have been injured for a dislocation to have occurred. Prompt reduction of the dislocation to its original anatomical position is required, following analgesia and/or a local anaesthetic or sedation. A competent clinician is required for this procedure.

The management of fractures and dislocations follows the standard primary and secondary survey for the trauma patient, but specifically consider:
- splinting the affected limb
- applying traction if the injury is an isolated shaft of femur fracture
- providing analgesia as these injuries can be very painful
- cover open fractures with a sterile dressing.

5.13.4 Fracture neck of femur

A fractured neck of femur (commonly referred to as a 'NOF'), also known as a fractured hip, is a very common injury in those aged over 65 (Figure 17.21). Around 65,000 people a year break their hip in the UK [NICE, 2017c] and it can have a huge impact on their future life. There is a 10% mortality at one month after injury and 30% at one year [Lisk, 2014]. The most common cause of a fractured hip is a fall from standing height and other conditions that make the bones weaker, such as osteoporosis, make it more likely for the injury to occur.

Signs and symptoms of a hip fracture include [NHS, 2016]:
- pain
- inability to lift, move or rotate the leg
- inability to stand or put weight on the leg
- a shorter leg on the injured side
- foot turning outwards on the injured side.

Treatment is the same as most other fractures including analgesia, immobilisation and conveying to hospital. Several hospitals now have direct 'NOF' pathways designed to support patients with hip fracture from the point they arrive in order to provide rapid diagnosis and treatment.

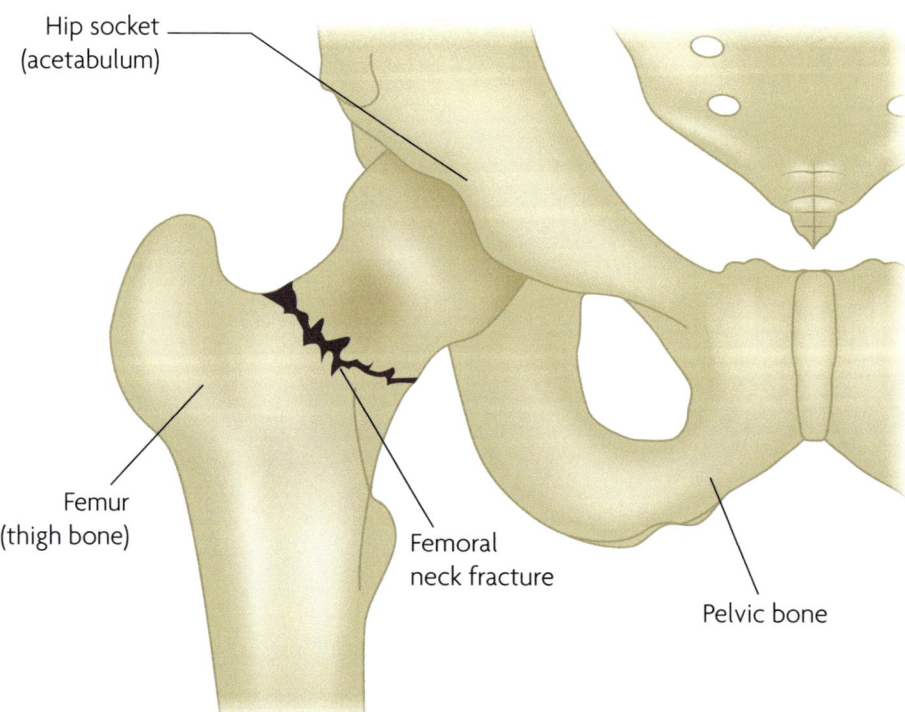

Figure 17.21 Fractured neck of femur.

5.13.5 Sprains and strains

Sprains are ligamental injuries that involve a partial or complete (depending on severity) tear of the ligament, whereas strains are tears in muscles. Their management is essentially the same [NICE, 2016h]:
- protect from further injury
- rest the injured limb
- ice wrapped in a damp towel should be applied to the injury for 15–20 minutes
- compress with a simple elastic bandage or elasticated tubular bandage, which should be snug, but not tight
- elevate the limb above the level of the heart.

6 Skeletal immobilisation

6.1 Learning objective

By the end of this section you will be able to:
- describe how to perform a range of skeletal immobilisation techniques.

6.2 Introduction

Skeletal immobilisation is an important skill to learn and remains a core concept in managing a large number of trauma patients. It has the following benefits when performed correctly [NAEMT, 2020; Greaves, 2019]:
- reduces pain
- reduces risk of further damage to soft tissues, nerves and blood vessels
- helps to control bleeding
- reduces risk of fat embolus.

In this section you will learn how to perform the following techniques and/or use the equipment listed:
- first-aid techniques
  - triangular bandages
- spinal immobilisation
  - manual methods
  - cervical collar application
  - crash helmet removal
  - orthopaedic (scoop) stretcher
- using splints:
  - box splint
  - vacuum splint
  - pelvic splint
  - traction splint.

6.3 First-aid techniques

Effective splinting does not have to require expensive equipment, which may or may not be available. Sometimes, it is preferable to use basic first-aid methods, such as triangular bandaging for the management of upper limb injuries.

6.3.1 Triangular bandages

Triangular bandages have three main uses:
- folded as a broad- or narrow-fold bandage to immobilise and support a limb or to secure a splint or bulky dressing
- opened to form a sling
- folded into a pad and used as a dressing.

In the ambulance service, it is probably most commonly used to make a sling to hold an injured limb close to the body and take some of the weight of that limb to prevent pain. Usually, the arm sling is used for injuries at the elbow or below and the elevated sling for injuries above the elbow. However, there is little evidence to support the benefit of either technique over the other and it is acceptable to adopt the technique that is most comfortable for the patient [Gregory, 2010b].

Procedure – Arm sling

Take the following steps to apply an arm sling [SJA, SAA, BRC, 2016]:

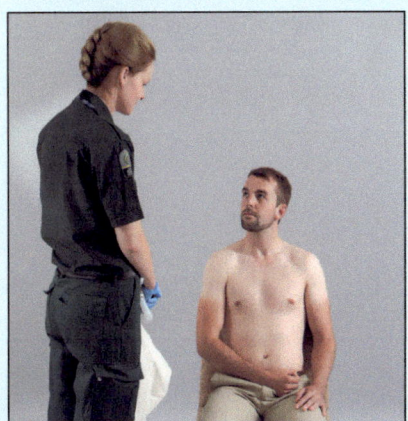

1. Explain the procedure to the patient and obtain valid consent. Provide analgesia as required to enable the sling to be applied. Prepare the triangular bandage.

Procedure – Arm sling – *cont*

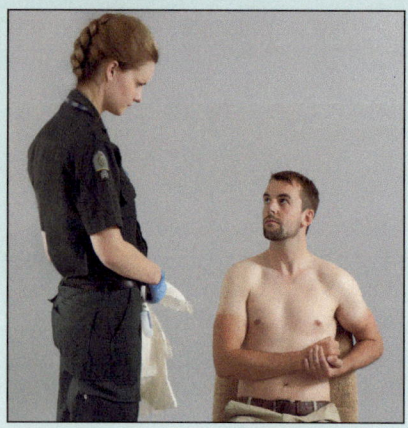

2. With the patient supporting their injured arm with the uninjured arm, ask them to flex the elbow to 90° if possible.

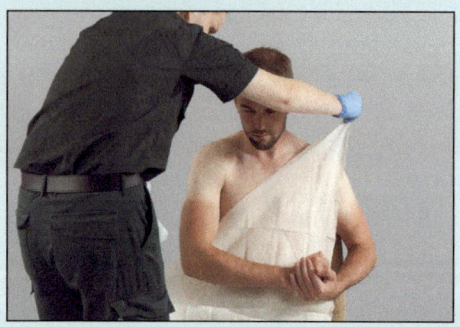

3. Slide the triangular bandage under the patient's arms so that the point is under the injured arm and the base (the long edge) is on the side of the uninjured arm.

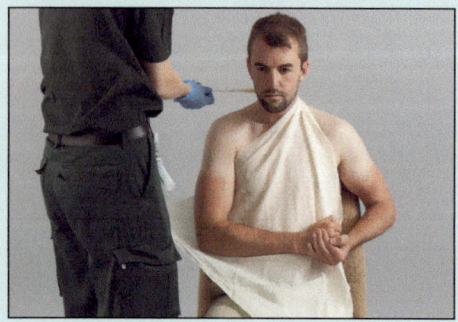

4. Slide the upper end of the triangular bandage around the neck towards the shoulder on the injured side.

Procedure – Arm sling – *cont*

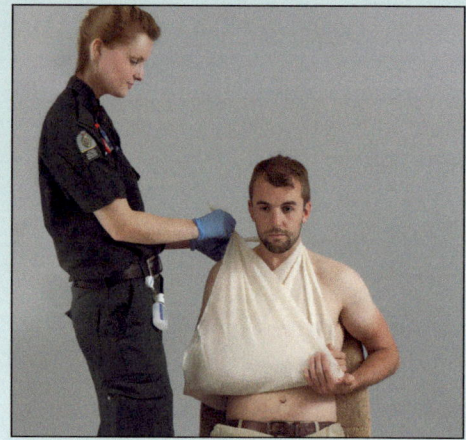

5. Fold the lower end of the bandage up over the forearm and bring it to meet the other end of the bandage at the shoulder.

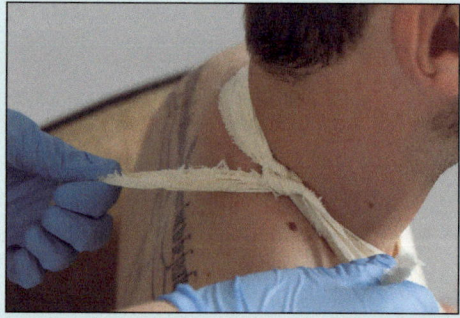

6. Tie the ends together using a reef knot. Consider applying a pad under the knot, if required.

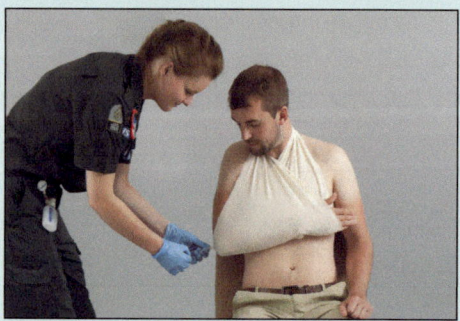

7. Holding the point of the bandage beyond the elbow, twist the point of the bandage until it fits the elbow snugly, then tuck it into the bandage. An alternative is to use tape or a safety pin.

Skeletal immobilisation

Procedure – Arm sling – *cont*

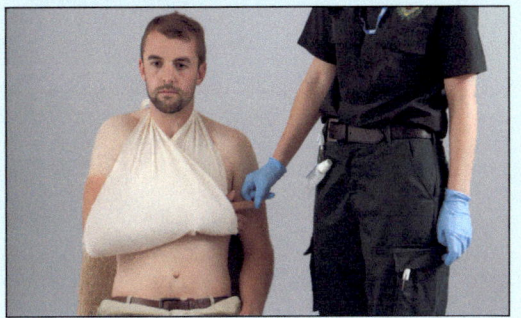

8. Re-check and record motor/sensory/circulation (MSC) function.

Procedure – Elevated sling

Take the following steps to apply an elevated arm sling [SJA, SAA, BRC, 2016; Gregory, 2010b]:

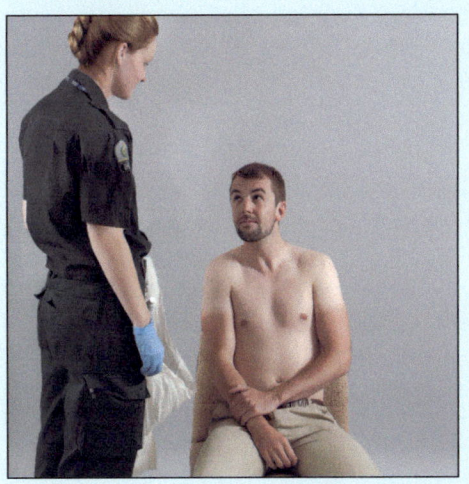

1. Explain the procedure to the patient and obtain valid consent. Provide analgesia as required to enable the sling to be applied. Prepare the triangular bandage.

Procedure – Elevated sling – *cont*

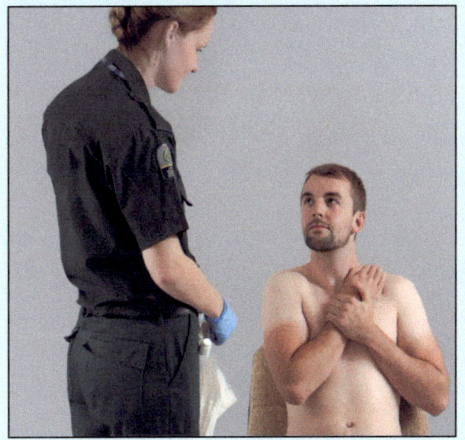

2. Ask the patient to support their injured arm across their chest, with the fingers of the injured arm resting on the opposite shoulder.

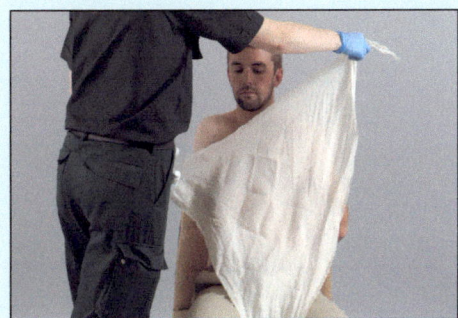

3. Place the sling over the injured arm so that the point of the bandage lies just beyond the elbow.

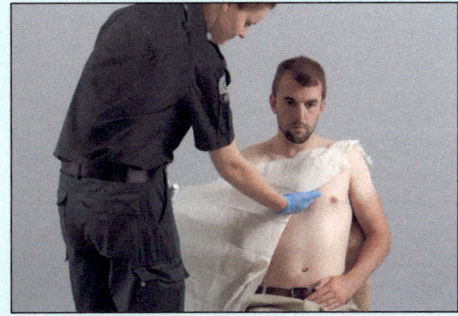

4. Ask the patient to let go of their injured arm. Tuck the base of the bandage under their lower arm.

Procedure – Elevated sling – cont

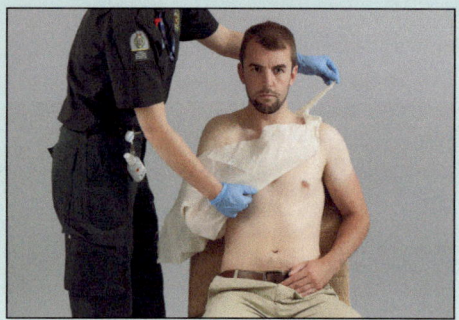

5. Bring the lower end of the bandage up diagonally across the patient's back to meet the other end at the shoulder.

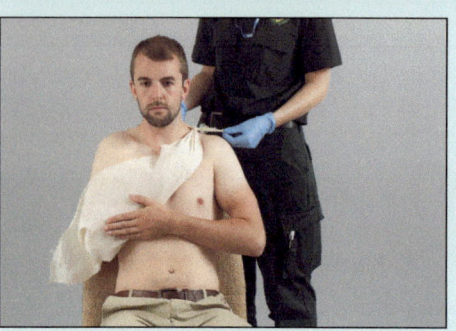

6. Tie the ends together using a reef knot. Consider applying a pad under the knot, if required.

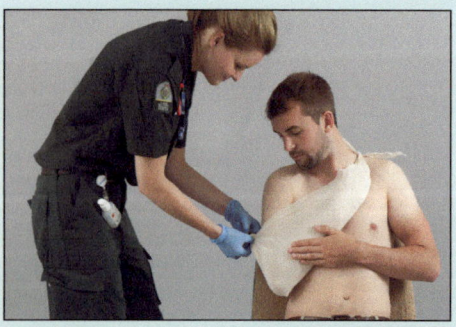

7. Holding the point of the bandage beyond the elbow, twist the bandage until it fits the elbow snugly, then tuck it into the bandage. An alternative is to use tape or a safety pin.

Procedure – Elevated sling – cont

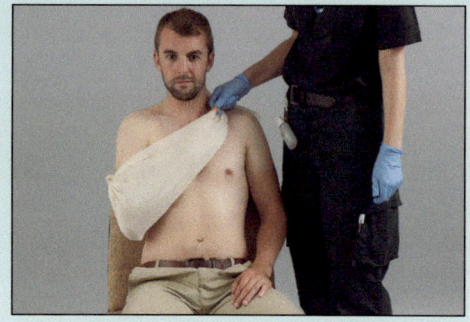

8. Re-check and record motor/sensory/circulation (MSC) function.

6.4 Spinal immobilisation

All patients with the possibility of spinal injury should have manual immobilisation commenced at the earliest opportunity so long as doing so does not delay other life-saving interventions. As part of the assessment of the patient, the senior clinician will consider whether spinal immobilisation is required and if so come up with a plan to apply other forms of immobilisation [JRCALC, 2019].

6.4.1 Manual in-line stabilisation

Manual in-line stabilisation (MILS) with adequate back support is one of two acceptable methods of immobilisation. The other requires the use of several items of equipment [JRCALC, 2019]. Therefore, MILS will almost always be the first form of spinal immobilisation to be applied to a patient with a suspected spinal injury.

Procedure – Manual in-line stabilisation

Take the following steps to apply manual in-line stabilisation [NAEMT, 2020]:

1. Use appropriate PPE as required. Advise the patient not to move their head, explain that you are about to hold their head, and gain their consent if possible.

Skeletal immobilisation

Procedure – Manual in-line stabilisation – *cont*

2. If the patient is supine (lying on their back) either kneel or lie on the ground behind the patient's head. If seated, move behind the patient. Hold the head firmly with both hands. Support the lower jaw with your fingers and support the head with your palms. Try to rest your lower arms on a surface (such as the ground or the back of a seat) as maintaining MILS can be tiring (Figure 17.22).

3. If the patient's head is not facing forwards and the patient is conscious, ask them to slowly move their head into a neutral, in-line position (eyes looking straight ahead and nose in line with umbilicus). If the patient is unconscious, gently move the head into a neutral position. In all patients, if there is any pain or resistance to this manoeuvre, stop immediately.

4. Do not let go until instructed to do so by a clinician.

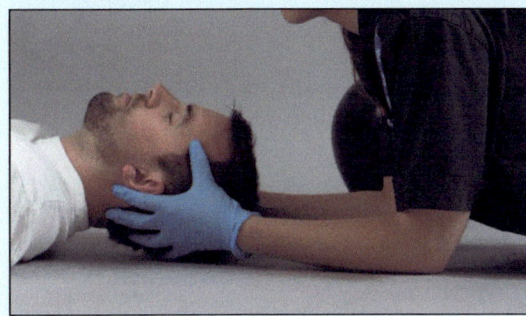

Figure 17.22 Manual in-line stabilisation.

6.4.2 Cervical collars

The most important thing to know about cervical (semi-rigid) collars is that they do not fully immobilise the cervical spine [NAEMT, 2020; Connor, 2013]. Until head blocks and a back support are in place, manual in-line stabilisation must be maintained. The evidence for the benefit of collars is uncertain and in some places their use is becoming less common, though you should still be familiar with the technique for those situations where you are asked to assist in applying one.

Procedure – In the sitting position – Ambu® Perfit adjustable collar for extrication (ACE)

Take the following steps to apply a cervical collar when the patient is in a sitting position [Ambu, 2011]:

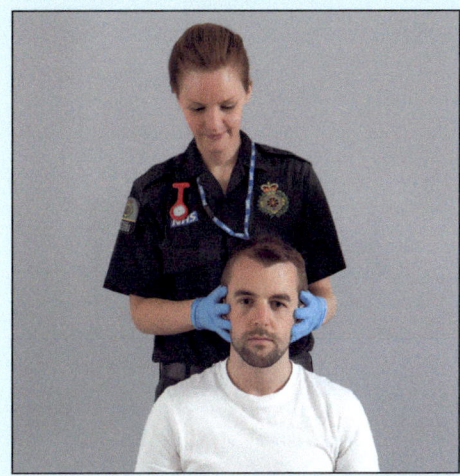

1. Use appropriate PPE as required. Inform the patient and obtain consent, if possible. One crew member should maintain manual in-line stabilisation while the other prepares the collar.

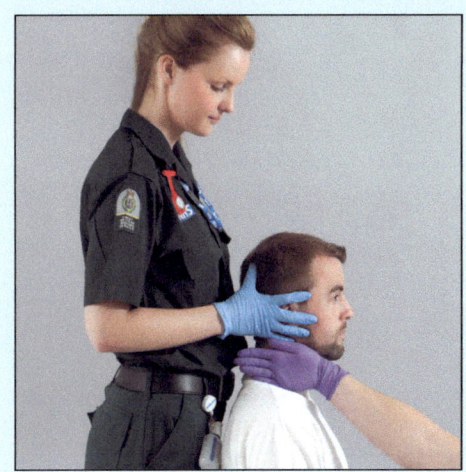

2. Ensuring the head is in a neutral position, size the collar by measuring the distance with your fingers between an imaginary line drawn horizontally and immediately below the patient's chin, and another immediately on top of the patient's shoulder.

Chapter 17 – *Trauma*

Procedure – In the sitting position – Ambu® Perfit adjustable collar for extrication (ACE) – *cont*

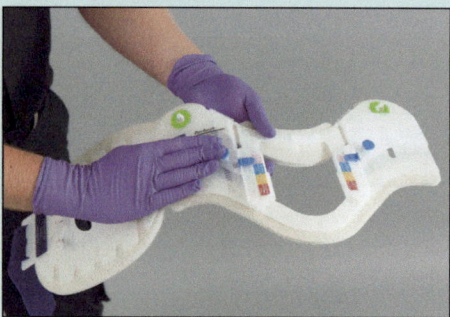

3. Compare this distance with the distance from the collar sizing line to the lower aspect of the plastic collar (NOT the foam).

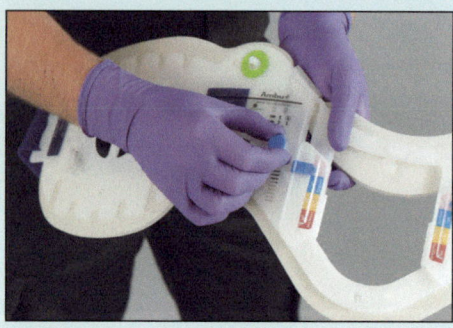

4. The Ambu® Perfit ACE collar is preset to size 3. If a larger size collar is needed, disengage the safety locks by pulling UP on the buttons.

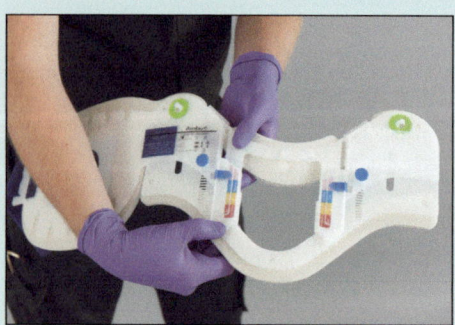

5. Adjust the collar to the correct size. There are 16 ratchet settings: simply pull the collar apart until the distance between the sizing line and the plastic collar body is the same as your finger measurement in step 2.

Procedure – In the sitting position – Ambu® Perfit adjustable collar for extrication (ACE) – *cont*

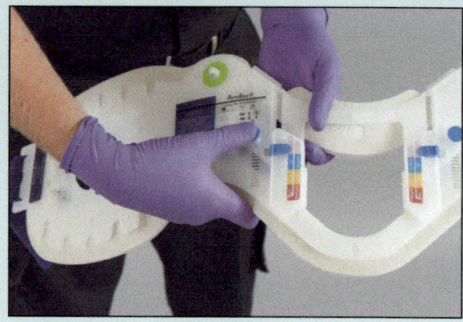

6. Engage the safety locks by pushing DOWN on the safety buttons.

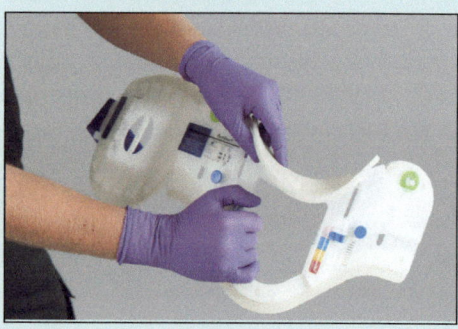

7. Assemble the collar by holding it near the tracheal opening and flip over the chin piece from the back of the collar to the front.

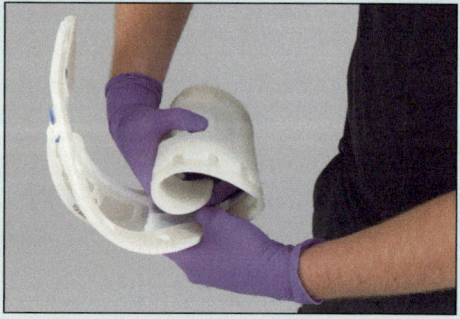

8. Preform the collar.

Skeletal immobilisation

Procedure – In the sitting position – Ambu® Perfit adjustable collar for extrication (ACE) – *cont*

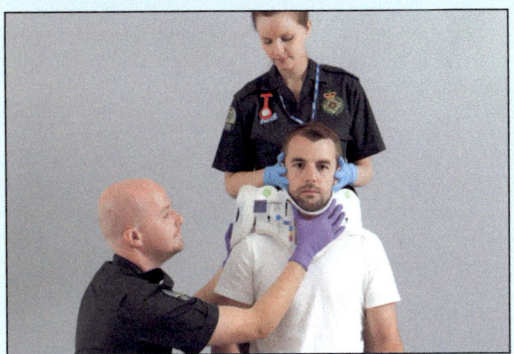

9. Slide the front of the collar along the patient's chest and position the chin piece so that the chin is supported. The collar body should rest on top of the patient's shoulder and against the sternum without gaps. The patient should remain in neutral alignment.

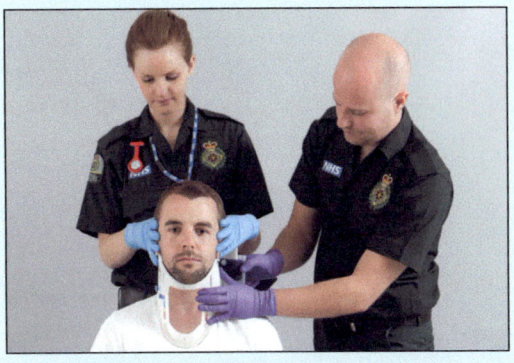

10. While holding the front of the collar in place, wrap the back of the collar around the back of the patient's head and neck and secure to the front of the collar with the Velcro tab. Maintain MILS.

Procedure – In the supine position – Ambu® Perfit adjustable collar for extrication (ACE)

Take the following steps to apply a cervical collar when the patient is in a supine position [Ambu, 2011]:

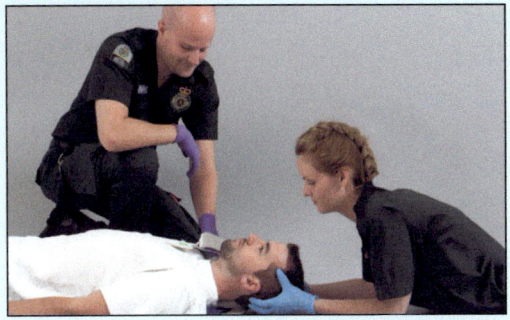

1. Follow steps 1 to 9 above. Slide the back portion of the collar directly behind the patient's neck until the Velcro can be seen on the opposite side of the patient's neck.

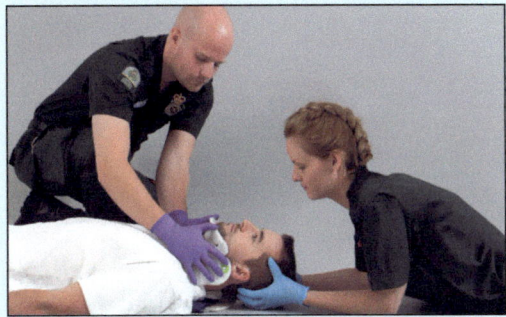

2. Position the chin piece under the chin.

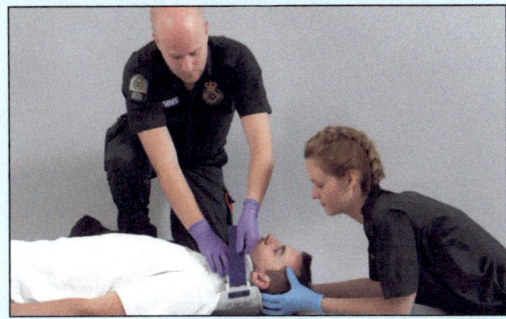

3. While maintaining proper positioning of the front of the collar with one hand, attach the Velcro with your other hand, to form a snug fit. Maintain MILS.

Chapter 17 – Trauma

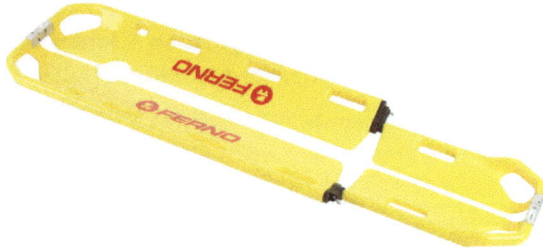

Figure 17.23 Orthopaedic stretcher.

6.4.3 Orthopaedic (scoop) stretcher

Orthopaedic stretchers (Figure 17.23) are the preferred tool to immobilise and transport patients who require spinal immobilisation [JRCALC, 2019]. This results in less movement of the spine while placing the patient onto the device, compared to the extrication board, and is also more comfortable [Krell, 2006].

Procedure – To apply the orthopaedic stretcher

Take the following steps to apply the orthopaedic stretcher [Ferno, 2006]:

1. Explain the procedure and obtain the patient's valid consent, if possible. In major trauma, you should remove the patient's clothes ('skin to scoop') and maintain in-line stabilisation (MILS). Assess distal motor, sensation and circulatory (MSC) function in each extremity. Apply a cervical collar if requested to do so.

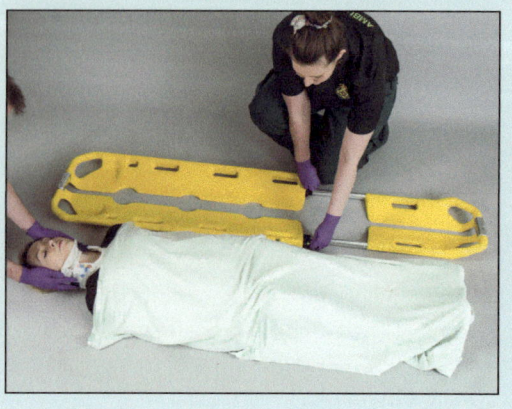

Procedure – To apply the orthopaedic stretcher – *cont*

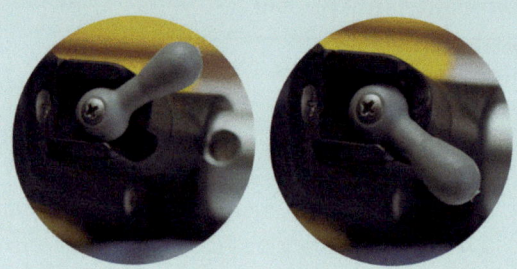

2. Adjust the length of the stretcher before uncoupling the halves. This ensures equal adjustment to both halves:
   - Move the lock-pin lever on each side of the frame to the unlocked position.
   - Pull the foot section outward to the desired length, stopping near one of the locking positions located at the holes along the foot-section frame.
   - Return both lock-pin levers to the locked position.
   - Push or pull the foot section a little until it locks into place
   - Make sure both sides are securely locked.

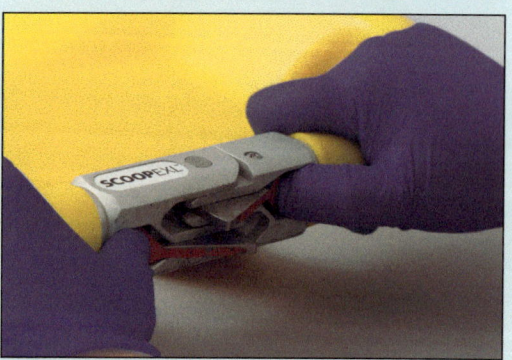

3. To separate the stretcher halves, unlock the Twin Safety Lock coupling by pressing both levers of the Twin Safety Lock and pull the coupling halves away from each other. Place one half on either side of the patient.

Skeletal immobilisation

Procedure – To apply the orthopaedic stretcher – *cont*

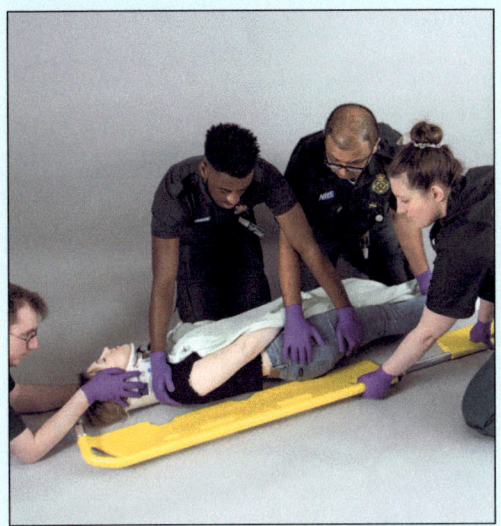

4. Gently insert each side of the orthopaedic stretcher under the patient. This may require a 10° tilt. If required and not already applied, then a pelvic binder should be inserted at this stage.

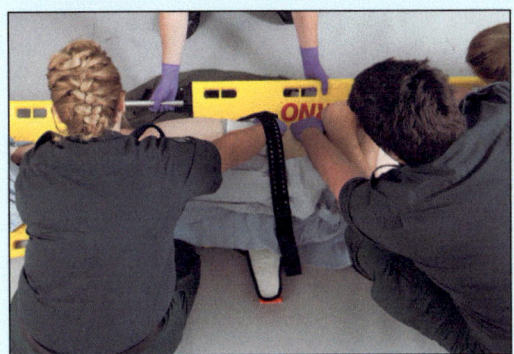

5. Return the patient to the supine position and repeat step 4 with the other half of the orthopaedic stretcher.
6. To rejoin the stretcher halves, align the right and left halves of the head and foot couplings and push them together until the Twin Safety Locks engage.

Procedure – To apply the orthopaedic stretcher – *cont*

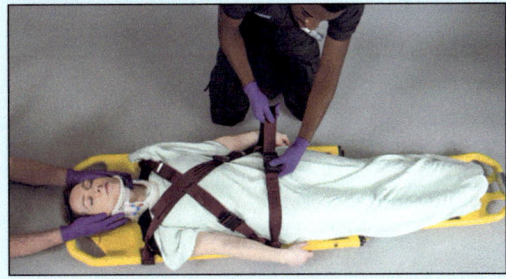

7. Secure the chest and hips with belts. Note the belts cross on the chest and the buckles should be off the chest and towards the hips if possible.

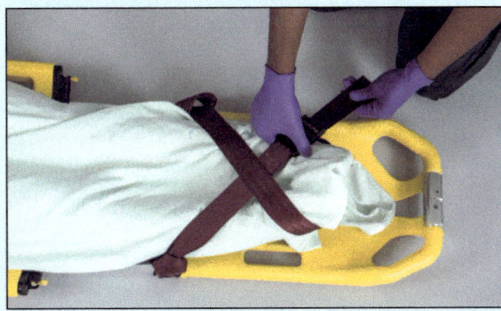

8. Secure the feet by wrapping the belt around the end of the feet in a figure of eight configuration.

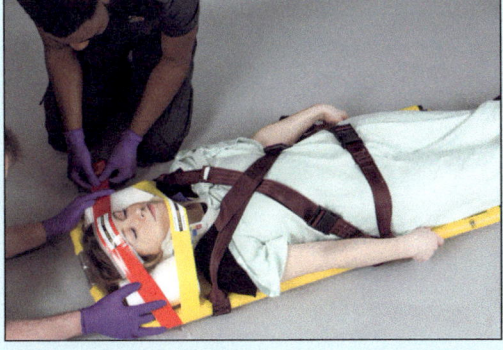

9. Immobile the head using a device designed for the purpose. Here a disposable device is used.
10. If the patient is more than 20 weeks pregnant, tilt the stretcher 15–30° to the left, or manually displace the uterus to the left.

6.4.4 Extrication board

Long extrication/extrication boards should only be used as an extrication device. Supine patients should be placed on an orthopaedic stretcher or vacuum mattress [Connor, 2013].

In the event that you need to use an extrication board to extricate a patient at a road traffic collision, you will be directed on what to do by a senior clinician. You should have received some training in extrication techniques and working with the Fire and Rescue Services as part of your core training.

6.4.5 Crash helmet removal

Patients who are wearing crash helmets need to have them removed in order to assess and manage their airway and ventilation. In addition, hidden bleeding at the back of the head can be identified and the head moved into a position of neutral alignment. Note that some degree of spinal motion will occur, even in optimal circumstances [NAEMT, 2020].

> **Procedure – Crash helmet removal**
>
> **Note:** Unless immediate airway intervention is required, a single rescuer should not attempt helmet removal [NAEMT, 2020].
>
> Take the following steps to remove a crash helmet [NAEMT 2020; QAS, 2018b]:
>
>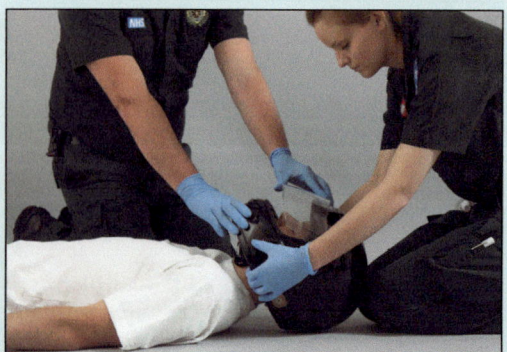
>
> 1. Explain the procedure and obtain the patient's valid consent, if possible. Rescuer one should position themselves above the patient's head. Their palms should be pressed on the sides of the helmet and

> **Procedure – Crash helmet removal –** *cont*
>
> fingertips curled underneath. The helmet, head and neck should be maintained in as near to an in-line neutral position as possible. Rescuer two should remove the face shield, glasses (if worn) and chin strap.
>
>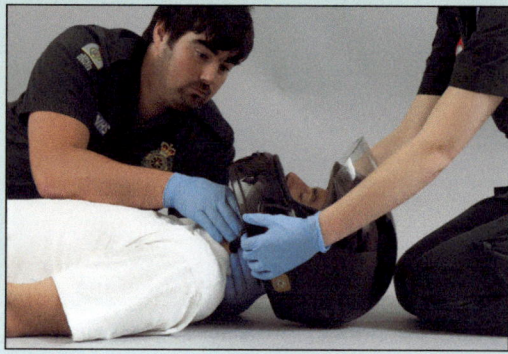
>
> 2. Rescuer two should move their thumb and first two fingers up to support the mandible. Their other hand should be placed behind the head at the back of the helmet. From this position, they can provide manual in-line stabilisation to keep the head and neck still.
>
>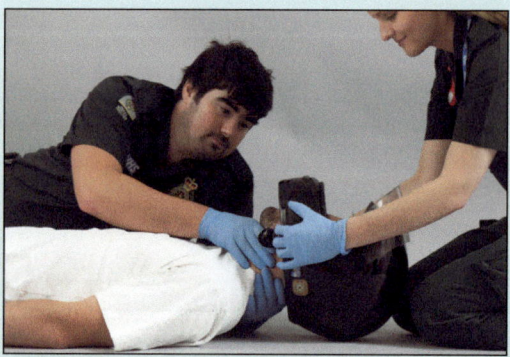
>
> 3. Rescuer one pulls the side of the helmet slightly apart and gently tilts the helmet up and down while applying traction to remove the helmet. This should be slow and deliberate. Take care as the helmet clears the patient's nose.

Skeletal immobilisation

Procedure – Crash helmet removal – *cont*

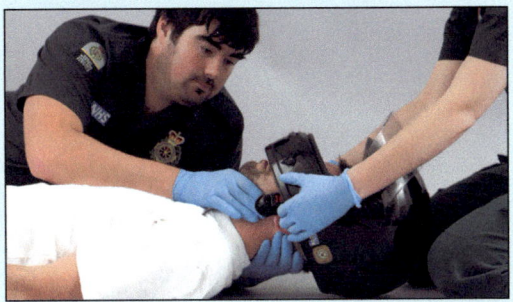

4. Once the helmet has reached the halfway point, rescuer one should stop moving the helmet, while rescuer two repositions their hands from the back of the helmet to the occiput. Take care, the head is heavy!

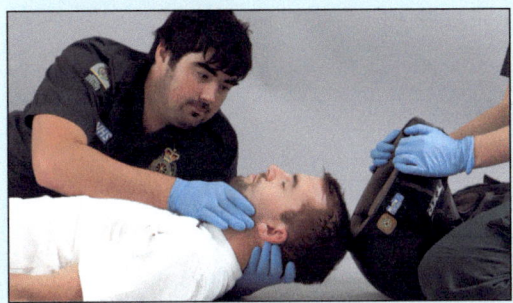

5. Once rescuer two has repositioned their hands and has control of the patient's head, rescuer one should continue to remove the helmet.

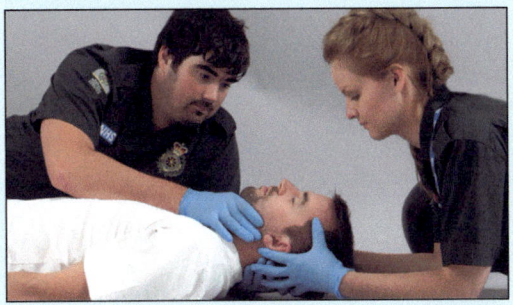

6. Rescuer one should reapply MILS and together rescuer one and two should lower the head into a neutral alignment position. This may require a small amount of padding to be placed under the occiput of the head.

Procedure – Crash helmet removal – *cont*

7. Be aware that the manufacture of helmets often design them in order to be easily removed by the emergency services. This includes being able to remove parts of the padding before removing the helmet, making it easier to slip off. Look out for obvious markings or instructions on the helmet or any such devices before removing them.

6.5 Splints

Splinting forms an important part of fracture management, particularly in the lower limbs. The benefits of splintage include reducing [Greaves, 2019]:
- pain
- blood loss
- pressure on skin
- pressure on adjacent neurovascular structures
- risk of fat embolism
- risk of further damage
- risk of infection if the fracture is open.

Basic principles of immobilisation should consist of assessment and reassessment of the neurovascular status before and after any manipulation or handling of the fracture, and immobilisation of the joints above and below the fracture.

Note: It is not possible to show the application of every type of splinting device in this text. Instead, a selection of commonly used devices is explained. This is not a substitute for hands-on training with your service's splints.

6.5.1 Box splints

Box splints are simple devices that are most commonly used for lower leg fractures (Figure 17.24). They are only suitable for the immobilisation of straight limbs as they will not conform to the shape of deformed limbs [Gregory, 2010b].

Chapter 17 – *Trauma*

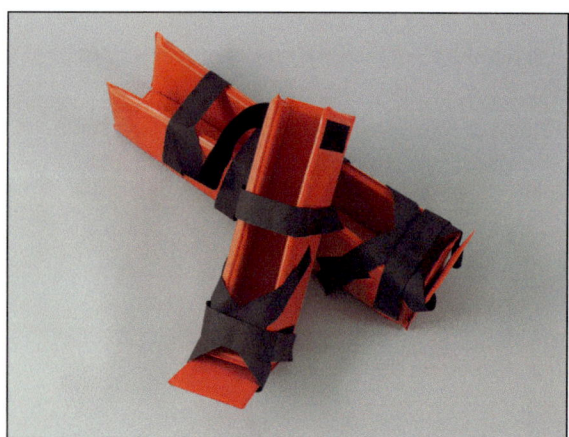

Figure 17.24 A box splint.

Procedure – To apply a box splint

Take the following steps to apply a box splint [EEAST, 2014; Gregory, 2010b]:

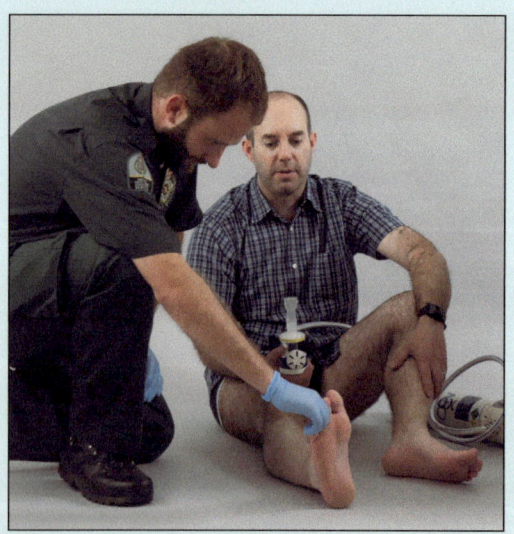

1. Gain the patient's valid consent. Provide analgesia if required prior to the procedure. Ensure the splint is clean and undamaged. Check motor/sensory/circulation (MSC) function.

Procedure – To apply a box splint – *cont*

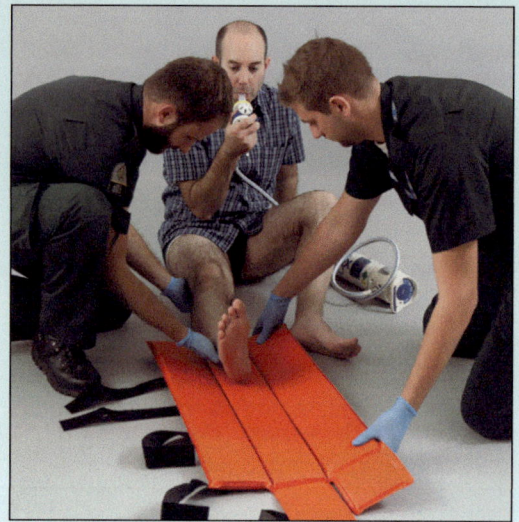

2. Expose the injured limb and remove footwear where possible. Support the limb manually and raise it carefully while the splint is passed under it.

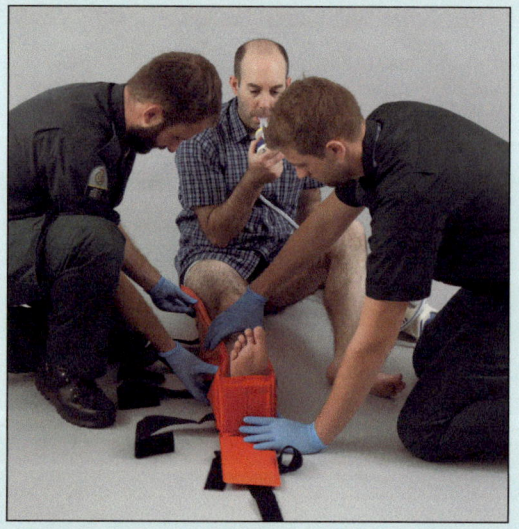

3. Fold the two sides of the splint around the limb to form a box to support the limb.

Skeletal immobilisation

Procedure – To apply a box splint – *cont*

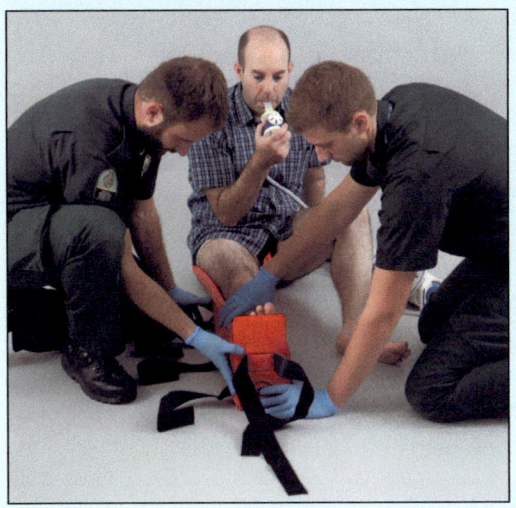

4. Ensure the foot piece is placed against the sole of the foot at 90° or in a position comfortable for the patient.

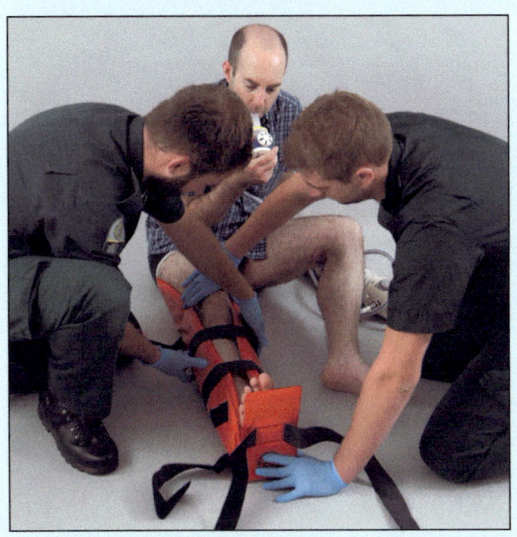

5. The Velcro straps should be carefully placed over the limb, avoiding the area of injury. The foot strap should be passed over the top of the foot.

Procedure – To apply a box splint – *cont*

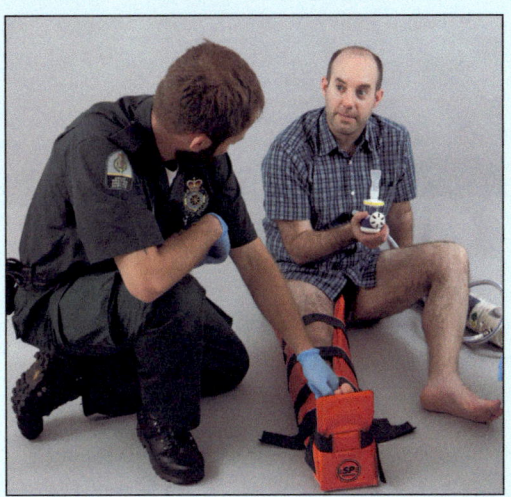

6. Re-check MSC function of the limb after application of the box splint.

6.5.2 Vacuum splints

Vacuum splints are made from a case of conformable plastic filled with small polystyrene beads. When air is in the splint, these beads are free to move around, but once the air has been vacuumed out the splint becomes hard and stays in the shape it has created. The advantage of vacuum splints is that they can be conformed to the shape of the patient's limb, which makes them more comfortable for the patient and results in less movement.

Procedure – To apply a vacuum splint

Take the following steps to apply a vacuum splint [Hartwell, 2016]:

1. Gain the patient's valid consent. Provide analgesia if required prior to the procedure. Ensure the splint is clean and undamaged.

2. Ensure the limb is exposed, any wounds have been dressed and check motor, sensory and circulation (MSC) function.

Chapter 17 – Trauma

Procedure – To apply a vacuum splint – *cont*

3. The correct size splint should be large enough to immobilise a joint above and below the suspected injury (the photos below show a suspected foot fracture).

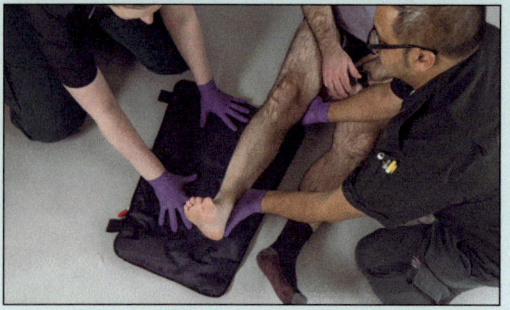

4. Support the limb manually and raise it carefully while the splint is passed under it.

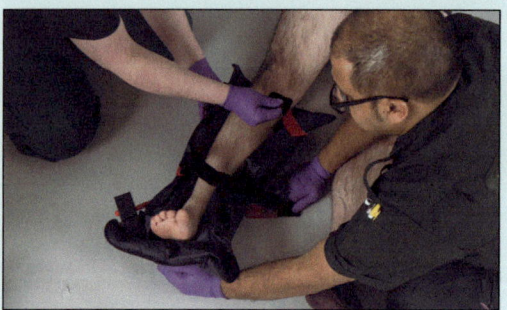

5. Conform the splint around the patient's leg so that the polystyrene balls inside take up any gaps. Once a good shape has been achieved the straps can be loosely placed to help hold the splint in position if needed.

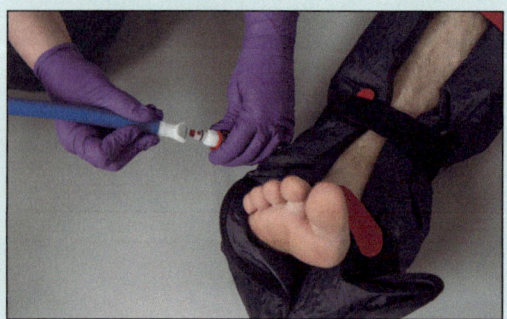

6. Once in position, the pump should be connected to the air valve on the splint. To do this, remove the red cap and push the

Procedure – To apply a vacuum splint – *cont*

valve and pump connectors together until a click is heard.

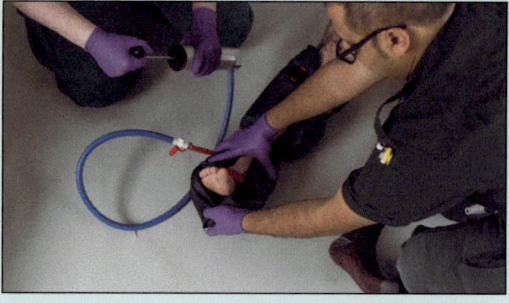

7. Suck the air out of the splint using the pump. Whilst this is happening another person should be confirming the splint around the suspected fracture site.

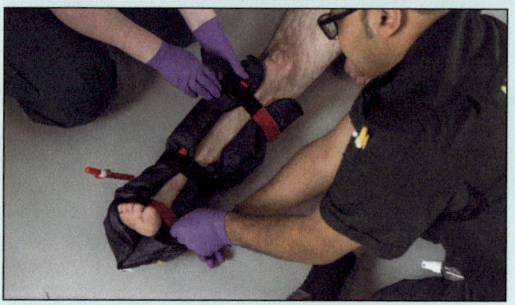

8. When all of the air has been removed, the splint can be released, and the straps tightened to apply slight tension. The splint should then be firm and prevent the limb from moving. Before moving the patient, you should recheck MSC function.

6.5.3 Pelvic splints

Serious pelvic fractures are associated with a high risk of death due to internal bleeding [Vaidya, 2016]. Commercial pelvic splints (commonly called pelvic binders) have been shown to reduce stable, 'open book' and rotational and vertically unstable fractures adequately (Figure 17.25), with no significant displacement of fractures, irrespective of device [Knops, 2011]. That said, there is no conclusive evidence that the use of pelvic binders reduces morbidity or mortality from serious trauma either [Stewart, 2013]. Despite this, their early

Skeletal immobilisation

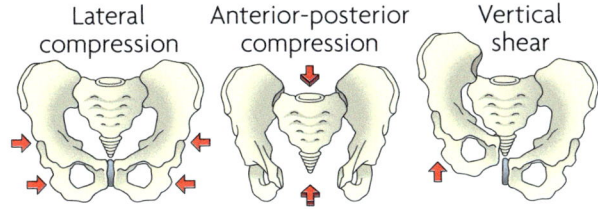

Figure 17.25 Types of pelvic fracture. The red arrows indicate the direction of the force.

application in suspected serious pelvic trauma with internal bleeding is recommended as a method for stabilising the fracture and helping to reduce further blood loss [NICE, 2017d]. Ultimately it will be the decision of the senior clinician at scene as to whether a patient requires a binder.

You will remember that earlier in this chapter we discussed how common it is for pelvic binders to be applied in the wrong place (normally too high), so be careful to get your landmarks right when applying a binder.

There is currently no reason to recommend one device over another, though two devices, the SAM pelvic sling and T-POD device have the most available evidence [Scott, 2013], both of which are covered below.

Procedure – To apply a SAM pelvic sling II

Take the following steps to apply the SAM pelvic sling II [SAM, 2019; Greaves, 2019]:

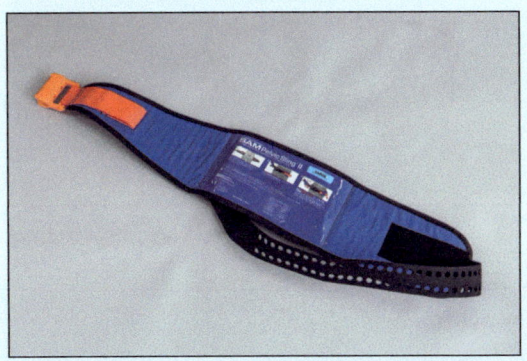

1. Use appropriate PPE as required. Inform the patient and obtain consent, if possible.

Procedure – To apply a SAM pelvic sling II – *cont*

Choose the correct size (three available) and prepare the SAM splint. Fully expose the patient as the splint needs to be placed directly on the patient's skin, which includes removing underwear. Cover the patient to preserve their dignity and prevent heat loss.

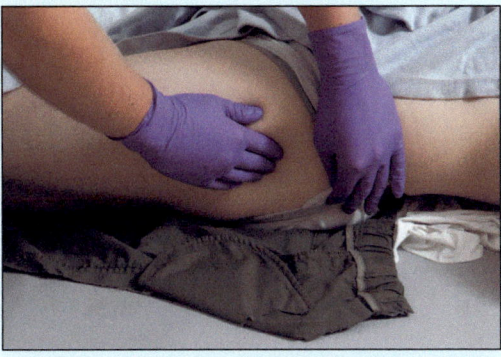

2. Identify the level of the greater trochanters.

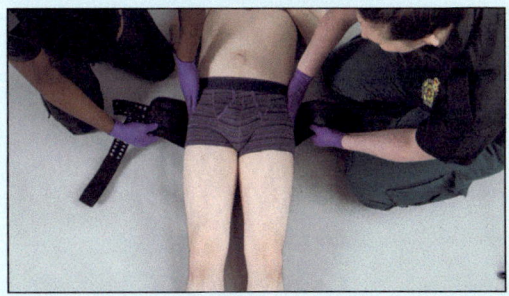

3. Insert the splint under the legs and move up into position so that the buckle is at the level of the greater trochanters. Ensure this is equal on both sides.

Chapter 17 – Trauma

Procedure – To apply a SAM pelvic sling II – *cont*

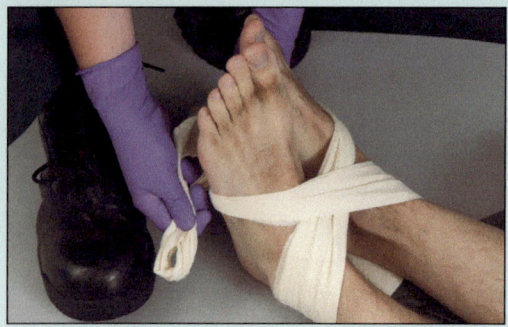

4. As long as there are no lower limb fractures, tie the patient's feet together in a figure of eight using a sling prior to securing the splint.

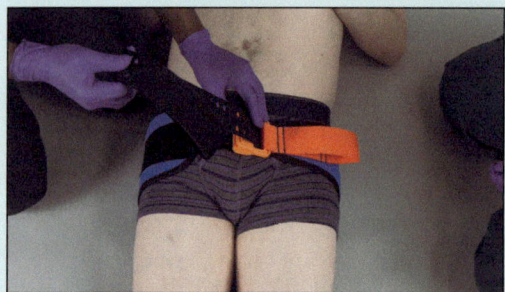

5. Place the black strap through the orange buckle and pull completely through.

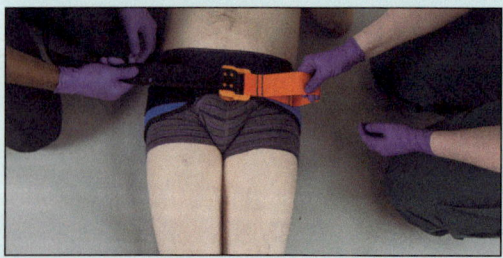

6. With someone else securing the orange strap, pull the black strap in the opposite direction until you hear and feel the buckle click. Maintain tension and immediately press the black strap onto the surface of the SAM splint to secure. You may hear a second click as the sling secures.

7. Re-cover the patient to maintain dignity and minimise heat loss.

Procedure – To apply a T-POD Device

Take the following steps to apply the T-POD Device [PYNG Medical, 2014; Greaves, 2019]:

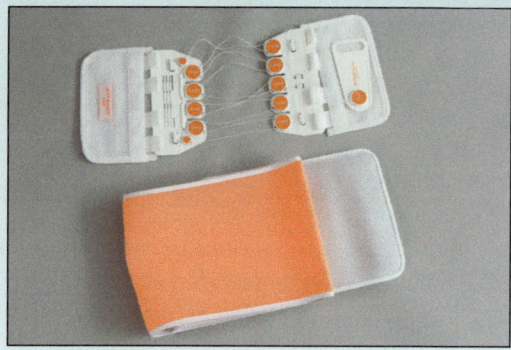

1. Use appropriate PPE as required. Inform the patient and obtain consent, if possible. Open the T-POD and get the belt and pulley system ready. Fully expose the patient as the splint needs to be placed directly on the patient's skin. Cover the patient to preserve their dignity and prevent heat loss.

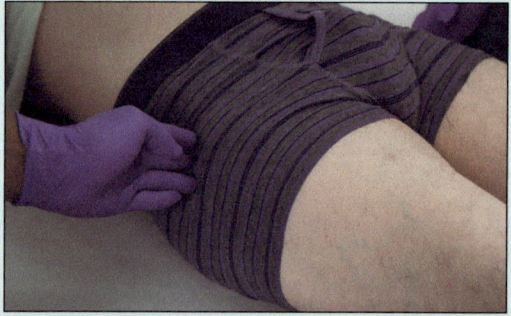

2. Identify the level of the greater trochanters.

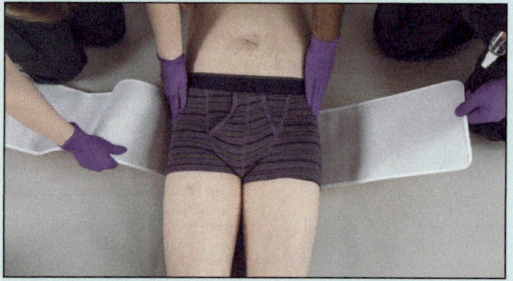

3. Place the belt under the patient so that the centre of the belt is at the level of the greater trochanters. The belt should be white side towards the patient.

Skeletal immobilisation

Procedure – To apply a T-POD Device – *cont*

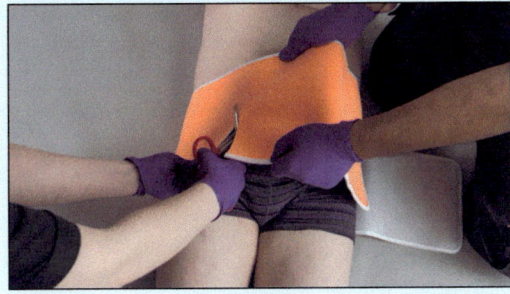

4. Trim the belt with shears, leaving a gap of approximately 15–20 cm over the centre of the pelvis. Do not fold the excess back towards the patient.

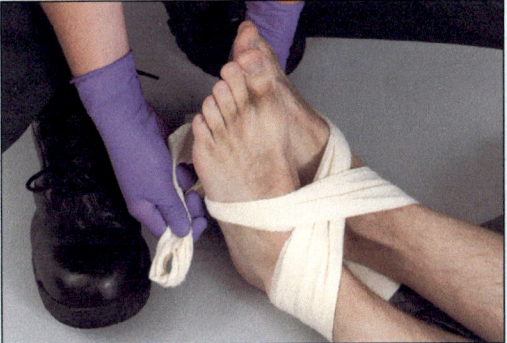

5. As long as there are no lower limb fractures, tie the patient's feet together prior to securing the splint.

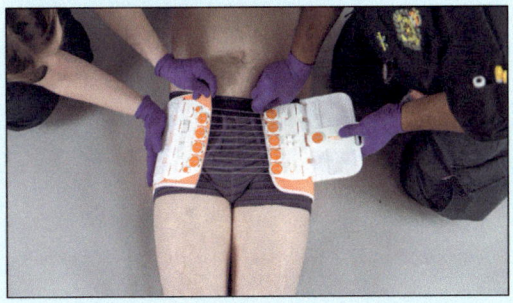

6. Apply the Velcro-backed pulley system to each side of the trimmed belt.

Procedure – To apply a T-POD Device – *cont*

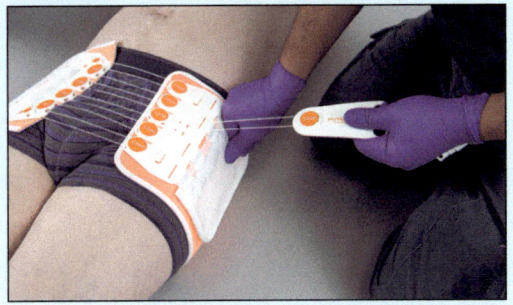

7. Place padding under the drawstring to avoid trapping skin/genitals. Gently draw tension on the pull tab to create circumferential pressure.

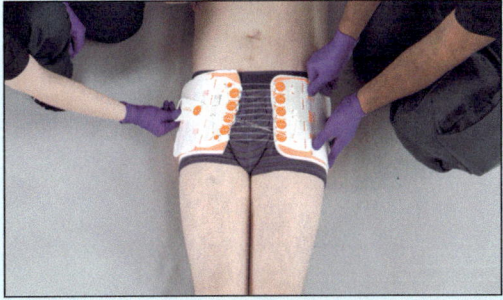

8. Secure the cord to the hooks and Velcro the pull tab to the belt.

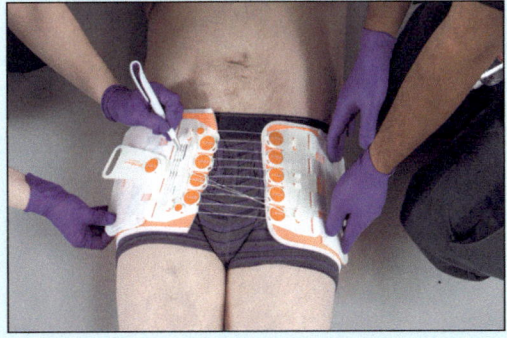

9. Record the date and time on the space provided on the pulley system.
10. Re-cover the patient to maintain dignity and minimise heat loss.

6.5.4 Traction splint

Traction splints apply longitudinal force to long bones (normally the femur). Correctly splinting the femur using this method helps to reduce [JRCALC, 2019]:
- pain
- haemorrhage and damage to blood vessels and nerves
- movement of bone fragments and the risk of a closed fracture becoming an open fracture
- the risk of a fat embolus
- muscle spasm.

Indication
- Suspected fracture of the femoral shaft.

Contra-indications [NAEMT, 2020]
- Suspected pelvic fractures (except the Kendrick Traction Device).
- Suspected femoral neck fracture.
- Avulsion or amputation of ankle and foot.
- Fractures close to, or below, the knee.
- Dislocated knee (not just patella).

Procedure – To apply a Kendrick Traction Device (KTD)

Take the following steps to apply the KTD or similar traction splints [Prometheus Medical, 2018]:

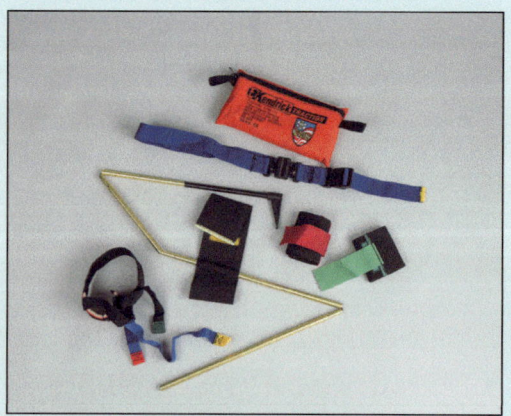

1. Use appropriate PPE as required. Inform the patient and obtain consent, if possible.

Procedure – To apply a Kendrick Traction Device (KTD) – *cont*

Remove the patient's shoes and clothing to expose the injured leg. Check motor, sensation and circulation (MSC) function below the injury. Prepare the splint.

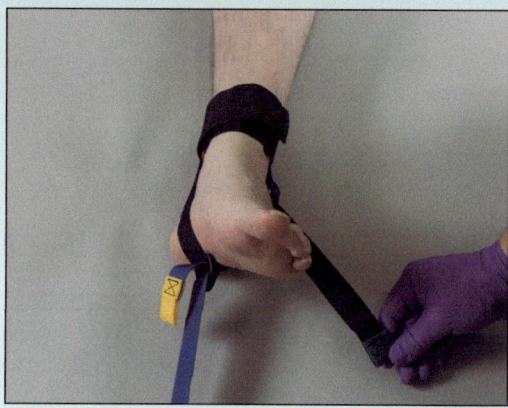

2. Apply the ankle hitch around the injured leg, just above the anklebone, and tighten the stirrup by pulling the green tabbed strip until snug under the heel.

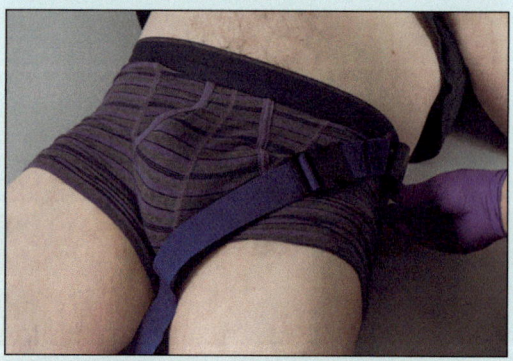

3. Apply the upper thigh strap by sliding the male buckle under the knee, 'see-saw' the strap upwards until it rests in the crotch area and click the ends together. Tighten the strap until the traction pole receptacle is positioned at approximately the level of the belt. Make sure male genitals are clear of the strap.

Procedure – To apply a Kendrick Traction Device (KTD) – *cont*

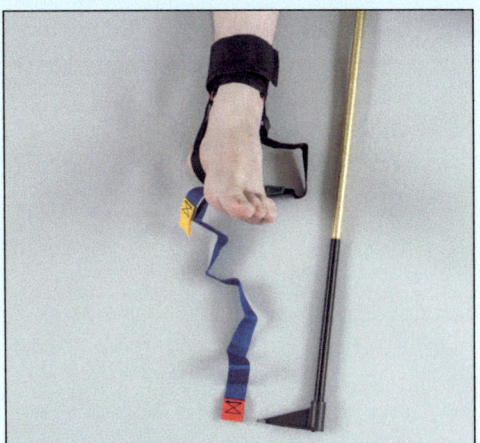

4. Snap out the traction pole, ensuring each joint is securely seated. Place the traction pole alongside the leg so that one section extends below the foot.

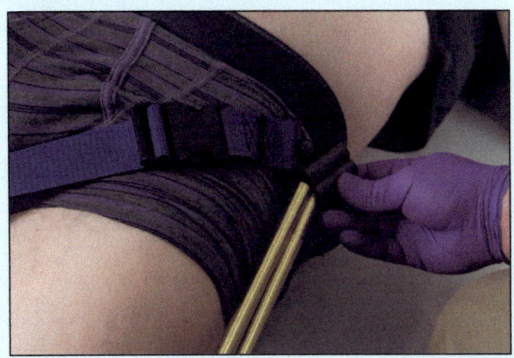

5. Adjust the length of the pole and place the ends into the traction pole receptacle.

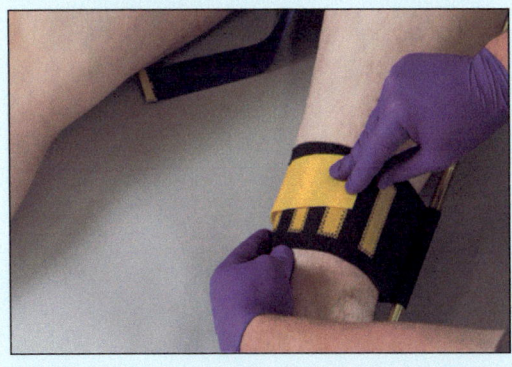

6. Secure the elastic strap around the knee.

Procedure – To apply a Kendrick Traction Device (KTD) – *cont*

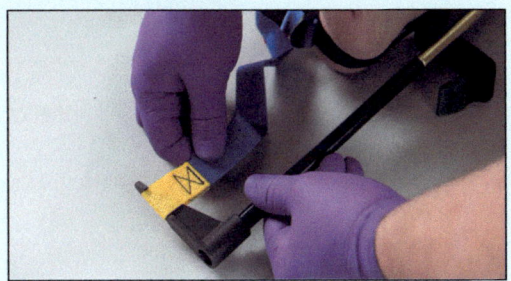

7. Place the yellow tab over the dart end.

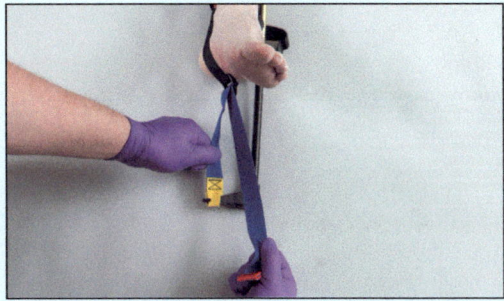

8. Apply traction by pulling on the red tab. As a guide, apply around 10% of body weight (up to 7 kg) tension. Use patient comfort as the main objective. Traction can be applied smoothly by grasping the strap either side of the buckle and simultaneously feeding and pulling with equal pressure.

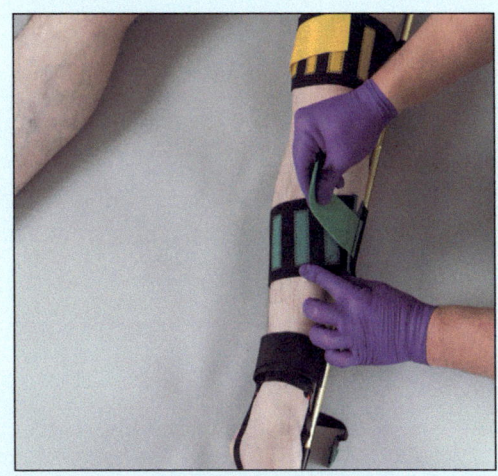

9. Finish packaging by applying upper and lower straps. Re-check and record MSC function.

7 Burns

7.1 Learning objectives

By the end of this section you will be able to:
- explain what is meant by the term 'burn'
- describe the types of burn and their causes
- explain the safety considerations when dealing with burns
- state the rules associated with estimating the size of burns
- explain time-critical factors that affect the management of burns
- explain the complications associated with burns
- explain the treatment of burns
- explain why burns patients are transported to definitive care.

7.2 Introduction

A burn is an injury caused by energy transfer to the body's tissues, causing necrosis and an associated inflammatory reaction [Greaves, 2008].

Approximately 130,000 people with burns injuries visit the ED each year in the UK, with approximately 10,000 being admitted to hospital [NHS England, 2013b]. In England and Wales, serious burn injury (defined as requiring at least a 72-hour stay in hospital) is responsible for 5.4% of all serious trauma [Kalson, 2012].

Burn injury most commonly occurs in the home (over 30%) with the kitchen being the favoured location. The most common sources of injury are [NBCG, 2008]:
- cup of tea in children
- petrol ignition in adults
- bathing, kettle spills and central heating radiators in elderly people.

Burns are commonly split into a number of types [JRCALC, 2019]:
- chemical
- cold
- electrical
- friction
- radiation
- thermal.

7.3 Assessment of burns

7.3.1 History

It is important to identify the mechanism, including the cause of the burn, how it came into contact with the patient and any first aid undertaken. Note when the injury occurred, how long the patient was exposed to the source and the duration of any cooling. Don't forget to be alert for signs of non-accidental injury.

7.3.2 Assessment

Pre-hospital estimation of total body surface area (TBSA) of burn injury is poor, with the 'rule of nines' (Figure 17.26) underestimating burns of less than 20% and overestimating burns over 40%; also, it is not suitable for children under 14 years of age [Hettiaratchy, 2004; JRCALC, 2019].

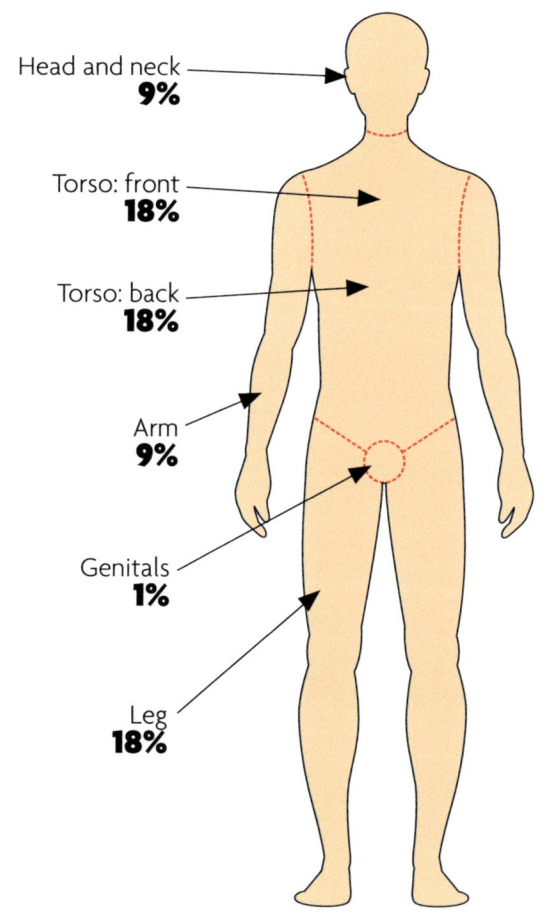

Figure 17.26 The 'rule of nines' in adults.

The whole hand (palm and fingers) represents about 0.82% TBSA in adults and 0.77% in children, making accurate calculations tricky. However, the palm alone is 0.5% TBSA [Muehlberger, 2010] and is suitable for estimating burns less than 15% or greater than 85% TBSA. Note that these methods will generally underestimate % TBSA in obese patients [Butz, 2015].

Lund and Browder charts are more accurate, but these are cumbersome to complete in the back of an ambulance. An alternative that has been advocated is serial halving [Allison, 2004]. This involves determining whether greater than or less than 50%, 25% and finally 12.5% of the TBSA is burnt. This approximation is sufficient to determine whether the patient requires referral to a burns unit (if direct access is an option) and the need for intravenous fluids. Erythema (reddening) should not be included when calculating TBSA of burn injury [Enoch, 2009].

A more novel way of calculating TBSA is by using apps, such as the Mersey Burns app, which allows you to shade in the amount of burn a patient has sustained and then calculates the TBSA for you, This technique is now recommended by NICE [2016g] and has been shown to be faster and more accurate when calculating TBSA and estimating patient fluid requirements [Barnes, 2015].

7.3.3 Classification

Although important for subsequent burns management, the depth of a burn does not affect pre-hospital treatment, but may provide some indication as to the cause (Table 17.5) [NZGG, 2007].

7.3.4 Burns requiring transport to hospital

The National Network for Burn Care (NNBC) has set out a suggested minimum threshold for patients who may require specialised burn care services. These patients will require transport to hospital [NNBC, 2012]:
- All burns > 2% TBSA in children or > 3% in adults.
- All full-thickness burns.

Table 17.5 Burns classification.

Classification	Other names	Example causes	Appearance	Sensation
Epidermal	Superficial, first degree	UV light, scalds	Dry and red, blanches with pressure, no blisters	May be painful
Superficial dermal	Superficial, partial thickness, second degree	Scald (spill or splash)	Pale pink, fine blisters, blanches with pressure	Very painful
Mid-dermal	Superficial, partial thickness, second degree	Scald (spill), flame	Dark pink with large blisters, delayed capillary refill	May be painful
Deep dermal	Deep, partial thickness, second degree	Scald (spill), flame	Blotchy red, may blister, no capillary refill	No sensation
Full thickness	Third degree	Scald (immersion), flame, steam, high-voltage electricity	White, waxy or charred, no blisters or capillary refill Children: dark lobster red with mottling	No sensation

Chapter 17 – Trauma

- All circumferential burns.
- Any burn not healed in two weeks.
- Any burn with suspicion of non-accidental injury.
- All burns to hands, feet, face, perineum or genitalia.
- Any chemical, electrical* or friction burn.
- Any cold injury.
- Any unwell/febrile child with a burn.

*May not apply to low (domestic) voltage injury.

7.4 Thermal burns
7.4.1 Pathophysiology

The most common type of thermal burns (sometimes referred to as thermal injuries) are flame, scald and contact. Flame burns are more common in adults and are often associated with smoke inhalation and other traumatic injuries. These are more likely to result in deep dermal or full-thickness burns.

Scalds are the most common cause of burn in children, usually due to spillages of hot drinks [Greaves, 2019]. They generally cause epidermal or superficial dermal burn injury [Hettiaratchy, 2004].

Direct contact burns are caused by brief contact with a very hot object, or (more commonly) prolonged contact with a cooler object. Typical patient groups include epileptics and those who misuse alcohol or drugs.

Irreversible damage to the epidermis can be caused by exposure to 44°C heat for six hours, or 65°C for one second [Moritz, 1947]. Burns injuries are characterised by a local response and, if the total body surface area (TBSA) burnt is greater than 20%, a systemic response [Greaves, 2008].

Local response
At skin level, burns form three zones of injury [Hettiaratchy, 2004] (Figure 17.27):
- **Zone of coagulation:** The point of maximal injury, with irreversible damage to tissue due to protein coagulation.
- **Zone of stasis:** Surrounds the zone of coagulation and is characterised by reduced tissue perfusion. Potentially salvageable with adequate resuscitation.
- **Zone of hyperaemia:** Surrounds the zone of stasis and is characterised by increased tissue perfusion. Usually recovers.

The zones spread out from the point of injury in three dimensions, including deeper into dermal tissue.

Systemic response
The level of inflammatory response is related to the % TBSA that is burnt. Once the burn covers more than 20% TBSA, the inflammatory response can exert systemic effects. Capillary permeability

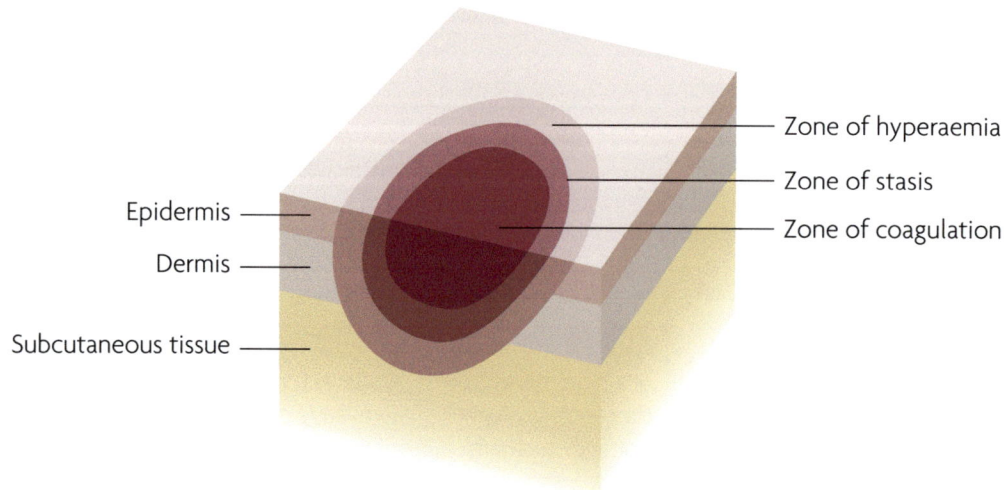

Figure 17.27 Zone of burn injury.

increases, leading to loss of intravascular proteins and fluid into interstitial space. Peripheral and splanchnic vasoconstriction occur and myocardial contractility decreases. Combined with fluid loss from the burn, this results in hypotension and end-organ hypoperfusion. In the lungs, there can be bronchoconstriction and the development of acute respiratory distress syndrome with any severe burns. Initially, there is a reduction in metabolic rate ('ebb phase'), but this can double in the days following burn injury ('flow phase') [Sheridan, 2012].

Acute smoke inhalation injury
Smoke inhalation is a killer, with the majority of fire fatalities either due to being 'overcome by gas or smoke', or a combination of 'burns and overcome by gas or smoke' [Home Office, 2017]. Naso-oropharyngeal and mucosal burns are common [Toon, 2010], but thermal injury below the vocal cords is rare since heat is effectively exchanged in upper airway passages [Prien, 1988]. When air, steam and/or smoke are at sufficiently high temperatures to cause thermal injury to the lower airways, rapid oedema of the glottis develops, resulting in fatal airway obstruction.

Systemic toxins are the products of incomplete combustion and include carbon monoxide (CO) and hydrogen cyanide. CO is an odourless, colourless gas that binds to haemoglobin with 250 times the affinity of oxygen. This results in a decrease in the oxygen-carrying capacity of the blood. Hydrogen cyanide adversely affects internal respiration by preventing aerobic production of adenosine triphosphate (ATP, the energy source for cells) [Toon, 2010].

Particulates and irritants have the greatest effect on the pathophysiological processes that occur due to smoke inhalation. Soot impregnated with toxins can reach the alveoli suspended in air. The types of chemicals vary, depending on what has been burning, but they trigger a cascade of events, resulting in pulmonary oedema and other respiratory problems [Murakami, 2003]. Water-soluble gases such as ammonia and hydrogen chloride react with the mucous membranes, producing strong alkalis and acids, leading to intense and prolonged inflammatory reactions. Lipid (fat) soluble irritants act more slowly as they dissolve into cellular membranes.

Friction burns
Although friction burns are strictly speaking a thermal burn, they are the result of heat production caused by friction between the skin and another object. This can result in not just a burn, but abrasions too (see the section on wounds and bleeding) [Gregory, 2010b].

7.4.2 Management
Safety first! The patient needs to be removed from the source of the burn if it is safe to do so, but don't get burnt yourself. Clothing should be removed unless it is sticking to the patient, as should jewellery, which may become constrictive as tissues swell.

Follow the <C>ABC approach for burns as you would any traumatic injury. However, inhalation injury is a particular concern and occurs in around 22% of all burns, and in 60% if facial burns are present [Toon, 2010].

Signs of inhalation injury include [Singer, 2010]:
- full-thickness or deep dermal burns to face, neck or upper torso
- singed nasal hair
- soot in sputum or oropharynx
- dyspnoea, hoarseness, cough or stridor
- cyanosis
- altered level of consciousness.

Administer high-flow oxygen via a non-rebreathe mask. CO poisoning may make pulse oximetry readings unreliable [JRCALC, 2019].

Cooling
Thermal burns should be cooled for 20 minutes [Bartlett, 2008], preferably with running water (between 8–15°C) [NZGG, 2007]. There is little evidence that ice causes damage to underlying tissues, but it runs the risk of making the patient hypothermic so is not recommended [Cuttle, 2008; Cuttle, 2009]. Cooling should commence immediately after the burn has occurred, but can be done up to three hours after injury if that is the first opportunity to do so [BBA, 2018].

If running water is not available or practicable, then gel-based body blankets can be used without causing hypothermia [NZGG, 2007; Singer, 2006; Martineau, 2006].

Covering/dressing
Patients with burns lose heat from non-epithelialised areas of skin due to evaporation. With the thermoregulatory function of the skin disrupted, patients are at risk of hypothermia, even on a warm day [AAOS, 2011]. Hypothermia is part of the lethal triad in trauma. For each 1°C reduction in body temperature the mortality rate increases significantly [Lonnecker, 2001], although there is no evidence currently to suggest that pre-hospital cooling causes hypothermia [Lonnecker, 2001; Singer, 2010]. Once cooling has been completed, cover the burn with a clean sheet or clingfilm, but take care not to apply it circumferentially as it can become constrictive as oedema develops [NZGG, 2007].

Time-critical features
A blue-light transfer to the most appropriate location is required for any of the following conditions [JRCALC, 2019]:
- any major ABCD problems
- airway burns
- history of hot air or gas inhalation
- respiratory distress
- evidence of circumferential (completely circling the neck, torso or limb) burns
- significant facial burns
- burns covering more than 15% TBSA in adults or 10% TBSA in children
- presence of other major injuries.

Note that transfer may not be to your nearest hospital, but to a major trauma or specialised burns centre. Check local guidance.

7.5 Chemical burns including acid attacks

Chemical burns generally result from exposure to acids, alkalis and other corrosive materials. This can be accidental, but increasingly commonly it is an intentional form of violence [NARU, 2017b] with 400 attacks reported in the six months leading up to April 2017 [UK Government, 2017b]. Alkali burns are generally more serious as they penetrate more deeply than other chemicals [NAEMT, 2020]. Their severity depends on the concentration of the chemical, the duration of exposure and the speed in applying first-aid measures [Greaves, 2008].

7.5.1 Management

Safety first! It is important that you do not become exposed to the chemical. If in doubt, do not approach the scene but wait for the hazardous area response team (HART) or the fire and rescue service to attend. If you do treat the patient wear full PPE, including apron, double gloves and eye protection.

The following first aid measures apply to chemical burns [FPHC, 2018]:
- evacuate the casualty to a clean area away from the hazard
- remove contaminated clothing (cut it off and avoid removing over the head)
- remove excess contamination:
  - brush off solid material
  - gently blot (not rub) excess and thickened liquids with absorbent material and discard
- rinse with copious amounts of water with the patient leaning forward so that contamination does not run over themselves any more.

Chemical burns should be irrigated for at least 15 minutes, and ideally for up to an hour (although alkali burns may require much longer periods of irrigation), but watch for hypothermia [NZGG, 2007].

Be aware of local policy. Some hospitals have specialist treatments available for chemical burns patients.

7.6 Radiation burns

Radiation burns are most commonly caused by UV radiation from the sun or sunlamps (sunburn). However, in rare cases, it can be caused by exposure to radioactive materials [Gregory, 2010b].

Approximately 80% of skin cancer is preventable, and avoiding sunburn is key [Simon, 2010]:
- Take care not to burn.
- Cover up with loose cool clothing, a hat and sunglasses.
- Seek shade during the hottest part of the day.
- Apply high-factor sunscreen (at least sun protection factor 15) to sun-exposed body parts.
- Take extra care to protect children in the sun.

7.6.1 Management

Safety first! If the burns are due to exposure to radioactivity, do not approach but wait for the hazardous area response team (HART).

Sunburn

Basic first-aid measures are usually sufficient [SJA, SAA, BRC, 2016]:
- Cover the patient's skin with light clothing or a towel. Move them out of the sun, preferably indoors.
- Encourage them to drink frequent sips of cold water while cooling the affected area with cold water. If the area of sunburn is large, it may be more practical for the patient to soak the area in a cold bath for ten minutes.
- If burns are mild, calamine or an after-sun lotion may help. Patients should be advised to stay inside or in the shade.

Most sunburn will manifest as reddening of the skin (erythema), but blistering is evidence of a partial-thickness burn and transport to hospital should be considered if it meets the criteria for review by specialised burns care services [NNBC, 2012].

7.7 Electrical injuries

Electrical injuries are uncommon, but they cause significant damage and even death when they occur. The majority of electrical injuries in adults occur in the workplace and involve high voltages, whereas in children most injuries occur in the home with domestic voltage. Electrocution from lightning strikes is very rare, leading to around 1,000 deaths each year worldwide [Nolan, 2010].

Electrical burns arise when a source of electrical power makes contact with the patient's body. They are frequently more serious than they appear, since rapid heat loss from the surface of the skin may leave it relatively undamaged, whereas the underlying tissues may have sustained serious injury, particularly between the entry and exit points (don't forget to look for both!).

7.7.1 Management

Safety first! Do not approach the patient until you are certain that the source of electricity has been cut off.

When dealing with electrical injuries, the thermal burns sustained may not be your highest priority. The patient may be in cardiac arrest, have airway or facial burns, have cardiac arrhythmias (also perform electrocardiogram monitoring) and be traumatically injured (fractures, serious internal injuries) that will need addressing first. Associated thermal burns can be managed as previously described.

7.8 The impact of burns

Without appropriate intervention and management, patients with serious burns can die due to [Sheridan, 2012]:
- burn shock due to excessive fluid loss in the first 24 hours
- respiratory failure in the subsequent 3–5 days
- burn wound sepsis in the following few weeks.

Thankfully, because of prompt transfer by ambulance staff to burn centres and the subsequent specialised management that patients receive, this is less common. However, it does underline the importance of transporting patients to definitive care.

There are four general phases of burn care, with the ambulance service only playing a small part in the initial management stage [Sheridan, 2012]:
- Initial evaluation and resuscitation (0–72 hours).
- Initial surgery and temporary closure of wounds created by removal of full-thickness burns (days 1–7).
- Definitive wound closure (weeks 1–6).
- Rehabilitation and reconstruction (up to two years).

Chapter

18 Assisting the Paramedic

1 Tracheal intubation

1.1 Learning objectives

By the end of this section you will be able to:
- explain your role in assisting the paramedic with tracheal intubation
- explain the function of equipment associated with tracheal intubation.

1.2 Introduction

Having completed Chapter 11, 'Airway', you already know about airway anatomy and have knowledge of a range of manual airway manoeuvres and adjuncts. This section will cover one other airway procedure in which you may be required to assist a paramedic:
- tracheal intubation.

1.3 Tracheal intubation

Tracheal intubation involves the insertion of a cuff-sealed tube into the trachea. This provides protection against aspiration of solid or liquid material, but without the assistance of drugs that are not currently in routine use by paramedics. Only patients who have a severely depressed level of consciousness (and, most likely, in cardiac arrest) can be intubated [Gowens, 2018]. Evidence of the benefit of performing tracheal intubation by paramedics is limited [Fouche, 2014].

When to do it (indication)
- Unconscious patients with no gag reflex, whose airway cannot be managed with more basic airway methods/adjuncts.

When not to do it (contra-indications)
- Patients with an intact gag reflex.
- In the first few minutes of a cardiac arrest (chest compressions have priority and usually a basic airway adjunct or a supraglottic airway device will be sufficient).
- If end-tidal carbon dioxide ($EtCO_2$) measurement by capnography is not possible.

Advantages
- Provides a secure airway that protects against aspiration.
- Allows for ventilation at higher airway pressures (e.g. in cases of life-threatening asthma).

Disadvantages
- Requires skill and frequent practice to remain competent.
- Bypasses physiological functions of the upper airway (filtering, warming and humidifying).
- Unrecognised oesophageal intubation will result in the death of the patient.

1.3.1 Equipment

Preparation is key to (tracheal) intubation and it cannot be done properly by one clinician. You are vital to the success of this procedure and it starts with assembling the equipment required (Figure 18.1). The airway is not sterile, but the equipment used should be clean, not damaged and disposable items such as the tracheal tube should be in date. Care needs to be taken to ensure that equipment that is going to end up inside the patient's airway is kept as clean as possible. Do not place items directly on to the floor, and where possible keep items in their packaging (although opened) until required for use.

Tracheal tube
The tracheal tube (Figure 18.2) consists of a bevelled end, which is inserted into the patient, and the opposite end with an adaptor that can be connected to a catheter-filter-capnography mount assembly and ventilation device such as a self-inflating bag.

The inflation port includes a one-way valve into which air can be injected by use of a syringe. The pilot balloon gives an indication as to whether the inflatable cuff is inflated or deflated once it has been inserted into the trachea.

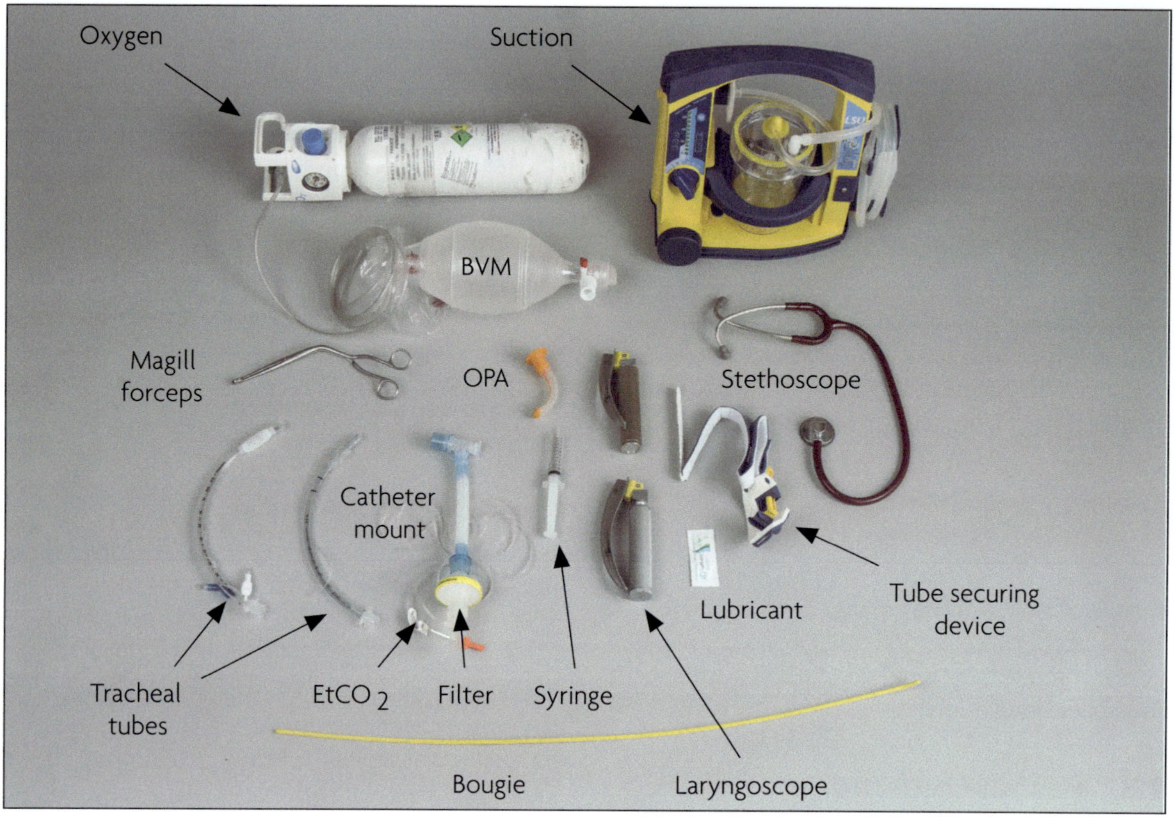

Chapter 18 – Assisting the Paramedic

Figure 18.1 Equipment required for an intubation attempt.

Tracheal tubes come in a variety of sizes with adult males typically requiring a tube with an internal diameter of 7.5–8.0 mm, and adult females requiring a tube with an internal diameter of 7.0 mm [Nolan, 2016].

Laryngoscope blades and handle

Blades also come in different sizes and it is helpful to have a selection available. Size 3 and 4 blades are typically required for adults. Blades can be straight or curved, but the curved variety (Macintosh) are most commonly used for adults. The blade usually has a light source and the handle contains batteries. The handle and blade are designed to connect together (Figure 18.3); when the blade is moved into a perpendicular position, the light should come on. In addition, video laryngoscopes, which have a camera mounted on the blade with a screen on top of the handle, are increasingly being used in the out-of-hospital setting.

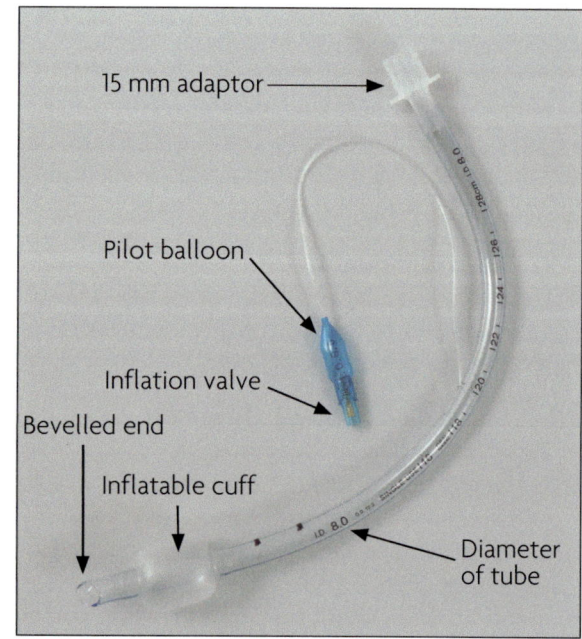

Figure 18.2 The tracheal tube.

Tracheal intubation

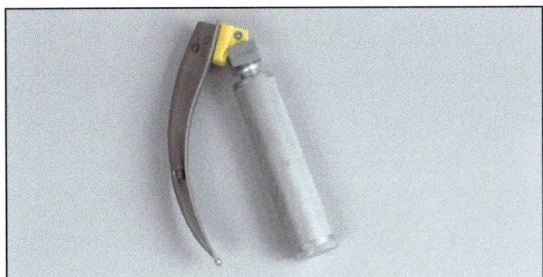

Figure 18.3 Laryngoscope blade and handle.

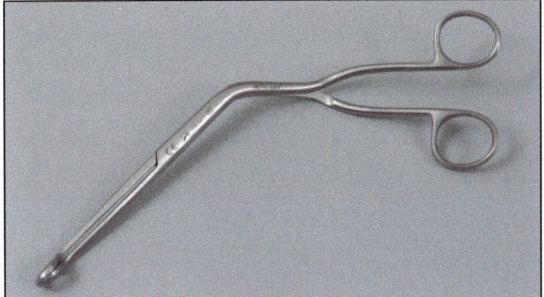

Figure 18.4 Magill forceps.

Magill forceps
These are curved forceps that enable the removal of foreign bodies from the airway without the operator's hands obscuring the view (Figure 18.4).

1.3.2 Procedure

Procedure – Tracheal intubation

The following steps are required to perform tracheal intubation. Note where you are required to assist [Walls, 2012]:

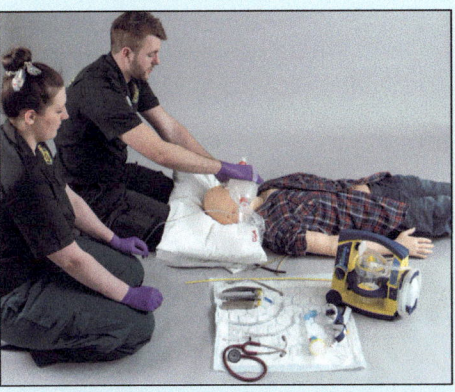

1. Adopt standard precautions (gloves and face shield). The patient will be pre-oxygenated

Procedure – Tracheal intubation – *cont*

for 2–3 minutes with a bag-valve-mask (BVM) and oxygen, unless the patient is in cardiac arrest.

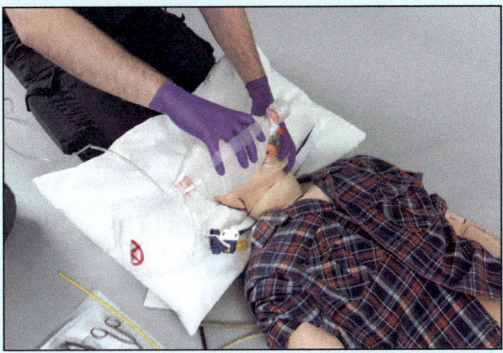

2. The patient's head should be in the 'sniffing the morning air' position (head extended and neck flexed) to give the best view, if they do not have a cervical spine injury. A good position will have been achieved when the external auditory meatus ('earhole') is at the same level as the sternal notch ('neck hole'). Use pillows/cushions/towels/books or anything else similar in the vicinity of your patient to maintain this position by placing the item under the patient's head.

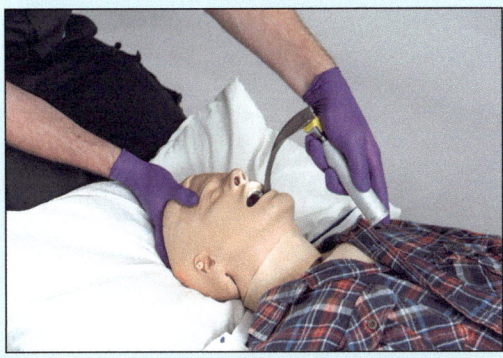

3. The paramedic will open the patient's mouth and insert the laryngoscope blade into the right side of the patient's mouth. The laryngoscope will then be moved to the midline, displacing the tongue to the left.

Procedure – Tracheal intubation – *cont*

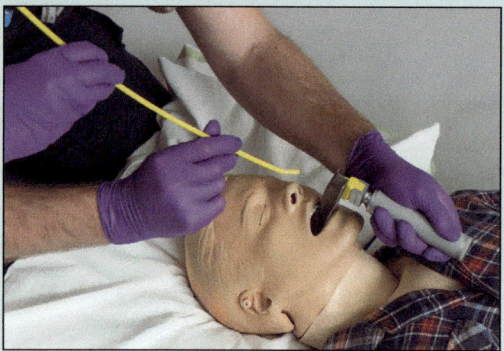

4. By gently lifting the laryngoscope handle, the glottic opening and vocal cords should be visualised. If this is not the case, you may be asked to perform the BURP manoeuvre. Once the glottic opening is visualised, you'll be asked for the bougie, so have it ready. The bougie will have a bent end, which goes into the mouth first, so present it to the paramedic with the bent end closest to the patient's mouth.

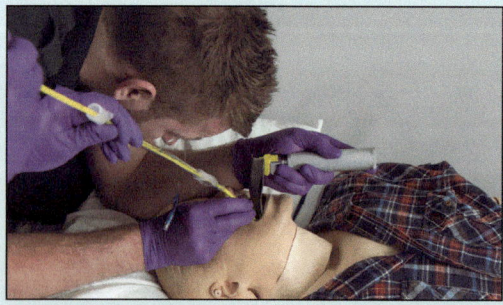

5. With the bougie inserted into the trachea, your next job is to thread the tracheal tube over the bougie, making sure the bevelled end enters the patient's mouth first. Once the tube is on the bougie, you'll be asked to hold the top of the bougie to prevent it moving while the paramedic inserts the tube into the trachea. Tell the paramedic when you have hold of the top of the bougie.

Procedure – Tracheal intubation – *cont*

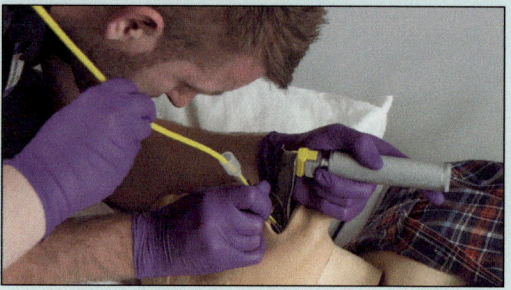

6. Once the paramedic is satisfied that the tube is in the trachea and at the right depth, you'll be asked to remove the bougie.

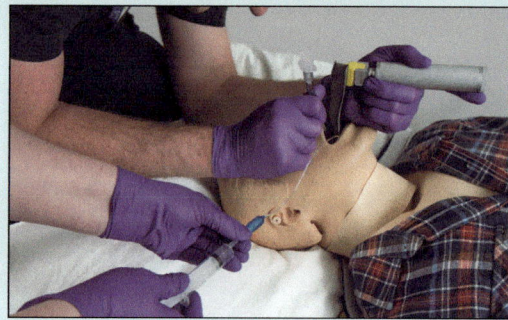

7. Inflate the tube cuff by injecting 6–8 ml of air into the inflation valve with a 10 ml syringe.

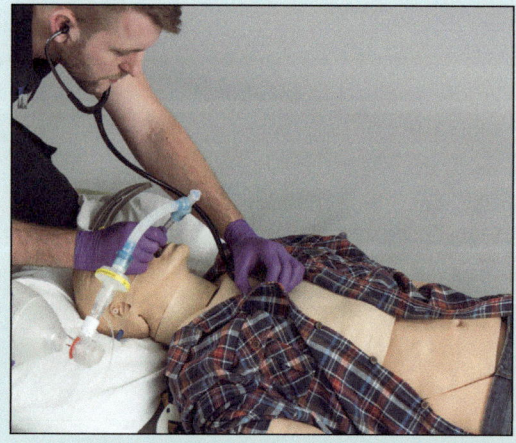

8. Attach the capnography, filter and catheter mount on to the tracheal tube. Once a capnography waveform has been seen on the monitor, the laryngoscope will be

Tracheal intubation

Procedure – Tracheal intubation – cont

removed from the patient's mouth, but the tube will be firmly held at all times to prevent it from becoming displaced. In addition to measuring $EtCO_2$, both lung fields should be auscultated to confirm correct tube placement.

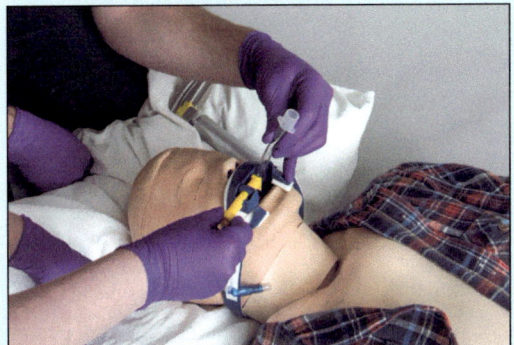

9. Once the paramedic is confident that the tube is correctly placed, it needs to be secured, preferably with a commercial device like the Thomas ET-tube holder, but tape will suffice if this is not available.

1.3.3 Additional manoeuvres/procedures

The BURP manoeuvre

In the event that the view of the glottic opening is poor, you may be asked to perform the BURP manoeuvre to improve the view. BURP stands for [Levitan, 2006]:
- backwards
- upwards
- rightwards
- pressure.

Place your thumb, index and middle fingers on the patient's thyroid cartilage and push firmly backwards, upwards (towards the head) and then rightwards (Figure 18.5). Alternatively, the paramedic may manipulate the thyroid cartilage themselves while looking for the glottic opening (bimanual laryngoscopy) and ask you to maintain the position of the thyroid cartilage once they have found the position that gives the best view [Walls, 2012].

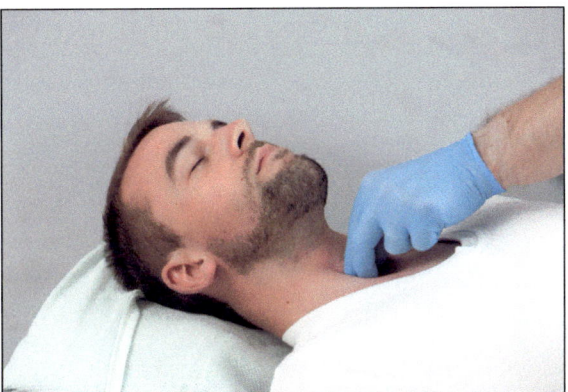

Figure 18.5 The correct hand position for the BURP manoeuvre.

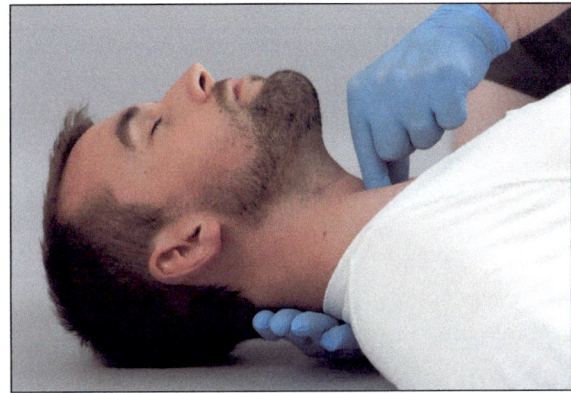

Figure 18.6 Sellick's manoeuvre.

Sellick's manoeuvre (cricoid pressure)

Paramedics sometimes ask for cricoid pressure (Figure 18.6) when they want an improved view of the glottic opening. Sellick's manoeuvre is actually meant to occlude the oesophagus to prevent air going into the stomach during positive-pressure ventilation. The technique involves placing your thumb and index finger on the cricoid cartilage and pushing firmly backwards (30–40 N of force should be applied) [May, 2007]. It actually worsens the laryngeal view and so should not be used for this purpose [Levitan, 2006]. Bimanual laryngoscopy or the BURP manoeuvre should be used instead.

Confirming tube placement

Since unrecognised oesophageal intubation will likely result in the death of the patient, it is vital that the correct tube placement is confirmed. This

should be done by ensuring all of the following are present [Nolan, 2016]:
- Waveform capnography: This is the best way of confirming correct tube placement.
- Direct visualisation of the tube passing through the vocal cords.
- Observing for bilateral chest movement and auscultating for bilateral air entry in the lungs and absence of air entering the stomach. Note that these are not completely reliable.

Following a coroner's action to prevent future deaths, the Association of Ambulance Chief Executives (AACE) set out guidance that the use of either a digital $EtCO_2$ monitoring device or waveform capnography should be used to assist in confirming placement. If either of these are not available, then intubation should not be performed [JRCALC, 2019].

1.4 DOPES

Assessment of the airway and ventilatory adequacy is a dynamic process. Inserting an oropharyngeal airway, supraglottic airway device or ET tube is just the start of the process. $EtCO_2$ can provide an early warning that something is wrong, but you need to be aware of problems that arise and how to troubleshoot them.

Although originally conceived for the paediatric airway, the DOPES mnemonic can help you to systematically work through possible causes of acute deterioration of A and B problems [Skellett, 2016]:
- **Displacement:** $EtCO_2$ can confirm that the patient is ventilating, but won't tell you if the tube is in the right main bronchus, so auscultation is still important. It will provide an early warning of displacement and reduced or absent ventilation, well before your pulse oximetry reading starts to fall.
- **Obstruction:** Thick pulmonary secretions can cause problems and, particularly in children, kinking of the ET tube can block airflow.
- **Pneumothorax:** A decreasing compliance and unilateral chest movement should have you reaching for your stethoscope. Your senior clinician may need to decompress the chest.
- **Equipment failure:** Check your oxygen flow, ventilation settings and tubing. Don't be afraid to go back to airway and ventilation basics while you find the cause.
- **Stomach:** Over-enthusiastic use of the BVM can lead to abdominal distension, which in children in particular can splint the diaphragm and impede ventilation. Your senior clinician may elect to insert a nasogastric tube or, if the patient is intubated, apply gentle pressure over the abdomen to expel the air.

2 Intravenous drug administration

2.1 Learning objectives
By the end of this section you will be able to:
- explain your role in assisting the clinician with cannulation and intravenous infusions
- explain the function of equipment used during cannulation and intravenous infusions
- describe the safety checks undertaken prior to cannulation and starting intravenous infusions
- explain your role in infection prevention and control in relation to cannulation and intravenous infusions.

2.2 Introduction
Many of the drugs in use by the ambulance service are given directly into a patient's vein. This intravenous method of administration requires the insertion of a cannula directly into the patient's blood stream; if this is not undertaken correctly, it can result in harm to the patient. Your assistance in these procedures can help reduce the risk of this occurring.

However, intravenous cannulation can be difficult to obtain, particularly in paediatric patients and those in cardiac arrest, for example. In these cases, intraosseous cannulation can be of great help in enabling the administration of drugs and fluids.

2.3 Intravenous cannulation
Intravenous cannulation is the technique of siting a cannula (a plastic tube) into a vein. This is undertaken to administer drugs and/or fluids.

Intravenous drug administration

This is a technical skill and needs to be as aseptic as possible. Your assistance will be helpful, but if you are not aware of the steps involved, you could inadvertently put you, your colleague and/or the patient at risk from a sharps injury and/or infection.

When to do it (indications)
- Intravenous (IV) drug or fluid administration.
- Prophylactically in unstable patients.
- To expedite ongoing care in hospital.

When not to do it (contra-indications)
- Patient unlikely to require IV drugs or fluids.
- Site contraindications:
  - presence of injury, inflammation or infection at the site
  - presence of arterio-venous fistula
  - right dorsum of the hand in patients who are going for primary percutaneous coronary intervention (pPCI).

Advantage
- Effective drug and fluid administration route, even if the patient is not conscious.

Disadvantages/complications
- Procedure is painful.
- Can delay on-scene times.
- Provides direct entry for infectious pathogens.
- Accidental damage to nerves, tendons and arteries can occur.
- Extravasation (leakage of fluid/drug out of vein) if cannula not sited properly.

2.3.1 Equipment

Figure 18.7 shows most of the equipment you will need. However, you will also require a sharps bin for safe disposal of the needle inside the cannula, and you may need to have several cannulas of differing sizes available.

2.3.2 Cannulas

Cannulas come in a range of sizes and types. Many ambulance services use safety cannulas, which will cover the sharp end of the cannula when the needle is withdrawn. However, they offer no protection until the needle is removed, and even afterwards you should treat them as a sharp that can puncture the skin.

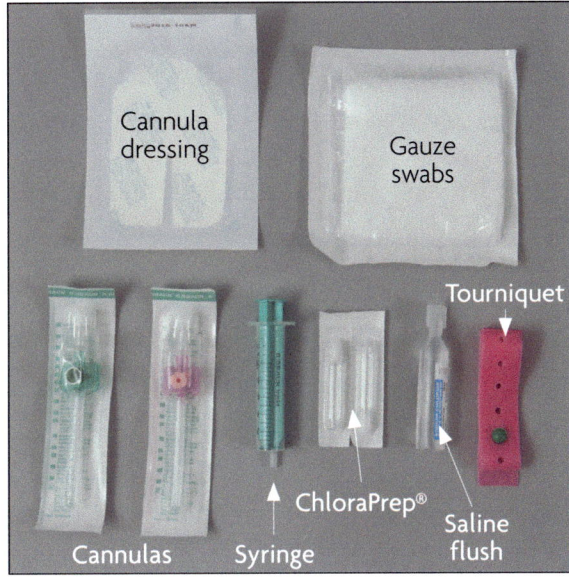

Figure 18.7 Equipment for intravenous cannulation.

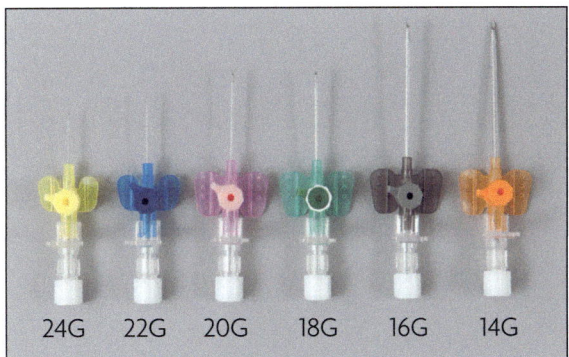

Figure 18.8 Cannulas.

Cannulas in common use by the ambulance service are sized from 24 gauge (G) to 14G. Somewhat counterintuitively, a 24G cannula has a smaller diameter than the 14G, which is the largest. Figure 18.8 shows the range of cannulas.

2.3.3 Procedure for intravenous cannulation

The following procedure outlines the steps that the paramedic will take when cannulating a patient and the actions that you may be required to take when assisting [Dougherty, 2008]:

Chapter 18 – *Assisting the Paramedic*

Procedure – Intravenous cannulation

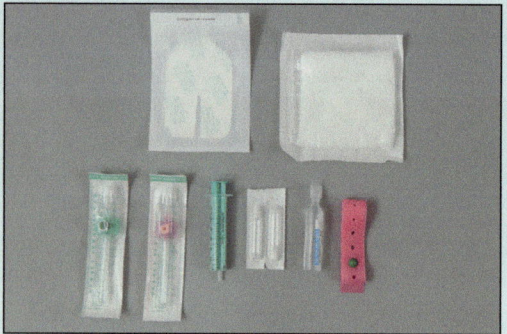

1. The paramedic will explain the procedure and obtain consent (unless the patient is not capable, such as when the patient is unconscious). You may be asked to prepare the equipment while the paramedic undertakes the next steps.

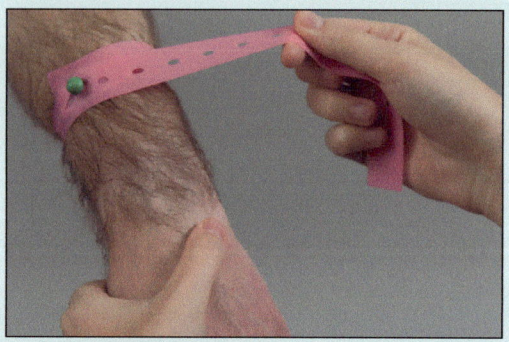

2. A tourniquet will be applied above the cannulation site in order to stop venous flow back to the heart and causing the veins to bulge.

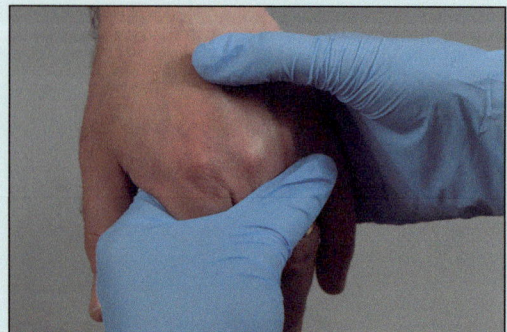

3. The paramedic will wash their hands (or use hand sanitiser) and put on disposable gloves.

Procedure – Intravenous cannulation – *cont*

You should too. They will then attempt to feel for a suitable vein.

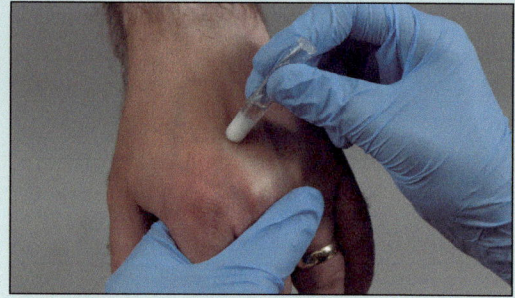

4. The vein will require cleaning with ChloraPrep®, so have one ready. Make sure you do not accidentally contaminate the cleaned area by touching it.

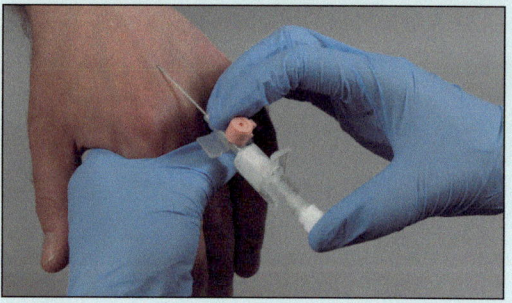

5. You may be asked to open the packaging the cannula comes in. Avoid touching the cannula inside. The paramedic will then insert the cannula.

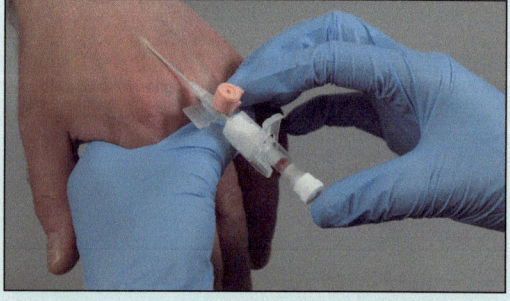

6. A 'flashback' should be observed. This is when blood enters the back chamber of the cannula. If you see a growing lump under the skin where the cannula has been inserted, it is likely that the cannula will need to

Procedure – Intravenous cannulation – *cont*

be removed. Have some gauze ready and remove the tourniquet if asked.

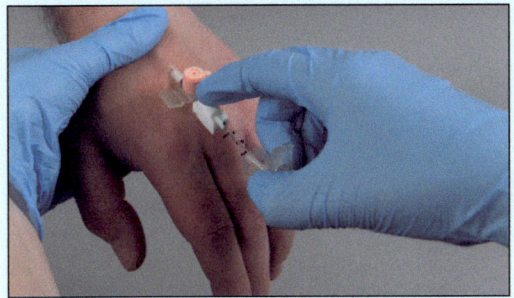

7. The cannula will be advanced over the needle. Make sure the sharps bin is nearby.

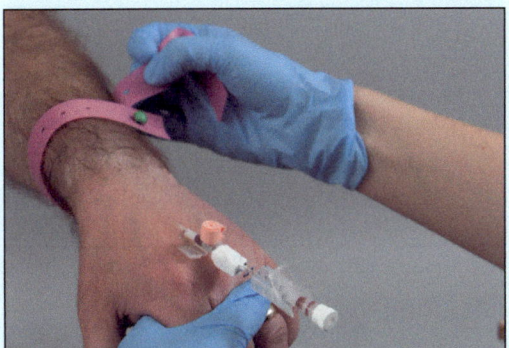

8. Before the needle can be removed, the tourniquet needs removing. You may be asked to do this.

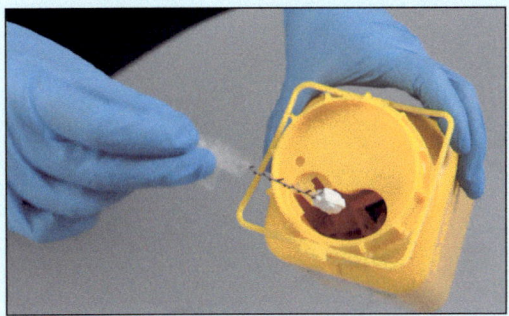

9. The needle will be removed by the paramedic and should go straight into a sharps bin. Try to avoid holding the bin if you can, but if this is unavoidable, ensure your hands are well away from the top of the bin so that you are less likely to

Procedure – Intravenous cannulation – *cont*

get injured if the needle misses the hole (because it is dropped, for example).

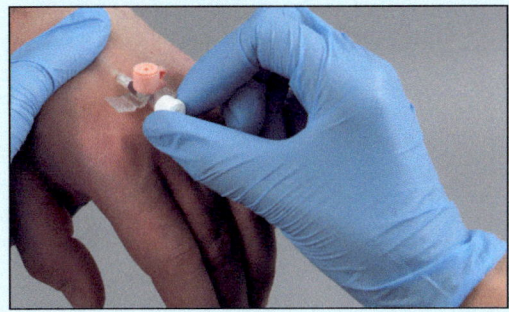

10. A bung needs to be placed on the end of the cannula to prevent blood from running out of the vein. This is sometimes dropped. Do not pick it up. Instead, obtain another one and pass it to the paramedic.

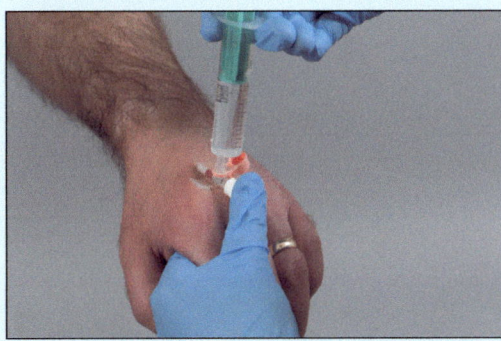

11. The cannula is flushed with 5–10 ml of saline to ensure it is patent. You may be asked to draw this up: the procedure is the same as for drug administration.

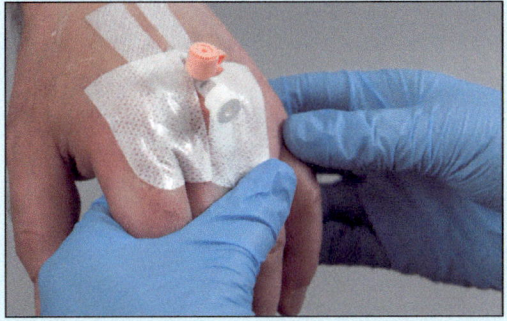

12. Finally, the cannula will then be secured with the cannula dressing.

Chapter 18 – *Assisting the Paramedic*

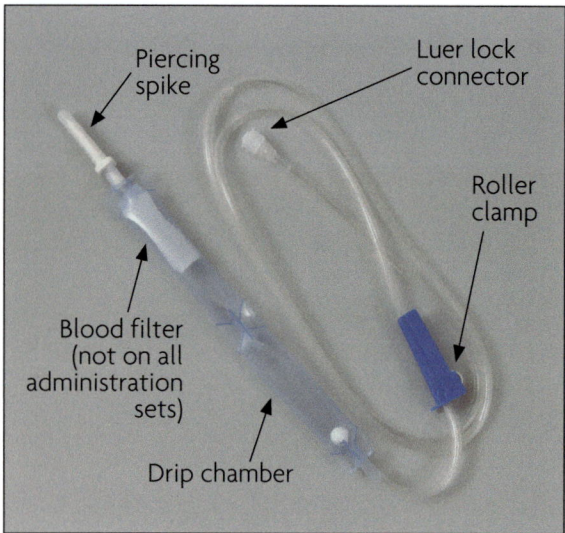

Figure 18.9 A fluid administration set.

2.4 Preparing an intravenous infusion

The equipment for an intravenous infusion consists of the administration set (also called a giving set; see Figure 18.9) and the fluid to be administered. You may be asked to assemble this while the paramedic is obtaining intravenous access.

2.4.1 Procedure

Take the following steps to prepare an intravenous infusion [Dougherty, 2008]:

Procedure – Intravenous infusion

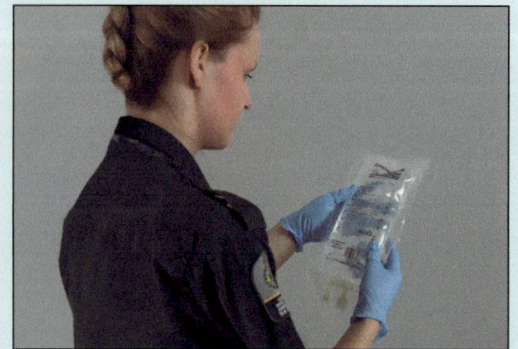

1. Take standard precautions. Confirm with the paramedic that the fluid to be administered

Procedure – Intravenous infusion – *cont*

is the correct type and concentration, has not expired, has intact packaging, looks clear and is free of contaminants.

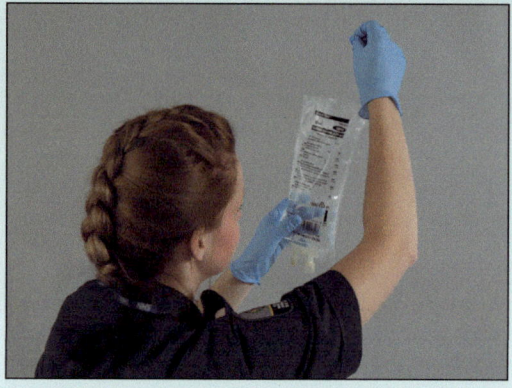

2. Remove the protective packaging and hang up the bag of fluid. This can be achieved using the ceiling-mounted hooks or holders in the ambulance, if available, but sometimes a bystander or ingenuity is required. Avoid placing sterile fluid bags on the floor or other contaminated surface.

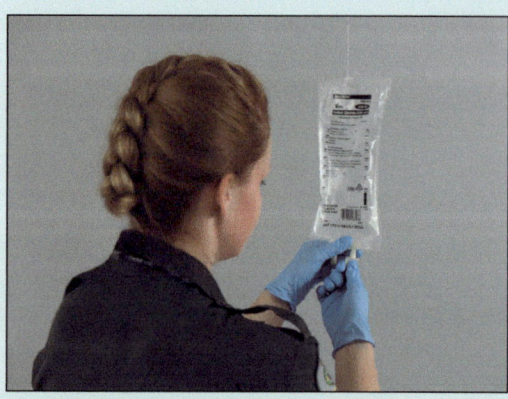

3. Twist and remove the rubber pigtail on the bottom of the bag of fluid. The bag will remain sealed until punctured by the piercing spike.

Intravenous drug administration

Procedure – Intravenous infusion – *cont*

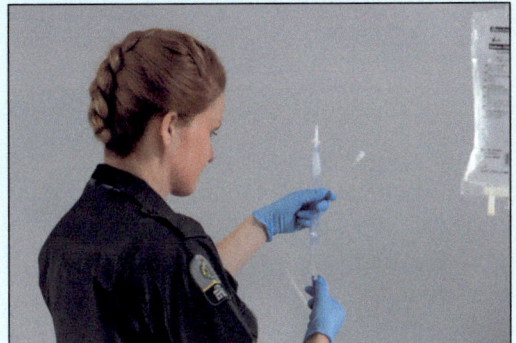

4. Check the administration set for damage and to ensure it has not expired. Open the packaging and close the roller clamp.

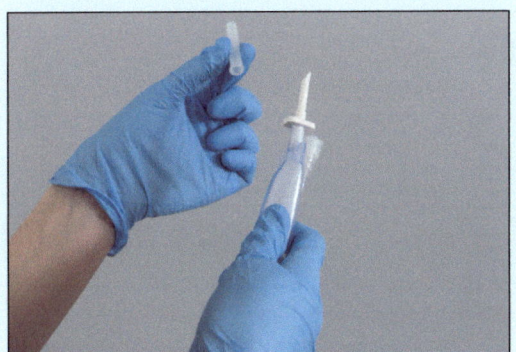

5. Remove the protective cover from the piercing spike. This is sharp and sterile, so don't stab yourself with it or let it come into contact with anything.

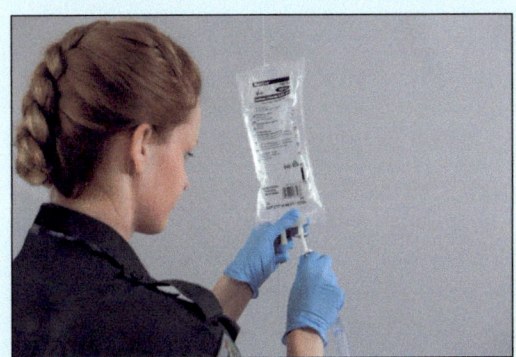

6. Slide the spike into the bag using the port exposed when you removed the rubber

Procedure – Intravenous infusion – *cont*

pigtail. You will need to hold the bag steady, but keep your fingers clear of the spike. A twisting motion sometimes helps to insert the spike into the bag. You can stop once you see fluid enter the drip chamber.

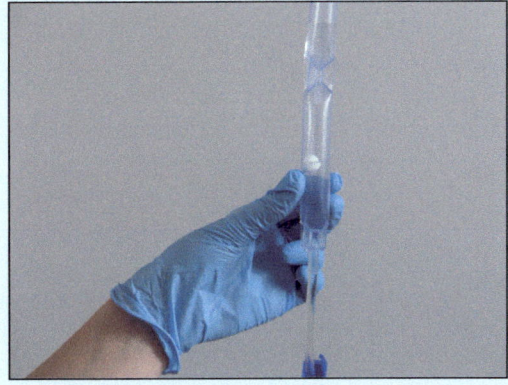

7. Squeeze the drip chamber to fill it halfway.

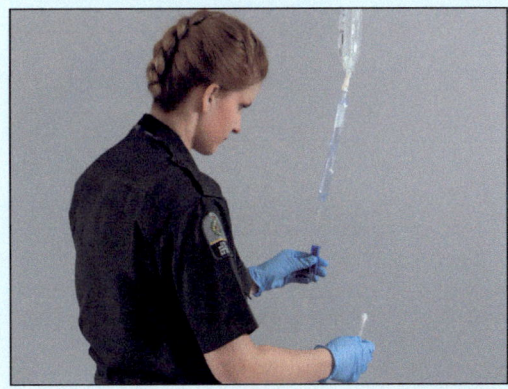

8. Open the roller clamp to allow the fluid to run slowly down the length of the administration set. This will prime the set and remove the air. If air bubbles can still be seen, then remove the protective cover from the Luer lock and run some of the fluid off. This is not ideal, because this end is also sterile and removing the cover increases the risk of infection.

Chapter 18 – *Assisting the Paramedic*

Procedure – Intravenous infusion – *cont*

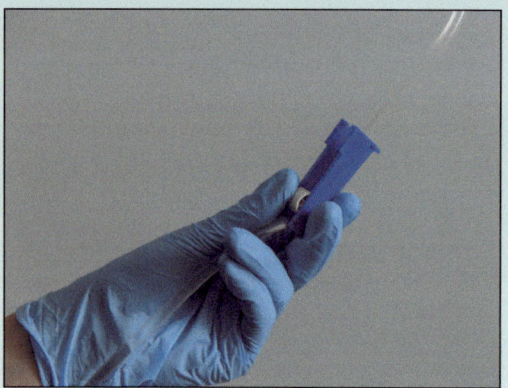

9. Once the tube is primed, stop the flow by closing the roller clamp. Re-check the drip chamber. If it is less than half-full, gently squeeze the chamber to fill it. If it is too full, invert the bag and administration set and squeeze the chamber to return some of the fluid back into the bag.

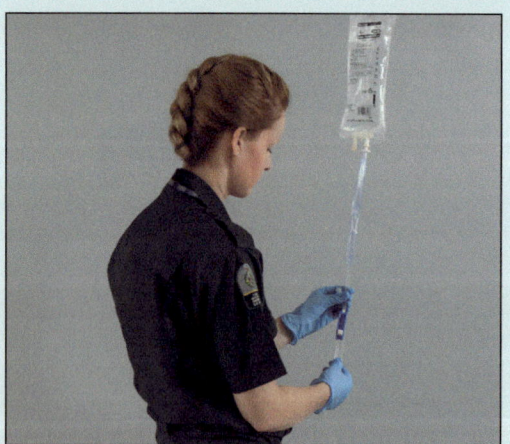

10. Hang up the bag and administration set. Do not let the tubing drop to the floor.

2.5 *Intraosseous cannulation*

Intraosseous (IO) cannulation is an alternative to intravenous (IV) cannulation when the IV route proves difficult or impossible to achieve, for example, during cardiac arrest [Soar, 2015]. IO is particularly useful in gaining fast vascular access in children [Skellett, 2016].

When to do it (indication)
- Vascular access is required urgently and IV cannulation has failed or is not possible to obtain.

When not to do it (contra-indications)
- Conscious patients (unless your senior clinician can administer local anaesthetic drugs).
- Fracture of the targeted bone.
- Previous, significant orthopaedic procedures at insertion site (e.g. prosthetic limb or joint).
- IO in the targeted bone within the past 48 hours.
- Infection at area of insertion.
- Excessive tissue or absence of adequate anatomical landmarks.

Advantages
- Fast vascular access in emergencies.
- Comparable peak drug concentrations to IV administration.
- All drugs and fluids typically found on an ambulance that can be administered via the IV route can be given IO.

Disadvantages/complications
- IO infusions are painful.
- Drugs and fluids need to be administered under pressure: they will not enter the vasculature under gravity (unlike IV).
- Extravasation of fluid is the most common complication of IO infusion.
- Compartment syndrome can result if a large extravasation goes undetected, which may require surgical intervention or amputation.
- Osteomyelitis is a rare but serious infection that can occur following IO insertion.

Although there are a range of IO vascular access devices available, a common one in use in UK ambulance services is the Arrow EZ-IO®, which is described here [Teleflex, 2017].

2.5.1 Equipment
You will require the following equipment for an EZ-IO® insertion (Figure 18.10):

Intravenous drug administration

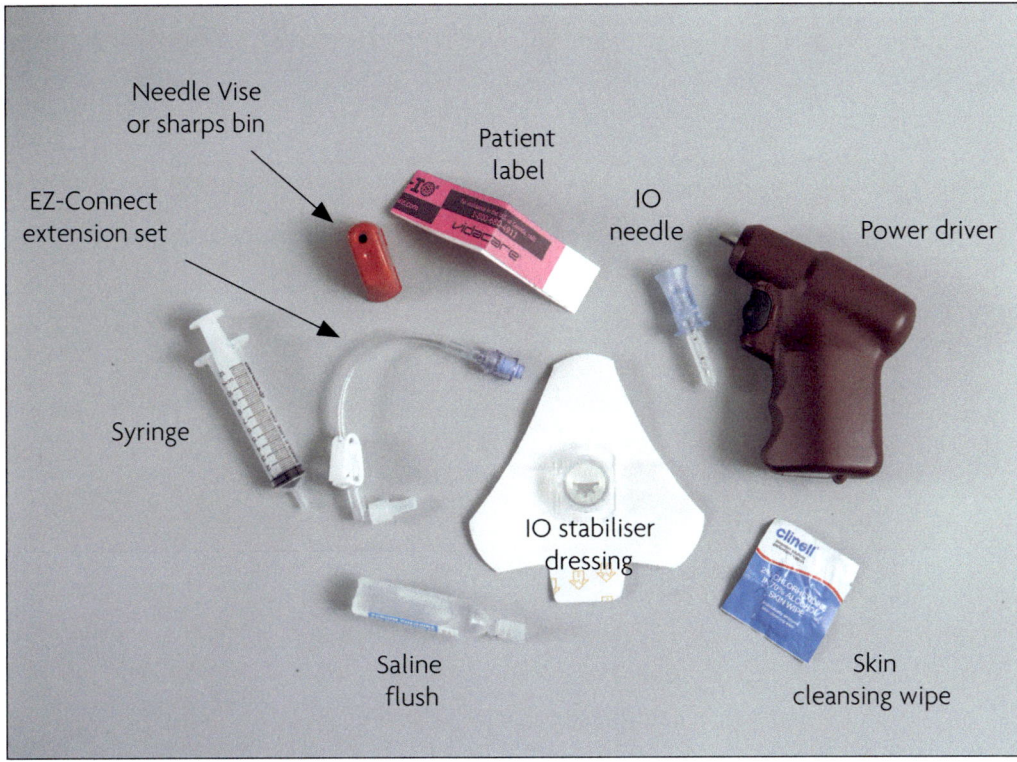

Figure 18.10 Equipment for EZ-IO® insertion.

- EZ-IO® Power Driver
- EZ-IO® Needle Set and EZ-Connect extension set
- EZ-Stabiliser® dressing
- cleansing agent of choice
- Luer lock syringe with sterile normal saline flush (5–10 ml for adults, 2–5 ml for infant/child)
- sharps container
- needle.

There are three needle sizes for the EZ-IO®. Choice of needle length is determined by clinical judgement, patient weight, anatomy and tissue depth over the insertion site (Figure 18.11).

It is important that at least 5 mm of the needle is visible once it has punctured the overlying tissue, but before entering the bone (the black mark closest to the hub (the coloured plastic; see Figure 18.12).

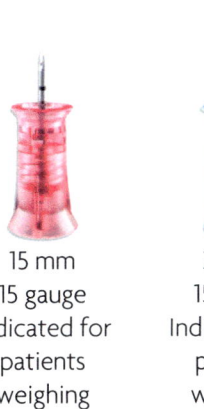

15 mm
15 gauge
Indicated for patients weighing 3–39kg

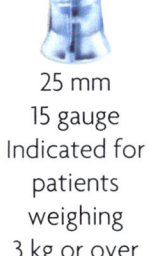

25 mm
15 gauge
Indicated for patients weighing 3 kg or over

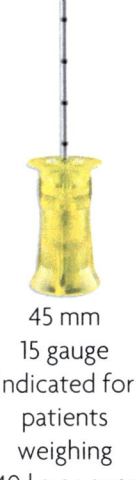

45 mm
15 gauge
Indicated for patients weighing 40 kg or over excessive tissue depth

Figure 18.11 EZ-IO® needles.

Chapter 18 – Assisting the Paramedic

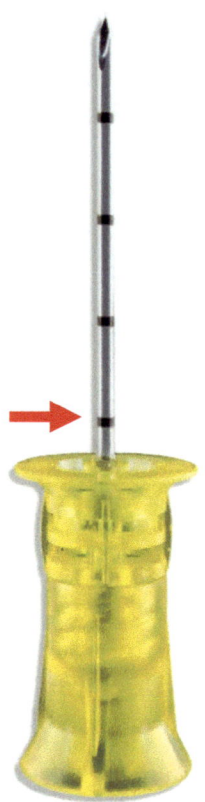

Figure 18.12   5 mm mark closest to the needle hub.

2.5.2 Procedure

> **Procedure – EZ-IO® proximal humerus**
>
> The following steps describe how to obtain IO access with the EZ-IO® in the proximal humerus [Teleflex, 2017]. Note that this is unlikely to be within your scope of practice and is included for information only.
>
> 1. Prepare the equipment while the senior clinician obtains consent. Clarify the needle length required. This is likely to be the 45 mm needle.

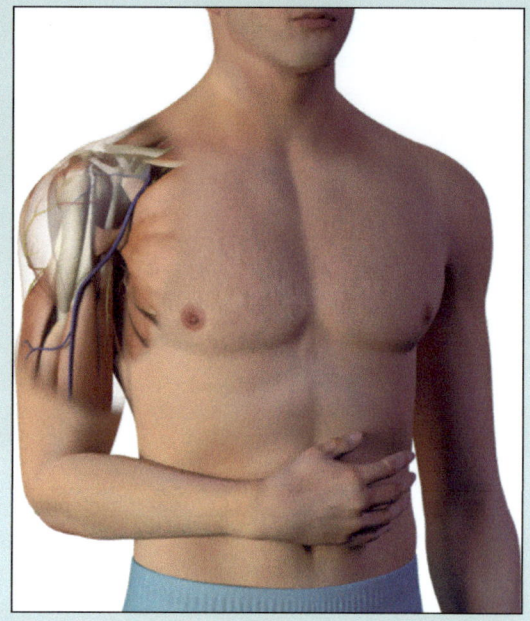

Procedure – EZ-IO® proximal humerus – *cont*

2. Place the patient's hand over the abdomen (elbow adducted and humerus internally rotated).

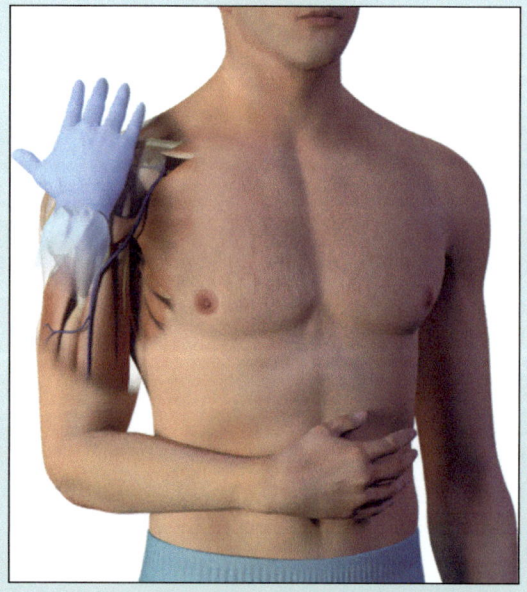

3. Place your palm on the patient's shoulder anteriorly. The area that feels like a 'ball' under your palm is the general target area. On obese patients, you should be able to feel this ball by pushing deeply.

Intravenous drug administration

Procedure – EZ-IO® proximal humerus – *cont*

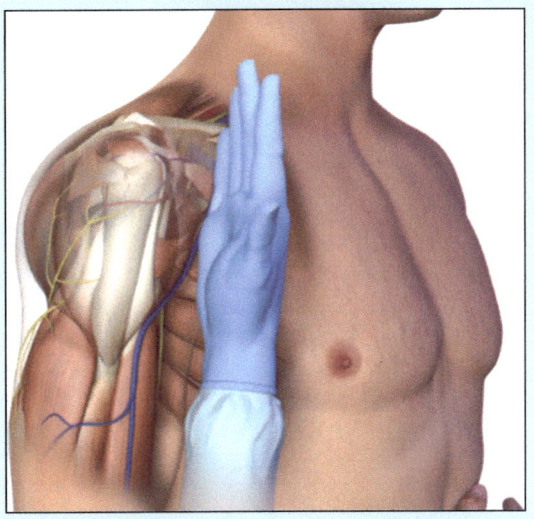

4. Place the ulnar aspect of one hand vertically over the axilla.

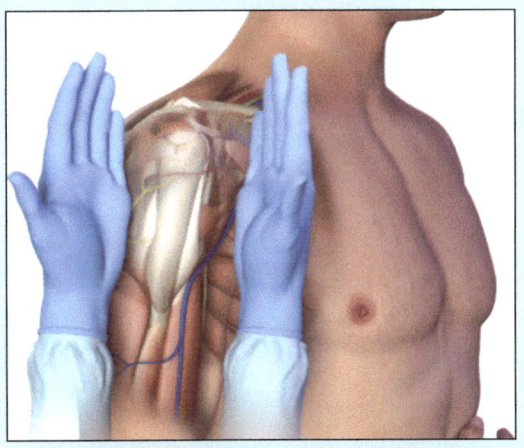

5. Place the ulnar aspect of the opposite hand along the midline of the upper arm laterally.

Procedure – EZ-IO® proximal humerus – *cont*

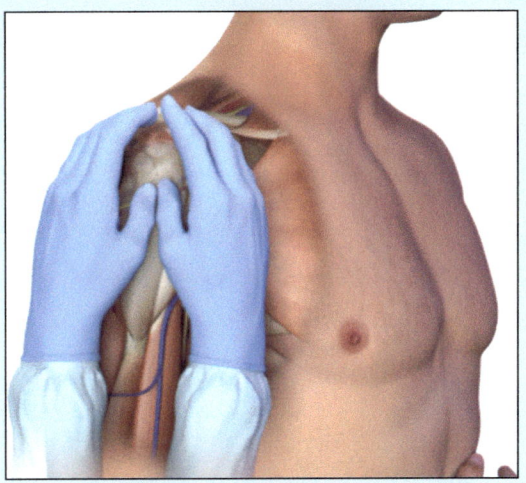

6. Place your thumbs together over the arm. This identifies the vertical line of insertion on the proximal humerus.

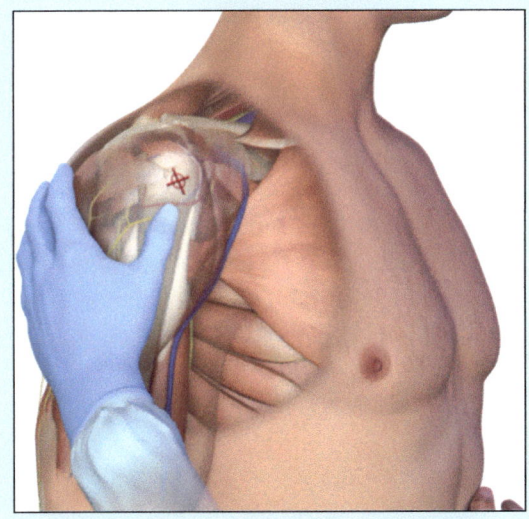

7. Palpate deeply as you climb up the humerus to the surgical neck. It will feel like a golf ball on a tee – the spot where the 'ball' meets the 'tee' is the surgical neck.

   The insertion site is on the most prominent aspect of the greater tubercle, 1–2 cm above the surgical neck.

Procedure – EZ-IO® proximal humerus – *cont*

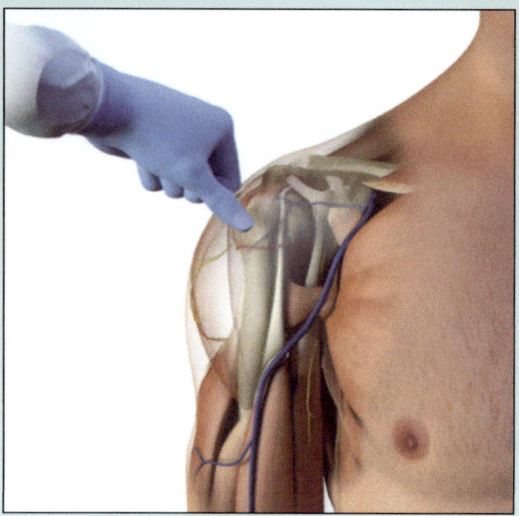

8. If necessary, for further confirmation, locate the inter-tubercular groove: with your finger on the insertion site, keeping the arm adducted, externally rotate the humerus 90°. You may be able to feel the inter-tubercular groove.

   Rotate the arm back to the original position for insertion. The insertion site is 1–2 cm lateral to the inter-tubercular groove.

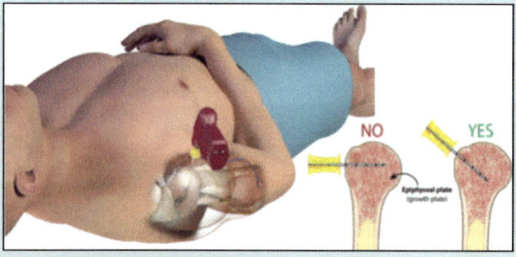

9. Prepare the site with ChloraPrep®.

   Remove the needle cap.

   Aim the needle tip downward at a 45° angle to the horizontal plane. The correct angle will result in the needle hub lying perpendicular to the skin.

   Push the needle tip through the skin until the tip rests against the bone. The 5 mm mark from the hub must be visible above the skin for confirmation of adequate needle length.

Procedure – EZ-IO® proximal humerus – *cont*

Gently drill into the humerus 2 cm or until the hub reaches the skin in an adult.

Stop when you feel the 'pop' or 'give' in infants and children.

Avoid recoil by actively releasing the trigger when you feel the needle set enter the medullary space – do not pull back on the driver when releasing the trigger.

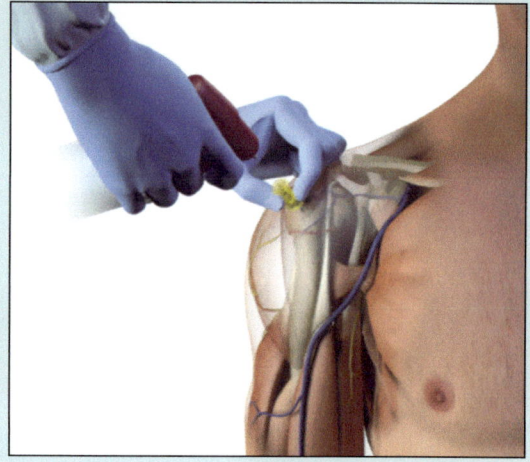

10. Hold the hub in place and pull the driver straight off.

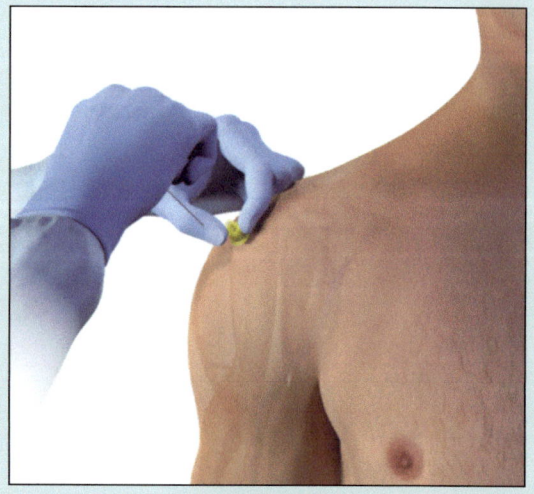

11. Continue to hold the hub while twisting the stylet off the hub with counter-clockwise rotations.

Intravenous drug administration

Procedure – EZ-IO® proximal humerus – *cont*

The needle should feel firmly seated in the bone (first confirmation of placement).

Place the stylet in a sharps container.

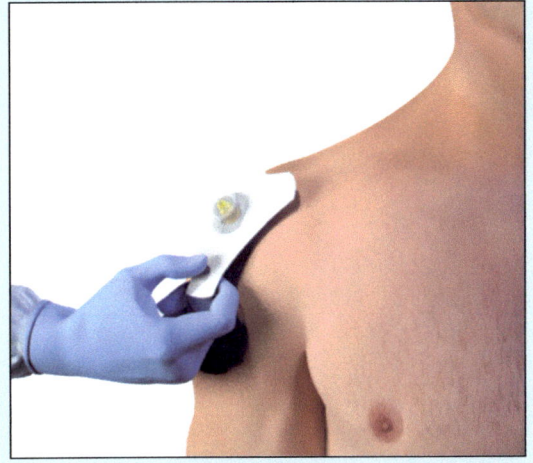

12. Place the EZ-Stabiliser dressing over the hub.

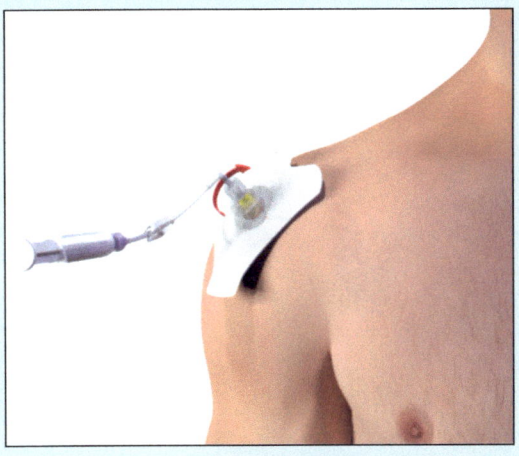

13. Attach a primed EZ-Connect extension set to the hub, and firmly secure by twisting clockwise.

    Pull the tabs off the EZ-Stabiliser dressing to expose the adhesive, and apply to the skin.

Procedure – EZ-IO® proximal humerus – *cont*

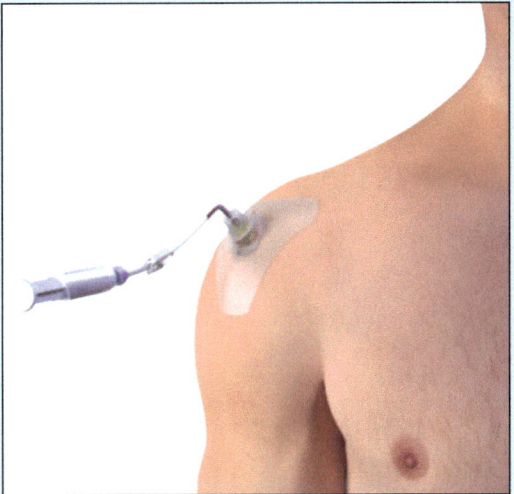

14. Aspirate for blood/bone marrow (second confirmation of placement).

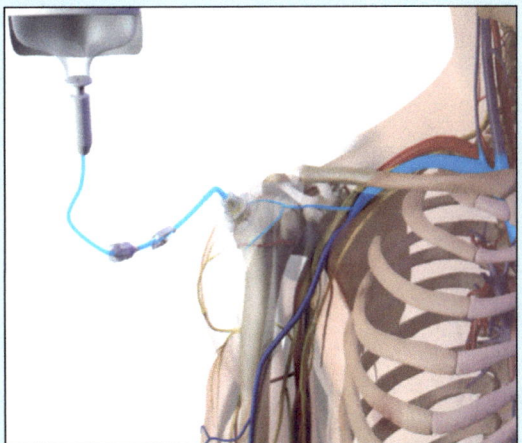

15. Flush the IO catheter with normal saline (5–10 ml adults, 2–5 ml for infants and small children).

    Secure the arm in place across the abdomen.

Chapter 18 – *Assisting the Paramedic*

2.5.3 Procedure

Procedure – EZ-IO® proximal tibia

The following steps describe how to obtain IO access with the EZ-IO® in the proximal tibia [Teleflex, 2017]. Note that this is unlikely to be within your scope of practice and is included for information only.

1. Prepare the equipment while the senior clinician obtains consent. Clarify the needle length required. This is likely to be the 25 mm needle.

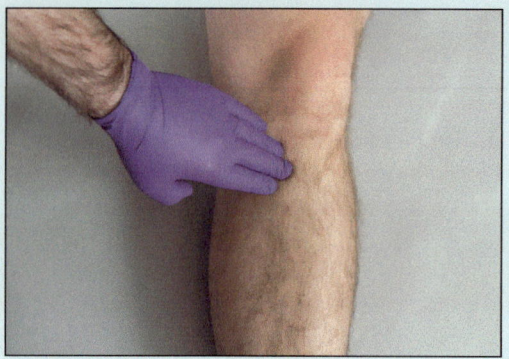

2. Identify the site. First, extend the leg. In adults, the insertion site is 2 cm medial to tibial tuberosity, or approximately 3 cm (two finger widths) below the patella and approximately 2 cm (one finger width) medial, along the flat aspect of the tibia.

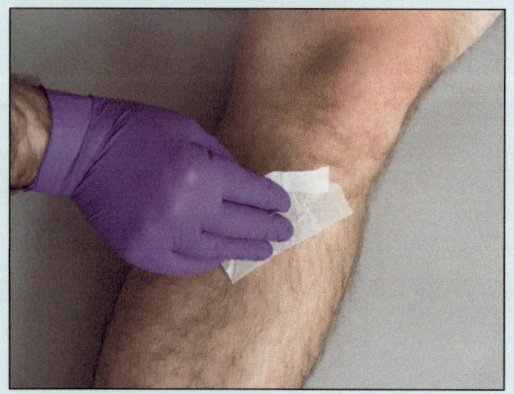

3. Prepare the site with ChloraPrep®.

Procedure – EZ-IO® proximal tibia – *cont*

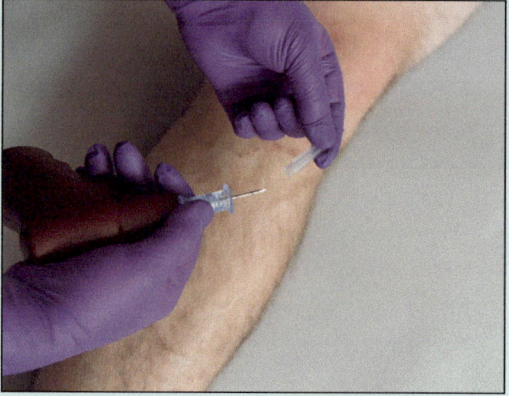

4. Attach the needle to the driver. While holding on to the base of the needle, remove the needle cap. Do not touch the needle.

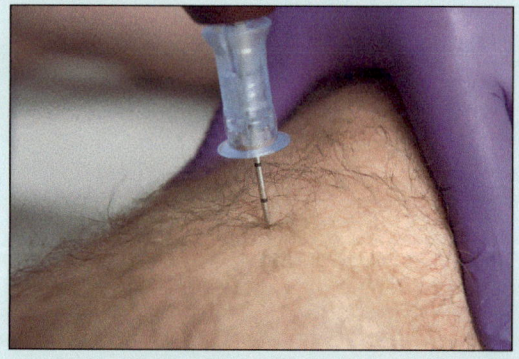

5. Stabilise the extremity. Aim the needle set at a 90° angle to the centre of the bone.

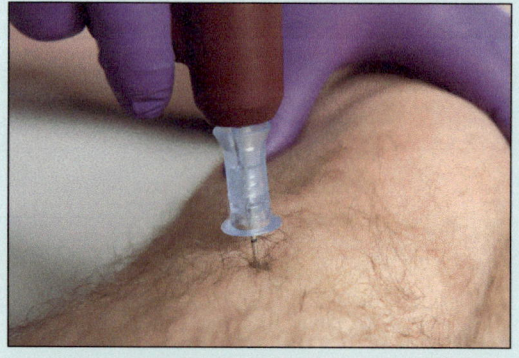

6. Push the needle tip through the skin until the tip rests against the bone. The 5 mm

Procedure – EZ-IO® proximal tibia – *cont*

mark from the hub must be visible above the skin for confirmation of adequate needle set length.

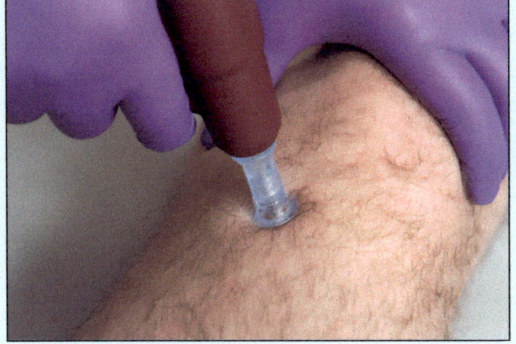

7. Gently drill, advancing the needle set approximately 1–2 cm after entry into the medullary space or until the needle set hub is close to the skin.
   - Infants and small children: Gently drill, immediately release the trigger when you feel the 'pop' or 'give' as the needle set enters the medullary space.
   - Do not pull/jerk back (recoil) on the driver when releasing the trigger.

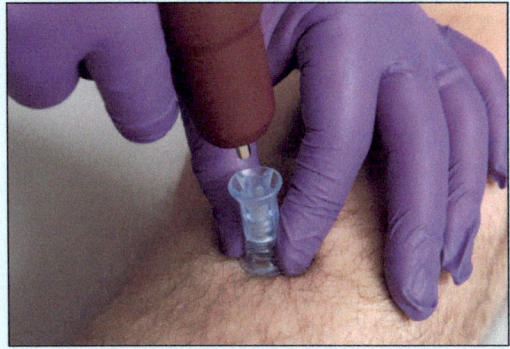

8. Hold the hub in place and pull the driver straight off needle set. The cannula should feel firmly seated in the bone (first confirmation of placement). Place the stylet in a sharps container.

Procedure – EZ-IO® proximal tibia – *cont*

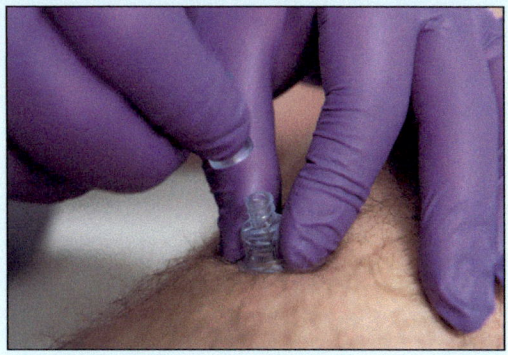

9. Continue to hold the hub while twisting the stylet off the hub with counterclockwise rotations.

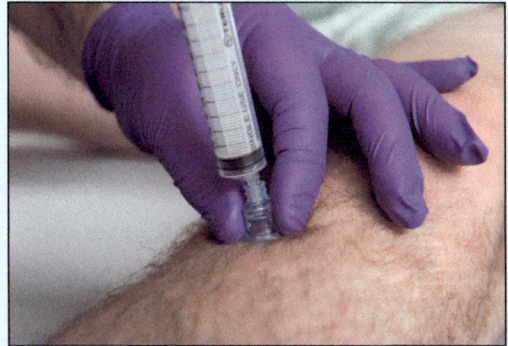

10. Aspirate for blood/bone marrow (second confirmation of placement).

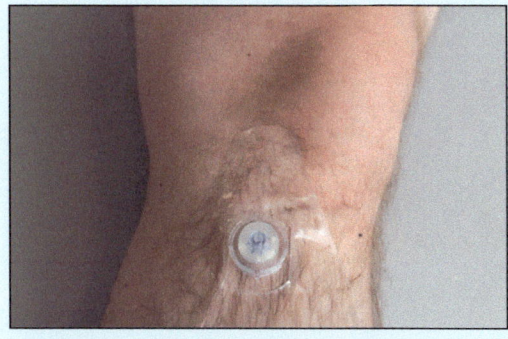

11. Place the EZ-Stabiliser dressing over the hub.

Chapter 18 – *Assisting the Paramedic*

Procedure – EZ-IO® proximal tibia – *cont*

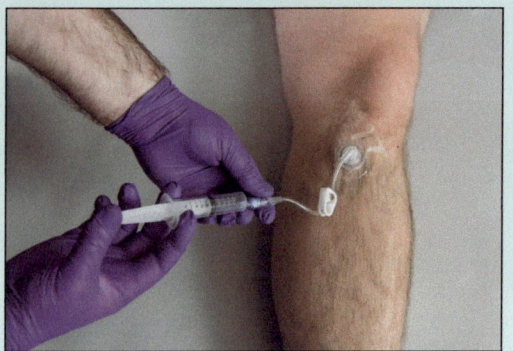

12. Attach a primed EZ-Connect extension set to the hub, and firmly secure by twisting clockwise.

Procedure – EZ-IO® proximal tibia – *cont*

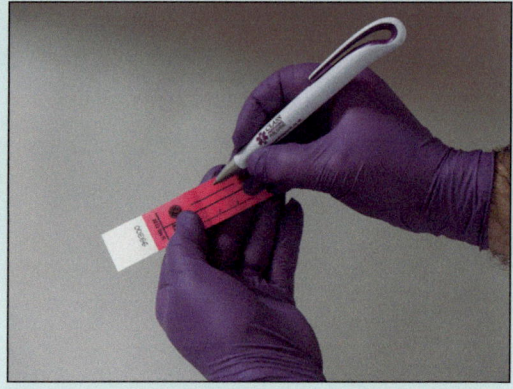

13. Document the time of insertion on the EZIO wrist label and place on patient's wrist.

Chapter 19 Obstetrics and Gynaecology

by Aimee Yarrington

1 Reproduction

1.1 Learning objectives

By the end of this section you will be able to:
- define obstetrics and gynaecology
- describe the anatomy and physiology of the reproductive system
- explain the terminology commonly used in pregnancy
- explain how to assess a pregnant woman.

1.2 Introduction

Obstetrics is the branch of medicine associated with childbirth and midwifery and gynaecology deals with the functions and diseases specific to the reproductive systems of women and girls. This chapter will explore your role in assisting women during pregnancy, birth and with other issues related to the reproductive system.

1.3 Anatomy and physiology

The female reproductive organs are divided into internal and external. The majority of the reproductive system lies internally, but knowing the normal appearance of external genitalia is important so that changes can easily be noted.

The vulva or vulval area is the term applied to the external genitals that can be seen [Coad, 2015]. It is important to have a knowledge of the 'normal' female anatomy (Figure 19.1) as inspection of this area during labour can often show signs of impending second stage as well as factors such as female genital mutilation.

The normal female external genitalia comprise the labia majora, which are the two folds of fatty tissue forming the boundary of the vulva. They join anteriorly at the symphysis pubis and posteriorly with the perineum. Hair grows on the mons pubis,

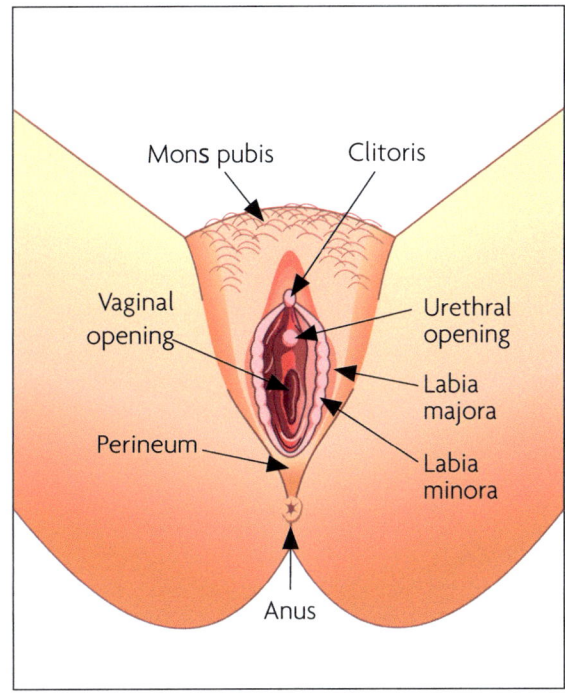

Figure 19.1   Vulva.

a fatty pad over the pubic bone, and on the lateral surface of the labia majora at the point of puberty [Fraser, 2012].

1.3.1 External genitalia

The labia minora are two smaller folds that lie between the labia majora. The cleft between the labia minora is the vestibule, which consists of the vagina, urethra and clitoris.

The clitoris is a highly sensitive body of erectile tissue that is similar in its properties to that of the male penis. Although it has no reproductive function, it has an important role in sexual arousal, causing the reaction of lubrication of the surrounding tissues [Coad, 2015].

Chapter 19 – *Obstetrics and Gynaecology*

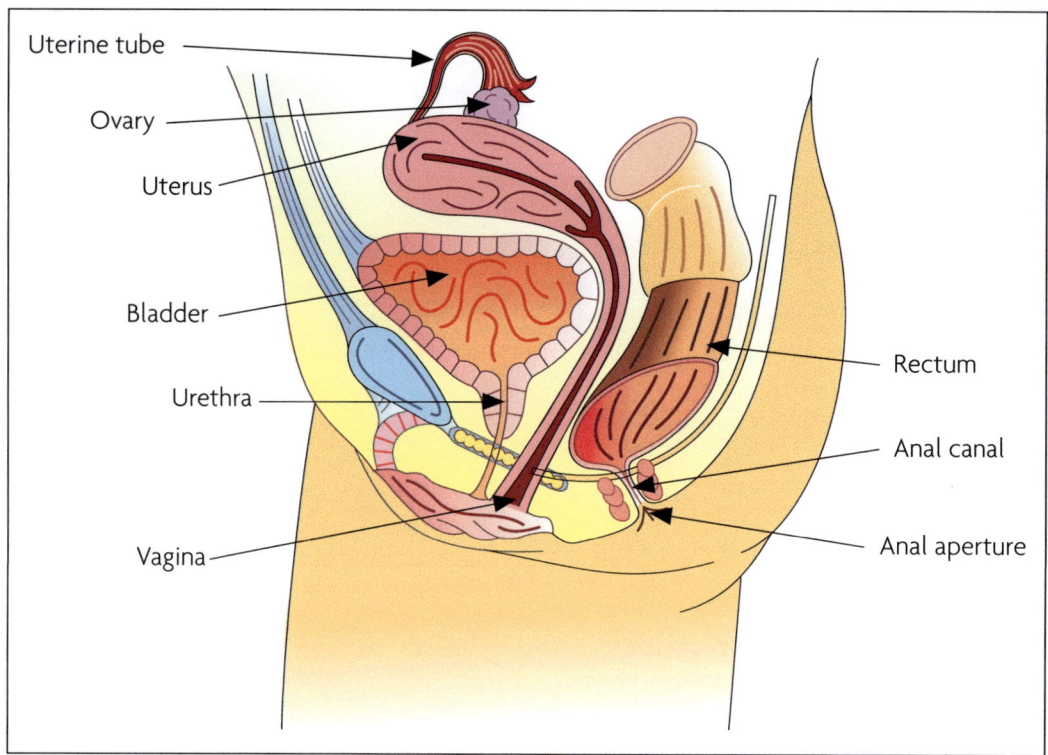

Figure 19.2 Female internal genitalia.

1.3.2 Internal genitalia

The vaginal opening marks the boundary between the external and internal genitalia (Figure 19.2).

Vagina

The vagina is a fibromuscular tube approximately 10 cm in length and capable of considerable distension during the process of childbirth. This is enabled by a lining of smooth muscle and folds on the surface known as rugae. The terminus of the vagina is met by the cervix of the uterus at its end. It is lined by moist epithelial cells and although it does not have glands it is kept moist by cervical glands and through vessels below the vaginal surface. The vaginal pH is strongly acidic (pH 4.5); this is because the vagina is a direct link between the internal and the external environments so this level of acidity helps to prevent the growth of many pathogens [Fraser, 2012].

Uterus

The uterus sits superior to the vagina and is a hollow pear-shaped muscular organ. It is made up of three areas: the fundus, body and cervix [Waugh, 2011] (Figure 19.3). Its position within the pelvic cavity is between the bladder, which lies anteriorly, and the rectum, to the posterior [Fraser, 2012]. In the non-pregnant state, it weighs approximately 30 g and when in a horizontal position is approximately 7.5 cm long and 5 cm wide; the walls are 2.5 cm thick [Waugh, 2011]. There are three distinct layers: the inner layer, the endometrium, which is shed each month during the menstrual cycle; the middle layer, the myometrium, composed of smooth muscle; and the outer layer, a covering of peritoneum called the perimetrium [Coad, 2015]. Blood supply is derived from a branch of the internal iliac artery as well as from the ovarian artery that supplies the ovary and uterine tubes before draining into the corresponding veins [Fraser, 2012]. Functions of the uterus include [Waugh, 2011]:

- preparing a suitable environment to receive and nourish a fertilised egg
- preventing expulsion of a fertilised egg prior to the end of the pregnancy
- providing strong rhythmical contractions to facilitate the expulsion of the fetus at birth.

Reproduction

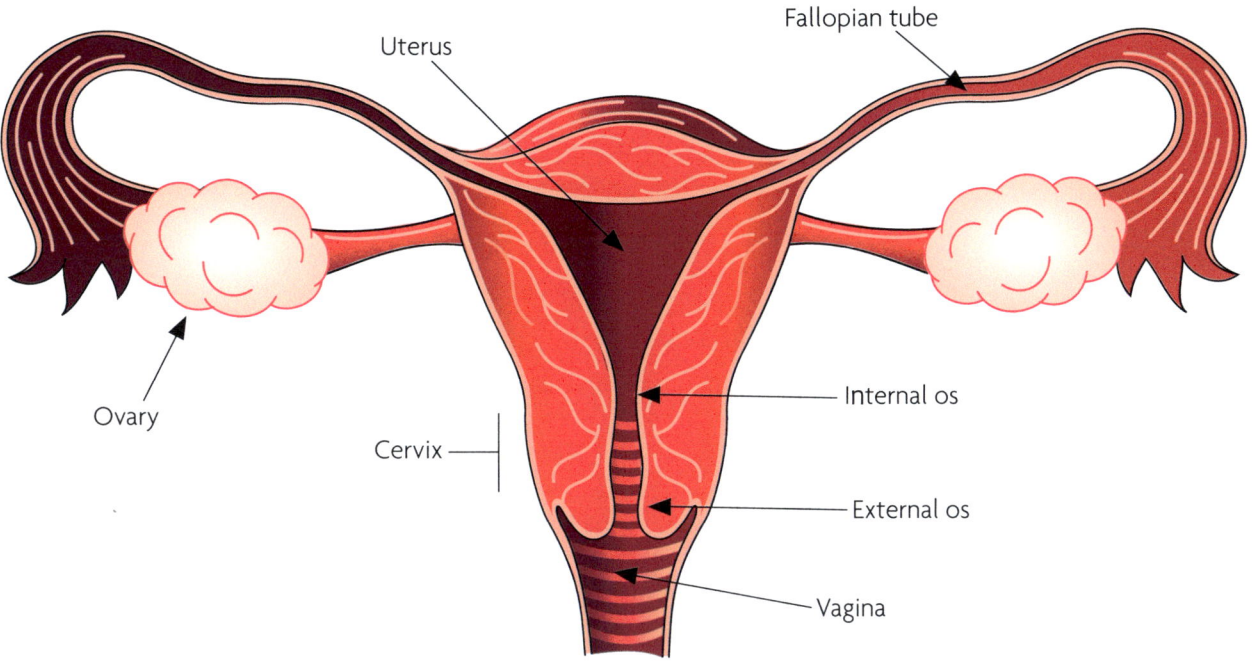

Figure 19.3 The uterine cervix.

The lowest portion of the uterus is the cervix and this connects the uterus to the vagina. It is approximately 2.5 cm long and contains the numerous mucus-secreting glands that help to keep the vagina moist [Magowan, 2014]. It is also the portion that opens up, or dilates, in labour to allow for the passage of the fetus from the uterus through the vagina into the outside world.

Fallopian or uterine tubes

Lying laterally to each side of the uterus from the fundal area are the uterine or fallopian tubes. They are approximately 12 cm in length and have walls of smooth muscle that are lined with ciliated cells [Coad, 2015]. They have a funnel-shaped end composed of fringed finger-like projections called fimbriae, which lie in close proximity to the ovary [Fraser, 2012]. The smooth muscle in combination with the ciliated lining allows for the egg, whether fertilised or not, to be moved utilising peristaltic movement towards the uterus. If a fertilised egg does not reach the body of the uterus it will result in an ectopic pregnancy.

Ovaries

The ovaries are positioned at the end of each fallopian tube. They lie very close to the fimbriae but are not attached directly to the tubes, with only one of the fine finger-like projections, the ovarian fimbria – which is the longest – being in close association with the ovary. The ovaries are referred to as the female gonads as they are responsible for the production of the female sex hormones (oestrogen and progesterone), which control the woman's menstrual cycle, and ova, or eggs [Waugh, 2011]. Their size is dependent on the woman's age and the stage of her menstrual cycle. They grow during puberty when they become almond-shaped, and are approximately 3 cm long, 1.5 cm wide and 1 cm thick [Monga, 2011]. Each month, an ovum or egg is released from either one of the ovaries. The process is controlled simultaneously by hormones from the ovaries, hypothalamus and pituitary gland. Each month from approximately 12 years of age, which is the average age to commence menarche (meaning first monthly bleeding), the uterus will go through changes to prepare it to potentially receive a fertilised egg. Although 12 is the average, between 8 and 16 years is considered normal [Fraser, 2012]. The uterus and ovaries work simultaneously in cycles to first prepare the uterus and second release the egg. The whole cycle takes place every 26–30 days, with the average woman's cycle taking 28 days. This process will continue from the menarche to the menopause (when the menstrual cycle will cease) and will be repeated every month unless pregnancy occurs.

1.3.3 Menstrual cycle

The menstrual cycle is the term used to describe the changes that occur within the uterus every month in order to prepare it should a fertilised egg be received. Should there not be a fertilised egg, then the cycle will start over again as the woman menstruates, or has her period. The cycle is split into three phases [Waugh, 2011; Fraser, 2012]:

- **Menstrual phase:** The starting point is when the woman will bleed or have her period and most women lose less than 80 ml of blood [NHS, 2018b]. During this phase the inner lining of the uterus, the endometrium, is shed down to the basal layer and blood along with the unfertilised egg will be lost. The bleeding normally lasts for 2–7 days, and some women will experience cramp-like pains during this phase as the muscle of the uterus contracts to expel the tissue. This is due to a drop in the hormone levels as they are not being maintained by the fertilised egg, so the corpus luteum, which produces progesterone to maintain the lining of the uterus for the fertilised egg, breaks down; as the progesterone level drops, the lining is then lost.
- **Proliferative phase:** A new layer of endometrium is formed, regenerating the layer that was lost in the menstrual phase in preparation for the next reception of a fertilised egg. The rise in hormone levels of oestrogen and luteinising hormone (LH) causes a follicle within the ovary to mature into a mature follicle capable of becoming fertilised if met by a sperm.
- **Secretory phase:** This phase is simultaneous with ovulation, when the mature egg is released from the ovary. The inner lining of the uterus thickens to approximately 3.5 cm and looks spongy because of the vast blood supply; however, this will only last for 7 days while awaiting the fertilised egg.

1.3.4 Female genital mutilation

Female genital mutilation (FGM) refers to the practice of deliberately harming a woman's genitals. The World Health Organization (WHO) defines FGM as 'all procedures that involve partial or total removal of the external female genitalia, or other injury to the female genital organs for non-medical reasons' [WHO, 2008]. It is classified into four types (Figure 19.4):

- **Type 1 – Clitoridectomy:** Removal of the prepuce (the fold of skin surrounding the clitoris) only (rare) or together with the partial or total removal of the clitoris.
- **Type 2 – Excision:** Partial or total removal of the clitoris and the labia minora, with or without excision of the labia majora.
- **Type 3 – Infibulation:** Narrowing of the vaginal opening through the creation of a covering seal. The seal is formed by cutting and repositioning the inner or outer labia (minora or majora, respectively), with or without removal of the clitoris.
- **Type 4 – Other:** All other harmful procedures to the female genitalia for non-medical purposes, e.g. pricking, piercing, incising, scraping and cauterising the genital area.

It is estimated that more than 200 million women worldwide have undergone a form of FGM (Figure 19.4), but this is likely to be grossly underestimated due to the nature of the procedure, and the fact it is often carried out in communities and not talked about publicly [UNICEF, 2013]. Around 1.5% of all women giving birth each year in England and Wales have FGM [Macfarlane, 2014]. The FGM mandatory reporting duty is a legal duty as required under the FGM Act 2003 (as amended by the Serious Crime Act 2015). The legislation requires regulated health and social care professionals and teachers in England and Wales to make a report to the police where, in the course of their professional duties, they either:

- are informed by a girl under 18 that an act of FGM has been carried out on her
- observe physical signs that appear to show that an act of FGM has been carried out on a girl under 18 and they have no reason to believe that

the act was necessary for the girl's physical or mental health or for purposes connected with labour or birth.

Complying with the duty does not breach any confidentiality requirement or other restriction on disclosure that might otherwise apply.

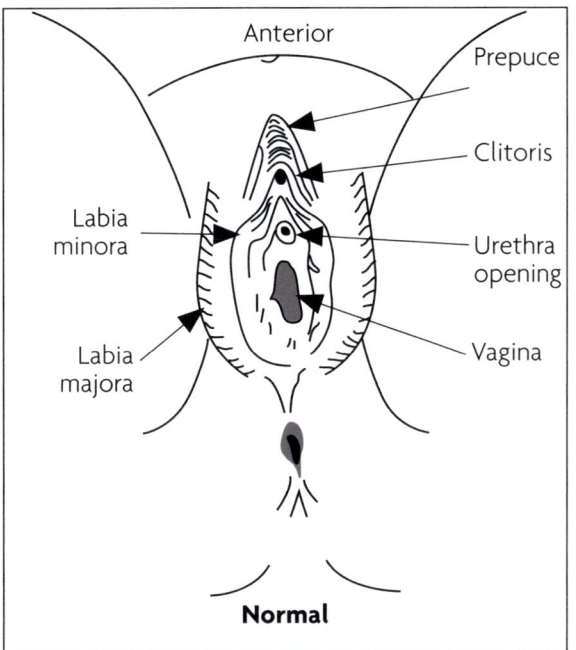
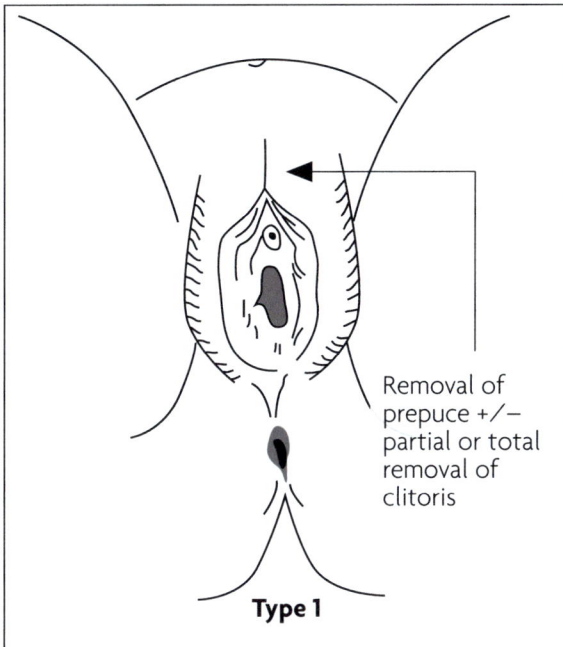
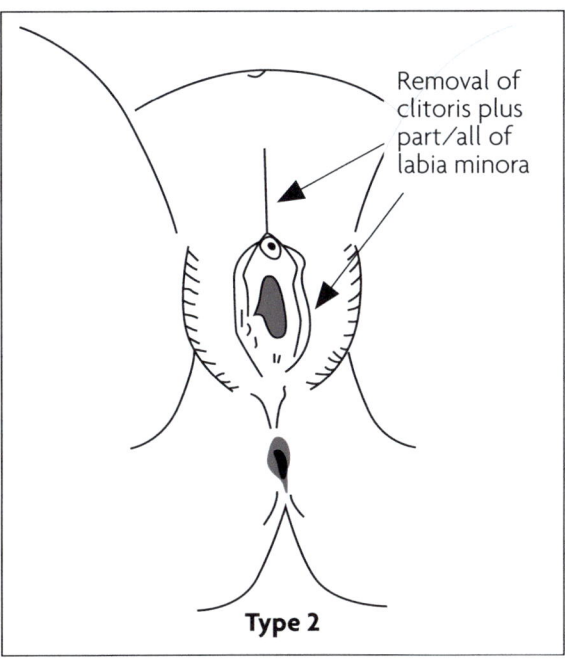
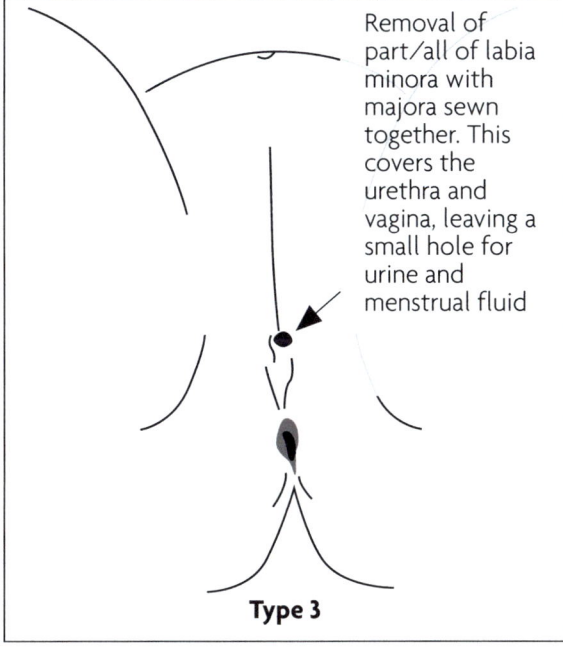

Figure 19.4 Types of FGM (Type 4 not shown).

Source: FGC_Types.jpg:Kaylima at en.wikipedia derivative work: Mouagip from Wikimedia Commons.

Chapter 19 – Obstetrics and Gynaecology

1.3.5 The male reproductive system

The male reproductive system is similar to the female in the fact that there are a number of internal as well as external organs. Externally lie the scrotum and penis, whereas the prostate and seminal vesicles, which link up with the testes within the scrotum to allow the transfer of sperm into the female for the purpose of reproduction, are found internally [Fraser, 2012] (Figure 19.5).

Scrotum

The scrotum is a soft muscular pouch of pigmented tissue that is located below the symphysis pubis behind the penis and between the thighs. It has several functions including forming a pouch within which to suspend the testes and keeping them outside the body at a temperature of approximately 34.4°C to allow the production of viable sperm [Fraser, 2012].

Testes

Testes are the male equivalent of the ovaries. They produce the male sex hormone testosterone and are responsible for the production of sperm. There are two testes, one sitting in each pouch of the scrotal sac. They are oval in shape, weigh around 25 g each and are approximately 5 cm long and 3 cm in diameter.

Spermatic cord

This is the link that provides the passageway for the sperm from the testes to the ejaculatory duct.

Seminal vesicles

These are two tubular glands that are positioned below the bladder. They produce a fluid that helps to keep the sperm alive and mobile and accounts for 60% of the fluid ejaculated from the penis (semen). Ejaculatory ducts carry the semen towards

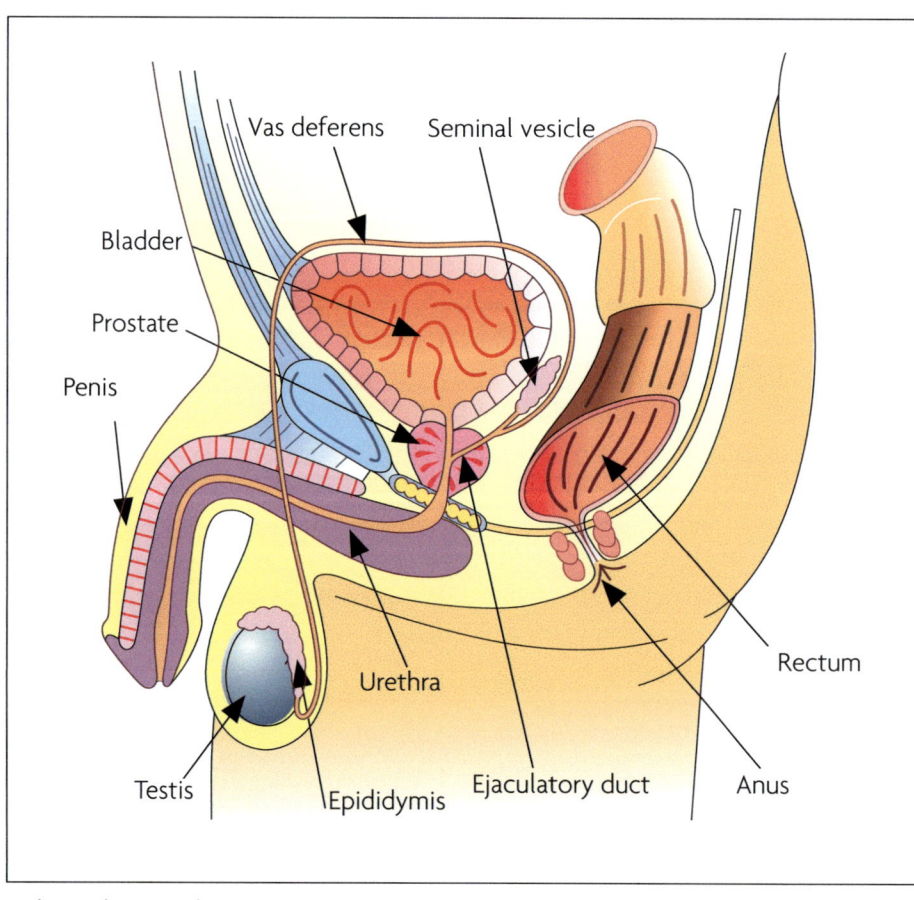

Figure 19.5 The male reproductive system.

the urethra, passing through the prostate gland, which produces a thin lubricating fluid. This fluid contains a clotting enzyme that causes it to thicken in the vagina, increasing the likelihood of it being retained and allowing the sperm passage into the cervix [Waugh, 2011].

Penis
The penis is the male reproductive organ, which sits externally and in front of the scrotum. The urethra running along the shaft of the penis allows for both urination and the passage of semen. It becomes engorged with blood during periods of sexual excitement due to large masses of erectile tissue causing it to stiffen and allow penetration of the woman's vagina and the deposit of semen near the cervix for fertilisation [Fraser, 2012].

1.4   Normal pregnancy
1.4.1   Normal fertilisation and implantation

Once a sperm has penetrated an ovarian egg, the egg is considered fertilised and makes its way along the fallopian tube to the uterus (womb). Around six days after fertilisation, it loosely attaches itself to the endometrium (the inner lining of the uterus), usually at the fundus of the uterus. As the egg (now called a blastocyst) invades the uterine wall, it divides into two distinct types of cells that form the placenta. One set of cells invade through the endometrial layer of the uterus until they reach the maternal arterioles. The cells constrict the flow through these vessels, digest the vessel wall and form blood-filled cavities called lacunae. Since the lacunae are still connected to the maternal circulation, blood passes through the maternal arterioles and the lacunae before returning via the maternal venules. The second set of cells from the blastocyst form into finger-like projections called chorionic villi. These project into the lacunae and allow diffusion of nutrients and gases to occur between the maternal and fetal circulations [Tortora, 2017].

Maternal blood flow through the placenta is mostly pressure-dependent and so is sensitive to reductions in maternal blood pressure and increases in venous pressure (for example, caval occlusion if a pregnant woman is laid supine).

The placenta affects fetal circulation by altering resistance to blood flow. Increases in placental resistance, due to pre-eclampsia for example, can have a negative impact on umbilical artery blood flow [Vause, 2005].

1.4.2   Maternal physiology
There are a number of maternal changes that occur in pregnancy including [JRCALC, 2019; ALSG, 2018]:
- Cardiac output at the end of pregnancy increases by 50%.
- Average maternal heart rate increases by 10–15 beats per minute.
- Systolic and diastolic blood pressures drop by 10–15 mmHg, although by the end of pregnancy, these values usually approach the normal range.
- Work of breathing increases, as does respiratory rate, while vital capacity reduces.
- Circulating blood volume increases by 50% (although there is a relative anaemia).
- The increase in blood volume results in the pregnant patient tolerating greater blood or plasma loss before showing signs of hypovolaemia. In fact, tachycardia may not develop until blood loss exceeds 1,000 ml and blood pressure is usually maintained well beyond this level of loss [Bose, 2006]. However, in order to maintain maternal blood pressure in hypovolaemic states, blood is shunted away from the uterus and placenta, compromising the fetus.

1.5   Terminology and abbreviations

There are many terms and abbreviations associated with obstetrics. Here is a list of the most common terms as well as abbreviations you may see written in the mother's hand-held records or hear spoken by midwives:
- **EDD:** estimated date of delivery
- **Gravid:** pregnant uterus
- **Parity:** number of live children born
- **G1P0:** shortened in notes to G and P, this woman would be on her first pregnancy and has no live children
- **G2P1:** this woman would be on her second pregnancy, having one child already

- **Fundus:** the top portion of the uterus that forms the landmark for assessing gestation
- **Ceph./Cephalic:** the baby is in the head-down position for birth
- **Br./Breech:** the baby is in the bottom or feet-first presentation
- **SROM:** spontaneous rupture of membranes
- **USS:** ultrasound scan
- **LSCS:** lower segment caesarean section
- **VBAC:** vaginal birth after caesarean section
- **HBAC:** home birth after caesarean section
- **Vent.:** ventouse delivery
- **NBFD:** Neville Barnes forceps delivery (a specific type of forceps; there are many)
- **/40:** the number above the /40 denotes the week of pregnancy the woman is in
- **APH:** antepartum haemorrhage
- **PPH:** post-partum haemorrhage
- **EBL:** estimated blood loss
- **AN/ANC:** antenatal/antenatal clinic
- **Cx:** cervix; for example, if a woman has been examined vaginally it may be written in her notes Cx = 2–3 cm, so her cervix is dilated 2–3 cm
- **NAD:** nothing abnormal detected
- **MLU:** midwife-led unit (low risk)
- **CU:** consultant-led unit (high risk).

1.6 Assessing the pregnant woman

The aim of the obstetric primary survey is to identify the existence of life-threatening problems so that management can be commenced as rapidly as possible. The <C>ABCDEFG approach is recommended by ALSG [2018].

1.6.1 Catastrophic life-threatening haemorrhage

- Is there a significant volume of blood visible?
- Is blood pooling on the floor?
- Is the woman's clothing soaked?
- Are there a number of blood-soaked pads in evidence?
- If this is present, in many antenatal causes it cannot be stopped as easily as with trauma cases as it is normally coming from the uterus or placenta to which pressure cannot be applied.

1.6.2 Airway

Is the woman able to talk? If she is, it tells the clinician two important things:
- The woman is alert (or responds to voice if not previously aware of presence).
- The woman has a clear airway.

1.6.3 Breathing

If the woman is speaking in full sentences, this indicates that there is no immediate respiratory or circulatory problem. If cyanosis is seen, this indicates severe hypoxia. Oxygen may need to be administered to the woman.

1.6.4 Circulation

The presence of a radial pulse does not indicate a minimum recordable blood pressure. Its presence does, however, indicate that the woman's blood pressure is sufficient to perfuse the major organs of the body. The physiological changes of pregnancy mean that the woman is unlikely to show changes in her vital signs until 35% of her circulating blood volume is lost, but you have to remember that absence of visual blood loss does not exclude internal haemorrhaging.

1.6.5 Disability

An AVPU score will have already been established by this point of the assessment, but reassess it now and establish a GCS level.

1.6.6 Expose

As with all patient assessment and treatment, it is important to gain informed consent from the patient. When assessing a pregnant woman who could possibly be close to giving birth, it is important to establish the following:
- Is there any blood loss? Visually assess for bleeding and, as long as patient consent is given, check:
  - the patient's clothing, including underwear
  - how many pads or towels have been used
  - if the surface the patient is sitting on has absorbed blood.
  - Ask the woman about bleeding:
    - If she has discarded pads, how saturated were they?

Reproduction

- How many pads has she used in what time period?
● Examine the vulval area if appropriate and consent can be gained (i.e. if she has an urge to push). If consent is gained, the vulval area should be examined for:
  - any evidence of bleeding
  - a visibly presenting part of the baby
  - a prolapsed loop of cord
  - whether the waters have broken
  - whether there is a perineum bulge with each contraction.
● If the baby has been born, the vulval area should be examined for:
  - a significant perineal tear
  - a visible part of the uterus.

1.6.7 Fundal height of uterus

Making a quick assessment of the uterine fundal height is something that is rarely done out of hospital, but is entirely relevant to the examination of a pregnant patient. After approximately 12 weeks of pregnancy, the fundus (top of the uterus) can be palpated above the symphysis pubis or pubic bone (Figure 19.6). This grows upwards during the pregnancy until it can be palpated just below the xiphisternum. In the emergency setting, the fundal height in relation to anatomical landmarks is probably the most useful as it is a quick and easy assessment to make. Its use as an indication of gestation could be highly informative in the emergency setting if a pregnant woman is unable to inform the clinician of the gestational age of the fetus. This could be for several reasons: she may not know she is pregnant, she may not speak English or she may not have a set of pregnancy hand-held records available.

The procedure to palpate the fundal height is as follows:
● First the woman must lie on her back with some support under the head and knees. Although it is important to be mindful of aortocaval occlusion, it is acceptable for the mother to remain on her back during this part of the assessment. Explain to her what you are going to do and gain consent before you begin touching the patient's abdomen. Palpation should be firm but gentle. Begin by walking the fingers up the side of her abdomen until the top of the uterus is felt under the skin.
● Moving the fingers to the top of the uterus will locate the fundus, which should feel like a hard ball.
● You can feel the top better by curving your fingers gently into the abdomen.
● At about 12–14 weeks, the top of the uterus is usually palpable just above the symphysis pubis.
● At about 20 weeks, the top of the uterus is usually at the level of the umbilicus. If, when palpated, the fundal height is below the umbilicus it would suggest that if the fetus were to be born at this point it would be unlikely to survive.
● At about 36–40 weeks, the top of the uterus is almost up to the xiphisternum. It can drop a few centimetres at around two weeks before birth; this is due to the fetus engaging (dropping its head into the pelvis).

1.6.8 Get to the point … quickly!

Remember the aim is to identify time-critical problems as quickly as possible, to allow for rapid management and, if appropriate, transportation for

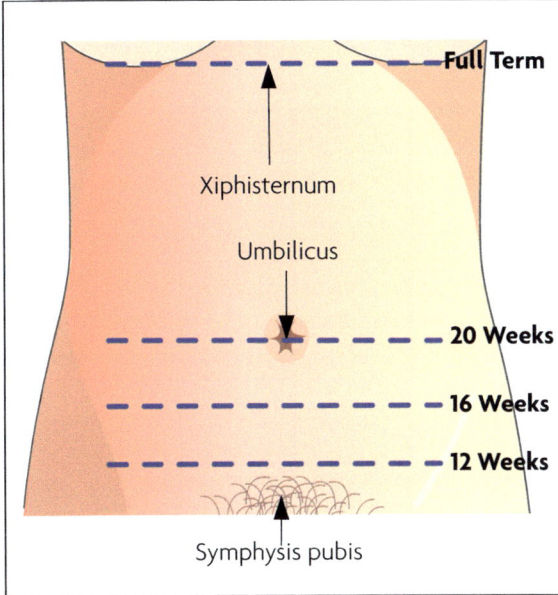

Figure 19.6 Fundal height.

definitive care to a suitable obstetric facility, which is not necessarily the unit to which the patient has been booked to have their baby.

2 Complications in pregnancy

2.1 Learning objectives
By the end of this section you will be able to:
- explain the following conditions and their management:
  - ectopic pregnancy
  - antepartum haemorrhage
  - miscarriage
  - pre-eclampsia.

2.2 Ectopic pregnancy
In an ectopic pregnancy, the egg implants itself somewhere other than the uterus. This occurs in 1–2% of all pregnancies; although fatality rates have lowered, there is still a significant risk of mortality and morbidity [Coad, 2015]. Risk factors increasing the chance of an ectopic pregnancy include [EPT, 2015]:
- pelvic inflammatory disease
- chlamydia
- smoking
- abdominal surgery
- tubal surgery
- intrauterine contraceptive device
- the 'mini pill' (progesterone-only pill)
- the morning-after pill
- fertility treatment
- previous ectopic pregnancy
- sterilisation or reversal of sterilisation
- endometriosis.

Signs and symptoms of an ectopic pregnancy typically present when the patient is 6–8 weeks pregnant, so the mother will usually have missed only one menstrual period. Remember that vaginal bleeding will only occur in 40–50% of extrauterine pregnancies [Gruenberg, 2008]. Signs and symptoms include [JRCALC, 2019]:
- acute lower abdominal pain
- small amounts of bleeding externally or a brownish vaginal discharge
- signs of blood loss inside the abdomen (signs of shock)
- unexplained fainting
- shoulder-tip pain.

2.2.1 Management
The management of an ectopic pregnancy will be the same if the tube is intact or has ruptured. The process of management of ectopic pregnancy includes [JRCALC, 2019; ALSG, 2018]:
- recognition of the time-critical nature of the event and that deterioration can occur quickly
- oxygen administration to maintain an SpO_2 of 94–98%
- intravenous access and fluids if the woman is hypotensive and paramedic assistance is present
- pain relief
- reassurance
- prompt (blue light) transport to the emergency department of an appropriate receiving hospital
- keeping the patient nil by mouth.

Many of these interventions, like most in time-critical situations, are likely to be performed en route to the hospital.

2.3 Antepartum haemorrhage
Antepartum haemorrhage (APH) is defined as bleeding from the genital tract after the 24th week of pregnancy and is primarily related to three conditions: placental abruption, placenta praevia and uterine rupture [Magill-Cuerden, 2011].

2.3.1 Placental abruption
This occurs when a normally sited placenta separates from the uterine wall, resulting in bleeding from the maternal sinuses. The exact cause (aetiology) of abruption is unclear, but there are a number of identified risk factors [Mukherjee, 2008; Walfish, 2009]:
- trauma to the abdomen, normally direct blunt force
- multiparity (multiple births previously)
- substance abuse
- smoking
- prior abruption
- hypertension (high blood pressure)

Complications in pregnancy

- pre-eclampsia
- pre-term prelabour rupture of membranes.

There are two types of placental abruption: concealed (Figure 19.7) and revealed (Figure 19.8).

Placental abruption often causes severe abdominal pain. If the patient is not already in labour, she is likely to start with contractions. The difference between contraction pain and the pain from an abruption is that the abruption pains will not subside like contractions, increasing and subsiding. Instead, the uterus will be constantly tense, feeling hard and woody, and the abdomen will be tender. The volume of visible blood loss is not likely to be an accurate indicator of actual blood loss. Any revealed blood loss is typically dark in colour. Suspect concealed haemorrhage if there is a good history and signs of altered mental status or increasing tachycardia, even if the systolic blood pressure is normal [ALSG, 2018]. Remember that the blood lost from an abruption can amount to several litres without maternal collapse, due to the physiological adaptations of pregnancy.

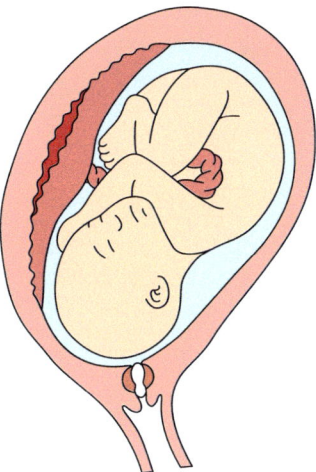

Figure 19.7 Concealed placental abruption.

2.3.2 Placenta praevia

This term refers to a placenta that is partially or completely sited in the lower part of the uterus (Figure 19.9), in some cases over the cervix, making a normal vaginal birth impossible. There are a number of risk factors including [Walfish, 2009]:

- multiparity
- advanced maternal age
- previous caesarean section or other uterine surgery
- previous placenta praevia.

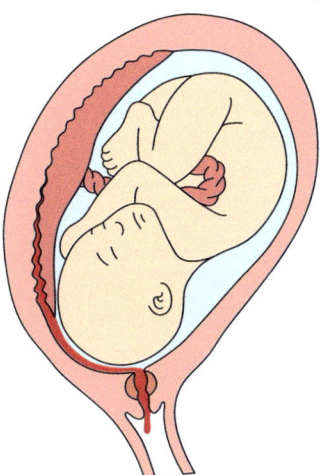

Figure 19.8 Revealed placental abruption.

Most blood loss is likely to be revealed and can be significant, particularly if the patient is in labour. Blood loss tends to be bright red. If the patient is not in labour, then the uterus will be relaxed, the abdomen non-tender and the patient may be pain-free. However, bleeding can cause uterine irritation which will result in contractions and associated discomfort. Placenta praevia is usually identified during antenatal scans and patients deemed at risk are booked in for an elective caesarean section. Recurrent bleeding is common. Other key differences between the two types of APH are shown in Table 19.1.

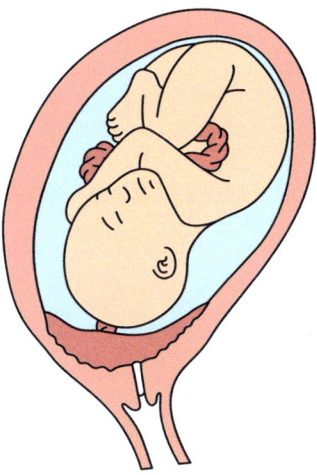

Figure 19.9 Placenta praevia.

Table 19.1 Key differences between placenta praevia and placental abruption.

Clinical sign	Placenta praevia	Placental abruption
Warning haemorrhage	Yes	No
Abdominal pain	Usually painless	Yes (often severe)
Blood loss and colour	Frank, fresh blood	Dark red-brown
Onset	At rest, postcoital	After exertion or trauma
Degree of shock	Proportional to loss	Disproportional to loss
Consistency of uterus	Soft, non-tender	Tense, hard, 'wooden'
Palpation	Fetus easy to palpate	Fetus difficult to palpate
Presentation	Malpresentation	Usually cephalic (head down)
Abdominal girth	Equal to gestation	Increased due to blood loss

2.3.3 Uterine rupture

This is a tear in the uterus and most commonly associated with previous caesarean section, but can occur in a first pregnancy (primigravida). It is rare and tends to occur during labour, but is very serious and can result in serious consequences, including death for mother and baby.

Uterine rupture can cause severe localised abdominal pain and rapid onset of maternal hypovolaemic shock. In labour, rupture may present with a sudden cessation of contractions and retraction of any presenting parts [Walfish, 2009].

2.3.4 Management

The management of APH includes [JRCALC, 2019; ALSG, 2018]:
- oxygen administration to maintain an SpO$_2$ of 94–98%
- positioning the mother in a full lateral tilt (Figure 19.10)
- intravenous access and fluids if the mother is hypotensive
- pain relief
- reassurance
- prompt (blue light) transport to an appropriate receiving hospital with obstetric theatres, blood transfusion, intensive care and anaesthetic services immediately available
- making an alert call to the receiving hospital stating the patient's EBL
- keeping the patient nil by mouth.

Many of these interventions, like most in time-critical situations, are likely to be performed en route to the hospital. According to ALSG [2018], time should not be wasted on scene cannulating and administering fluids; there is no evidence that administration of pre-hospital fluids saves lives whereas short on-scene times and quick transfer to an obstetric unit do save lives.

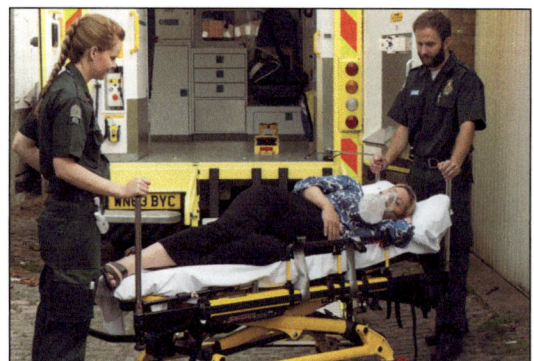

Figure 19.10 A woman who is more than 20 weeks pregnant in the left-lateral position on an ambulance stretcher.

Complications in pregnancy

2.4 Miscarriage

A miscarriage (previously called a spontaneous abortion) is defined as the loss of a pregnancy before 24 weeks' gestation. It is more common, however, in the first 12 weeks [ALSG, 2018]. If the products of conception are not completely passed through the cervix, they can become trapped and lead to cervical shock. This is a life-threatening emergency.

Risk factors for miscarriage include [JRCALC, 2019]:
- previous miscarriages
- smoker
- obesity.

2.4.1 Signs and symptoms

- Bleeding can be light or heavy and there may be clots or jelly-like tissue present.
- The patient is likely to have pain, which is typically located in the suprapubic region of the abdomen or the lower back. It may radiate down the back of the patient's legs.
- The patient may note that the signs of pregnancy (morning sickness or breast tenderness) have been improving.

2.4.2 Management

The management of a miscarriage includes [JRCALC, 2019; ALSG, 2018]:
- oxygen administration to maintain an SpO_2 of 94–98%
- positioning the mother in a full lateral tilt, if over 20 weeks
- intravenous access and fluids if the mother is hypotensive
- pain relief
- reassurance
- prompt (blue light) transport to an appropriate receiving hospital
- making an alert call to the receiving hospital
- keeping the patient nil by mouth.

2.5 Pre-eclampsia

Pre-eclampsia is defined as new hypertension presenting after 20 weeks of pregnancy with significant proteinuria (protein in the urine) [NICE, 2019]. It can be classified into mild, moderate and severe based on the mother's blood pressure [JRCALC, 2019]:

- **Mild:** Systolic blood pressure 140–149 mmHg and diastolic blood pressure 90–99 mmHg.
- **Moderate:** Systolic blood pressure 150–159 mmHg and diastolic blood pressure 100–109 mmHg.
- **Severe:** Systolic blood pressure 160 mmHg or greater and diastolic blood pressure 110 mmHg or greater.

Pre-eclampsia and eclampsia (generalised convulsions in the pre-eclamptic patient) are the second most common cause of maternal death after sepsis [Cantwell, 2011]. Risk factors for pre-eclampsia include [ALSG, 2018]:
- primiparity, or first baby with new partner
- previous severe pre-eclampsia
- pre-pregnancy hypertension
- diabetes
- obesity
- twins or higher multiple pregnancies
- kidney disease
- mother over 40 or under 16 years of age.

Mild and moderate pre-eclampsia are unlikely to require intervention from the ambulance service, but you may be called to a patient with severe pre-eclampsia. In addition to a raised blood pressure, they may also have signs and symptoms of [JRCALC, 2019]:
- headache: severe and frontal
- visual disturbances
- epigastric and/or right-sided upper abdominal pain
- muscle twitches or tremor
- nausea and vomiting
- confusion
- rapidly progressing oedema.

2.5.1 Management

The management of severe pre-eclampsia includes [JRCALC, 2019; ALSG, 2018]:
- oxygen administration to maintain an SpO_2 of 94–98%
- intravenous access, but no fluids
- reassurance
- preparing for eclampsia (convulsions)
- prompt transport to an appropriate receiving hospital with a consultant-led obstetric unit, although note that strobe lights and loud sirens can lead to eclampsia.

2.6 Trauma in pregnancy

The pregnant trauma victim is one who requires specific modifications to management in order to preserve the life of both the mother and the unborn child. Trauma is not limited to the confines of road traffic collisions, but can be a result of domestic violence and suicide. Thankfully the incidence of major trauma in pregnancy is very rare, but it is the leading cause of non-obstetric-related deaths and fetal demise [Battaloglu, 2016].

It is only by delivering optimal care to the woman that there is a chance the fetus may be saved. Placental abruption is the leading cause of isolated fetal death due to the elastic nature of the uterine muscle and the inelastic nature of the placental tissue [Battaloglu, 2015]. This separation of the placenta, be it total or partial, may not only cause demise of the fetus, but torrential internal maternal haemorrhage (see section 2.3.1, 'Placental abruption').

One of the under-reported causes of trauma in pregnancy is domestic abuse. Although the exact incidence of abuse is not known, it is estimated to be around 1–20% [Bailey, 2010; WHO, 2012]. If you suspect domestic abuse, ensure you report your concerns through local safeguarding arrangements and while handing over to the receiving clinician.

2.6.1 Management

As you approach the woman you should quickly scan the patient and scene as you approach to obtain a general impression. Undertake a primary survey <C>ABCDEF [JRCALC, 2019]:

- **Catastrophic haemorrhage:** Control external catastrophic haemorrhage using direct and indirect pressure or tourniquets where indicated. Remember, catastrophic bleeds can be internal.
- **Airway with cervical spine consideration:** Open, maintain and protect the vulnerable airway if required. If you are working with a paramedic, they may want to intubate the unconscious, pregnant trauma victim as this is recommended to help prevent the risk of aspiration. Provide cervical spine protection if indicated.
- **Breathing:** Closely monitor the respiratory rate, as this may be the first indication of impending respiratory failure. In the event that manual ventilation is required, avoid excessive ventilation pressure as pregnant women are more likely to aspirate. Administer high levels of supplemental oxygen and aim for a target saturation within the range of 94–98% and provide assisted ventilation as indicated.
- **Circulation:** If the woman is unable to position herself, e.g. if she is unconscious or requires spinal immobilisation, she should be tilted 15–30 degrees to the left, or the uterus manually displaced to prevent aortocaval compression. If the airway is compromised and the paramedic needs to closely monitor, the right lateral position may also be utilised. If using right lateral, however, be cautious that the tilt may need to be further over to ensure the vena cava is not occluded. Intravenous cannulation should be undertaken en route by the paramedic.
- **Disability:** Record the Glasgow Coma Scale (GCS) score and a blood sugar.
- **Expose:** Check for vaginal blood loss with consent. Note that abruption can occur 3–4 days after an initial traumatic incident.
- **Fundus:** Assess the fundal height and determine whether the pregnancy has been complicated. Ask whether the mother has her pregnancy record.
- **Abdominal pain:** This should be presumed to be significant and may be associated with internal unseen blood loss. Check whether the woman was wearing a seatbelt and, if she was, enquire whether it was correctly worn. The correct position for a seatbelt is between the breasts around the side of the abdomen, and the lap strap worn as low as possible across the hips and not directly over the abdomen. An incorrectly worn seatbelt can cause abdominal bruising.

To summarise:
- Correct and prompt treatment of the mother will ensure that the fetus has the best chance of survival. Compression of the inferior vena cava by the pregnant uterus after 20 weeks is a serious potential complication of supine hypotension syndrome. To avoid this, tilt the patient 15–30 degrees to the left side or manually displace the uterus.

- Signs of shock appear very late and hypotension is an extremely late sign. Any signs of hypovolaemia during pregnancy are likely to indicate a 35% blood loss. However, around 50% of women with significant trauma will have no sign at all of intra-abdominal haemorrhage [Paterson-Brown & Howell, 2016].
- All trauma is significant, regardless of how minor it may seem.
- If the mother is found in cardiac arrest or develops cardiac/respiratory arrest en route, commence life support and alert the hospital so that an obstetrician should be on standby in the ED for an emergency resuscitative hysterotomy.
- The use of a pelvic binder is not contra-indicated in pregnancy. In addition, pelvic fractures may also cause fracture to the fetal skull, a particular risk at the end of pregnancy when the fetal head becomes engaged [Paterson-Brown & Howell, 2016].

3 Normal childbirth

3.1 Learning objectives

By the end of this section you will be able to:
- outline the stages of labour
- identify the equipment required for birth
- explain your role in the management of labour
- describe how to support a woman in labour
- state the components of the APGAR assessment for newborn babies.

3.2 Stages of labour

Labour is deemed 'normal' if it starts spontaneously after 37 completed weeks of pregnancy with the baby in the head down, or cephalic, position [WHO, 1996].

Normal labour follows a sequence of progressively painful contractions of the uterus that cause the cervix to shorten and dilate, which enables the descent of the fetus through the maternal pelvis, leading to spontaneous vaginal birth of the baby. Afterwards, the placenta and membranes are expelled. Typical time frames are shown in Table 19.2 [Magill-Cuerden, 2011].

Table 19.2 Typical time frames in labour.

Stage of labour	First pregnancy	Subsequent pregnancies
First	12–14 hours	6–10 hours
Second	60 minutes	Up to 30 minutes
Third	20–30 minutes	20–30 minutes

3.2.1 First stage

This stage commences with the onset of regular contractions, which cause cervical dilation from 0 to 10 cm. Established labour is signified by regular contractions (about 3–4 in ten minutes) lasting around one minute each. By 8 cm dilated, women typically become vocal, requesting epidurals and demanding that the baby be delivered, for example [ALSG, 2018].

Clinical signs and symptoms that can assist in identifying the first stage of labour include:
- There will be 3–4 contractions in ten minutes.
- No pressure will be felt in the rectum.
- The woman will be able to rest and speak between contractions.

3.2.2 Second stage

This stage starts once the cervix is fully dilated and ends with the birth of the baby. Women may have a strong urge to push, which can feel similar to the sensation of wanting to open their bowels … which might also happen, so be prepared!

Clinical signs and symptoms that can assist in identifying the second stage of labour include [ALSG, 2018]:
- The woman will have pressure in the rectum, with strong urges to push.
- The presenting part will be visible.
- There are also several features that may or may not be present (time-dependent!):
  - vomiting
  - heavy blood-stained show
  - bulging of the vaginal entrance and anus.
- Women at this point of transition often become very distressed and will become unco-operative.
- Rupture of membranes. This is the optimum time for the membranes to rupture. However, if they do not, they may be seen protruding at the

vaginal opening and the baby may even be born still encased within them, known as being born in the 'caul' [Fraser, 2012].

If the waters fail to break before the birth of the baby and the baby is born in the membranes, take your fingers and break open the bag, either under the baby's arm or by the neck. Do not use scissors as you will risk injury to the baby. The membranes have the consistency of tough cling film and are comprised of two layers. Don't rush this procedure as it's not time critical. The baby will still be oxygenated via the blood supply from the umbilical cord.

3.2.3 Third stage

After the birth of the baby, the third stage commences, ending with the delivery of the placenta. If this stage lasts more than 60 minutes, the placenta is classed as being retained. In addition, if the placenta partially separates, life-threatening haemorrhage can ensue (post-partum haemorrhage) [ALSG, 2018].

Keep an eye out for blood loss: women in late pregnancy typically have a circulating blood volume of around 6–7 litres (compared with the normal 5 litres) to allow for blood loss during birth. However, while some women can tolerate losses up to 1 litre with no apparent effect on their circulation, others will become symptomatic with much smaller volumes. Alert the clinician to all blood loss you identify [PROMPT, 2017].

Identifying the third stage of labour
Once the baby is born, the third stage starts. In the case of twins or higher-order births, the third stage does not commence until the last fetus is born. In the case of concealed pregnancies, care must be taken in the administration of oxytocics (Syntometrine or misoprostol) if used to prevent the demise of unknown twins [ALSG, 2018].

3.3 Equipment for childbirth

When assisting a clinician with a birth, either in the community or in the back of an ambulance, an important task is preparing the area for birth and having the correct equipment to hand.

If birth is imminent, prepare the area:
- Drape the bed/sofa, etc. (or the ambulance stretcher if things have gone quicker than expected) with incontinence pads as childbirth is messy!
- Open the maternity pack and lay out the contents so they are easily to hand, but not too close that they may get contaminated.
- Towels: These should be warm and dry. You'll need at least two, but more if possible.
- Blankets: To cover the mother to keep her warm and protect her modesty.
- Heat: The birthing area should be around 25°C, which is generally uncomfortably hot for you and your colleagues, but is essential to avoid the newborn becoming hypothermic.

3.3.1 Maternity packs

The contents of maternity packs vary, so make sure you are familiar with the contents of your service's packs. Typical equipment found in maternity packs as shown in Figure 19.11 consists of:
- **Towels:** These often have an insert so that it can be placed over the baby's head. If you have plenty of warm towels, you may not need this.
- **Clinical waste bag**
- **Umbilical cord clamps:** These are used to prevent blood loss from either the baby or the mother via the placenta following birth.
- **Maternity pad:** Multiple uses, but helpful for applying direct pressure during excessive blood loss following childbirth.
- **Clear polythene bag:** To put the placenta in for transport.
- **Scissors:** To cut the cord.
- **Shallow dish:** Usually used to catch or place the placenta in. It is important that a midwife checks the placenta to ensure it is complete and no parts have been retained inside the mother.
- **Suction catheters:** Not usually required, but useful for removing excessive secretions from the baby's mouth and nose.

3.3.2 Resuscitation equipment

Most childbirths end with a screaming baby and a happy mother, but ensure you have the following equipment to hand in case there is a need to

Normal childbirth

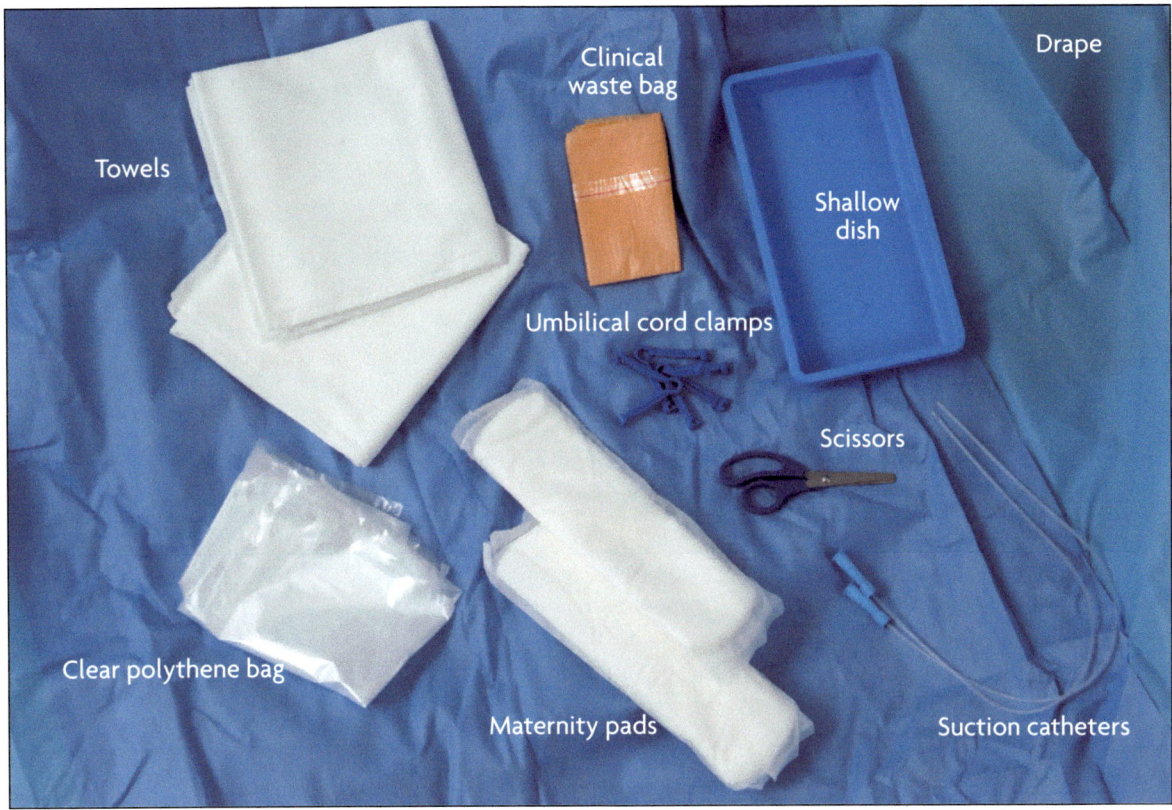

Figure 19.11 A maternity pack.

resuscitate the newborn or support the mother in the event of large blood loss.

For the baby:
- paediatric bag-valve-mask
- a selection of masks
- a selection of OPAs
- more towels
- stopwatch.

For the mother:
- oxygen
- suction unit
- cannulation equipment (adult)
- intravenous fluids (usually sodium chloride).

3.4 *Management of the first stage of labour*

- Provide support and reassurance: labour and childbirth can be frightening for women.
- Help the mother to adopt whichever position she finds comfortable, although make sure she does not lie on her back. In this position, a pregnant uterus can compress the inferior vena cava, reducing cardiac output and making the mother's blood pressure drop. The best position for the woman to labour and give birth in is in a standing or squatting position [Dekker, 2018], but allow her to make that decision.
- Provide analgesia, ensuring that pain relief is to hand: Entonox is safe to use in labour (Figure 19.12) and will not speed up delivery if it is not imminent; if it is, nothing will stop that!
- Observe and monitor contractions.
- Monitor any vaginal loss.
- Record all findings.

3.5 *Management of the second stage of labour*

The main thing to remember is to try to avoid the woman giving birth in the ambulance. There are several reasons for this:

Chapter 19 – Obstetrics and Gynaecology

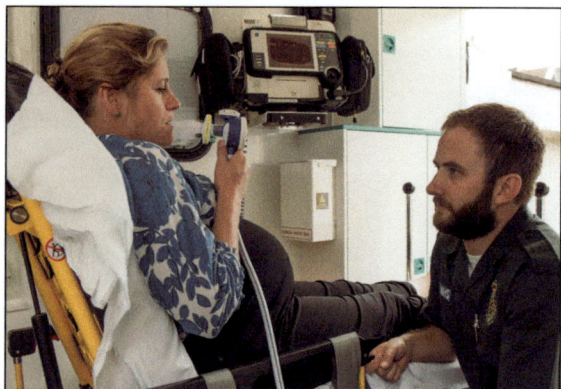

Figure 19.12 Entonox is safe to use in labour.

- **Limited space:** This results in restriction of maternal position and she will be unable to get into the most comfortable positions.
- **Temperature:** Most ambulance heaters work well, but as soon as the doors are opened, the heat is lost and the baby is at risk of hypothermia.
- **Infection control:** Ambulance interiors are not the most hygienic of areas.
- **Lack of modesty:** There is a risk that the woman will be exposed if the rear doors are opened without warning.

Any decision to move during labour should be based on:
- any complications seen or expected
- gestation of the baby
- frequency of contractions
- the number of babies the woman has had previously
- whether the membranes have ruptured
- whether there is a known malpresentation
- whether this is a multiple pregnancy
- any maternal/fetal medical conditions
- distance to the nearest maternity unit, weather conditions and the time of day traffic.

Do not move a woman in the second stage of labour if she is having regular contractions (every 1–2 mins or more frequent) and has an urge to push or bear down or if any part of the baby is visible. You should call for a midwife and a second crew.

3.5.1 Procedure for childbirth

Procedure – Childbirth

Take the following steps to prepare for childbirth:

1. Make preparations for the birth of the baby: Put the central heating on, close windows and warm the birth environment as much as possible.
2. Prepare all equipment (maternity pack, extra towels/sheets, neonatal resuscitation equipment).
3. Maintain the mother's dignity as much as possible, close curtains if ground level, keep her covered with a blanket.
4. Only encourage pushing when the presenting part is visible. This is to prevent the woman pushing prior to the full dilatation of the cervix, as some malpresentations of the fetus can cause a premature urge to push if the baby is in the back-to-back position [Chapman, 2013].
5. Anticipate the movement of the baby through the birth canal [ALSG, 2018]:
   - **Descent:** The fetus descends into the pelvis due to the contractions shortening the fibres of the uterine muscle, causing the uterus to shrink in size forcing the fetus down into the vagina.
   - **Flexion:** The fetal head flexes downward to allow the narrowest diameters of the fetal skull to present into the vagina for birth. Malposition at this stage can cause delay to the birth.
   - **Internal rotation:** As the head meets the resistance of the pelvic floor muscles, it causes the head to twist in order to allow the narrowest diameters to present through the natural diameters of the pelvis. The presenting part, either the head or bottom, will now be visible to you. The presenting part will 'bob' forwards and backwards as the woman pushes, due to the resistance of the pelvic floor. This is normal; once the head does not slip backwards and

Normal childbirth

Procedure – Childbirth – *cont*

continues to advance, the mother should be encouraged to breathe through and the head should be born slowly. A hand should be placed on to the head and gently pressed downward to ensure the slow birth of the head [JRCALC, 2019]; this is not only to protect the fetal head from rapid birth but also to help to protect the perineum from excessive tearing.

- **Crowning:** This is the point at which the widest portion of the fetal head is born, as if the infant is wearing a crown. It is at this point that the mother may become very distressed as the perineum is at maximum stretch and is at risk of tearing. The mother should be encouraged to make slow small pushes to minimise trauma and assist with the slow release of the fetal head to prevent rapid expansion of the fetal skull.
- **Extension:** The head will be delivered by a process of extension of the neck, causing the face and chin to be delivered over the perineum. It is not necessary to check whether the cord is around the neck.
- **Restitution:** There is normally (although not always!) a pause while the shoulders internally rotate into the correct pelvic diameter, allowing the anterior shoulder to be born.
- **External rotation:** The fetal head rotates to meet with the shoulders, allowing the birth of the baby. It is very important during this stage that there is no twisting or pulling of the baby's head. It must be allowed to follow the natural curves of the pelvis by itself.

6. The baby is now in the correct position to allow the anterior shoulder to slip under the symphysis and is born through the process of lateral flexion. Gentle axial traction may be applied to the fetal head if required, but care needs to be taken this is not excessive as extension upon the fetal neck can cause irreparable damage to the brachial plexus nerves. The baby should then be lifted onto

Procedure – Childbirth – *cont*

the mother's abdomen once born, dried fully and the mother encouraged to have skin-to-skin contact. Skin-to-skin contact between mother and baby is beneficial as it:
- provides thermoregulation for the baby as well as regulating the baby's heart and respiratory rate and blood sugar
- assists with bonding between mother and baby
- helps to increase hormone levels in order to help expel the placenta and initiate lactation
- makes breastfeeding more likely [Mercer, 2007].

3.5.2 Management of the umbilical cord

The cord must be left with minimal handling until pulsation has stopped. Delayed cord clamping is beneficial because it:
- increases neonatal circulating blood volume
- reduces neonatal anaemia
- provides the baby with an oxygenated blood supply while the baby is transitioning to extrauterine life
- provides vital stem cells.

There is also evidence to show that there is a clear improvement in neurodevelopment with waiting [Rana, 2018].

Once pulsation has ceased, place two cord clamps 3 cm apart at approximately 15 cm from the umbilicus, ensuring that both clamps are locked fully and all fingers and genitalia are clear. Make the cut between the two clamps [JRCALC, 2019]. If the cord snaps prior to the application of any clamps or there is failure of the clamps in any way, ensure the baby's clamp is the priority as maternal volume is easier replaced; blood loss from the fetal circulation can put the fetus into severe cardiovascular compromise.

3.5.3 FGM during the second stage of labour

The issues that can arise during childbirth are very much dependent on the type of FGM that is performed. There will not only be the physical scars to deal with, which will be greater in type 3, but there are the mental scars to be considered. These will be present in every woman, no matter which type she had performed. Women who declare at booking that they have had any form of FGM performed on them will be assessed by a specialist to ensure that they are able to give birth vaginally. Within the UK there are 15 specialist centres that will receive women with FGM, provide counselling and a procedure known as de-infibulation. This procedure is done not just for pregnant women but also for women who have suffered the trauma of undergoing type 3 FGM. The procedure is done under local anaesthetic and involves cutting upwards through the scar tissue, then stitching back over the edges to form labia that would have been removed [Daughters of Eve, 2018]. The procedure is done antenatally in preference to labour as there is a risk of damage to the underlying structures (such as perineal and vaginal tears) and complications such as haemorrhage [Paliwal, 2014].

Out-of-hospital, if the case arises where a woman has not been seen and a plan not been made antenatally, then there are a few issues the clinician needs to bear in mind. In cases of type 1 FGM, there is little difference with regard to managing a normal birth as there is no involvement of the major structures. With type 2 FGM, there may have been damage to the outer labia, although this should not affect the birth as greatly as with type 3. If dealing with cases of the latter, unless there is a midwife present who is able to perform the de-infibulation process quickly, the baby cannot be managed out-of-hospital, and you should transport the mother to the nearest consultant-led maternity unit without delay. It is likely that once the woman reaches the obstetric unit, de-infibulation will take place in order to facilitate the birth. Caesarean section is not routinely offered to women who have undergone FGM as this is not beneficial in the long term for mother or baby [Clarke, 2015].

3.5.4 APGAR

Once a baby has been born, he or she requires assessment to identify the need for intervention, up to and including newborn life support. A commonly used tool is the APGAR score, which was devised by Virginia Apgar in 1953 [Apgar, 1953]. APGAR is a mnemonic consisting of five elements that are helpful in assessing the newborn baby [JRCALC, 2019]:

- **A:** Appearance (skin colour).
- **P:** Pulse rate.
- **G:** Grimace (response to stimulation).
- **A:** Activity or muscle tone (whether moving spontaneously, or floppy).
- **R:** Respiratory rate.

APGAR scores are recorded at one and five minutes following birth and each element is awarded a score of 0–2 (Table 19.3) [AAP, 2006; JRCALC, 2019]. An APGAR score of 8 or more generally means that the newborn baby is in good condition [Magill-Cuerden, 2011].

Table 19.3 APGAR score.

Score	0	1	2
Appearance	Blue or pale all over	Blue extremities, body pink	Body and extremities pink
Pulse rate	Absent	< 100	≥ 100
Grimace or response to stimulation	No response to stimulation	Grimace/feeble cry when stimulated	Cry or pulls away when stimulated
Activity or muscle tone	None	Some flexing of arms and legs	Flexed arms and legs that resist extension
Respiration	Absent	Weak, irregular, gasping	Strong cry

3.6 Management of the third stage of labour

- Allow the cord to fully cease pulsating before it is clamped and cut – wait for white.
- When the placenta separates there are several features you may see:
  - The cord will lengthen at the vaginal entrance.
  - The uterus may rise up on abdominal palpation, making it easier to palpate.
  - There will be a gush of blood which can be 100–200 ml – this is normal as the placenta separates from the wall of the uterus.
  - The mother may get an urge to push as the placenta descends into the lower segment of the uterus.
- Assist the mother into an upright position as gravity will assist with the delivery.
- Encourage the mother to empty her bladder if this is possible, although the toilet is not recommended unless you have a bedpan.
- Do NOT pull on the cord in any way; if the placenta has not separated, the uterus can be inverted.
- Encourage the mother to push with the contraction to assist with the delivery.
- This stage can be very painful so appropriate analgesia should be provided.
- Place the delivered placenta into a suitable bag, ensuring the woman's name is on the bag.
- Note the time of the delivery and document all findings.

4 Childbirth complications

4.1 Learning objectives

By the end of this section you will be able to:
- explain the following conditions and their management:
  - cord prolapse
  - shoulder dystocia
  - breech presentation
  - post-partum haemorrhage
  - multiple births
  - pre-term labour.

4.2 Cord prolapse

If the umbilical cord descends below the presenting part, it is said to be prolapsed. However, the presenting part does not actually have to be visible from the entrance to the vagina (introitus). If the cord prolapses, it can become occluded by pressure from the presenting part, resulting in serious fetal morbidity or death. In the absence of a midwife, the only way to know that the cord has prolapsed is if someone checks the introitus, the vulval area, which is why it is vital to perform a visual check to see if the mother's waters have broken (i.e. the membranes have ruptured) [ALSG, 2018].

4.2.1 Management

This is a time-critical emergency. If the woman has been on the phone to a midwife, she may have been advised to adopt a knees-to-chest position (Figure 19.13), but this is not a practical position to transport the mother in an ambulance.

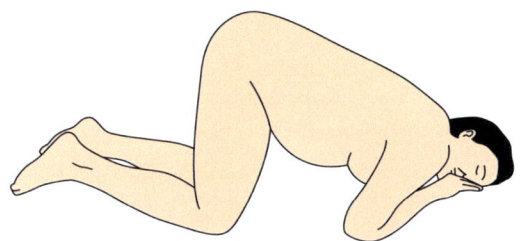

Figure 19.13 Knees-to-chest position.

Assuming birth is not imminent, get the mother on to the ambulance trolley as quickly as possible. If you can get the trolley alongside the mother that is great; otherwise walk her to the ambulance. Do not use a carry chair as this can compress the cord.

Once on the trolley (in or out of the ambulance), place the mother in the lateral position with hips raised, either with blankets under her hips (Figure 19.14), or by placing the trolley in the Trendelenburg position (i.e. foot end of the trolley raised and head lowered) [ALSG, 2018].

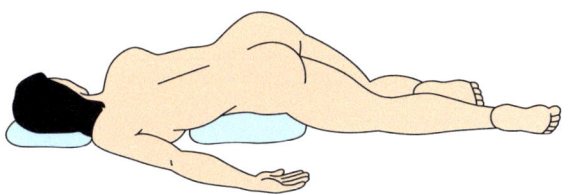

Figure 19.14 Left-lateral position with hips raised.

You as the clinician should make one attempt to reinsert small loops into the vagina using two fingers. Once this has been completed, cover the vagina with dry pads to prevent further prolapse [JRCALC, 2019].

The patient should be rapidly conveyed (blue light) to the nearest consultant-led obstetric unit. Make sure an alert call, including notification of a visible cord prolapse, is made.

If there is a midwife present or this case is a transfer from a midwife-led unit, then the midwife, if equipment is available, will fill the woman's bladder. By filling the bladder with 500 ml of normal saline the uterus will be pushed upwards, taking pressure off the cord. Many community midwives will carry the catheter to catheterise but not fluid to fill the bladder, so the midwife may ask you for a giving set and a bag of fluid as a priority [PROMPT, 2017].

Once you reach the obstetric unit, the doctor will use an ultrasound scanner to detect a fetal heartbeat. If the heartbeat is present, the woman will be taken immediately for a caesarean section; if it is absent, the woman will be allowed to labour and birth naturally.

4.3 Shoulder dystocia

Shoulder dystocia is a vaginal, head-first birth that requires additional obstetric manoeuvres after the head has been born, and there is delay between the birth of the head and the body [RCOG, 2012]. Shoulder dystocia is difficult to predict prior to birth, with around 50% of cases having no risk factors and occurring in babies of normal birth weight [ALSG, 2018].

In the late second stage of labour, a clue that shoulder dystocia is a possibility is head bobbing, where the fetal head is visible during contractions, but retracts in between. At the time of the birth of the head, you may see the 'turtle neck sign', where the fetal chin retracts tightly onto the mother's perineum and the fetal neck is not visible at all [RCOG, 2012].

4.3.1 Management

Shoulder dystocia is diagnosed when the baby fails to be born after two contractions once the head is born. If shoulder dystocia is diagnosed, immediately call for back-up and a midwife. The senior clinician will attempt to deliver the anterior shoulder by applying gentle axial traction. If this is not successful, place the mother flat on her back with a pillow under her head and ask her to bring her knees towards her chest (the McRoberts position; see Figure 19.15). Due to the size of the mother's uterus, this will cause flexion and abduction of her hips, increasing the anterior–posterior diameter of the pelvis [RCOG, 2012]. In 60–70% of cases, this position alone will result in successful delivery with gentle axial traction while the mother is encouraged to push for 30 seconds.

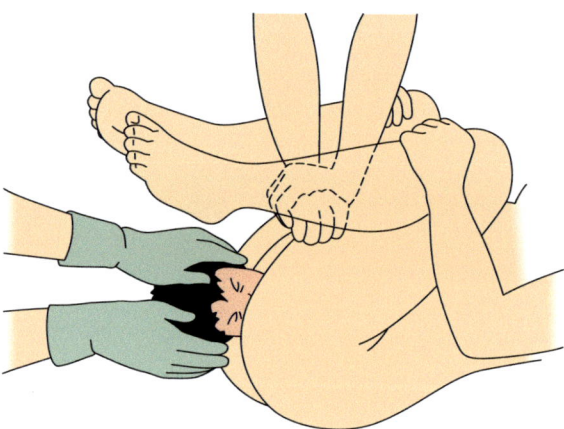

Figure 19.15 The McRoberts position with an assistant applying suprapubic pressure.

If after 30 seconds the baby has still not been born, you will be asked to apply suprapubic pressure to aid the birth. The procedure is as follows [JRCALC, 2019]:
- The clinician will identify the fetal back (usually the opposite side to the way the fetus is facing).
- You will be asked to stand on the same side as the fetal back and adopt a CPR-style hand technique with your hands positioned two finger-breadths above the symphysis pubis, behind the fetal shoulder.
- Do not push on the fundus (the superior portion of the uterus) as this could rupture the uterus.
- You will be instructed to press down and away to dislodge and rotate the shoulder.

Childbirth complications

- While this is being done, the clinician will apply gentle axial traction on the head.
- If the baby has not been delivered after a further 30 seconds:
  - The mother should be encouraged to empty her bladder.
  - You will be asked to continue applying pressure on the symphysis pubis but, in addition, gently rock backwards and forwards on the symphysis pubis.
- If the baby has not been born after a further 30 seconds:
  - Assist the mother on to all fours (hands and knees). The clinician will apply gentle axial traction to deliver the posterior shoulder (i.e. the shoulder nearer the mother's back).
- If the baby has not been born after a further 30 seconds:
  - It is time to go!
  - The mother should be rapidly transported to the nearest consultant-led obstetric unit. If you cannot get the ambulance stretcher next to the patient, it is acceptable to allow the mother to walk a short distance. If you have to walk down the stairs, the best way to position the mother is walking her backwards down the stairs using a bath towel or sheet between her legs to catch the baby should it be born.
- Place the mother in the lateral position with hips raised.
- Alert the nearest obstetric unit ensuring you tell them it's a shoulder dystocia.

4.4 Breech presentation

In a breech presentation, the fetus enters the birth canal with buttocks or feet first, rather than with the more usual head first. The most common presentations are shown in Table 19.4 [Magill-Cuerden, 2011]. A woman birthing a baby in the breech presentation will present in labour exactly the same as a cephalic, head down birth, except that you may see buttocks, feet or the soles of the feet during your assessment of the introitus. In addition, the genitals may look bruised and swollen, and meconium may be present (looking a bit like black toothpaste) [ALSG, 2018].

4.4.1 Management

If birth is not in progress and the clinician is confident that you can get the mother to hospital, transport the mother to the nearest obstetric unit, but continually reassess en route.

If birth is imminent, call for a second ambulance and community midwife and adopt the following principles [JRCALC, 2019]:
- The golden rule is that breech births should be as hands-off as possible. However, intervention must be undertaken if delay occurs.
- Ask the mother to adopt a comfortable position, but standing, all fours, squatting or upright is recommended for a breech presentation. If the mother chooses a semi-recumbent position i.e. if she is sitting on a bed, chair or sofa, get her to manoeuvre to the edge and support her legs (Louwen, 2016).
- The baby's body should be born spontaneously without intervention and should rotate so that the baby's tummy, if the mother is in all fours, should face upward. If the mother is sitting on the edge of the bed, you will see the baby's back. If this does not happen, the clinician should gently rotate the baby, holding on to the pelvis (not the legs or abdomen) and the baby must then be released to 'hang' without being aided or held on to. This is key; the baby must be free and not held on to.
- Do NOT clamp the cord until the head has been born.
- Once the body has been born, with the mother in all fours, the head should follow after the baby conducts 2–3 abdominal crunches. These will be spontaneous and must not be interfered with. If the mother is in a recumbent position, the clinician will need to lift the baby to assist in the birth of the head.

According to local policy, you may be authorised to use this method for the birth of the baby's head if the mother is in the recumbent position as this will occur spontaneously if the mother is in all fours [ALSG, 2018]:
- Once the baby is born up to the nape of the neck, the Mauriceau-Smellie-Veit manoeuvre can be used. This consists of laying the baby on one arm and hand, placing the first and third fingers

Chapter 19 – Obstetrics and Gynaecology

Table 19.4 Common breech presentations.

Presentation	Incidence	Explanation	
Frank	65%	Bottom first with legs flexed at the hip and extended at the knees	
Complete	25%	Hips and knees are flexed resulting in the fetus sitting cross-legged, with feet beside the bottom	
Footling	10%	One or both feet come first, with bottom higher up Rare presentation at term, but common in premature births	

Childbirth complications

of the same hand on the baby's cheekbones and the middle finger on the chin. The other hand hooks the baby's shoulders with index and ring fingers, and the middle finger applies flexion to the baby's occiput. In this way, delivery of the head occurs through flexion of the head and lifting of the baby's body.
- By providing this flexion and support of the baby, spontaneous delivery of the head should occur. If this is not effective, place the mother in the McRoberts position and repeat the flexion as described above.

Once the baby has been born, the mother and baby are managed as for a normal childbirth, but breech babies are more likely to be covered in meconium and require newborn life support.

4.5 Post-partum haemorrhage

Primary post-partum haemorrhage (PPH) is defined as a blood loss greater than 500 ml within 24 hours of birth [WHO, 2012]. It affects around 18% of vaginal births, although only 1.3% involve major PPH, which is a blood loss of over 1,000 ml [PROMPT, 2017]. Massive PPH is defined as loss of 50% of the mother's circulating blood volume within three hours of birth [JRCALC, 2019].

4.5.1 Risk factors

As with many aspects of obstetrics, there is no definitive list as to who will suffer from a PPH and who will not, but there are a number of risk factors that make a PPH more likely [ALSG, 2018]:
- multiparity greater than five
- advancing maternal age
- previous PPH or antepartum haemorrhage (APH)
- long labour
- obesity
- anything that increases the size of the uterus (multiple pregnancy, large baby, excess amniotic fluid)
- uterine fibroids
- partial separation of the placenta.

4.5.2 Management

The management of the PPH depends on the cause of the bleeding, so it is important to determine this early on in your assessment. There are four main causes of PPH, known as the four Ts [AAFP, 2012]:
- tone
- tissue
- trauma
- thrombin.

Tone

Uterine atony (poor tone of the uterus) is the cause of 70–90% of PPHs [AAFP, 2012]. Usually the uterus contracts after birth, occluding the spiral arteries that have provided the blood supply to the placenta during pregnancy.

In order to control the blood loss from an atonic uterus, the upper portion of the uterus (called the fundus) must be massaged to encourage the uterine fibres to contract. If you are asked to perform fundal massage, start at the umbilicus and apply firm pressure backwards towards the aorta and then downwards towards the uterus in a circular cupping motion. This will encourage the contraction of the uterus (Figure 19.16). As this is an uncomfortable procedure, it is important to remember to inform the patient of what you are about to perform and why, gain consent and ensure appropriate analgesia is used. The clinician may elect to use oxytocic drugs such as syntometrine or misoprostol [JRCALC, 2019].

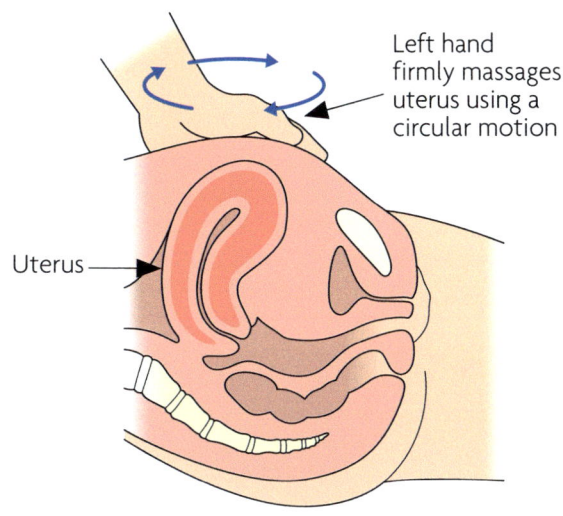

Figure 19.16 Fundal massage.

Tissue

If there are any tissues left behind after the birth, such as the placenta or membranes, the uterus will continue bleeding in order to remove them. This mechanism is responsible for around 10% of PPHs [AAFP, 2012]. These patients should not receive fundal massage as this might cause partial separation of the placenta, causing further bleeding [JRCALC, 2019]. The completeness of the placenta and membranes is important, so keep the placenta with the mother so that it can be checked to ensure it is complete.

Trauma

Trauma to the genital tract during childbirth occurs in approximately 85% of births [Smith, 2013]. These are wide-ranging in terms of severity, from small tears that only involve the skin of the perineum, to deeper tears that affect the muscle layers. Due to an abundant vascular supply, 20% of PPHs are caused by tears [AAFP, 2012]. The bleeding can originate from the tear or from ruptured vessels within the tissue. Definitive management is suturing of the perineum, but direct external pressure with a maternity pad or gauze and the administration of oxytocic drugs such as Syntometrine and misoprostol is the mainstay of pre-hospital treatment.

Thrombin

Clotting problems are rare, being responsible for only 1% of PPHs. These can lead to life-threatening clotting disorders that require urgent hospital management.

4.6 Multiple births

Multiple births (twins or greater) occur in about 1.6% of births in England and Wales each year [ONS, 2013]. It is uncommon for women with multiple pregnancies to give birth outside of hospital, but premature delivery (before 37 weeks) is more common, increasing the risk of parents being caught out [JRCALC, 2019].

Complications during a multiple pregnancy are also more likely and include [ALSG, 2018]:
- pregnancy-induced hypertension, including pre-eclampsia
- placental abruption
- placenta praevia
- post-partum haemorrhage
- pre-term birth.

Risk factors for multiple pregnancy include [ALSG, 2018]:
- fertility treatment
- previous history of twins
- family history of multiple pregnancies
- multiparity (having previously given birth twice or more).

4.6.1 Management

If birth is not imminent, then the mother should be transported rapidly to the nearest consultant-led obstetric unit [JRCALC, 2019].

If birth is in progress, however, follow local guidelines to request a community midwife and assist the clinician with the birth of the first baby.

Once the first baby has been born, mother and baby need to be transported rapidly to the nearest obstetric-led unit if the second baby is not imminently birthing. If the second baby is coming, remain on scene and contact the emergency operations centre (EOC) for an additional ambulance. Remember to make an alert call and ensure the unit knows that it is a multiple pregnancy [JRCALC, 2019].

4.7 Pre-term labour

Pre-term labour is defined as labour occurring before 37 weeks' gestation. It is a significant cause of neonatal morbidity and death, with survival unlikely (although not impossible) in babies born before 24 weeks [ALSG, 2018].

Risk factors for pre-term labour include [ALSG, 2018]:
- previous pre-term labour
- multiple pregnancies (twins or more)
- maternal smoking
- lower socioeconomic groups
- spontaneous rupture of membranes in the current pregnancy.

4.7.1 Management

The destination depends on the gestation (how many weeks pregnant the mother is). If the woman is fewer than 22 weeks pregnant, she should be taken to the nearest ED or gynaecology unit. After 22 weeks, the mother should ideally be transported to an obstetrician-led unit [JRCALC, 2019].

These babies are best born in hospital and the clinician will try to achieve this by asking you to promptly transport the patient. Confirm the destination hospital.

If it is clear that birth is imminent, either at the scene or en route to hospital, contact the emergency operations centre (EOC) and request a midwife and additional ambulance to your current location.

Once the baby has been born, it should be transported by the second crew immediately. Remember that babies born under 35 weeks are likely to be in need of resuscitation, and equipment for this should be prepared and available.

The mother should be transported in your ambulance to the same hospital as the infant.

5 Newborn life support

5.1 Learning objectives

By the end of this section you will be able to:
- demonstrate the resuscitation of the newborn in line with current national guidelines
- explain the pathophysiology of the pre-term baby.

5.2 Introduction

The resuscitation of babies at birth is different from that of infants and children, because of the transformation, usually within seconds, from being a fetus with fluid-filled lungs, with all respiratory work undertaken by the mother's placenta, to a baby with air-filled lungs who is capable of ventilating themselves. Childbirth is a hypoxic process for the fetus, but it is resilient and usually will not require intervention. However, if the normal physiological processes fail, then you will need to intervene [Wyllie, 2015].

5.3 Management

Although you can undertake the following steps on your own, you will require assistance with manoeuvres (such as maintaining a patent airway) that can be performed more effectively with two people. In some circumstances (such as post-partum haemorrhage) you may need to start resuscitation of a newborn until the mother can be stabilised or further help arrives.

There are five stages that the resuscitation moves through systematically (Figure 19.17):
- drying and covering the baby
- assessing the need for intervention
- airway
- breathing (aerating the lungs and positive-pressure ventilation)
- chest compressions.

When a baby is born, unless the clinician feels there is a need for immediate resuscitation, wait until the umbilical cord stops pulsating. Keep the baby warm during this period and then [Wyllie, 2015]:
- Dry the baby quickly. Discard the towel used to dry the baby and wrap it in another warm and dry towel.
- Assess the baby:
  - **Respiration:** Most babies will spontaneously breathe effectively, such that the heart rate rises above 100 beats/minute and leads to 'pinking up' of the torso within three minutes of the birth. If the baby is not breathing or is only making occasional gasps, then further intervention is required.
  - **Heart rate:** This is best undertaken by auscultating over the cardiac apex (near the baby's left nipple). To obtain a rapid and continuous heart rate reading, apply ECG leads and monitor. The exact rate is not necessary, just note whether it is very slow (less than 60 beats/minute), slow (60–100 beats/minute) or fast (over 100 beats/minute). Anything under 100 beats/minute is abnormal and will require intervention.
  - **Colour:** This is not a reliable sign, but improvements in colour are encouraging.
  - **Muscle tone:** Babies should be moving spontaneously and should resist gentle

Chapter 19 – Obstetrics and Gynaecology

Dry the baby
Maintain normal temperature
Start the clock or note the time

↓

Assess (tone), breathing and heart rate

↓

If gasping or not breathing:
Open the airway
Give 5 inflation breaths
Consider SpO_2 and ECG monitoring

↓

Reassess
If no increase in heart rate look for chest movement during inflation

↓

If chest not moving:
Recheck head position
Consider two-person airway control and other airway manoeuvres
Repeat inflation breaths
Consider SpO_2 and ECG monitoring
Look for a response

↓

Reassess
If no increase in heart rate look for chest movement

↓

When the chest is moving:
If the heart rate is not detectable or slow (< 60 beats/min) ventilate for 30 seconds

↓

Reassess heart rate every 30 seconds
If the heart rate is not detectable or slow (< 60 beats/min) start chest compressions at a ratio of 3:1 compressions to ventilation breaths

Figure 19.17   Newborn life support algorithm.
Source: Reproduced with kind permission of the Resuscitation Council (UK).

attempts to move their limbs. A floppy baby is not a good sign.

- **Airway:** A newborn baby's head is disproportionately large compared to its body, which leads to flexion of the neck and occlusion of the airway. Worse, overextension of the head can also lead to obstruction. Place the newborn on their back with their head in the neutral position, using a folded towel (to about a thickness of 2 cm) to support the shoulders (Figure 19.18). A jaw thrust may be required to open the airway.
- **Breathing:** The first five breaths are known as inflation breaths. These are prolonged (2–3 seconds in duration) and are best performed with a 500 ml paediatric bag-valve-mask (BVM) with a blow-off valve set at 30 cmH_2O to prevent excessive airway pressures from being generated. Note that the chest may not move for the first to third ventilations as fluid in the lungs has to be displaced. Successful ventilation can be gauged by either a rapidly increasing heart rate after the first five breaths, or a heart rate > 100 beats/minute. Note that you should ventilate with air not oxygen initially.
- **Chest compressions:** If the heart rate remains very slow (< 60 beats/minute) despite

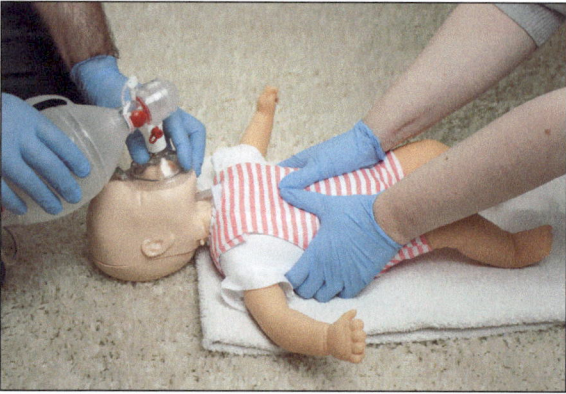

Figure 19.18   Resuscitation of the newborn. Note the use of a towel to help with positioning, the neutral position of the newborn's head, and the use of the encircling technique to provide chest compressions. Care must also be taken to prevent hypothermia at this stage of resuscitation.

30 seconds of ventilating the baby and seeing a visible chest rise with each inflation, you will need to start chest compressions. The best way to perform compressions on a neonate is to use the two-thumb encircling technique (Figure 19.18). Compress the chest quickly and firmly by one-third of its depth with a compression-to-ventilation ratio of 3:1. Once the heart rate rises above 60 beats/minute, compressions can be discontinued.

5.4 The pre-term infant

The pre-term infant is one born after 24 weeks and before 37 completed weeks and occurs in approximately 6–10% of births [Magowan, 2014]. This can be further divided into [WHO, 2014a]:
- extremely pre-term (< 28 weeks)
- very pre-term (28 to < 32 weeks)
- moderate to late pre-term (32 to < 37 weeks).

Globally, prematurity is the leading cause of death in children under the age of five and in almost all countries with reliable data, pre-term birth rates are increasing [WHO, 2014a]. The breakdown of causes of pre-term births is as follows [Magowan, 2014]:
- causes unknown: 35%
- elective birth, i.e. for maternal condition, hypertension, APH: 25%
- pre-term premature rupture of membranes: 25%
- multiple pregnancy: 15%.

Pre-term infants face a range of challenges [WHO, 2013]:
- The earlier in a pregnancy that babies are born, the less prepared their bodies are for the outside world.
- Staying warm: Pre-term babies lose body heat more easily, putting them at risk of life-threatening hypothermia. They need extra energy and care to stay warm and grow.
- Feeding: Pre-term babies can have trouble feeding because the co-ordinated suck and swallow reflex is not yet fully developed. They may need additional support for feeding.
- Breathing: Many pre-term babies start breathing on their own when they are born, but others need to be resuscitated. If the lungs are not fully developed and lack surfactant (a substance that helps keep the lungs expanded), pre-term babies may have difficulty breathing. Sometimes, premature babies that start off breathing are not strong enough to continue on their own. They exhaust themselves and may stop breathing (apnoea).
- Infections: Severe infections are more common among pre-term babies. Their immune systems are not yet fully developed and they have a higher risk of dying if they get an infection.
- Brain: Pre-term babies are at risk of bleeding in the brain, during birth and in the first few days after birth; about 1 in 5 babies weighing less than 2 kg has this problem. Pre-term babies can also have brain injuries from a lack of oxygen. Bleeding or lack of oxygen to the brain can result in cerebral palsy, developmental delays and learning difficulties.
- Eyes: Pre-term babies' eyes are not ready for the outside world. They can be damaged by an abnormal growth of blood vessels in the retina. The condition is usually more severe in very premature babies and if they are given too high a level of oxygen. This can result in visual impairment or blindness.
- Pre-term babies are at risk of developing disabilities that will affect them for their entire lives. The extent to which this will affect their life strongly depends on how early they were born, the quality of care they received during and around birth, and the days and weeks that followed.

6 Gynaecological emergencies

6.1 Learning objectives

By the end of this section you will be able to:
- Explain the following conditions and their management:
  - vaginal tissue damage
  - heavy menstrual bleeding (menorrhagia)

Chapter 19 – Obstetrics and Gynaecology

- termination of pregnancy
- uterine prolapse
- gynaecological cancers.

6.2 Introduction

Gynaecological issues can affect any woman at any point within her life. In this section, the common issues with the female reproductive system are discussed.

6.3 Vaginal tissue damage

The main cause of damage to the vaginal tract is from the childbirth process. Approximately 85% of women will have some degree of perineal trauma during childbirth [Smith, 2013]. The management of this trauma is recognition and removal to a suitable midwifery or obstetric facility so that suturing can take place. If vaginal tissue damage is associated with severe bleeding, follow the guidelines for the management of post-partum haemorrhage.

Outside of childbirth, injury to the genitals, such as abrasions or tears, without a clear indication that it was accidental injury or caused by consensual sexual activity, sexual abuse should be considered and local safeguarding procedures followed [RCPCH, 2015]. It must also be remembered that a high proportion of children who have been sexually abused do not have physical signs of abuse. Signs of abuse are more common after penetrative abuse and if the examination happens promptly (within 72 hours) following the episode(s) of abuse having taken place [RCPCH, 2015].

6.3.1 Management

Management depends on the cause of the trauma. In childbirth, the mother will need to be transported to the nearest obstetric facility. In the case of any other trauma, transport to the nearest emergency department, ensuring that any concerns about suspected abuse are passed on to a member of the nursing staff, is followed by a safeguarding referral. If the patient declares that they have been the victim of sexual abuse, enquire whether a local sexual assault referral centre (SARC) is available. They can provide help and support to victims of rape or sexual assault whether they report the offence to the police or not [Survivors Trust, 2012].

6.4 Heavy menstrual bleeding (menorrhagia)

Heavy menstrual bleeding or menorrhagia is when a woman experiences an excessive amount of bleeding during consecutive periods [Smith, 2018]. The average amount of blood a woman will lose during a period is 30–40 ml, with nine out of ten women losing less than 80 ml. Heavy menstrual bleeding is considered to be 60–80 ml or more in each cycle. About one-third of women describe their periods as heavy, and 1 in 20 women aged 30–49 years consults their GP each year regarding heavy menstruation. However, in 40–60% of women with menorrhagia, no underlying cause is found [NICE, 2015a]. However, there are certain conditions that can make menorrhagia more likely, such as:

- fibroids or polyps (growths of tissue) in the uterus
- endometriosis
- pelvic inflammatory disease – usually caused by a sexually transmitted infection (STI)
- polycystic ovary syndrome
- underactive thyroid.

6.4.1 Management

This will depend on the amount of bleeding and the clinical condition of the patient as this is normally a chronic condition managed with medication by the woman's GP. If there is excessive haemorrhage, where there may be a possibility of shock, immediate transport to the nearest emergency department is required. However, according to your local policy, referral to the woman's GP may be appropriate.

6.5 Termination of pregnancy

As a pre-hospital clinician, you may not think you need to be aware of termination of pregnancy. However, there may be occasions where there are complications following the procedure that need to be dealt with in a sensitive and delicate manner. A termination of pregnancy is also called

Gynaecological emergencies

an abortion, but care must be taken when using different terminology since there are a number of reasons for a pregnancy to be ended. Avoid being judgemental. A pregnancy can be terminated legally up to the 24th week of pregnancy [BMA, 2014b] and in two different ways:
- medical abortion
- surgical abortion.

6.5.1 Medical abortion
As the name implies, this requires the administration of drugs that make the uterus contract and expel the fetus. With this type of termination, the woman is allowed home and sometimes has to return for further medication to be administered [BPAS, 2015].

6.5.2 Surgical abortion
A surgical abortion involves a minor operation that can be done under a local or general anaesthetic. Up to 15 weeks' gestation, it is carried out by vacuum aspiration. From 15 to 24 weeks, a general anaesthetic is used and the pregnancy is removed by using forceps in a process of dilatation and evacuation, also referred to as a D&E or D&C [BPAS, 2015].

Side-effects are usually minimal from the termination process. Women are told to expect bleeding and most women bleed for around 1–2 weeks after treatment. They are told to use sanitary towels during this time in order to check the loss, which is like a normal menstrual period, but containing some small blood clots. Pain is also to be expected for about a week after the procedure, which is typically cramping in nature [Marie Stopes, 2019].

6.5.3 Complications
Unexpected or unusual symptoms that may lead to women seeking assistance include [BPAS, 2015]:
- heavy bleeding that soaks through two large sanitary pads an hour for two hours or more in a row
- abdominal tenderness, pain or discomfort that is not helped by medication, rest, a hot water bottle or heating pad
- a fever of 38°C or higher
- an unpleasant-smelling discharge from the vagina
- no bleeding at all after 24 hours of taking the medication.

6.5.4 Management
- Undertake a primary survey to eliminate major <C>ABCDE features. If any of these are present, undertake a time-critical transfer with alert call.
- Monitor oxygen saturations and administer oxygen if required.
- Assess blood loss. If there is a suitable clinician on scene, they will gain IV access. It is also important to take any blood-soaked pads to hospital.
- Assess the patient's level of pain and administer pain relief accordingly.
- Measure the patient's temperature.
- Keep patient nil by mouth.
- Position the patient for comfort.
- Transfer to further care for assessment.

6.6 Uterine prolapse
Uterine prolapse occurs when the uterus descends into, and sometimes through, the vagina. It can drastically affect a woman's quality of life by causing symptoms of pressure and discomfort, and can affect her urinary, bowel and sexual functions [NICE, 2009]. It is difficult to know exactly how many women are affected by uterine prolapse as many do not consult their doctor about it. However, it does appear to be very common, especially in older women. Half of all women over 50 will have some symptoms of pelvic organ prolapse, either uterus, bladder or bowel, and by the age of 80 more than 1 in 10 will have had surgery for prolapse [RCOG, 2013].

The causes of a uterine prolapse include the ageing process, pregnancy, delivery and previous pelvic surgery. It is associated with conditions that increase intra-abdominal pressure, such as chronic obstructive pulmonary disease, constipation, obesity and heavy manual labour. These lead to weakening of the pelvic floor muscles and ligaments that support the bladder, urethra, uterus and rectum, and can result in detachment from the ligaments or pelvic bone where the muscles were attached [Choi, 2014].

The symptoms will depend on the type and severity of the prolapse and can include [RCOG, 2013]:
- No symptoms at all, which may only be discovered following a vaginal examination by a healthcare professional, for example when a smear test is performed. A small amount of prolapse can often be normal.
- The most common symptom is the sensation of a lump 'coming down'. There may also be backache, heaviness or a dragging discomfort inside the vagina. These symptoms are often worse if the woman has been standing (or sitting) for a long time or at the end of the day. These symptoms often improve on lying down.
- The woman may be able to feel or see a lump or bulge. This should always be seen by a doctor (normally the patient's own GP) because there is a risk of the prolapse becoming sore, ulcerated or infected.
- Sex may be uncomfortable and the woman may also experience a lack of sensation during intercourse.

6.6.1 Management

There are two methods of management: conservative and surgical. The method will be determined by testing and discussion with the patient's GP. Transport the woman to the nearest treatment facility to ensure that an accurate diagnosis and management plan can be made.

6.7 Gynaecological cancers

The term 'gynaecological cancer' refers to the five cancers that start in the female reproductive system:
- uterine
- ovarian
- cervical
- vulval
- vaginal.

With the exception of cervical cancer, most are found in women aged over 50. However, there is some evidence that the age at which women are affected by gynaecological cancers is reducing [Eve Appeal, 2019]. The signs and symptoms of cancer, like all forms of cancer, are often non-specific. However, there are seven signs that are indicative of gynaecological cancers [CDC, 2017]:
- abnormal vaginal bleeding or discharge
- pelvic pain or pressure
- abdominal or back pain
- bloating
- changes in gastrointestinal or genitourinary symptoms (increased urination, constipation, diarrhoea)
- itching or burning of the vulva
- changes in vulva colour or skin (rash, sores, warts, ulcers).

6.7.1 Management

Diagnosis of these cancers is not going to be made by you, but you may need to care for women who are undergoing treatment.
- Undertake a primary survey <C>ABCDE.
- Evaluate whether the patient has any time-critical features or any signs of hypovolaemic shock.
- Assess blood loss: ask about clots, blood-soaked clothes or bed sheets, number of soaked tampons/towels/pads.
- If there are no time-critical features, perform a more thorough patient assessment with brief secondary survey for lower abdominal tenderness or guarding.
- Measure the patient's temperature.
- Check the patient's age: women over 50 years old are more at risk of cancers of the uterus/cervix.
- Monitor oxygen saturations and aim for a target range of 94–98%.
- Assess the patient's level of pain and administer analgesia as required.

Chapter

20 Children and Infants

1 Why paediatric patients are different

1.1 Learning objective

By the end of this section you will be able to:
- explain how paediatric patients are anatomically, physiologically and developmentally different from adults.

1.2 Introduction

Paediatrics is a speciality of medicine that looks after people from birth to 18 years of age. Children are generally divided into five main groups [Lissauer, 2007]:
- **Infants:** From birth to 12 months of age. In the first four weeks after birth, infants may also be called neonates.
- **Toddler:** Approximately 1–2 years of age.
- **Pre-school:** This is a young child aged 2–5 years.
- **School-age:** Generally, 5–12 years (or the onset of puberty).
- **Teenager:** Also called adolescents. Generally, from onset of puberty to 18 years, when, in the UK, they become an adult. Some guidance (such as for resuscitation or the administration of some drugs) treats this group the same as adults.

Note that for the purposes of resuscitation, an infant is a patient under 12 months of age and a child is a patient who is one year old to the onset of puberty (around 12 years) [Skellett, 2016].

1.3 Anatomy and physiology

As children get older, their bodies change anatomically and physiologically. This is important to remember when undertaking your assessment as you may need to modify your plan for their management.

1.3.1 Airway

Most of the changes in the infant and child airway have been covered in Chapter 11, 'Airway'. However, some extra points to consider are provided here.

Face and mouth

Infants' faces are small. This makes sizing of a face mask for resuscitation important if a good seal is to be achieved. It is important that pressure on the eyes is avoided as this can result in damage and a reflex bradycardia. The floor of the mouth is also easy to compress, so care must be taken not to apply pressure to the soft tissues under the mandible during airway opening and positive-pressure ventilations (Figure 20.1) [Skellett, 2016].

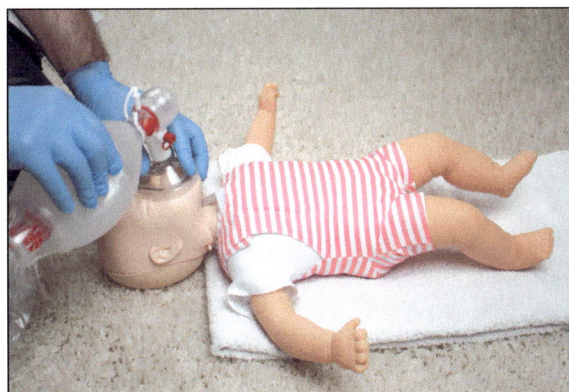

Figure 20.1 Infant positive-pressure ventilation.

Nose and pharynx

In the first six months, infants breathe through their nose, meaning that any nasal obstruction can result in increased work of breathing and respiratory compromise [AAP, 2018].

1.3.2 Breathing

Infants and small children have relatively small resting lung volumes, which means they have less oxygen capacity in reserve than adults and have a higher oxygen consumption. In cases of respiratory compromise, therefore, the blood oxygen levels in these infants and small children will rapidly decline, making the prompt administration of supplemental oxygen crucial [Skellett, 2016].

The ribs of infants are cartilaginous and so are very pliable. In addition, they have weak intercostal muscles, which means that the diaphragm is their main muscle of respiration. If the diaphragm is impeded in any way, such as by gastric distension, for example, their ventilation may become ineffective [AAP, 2018].

As children get older, their intercostal muscles become more developed, contributing more to mechanical ventilation. Their ribs ossify, hardening and acting as an anchor for the developing intercostal muscles, making them less likely to collapse during periods of respiratory distress. As a result, intercostal recession in any child over the age of five years should be seen as an ominous sign of severe respiratory distress [Skellett, 2016].

Infants have a relatively high metabolic rate, oxygen consumption and carbon dioxide production, requiring a higher respiratory rate than older children. This can be further increased by pain, fever and anxiety, resulting in changing 'normal' respiratory rates for infants and children (Table 20.1) [Skellett, 2016].

Table 20.1 Respiratory rate ranges in infants and children.

Age (years)	Respiratory rate (breaths/minute)
<1	30–40
1–2	26–34
2–5	24–30
5–12	20–24
>12	12–20

1.3.3 Circulation

The circulating blood volume in an infant is about 80 ml/kg, which means that in a newborn baby weighing 3 kg, their blood volume is only 240 ml, making small blood losses significant.

Another important point to note is that oxygen delivery to the tissues is dependent on the arterial blood oxygen content multiplied by the cardiac output. In respiratory failure, a reduction in arterial blood oxygen can be compensated by increasing cardiac output. However, in circulatory failure, it is not possible to increase arterial blood oxygen content, so tissue oxygen delivery falls immediately [Fuchs, 2012].

The stroke volume at birth is small, only 1.5 ml/kg, so increasing cardiac output is mainly achieved by increasing heart rate. Thus, heart rates in infants and small children are higher than in older children (Table 20.2). In addition, systemic vascular resistance increases as children get older, a change reflected by increased 'normal' blood pressures (Table 20.3) [Skellett, 2016].

Table 20.2 Paediatric heart rate ranges.

Age	Awake (beats (beats/minute)	Deep sleep (beats/minute)
0–3 months	85–205	80–140
3 months to 2 years	100–180	75–160
2–10 years	60–140	60–90
>10 years	60–100	50–90

Table 20.3 Paediatric blood pressure ranges.

Age	Systolic blood pressure (mmHg)
0–1 month	>60
1–12 months	80
1–10 years	90 + (2 × age in years)
>10 years	120

1.4 Cognitive development

Children are also challenging because their brain develops as they age. This means that during your assessment of a child, you will expect different levels of interaction and abilities in a one-year-old compared to a 12-year-old child [Lissauer, 2007; AAP, 2018; Fuchs, 2012].

1.4.1 Infants

Under two months
Infants in this age group will spend the majority of their time feeding and sleeping. They are unable to tell the difference between their parents/carers and others, so do not display stranger anxiety. They will exhibit primitive reflexes such as grasping objects placed in the palm of their hand or turning their head towards a gentle stimulation of the side of their mouth (rooting).

2–6 months
Infants become more active during this period, making assessment a little easier. They begin to make eye contact, will smile and follow the light of your pen torch or a toy with their eyes. They will also turn their head in response to a loud noise or the voice of their parent/carer. Their motor skills develop and they will start to roll over and reach for objects. They will vocalise with coos and laughs when spoken to.

6–12 months
Infants are much more socially interactive at this age. They may be able to say single words such as 'mama' or 'dada', but will also develop stranger anxiety in the latter stages (typically after nine months), so keep the infant with their parent/carer if possible. They will be able to feed themselves, sit unsupported, reach for objects and pass them between hands.

1.4.2 Toddlers

There is a rapid change in growth and cognitive development at this age. By 18 months, children will have a vocabulary of around 6–10 words, and will know the name of, and be able to point to, several parts of their body. They should be able to walk steadily and feed themselves with a spoon.

As they reach two years of age, children may be able to combine several words together to make a simple phrase. They will start to engage in symbolic play, feeding their teddy for example. Stranger anxiety may be extreme and they are typically illogical thinkers, learning by trial and error, but have no sense of danger. They are self-centred and will be able to label objects as 'mine'. Toilet training may lead to children being dry during the day.

1.4.3 Pre-school

These children are creative and illogical thinkers, often confusing fantasy and reality. They are likely to have misconceptions about illness, injury and bodily functions. In addition, they may fear the dark, being left alone and the presence of monsters under the bed. They have good language skills and can participate in parallel play, taking it in turns with others, but their attention span is short.

1.4.4 School-age

Children at this age understand cause and effect and are capable of abstract thought. They can tell you about the progress of their current illness or injury, but their ability to understand the seriousness of the situation is limited. They can be involved with their care if explanations are kept simple and clear. Peer-group support becomes important at this age, but they will still suffer from anxiety when separated from their parents/carers when ill, and fear pain and loss of control.

1.4.5 Teenagers

Teenagers (adolescents) are sometimes compared to toddlers: highly mobile but lacking common sense! However, they are able to rationalise and express themselves and their feelings in words. This is also a period of experimentation and risk-taking. Children at this age will typically transition from relying on their parents/carers for psychological support and development to their friends and peers. This typically leads to feelings of anxiety if they are 'different' from their peers. In addition, they may struggle with anxiety of independence, body image, sexuality and peer pressure.

2 Initial assessment and management of the paediatric patient

2.1 Learning objectives
By the end of this section you will be able to:
- conduct an initial assessment of the paediatric patient
- identify problems with a paediatric patient's airway, breathing, circulation and neurological status
- describe the principles that underpin the support of a seriously ill paediatric patient
- demonstrate the procedures to support a clinician to manage a seriously ill paediatric patient.

2.2 Introduction
The assessment of the paediatric patient is much the same as for adults, and you will follow the standard procedure you learnt about in Chapter 10, 'Patient Assessment'. As before, the primary survey is a chance to identify and correct life-threatening problems. In infants and children, prompt recognition and intervention when there are signs of respiratory and/or circulatory failure can prevent the majority of paediatric cardiorespiratory arrests [Skellett, 2016].

2.3 Developmental approach to the paediatric patient
A child's cognitive development changes as they age, which requires modification to your method of assessment. In this section, you will be provided with some suggestions about how to conduct an assessment of the paediatric patient. Don't forget that you will also need to manage and reassure an often anxious and distressed parent/carer.

2.3.1 Infants
Conduct your assessment by taking account of the following principles [AAP, 2018]:
- Keep the environment comfortable in terms of temperature and security for the infant. Familiar toys and blankets can help.
- Use the name of the patient while conducting your assessment.
- Where possible, assess an infant in the arms of a parent/carer.
- Approach the infant slowly and calmly. Loud voices and fast movements may scare them.
- Do not stand over an infant, but sit or kneel at their eye level.
- Look, listen and feel, in that order, to minimise infant distress.
- Warm your hands and tools such as stethoscopes.
- Be flexible in your assessment. If the infant is calm, count the respiratory rate and listen to the chest first. This is not possible to do accurately when the infant is crying.
- Observe the interaction between parent/carer and the infant. Consider if child abuse is a possibility.
- Toys can be used to distract the infant.
- Older infants may display stranger anxiety, so if you need to expose the infant, ask the parent/carer to do this. Don't let the infant get cold, though.
- Save painful procedures (such as blood sugar measurement) until last.

2.3.2 Toddlers
Conduct your assessment taking account of the following principles [AAP, 2018]:
- Use the name of the patient while conducting your assessment.
- Approach slowly and don't touch them until they are familiar with you.
- Communicate using a firm, but friendly, tone of voice.
- Do not stand over a toddler, but sit or kneel at their eye level.
- Where possible, place the toddler on the lap of a parent/carer.
- Use play and distraction to help you conduct your assessment.
- If you need to use equipment, such as a stethoscope, let them hold it and become familiar and comfortable with it.
- Communicate directly with the toddler. Admire their clothes or ask about pets. Remember they are self-centred at this age.

- Provide limited choices. For example: 'Do you want me to listen to your belly or chest first?'
- Avoid questions that can be answered with a 'No'.
- Examine a toddler from toe-to-head.
- Involve the parent/carer. For example, place the pulse oximeter probe on their finger first and ask them to remove the toddler's clothes or hold an oxygen mask near the toddler.
- Do not expect toddlers to sit still and co-operate. Be patient and opportunistic.

2.3.3 Pre-school

Conduct your assessment taking account of the following principles [AAP, 2018]:
- Use the name of the patient while conducting your assessment.
- Use simple terms to explain what you are going to do.
- Choose your words carefully. Use age-appropriate language and avoid scaring the child.
- A teddy or dolls can be helpful to explain what you are going to do.
- Set limits on behaviour, if required. For example: 'You can cry or scream, but not kick or bite'.
- Praise good behaviour.
- Use games and toys to provide distraction. Ambulance bandages can be useful for this.
- Focus on one thing at a time and minimise the time between explaining a procedure, especially a painful one, and carrying it out.

2.3.4 School-age

Conduct your assessment taking account of the following principles [AAP, 2018]:
- Use the name of the patient while conducting your assessment.
- Privacy becomes important in this age group. Make sure the environment is appropriate; if you need to expose the child to examine them, cover them up afterwards.
- Speak directly to the child first, then include the parent/carer. Ask older children if they would like their parent/carer present.
- Involve the child in their care if they want this. Feeling out of control can distress children in this age group. However, do not negotiate unless the child really does have a choice.
- Anticipate the fears that the child has and address them straight away. Assure them that becoming ill or injured is not a punishment.
- Explain in simple terms what is wrong and what is going to be done.
- Explain procedures just prior to undertaking them. Don't lie to the child, for example telling them a procedure won't hurt when it will.
- Praise the child for being co-operative, but do not chastise them if they are not.
- Physical assessments in this age group can usually be conducted head-to-toe.

2.3.5 Teenagers

Conduct your assessment taking account of the following principles [AAP, 2018]:
- Use the name of the patient while conducting your assessment.
- Speak directly to the teenager and ask them first for information. If they do not know the answer, for example the name of their GP, check with them if it is OK to ask their parent/carer.
- Respect their modesty and privacy. Be confidential unless you have a duty to report or pass on their disclosures.
- Be honest and non-judgemental. Provide accurate information and allay fears, particularly concerns over body image or being 'different' as a result of their current illness or injury.
- Do not mistake the size of the teenager as a measure of their maturity.
- Avoid becoming frustrated or angry if the teenager does not want to communicate or is unco-operative.
- Enlist the help of their friends to assist when the teenager is being unco-operative, although keep in mind the teenager's right to confidentiality.

2.4 Recognising the sick infant and child

Unlike adults, infants and children generally have a cardiac arrest secondary to respiratory and/or circulatory failure. Outcome from cardiac arrest in infants and children is significantly worse than adults; intervening early on can prevent this from occurring.

2.4.1 Respiratory failure

Respiratory failure can be either compensated or decompensated. Compensated respiratory failure (sometimes known as respiratory distress) is characterised by increased work of breathing to overcome a respiratory problem, e.g. bronchiolitis. Respiratory failure is termed decompensated when the respiratory system can no longer maintain appropriate blood levels of oxygen (O_2) and carbon dioxide (CO_2). Since blood gases are not available out-of-hospital, a rough equivalent is a pulse oximetry (SpO_2) reading of less than 90% when breathing room air [Skellett, 2016].

Occasionally, respiratory failure can be present in the absence of increased work of breathing, e.g. due to decreased level of consciousness or a morphine overdose.

2.4.2 Cardiac failure

As with respiratory failure, cardiac failure can also be compensated or decompensated. In compensated failure, vital organ (heart and brain) perfusion is maintained and blood pressure remains within normal limits. This is mostly achieved by peripheral vasoconstriction. Once there is insufficient circulation to deliver O_2 to the tissues (i.e. in shock), the infant or child will become hypotensive and their level of consciousness will reduce.

2.5 Primary survey

The primary survey in the infant and child is the same as for adults, except for the general impression component, which should include use of the paediatric assessment triangle (PAT). The PAT is advantageous in children because it can be undertaken without actually touching the child and can be performed 'across the room' to avoid increasing a child's anxiety by getting too close initially [AAP, 2018].

2.5.1 General impression

It is important to gain a general impression of the health of an infant or child from 'across the room', before your presence has an adverse effect on their level of anxiety or distress. To help you achieve this, use the paediatric assessment triangle (PAT) [Dieckmann, 2010]. As the name suggests, it consists of three key components:
- appearance
- work of breathing
- circulation to skin.

Appearance

The child's general appearance is probably the most significant aspect of the PAT as it provides information about the perfusion of the brain. The parts of this component can be remembered using the mnemonic TICLS [AAP, 2018]:
- **Tone:** Is the infant/child moving spontaneously or are they floppy and listless?
- **Interactiveness:** Does the infant/child respond to people, objects and sounds or are they uninterested in their surroundings?
- **Consolability:** Can the infant/child be consoled by their parent/carer?
- **Look/gaze:** Does the infant/child look at you or do they have a 'glass-eyed' stare into the distance?
- **Speech/cry:** Is their speech or cry strong or weak, muffled or hoarse?

Work of breathing

In children, it is their work of breathing that provides a better indication as to the adequacy of oxygenation and ventilation rather than the more traditional respiratory rate and/or auscultation in adults [AAP, 2018]. Look for signs of increased work of breathing as well as listening for abnormal airway sounds:
- **Abnormal airway sounds:** These include snoring, muffled or hoarse speech, stridor, grunting and wheezing.
- **Abnormal positioning:** Children who can sit up may adopt a 'sniffing the morning air' position, tripod position and/or refuse to lie down.
- **Recession:** Recession of the chest muscles provides an indication of increased work of breathing, as does head-bobbing in infants. Beware the child over five years who has signs of recession, as this is a sign of serious respiratory compromise [Skellett, 2016].
- **Flaring:** Look for nasal flaring, an exaggerated opening of the nostrils during laboured inspiration.

Circulation to skin

When cardiac output is not sufficient to meet the body's metabolic demands, the circulation to non-essential organs, such as the skin, reduces. This can manifest in children as [AAP, 2018]:

- **Pallor:** White or pale skin indicating a reflex shunting of blood away from the skin. This may be the only sign of compensated shock.
- **Cyanosis:** This is a blue discolouration of the skin caused by inadequate oxygenation. Note that blue hands and feet in newborns and infants under the age of two months (acrocyanosis) is a finding.
- **Mottling:** This is caused by abnormal blood vessel tone in the capillary beds of the skin. There are patchy areas of pallor and cyanosis. This can be normal when the child is exposed to a cold environment.

2.5.2 Airway

Obstruction of the airway is common in seriously ill children, causing hypoxia, which can lead to unconsciousness and cardiorespiratory arrest (such as in cases of choking) [Skellett, 2016]. The section on choking in the paediatric patient in Chapter 11, 'Airway,' covered the former, so will not be revisited here, but it is important to remember that chest movement does not imply a clear airway: you need to listen and feel for air movement.

Look for apparent difficulty in breathing or increased work of breathing. In conscious children, they may be in visible distress. Listen for additional noises, such as stridor, a high-pitched (usually) inspiratory sound [Skellett, 2016].

Management

Children who are conscious should be allowed to adopt a position of comfort, ideally one that they themselves adopt to maximise the efficiency of their airway, and supplemental high-flow oxygen via a non-rebreathe mask should be administered.

For unconscious children, their head needs positioning appropriately to open the airway and prevent the tongue from falling backwards and occluding the airway. This can be achieved in children using a head tilt–chin lift, or jaw thrust

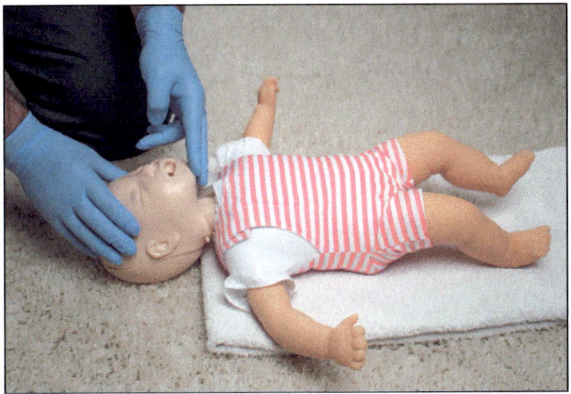

Figure 20.2 An infant, with their airway in neutral alignment.

manoeuvre as described in Chapter 11, 'Airway'. Remember that in infants, their head should be placed in the neutral position, with padding under the shoulders to account for their proportionally larger head (Figure 20.2). Care must be taken not to compress the soft tissues under a child's jaw as this can also occlude the airway [Skellett, 2016].

Suction is useful in children, as in adults, but in infants suction pressures should not exceed 120 mmHg.

Oropharyngeal airways (OPAs) can be used in children as for adults. For small children and infants, it is generally recommended that the OPA is introduced the 'right way round' and not rotated 180°. This is likely to require a tongue depressor or, if that is not available, a laryngoscope [Skellett, 2016].

2.5.3 Breathing

Assessment

The most effective way of determining whether the airway is obstructed is to look, listen and feel [Maconochie, 2015]:

- Look for chest (and abdominal) movements.
- Listen at the child's mouth and nose for breath (plus added) sounds. Auscultate the chest: Breath sounds should be audible in both lung bases.
- Feel for air movement on your cheek.

Note that the chest may move in children, even with an obstruction, making it important to listen and feel.

As part of gaining a general impression, you will already have considered the patient's work of breathing, which includes [AAP, 2018]:
- abnormal airway sounds
- abnormal positioning
- recession
- flaring.

Other signs of increased work of breathing include elevated respiratory rates and accessory muscle use.

Abnormal airway sounds

Stridor is a high-pitched inspiratory sound, which indicates an upper airway obstruction. This may be an object, or swelling due to infection. In severe cases, it can also occur on expiration. A wheeze, on the other hand, is usually an expiratory sound and is a sign of lower airway obstruction. You may be able to hear it with just your ears, but often it will only be heard on auscultation [AAP, 2018].

Grunting is usually heard in neonates and small infants, although it can occur in small children. It occurs when the infant exhales against a partially closed glottis. This generates a small amount of end-expiratory pressure, keeping the small airways from collapsing at the end of expiration. It is an indication of severe respiratory compromise [Skellett, 2016].

Abnormal positioning

Children in respiratory distress typically adopt a position that maximises their respiratory efficiency. In upper airway obstruction, this will be a 'sniffing the morning air' position. In lower respiratory problems they may adopt a 'tripod' position, sitting forward with their arms outstretched and resting on their knees [Skellett, 2016].

Recession

Recession can be sternal, subcostal and/or intercostal. Note that significant recession can be seen in infants and young children, even in mild respiratory distress, due to their compliant chest wall (Figure 20.3). However, as previously mentioned, it is a serious sign in children over 5 years of age [AAP, 2018].

Flaring

Nostril flaring in infants and young children is a sign of increased respiratory effort.

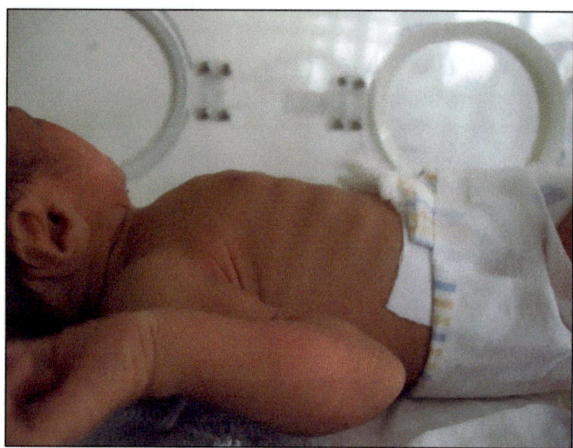

Figure 20.3 A newborn with intercostal recession.
Source: Bobjgalindo (Own work) [CC-BY-SA-3.0-2.5-2.0-1.0], via Wikimedia Commons.

Respiratory rate

An increased respiratory rate (tachypnoea) is often the first sign of respiratory problems, although it can be difficult to assess in the crying infant/child (Table 20.4) [Skellett, 2016].

Accessory muscle use

Additional muscles are often recruited when the work of breathing increases. One group is the sternocleidomastoid muscles in the neck. These cause 'head bobbing' in infants, who will nod their head up and down with each breath. However, this is not an efficient method of breathing [Skellett, 2016].

Table 20.4 Respiratory rate ranges in infants and children.

Age (years)	Respiratory rate (breaths/minute)
<1	30–40
1–2	26–34
2–5	24–30
5–12	20–24
>12	12–20

Initial assessment and management of the paediatric patient

Pulse oximetry
This can be unreliable when a child has poor peripheral circulation, but, if obtainable, a reading of less than 90% on air, or 95% on high-flow oxygen, is a sign of decompensated respiratory failure and urgent intervention is required [Maconochie, 2015].

Management
All seriously ill children should receive high-flow oxygen via a non-rebreathe mask, unless their ventilation is insufficient. In this case, assistance should be provided with bag-valve-mask ventilation. For children who are conscious, placing a mask over the child may be distressing. In this case, attempt administration using the least-threatening method, for example by asking the parent/carer to hold an oxygen mask close to the patient's mouth and nose [JRCALC, 2019].

Watch for signs of decompensation, which include:
- changes to respiratory rate: increasing or sudden decrease
- reducing level of consciousness/interaction with ambulance staff and parents/guardians
- exhaustion.

Unconscious children and infants whose airway is clear and who are breathing normally should be turned on their side into the recovery position [Maconochie, 2015]. While the adult recovery position can be used in children, modification is required for infants. Adopt the following principles when placing an infant in the recovery position:
- Place the child in as near true lateral position as possible, with their mouth suitably positioned to assist in the free drainage of fluid.
- The position needs to be stable. This may require a small pillow or a rolled-up blanket to be placed along the infant's back to maintain the position and prevent the infant from rolling on to their back or front.
- Avoid any pressure on the infant's chest that might impair breathing.
- Whatever the position, it should be possible to turn the infant from their side on to their back (and vice versa) easily and safely.

2.5.4 Circulation
Assessment
When assessing circulation, look for signs of blood and other fluid losses, which are causing shock. Children can compensate very well, maintaining their blood pressure until they have significant fluid losses. However, you can spot the child in compensated circulatory failure by examining the following [Skellett, 2016]:
- heart rate
- pulse volume
- capillary refill time.

Heart rate
Tachycardia is common in children and has a number of causes including pain, anxiety and fever. It is also often the first sign of circulatory failure. Bradycardia, defined in an infant as a heart rate of less than 80 beats/minute and in a child as a heart rate of less than 60 beats/minute, is a serious sign [Skellett, 2016]. A heart rate of less than 60 beats/minute in infants and children is normally an indication to start chest compressions.

Pulse volume
When a child develops shock, peripheral pulses will become weak and thready. If central pulses (such as a carotid pulse) become weak and thready, the child is in cardiorespiratory failure and arrest is imminent [Skellett, 2016], so always ensure you compare central and peripheral pulses.

As children become peripherally vasoconstricted in response to shock, their extremities will become cool. Sometimes there is a clear demarcation line between cool skin and warm skin that will either move towards the torso if shock progresses or move distally if perfusion and circulation improve [JRCALC, 2019].

Capillary refill time
Capillary refill time (CRT) can be a useful indicator of circulatory status and was covered in Chapter 13, 'Circulation'.

Skin
Skin perfusion can provide valuable clues as to the infant's or child's circulatory status. Note the temperature of the skin, particularly the level

of warm/cold demarcation lines on the limbs. Monitor this level frequently to see whether things are improving or heading to circulatory failure. The colour of the skin should also be assessed if it wasn't covered in the PAT.

End-organ perfusion

Although you will conduct a formal assessment of level of consciousness (LOC) in 'Disability' (see section 2.5.5 of this chapter), consider if there are any signs of poor cerebral perfusion. Early signs of compromise include a loss of interaction with the infant's or child's surroundings and irritability and agitation. Late signs include a loss of consciousness and loss of tone (e.g. a 'floppy' baby).

The kidneys are an essential organ and one clue that they are not being adequately perfused is a reduction in urine output. A simple way of assessing this is to ask about the number of wet nappies or the number of times the child has passed urine.

Management

The principal method of maintaining circulation is to ensure that airway and breathing are adequately addressed and any life-threatening conditions, such as tension pneumothorax, are identified and treated. However, for seriously fluid-depleted infants or children, intravenous access will be required and fluid replacement in 20 ml/kg boluses of normal saline will be required [JRCALC, 2019].

As with breathing, watch for signs of decompensation:
- changes in heart rate: increasing or sudden fall
- increasing peripheral vasoconstriction:
  - CRT increasing
  - warm/cold demarcation line moving up the limb towards the body
  - loss/reduction of peripheral pulses
- reduced level of consciousness
- hypotension (late sign).

2.5.5 Disability

Assessment

Often, you will already have an idea about the patient's level of consciousness (LOC) from the general impression. Use the AVPU mnemonic to quickly gauge the infant's or child's LOC:

- **A:** Alert
- **V:** Responds to voice
- **P:** Responds to pain
- **U:** Unresponsive.

As with adults, a more formal Glasgow Coma Scale (GCS) score can be calculated. For children under four years of age, a modified GCS has been proposed (Table 20.5) [JRCALC, 2019]. Children four years of age and older should be assessed using the adult GCS score (see Table 13.1 in Chapter 13, 'Disability').

Pupils should be checked for dilation, equality and reactivity. Seriously ill infants or children are typically hypotonic and floppy, but in cases of

Table 20.5 Modified Glasgow Coma Scale score for children under four years of age.

Component	Level of response	Score
Eye opening	Spontaneous	4
	To speech	3
	To pain	2
	None	1
Best verbal response	Appropriate words or social smiles, fixes on and follows objects	5
	Cries, but is consolable	4
	Persistently irritable	3
	Restless, agitated	2
	Silent	1
Best motor response	Obeys commands	6
	Localises	5
	Withdraws	4
	Abnormal flexion	3
	Extension	2
	None	1

serious brain dysfunction, posturing (particularly in response to pain) such as abnormal flexion and extension may be seen [Skellett, 2016].

Management
Ensure that airway, breathing and circulation are managed adequately. Don't forget to check blood glucose and during the history determine whether there is a risk of poisoning or meningococcal septicaemia [JRCALC, 2019].

2.5.6 Exposure/environment
In order to complete the primary survey, it may be necessary to remove some of the child's clothing, but be mindful that children lose heat rapidly, particularly infants. Use this time to thoroughly examine infants and children who are ill for rashes. Keep in mind the possibility of a non-accidental injury and check for bruises and other signs of injury (see Chapter 5, 'Safeguarding', for more detail on non-accidental injury).

Chapter 21 Mental Health

1 Mental health legislation and codes of practice

1.1 Learning objectives
By the end of this section you will be able to:
- define mental health and mental disorder
- explain a number of important roles specified by the Mental Health Act
- explain the guiding principles that are used when applying the Mental Health Act
- outline how a person is detained under the Mental Health Act
- define the terms 'community treatment orders', 'recall' and 'place of safety'
- describe your role and responsibilities when transporting a patient who has an application made under the Mental Health Act.

1.2 Introduction
Mental health is defined by the World Health Organization as 'a state of well-being in which every individual realises his or her own potential, can cope with the normal stresses of life, can work productively and fruitfully, and is able to make a contribution to her or his community' [WHO, 2014b].

However, around one in six people in England will suffer from mental ill health at some point in their lifetime. Common mental disorders include anxiety, depression, phobias, obsessive compulsive disorder (OCD) and post-traumatic stress disorder. The majority of these are managed by general practitioners (GPs) [NHS Digital, 2016].

1.3 The Mental Health Act 1983 (as amended 2007, MHA)
If a person has a mental disorder (defined as any disorder and disability of the mind) and is required to be detained against their wishes, specific sections of the MHA will be used to admit patients, potentially without their agreement. You will commonly hear these patients being referred to as being 'sectioned' or 'detained' under the MHA. This is in contrast to patients who agree to attend a psychiatric ward, whose admission may be referred to as 'informal' or 'voluntary' [UK Government, 1983].

1.3.1 Roles defined by the MHA
Approved mental health professional
An approved mental health professional (AMHP) is usually a social worker who has been approved by the local social services authority to carry out a number of activities specified in the MHA [DoH, 2015c]. Since the amendment to the MHA in 2007, nurses, occupational therapists and psychologists can also become an AMHP [UK Government, 2007].

The role of an AMHP includes the following [Dimond, 2015]:
- informing the nearest relative about the admission of the patient and their right to discharge
- consulting the nearest relative about admission for treatment or guardianship and discontinuing the application (in the case of detention under Section 3 of the MHA) if the relative objects
- applying for admission or guardianship if they are satisfied that the application is necessary
- interviewing patients to determine that detention in hospital is the most appropriate way to care for the patient
- reporting on the patient's social circumstances.

Section 12 doctor
This is a senior doctor (typically a middle-grade or higher psychiatrist, a doctor who specialises in mental health problems) who is an approved clinician, (i.e. has been approved by the Secretary of State (England) or Welsh minister (Wales)) [MIND, 2019a].

Nearest relative
This is a really important role in the MHA. The nearest relative is defined as the highest in the following hierarchy [UK Government, 1983]:
- relative who usually resides with or cares for the patient
- husband, wife or civil partner
- son or daughter
- father or mother
- brother or sister
- grandparent
- grandchild
- uncle or aunt
- nephew or niece.

They have a range of powers including [Dimond, 2015]:
- to apply for admission of the patient for assessment, treatment and guardianship (although this is unlikely; this is virtually always undertaken by an AMHP)
- to object to an AMHP's proposed application for treatment under Section 3
- to discharge the patient having given 72 hours' notice in writing to hospital managers
- to apply to a mental health review tribunal.

1.3.2 Guiding principles
When deciding on a course of action to take using the MHA, AMHPs must take into account the five overarching principles [DoH, 2015c]:
- **Least restrictive option and maximising independence:** This may include home treatment, staying at a crisis house, staying with a relative or friend, for example, or offering the patient the chance to attend hospital informally.
- **Empowerment and involvement:** Patients should be involved in decisions about their care. In addition, the views of family members, carers and others, if appropriate, should be taken into consideration.
- **Respect and dignity:** Patients, their families and carers should be treated with respect and dignity and listened to by professionals.
- **Purpose and effectiveness:** Care and treatment need to conform to current best practice guidelines and have clear therapeutic aims.
- **Efficiency and equity:** Provision of services should be of a high quality and be given the same priority as physical ill health.

1.3.3 MHA sections
Section 2
This section provides the power to admit a patient to hospital and detain them for up to 28 days for the purposes of assessment on the grounds that they are suffering from a mental disorder severe enough to warrant the admission, and that detention is appropriate for maintenance of the health and safety of the patient and others. The applicant needs to be an AMHP or the nearest relative and requires the agreement of two doctors, one of whom must be approved under Section 12 of the MHA [UK Government, 1983].

Section 3
This section provides the power to admit a patient to hospital and detain them for a period of six months initially (although it can be renewed) for the purposes of treatment, on the grounds that they are suffering from a mental disorder severe enough to receive treatment in hospital, that detention is appropriate for maintenance of the health and safety of the patient and others, and that an appropriate treatment is available. As before, the applicant needs to be an AMHP or nearest relative and requires the agreement of two doctors, one of whom must be approved under Section 12 of the MHA.

Section 4
This section is rarely used as it is viewed as an incomplete Section 2 or 3 by mental health professionals. It allows for the emergency admission of a patient for the purposes of assessment, requires the applicant to be an AMHP or nearest relative, but only requires one Section 12-approved doctor to recommend detention. The criteria for admission are the same as for Section 2.

Section 135
If a patient believed to have a mental disorder is being ill-treated, neglected or not kept under proper control, or is unable to care for themselves and living alone, an AMHP can obtain a warrant from a

magistrate to enter any property where the patient is believed to be located, and, if necessary, remove them to a place of safety. This requires a police officer to execute the warrant and gain access to a property, with force if necessary, but they must be accompanied by a doctor and AMHP [MIND, 2019b].

Section 136
If a police officer encounters a person in a public place who appears to be suffering from a mental disorder and is in immediate need of care or control, they can remove that person to a place of safety [UK Government, 1983]. This should be a hospital or other health-based location where mental health services are provided. However, other locations, such as residential care homes, may be appropriate, as is staying with a relative or friend of the patient. Police stations should not be used as a place of safety other than in exceptional circumstances. You are likely to be called to assist in transporting the patient to a suitable location, such as a Section 136 suite at a local psychiatric hospital [DoH, 2015c].

1.3.4 Community treatment orders

The purpose of a community treatment order (CTO) is to allow suitable patients to be treated in the community rather than being detained in a hospital [DoH, 2015c]. Only patients who are under Section 3 of the MHA can be considered for a CTO: it does not apply to patients detained under Section 2.

Patients under a CTO may be recalled back to hospital if the patient requires treatment for their mental disorder in hospital, there is a risk of harm to the health or safety of the patient or other people if the patient were to remain in the community, or the patient breaks any of the mandatory conditions imposed as a result of the CTO.

1.4 *Transporting patients*

The sections of the MHA typically require three healthcare professionals, including an AMHP, to make the application and two doctors, one Section 12-approved, to detain a patient under Sections 2 and 3 of the MHA. This is usually impractical in the community, so there is provision in the MHA for the detention (if necessary) and transport of patients for whom an AMHP has made an application under the MHA.

This limbo period in between deciding upon detention and the patient arriving at the ward is covered by Section 6 of the MHA. This allows the applicant (i.e. the AMHP) or someone (such as you) authorised by the applicant to take the patient to hospital, forcibly if necessary [UK Government, 1983]. Under Section 137(2), as an authorised person, you have the same powers, authorities, protection and privileges as a police officer! In reality, if there is a risk of physical violence, the police are likely to be involved following a risk assessment by the AMHP. You are also protected from civil and criminal proceedings (i.e. prosecution) under Section 139(1) of the MHA unless you act in bad faith or do not take reasonable care [UK Government, 1983]. Always make sure you take the documentation relating to the application for admission and treatment under the MHA with you, even if (in most cases) the AMHP does not travel with the patient.

Generally, it falls to the ambulance service to transport patients, as use of police personnel and vehicles has been highlighted as bad practice, and their use should be reserved for physically violent patients [DoH, 2014].

2 Mental disorders

2.1 *Learning objectives*

By the end of this section you will be able to:
- describe a range of mental disorders
- explain the aims and components that make up mental health first aid
- state some general principles to consider when assisting a patient with a mental disorder
- briefly outline the ABC model of emotion.

2.2 *Introduction*

Traditionally, mental disorders were divided into neuroses: illnesses that are severe forms of 'normal' experiences, such as anxiety and depression, and psychoses: illnesses that result in misperception of thoughts that arise from the patient's own mind/imagination as reality, and include delusions and hallucinations, such as schizophrenia [Kumar, 2012].

Although the terms are still used, definitions provided by the International Classification of Diseases version 10 (ICD-10) organise disorders according to common themes. Disorders covered in this chapter include [Cooper, 2012]:
- organic disorders
- schizophrenia and delusional disorders
- mood (affective) disorders
- neurotic, stress-related and somatoform disorders
- disorders of adult personality and behaviour.

2.3 Organic disorders

Organic disorders occur as a result of physical brain disease, such as occurs in dementia (see Chapter 23, 'Older People'), or from disturbed central nervous system (CNS) function, for example a fever-induced delirium [Kumar, 2012].

2.3.1 Delirium

Delirium is a common form of psychosis and is characterised by incoherent thoughts and speech, impaired memory and episodes of hallucinations and delusions. Common causes of delirium include systemic infection, metabolic disturbances, endocrine diseases and intracranial causes such as trauma, haemorrhage or epilepsy, for example. In addition, toxic doses of the patient's usual medication as well as drug and/or alcohol withdrawal can cause delirium.

2.4 Schizophrenia and delusional disorders

The most common type of schizophrenia is the paranoid subtype, which includes delusions and auditory hallucinations. Delusions are frequently [Cooper, 2012]:
- **Persecutory:** Someone or some group is out to harm the patient.
- **Delusions of reference:** The patient is mentioned on the TV news or in a newspaper.

Disorders of thought can occur including:
- **Derailment:** Seemingly random connections between verbal statements in conversation.
- **Neologisms:** The patient uses made-up words or uses words in a special way.
- **Word salad:** Mixed-up words, phrases or sentences.
- **Concrete thinking:** Inability to deal with abstract ideas.

Symptoms are often split into:
- **positive:** hallucinations and delusions
- **negative:** withdrawn, uncommunicative, unemotional, e.g. monotonic speech.

2.5 Mood (affective) disorders

Mood can be thought of as a temporary state of mind or feeling. Patients with mood disorders sit somewhere on a continuum from severe depression to severe mania, with 'normal' mood in the middle. Mood disorders can be bipolar or unipolar [Kumar, 2012].

2.5.1 Bipolar affective disorder

This disorder (formerly called manic depression) is characterised by recurring episodes of altered mood and activity, typically swinging between depression and mania.

The classic features of a manic episode are an elevated mood (although the patient can become irritable too) and the presence of the following associated features [Cooper, 2012]:
- exaggerated optimism and inflated self-esteem
- decreased social inhibition, e.g. sexual overactivity, reckless spending, dangerous driving
- rapid thinking and speech (flight of ideas)
- lack of insight into disorder.

2.5.2 Depression

Everyone experiences a low mood from time to time, but this is not depression. Depressive illness occurs when symptoms become severe enough to affect a person's ability to carry out daily activities or go to work, for example, and lasts for more than two weeks.

Patients often describe symptoms in physical terms and complaints of fatigue and headache are common. Other descriptions used by patients include describing the world as looking grey and of being without anything pleasurable or interesting to do or look forward to. Anxiety attacks are common and phobic and/or obsessive disorders can also result [Kumar, 2012]. In more severe forms, suicide can become a persistent and intrusive thought.

2.6 Neurotic, stress-related and somatoform disorders

Disorders in this category range from phobic and general anxiety disorder, panic disorder, obsessive compulsive disorder and post-traumatic stress disorder to somatoform disorders (whereby the patient complains of physical symptoms that are medically unexplained) such as hypochondriasis (a belief that you have a serious or life-threatening illness despite having no, or only mild, symptoms).

2.6.1 Panic disorder

This mental disorder is characterised by episodes of severe panic (anxiety) attacks, which can occur without an obvious trigger. These can be very frightening for patients, who experience fear and feelings of impending doom and have signs of sympathetic nervous stimulation (fight or flight), such as palpitations and sweating, chest pain and nausea and can experience feelings of 'losing control' or dying [Cooper, 2012].

2.7 Personality disorders

Personality-disordered (PD) patients make frequent contact with emergency services (police and ambulance), GPs and emergency departments. Although making up only 3.4–5.3% of the general population, prevalence is closer to 40% in psychiatric inpatients. They can be chaotic and challenging patients as they have a tendency to experience many pseudo-psychiatric symptoms and so are often referred to as 'borderline', which implies a condition that is fleeting in nature but not chronic. They are usually worse when there is some form of social/relationship stressor as a backdrop [Cooper, 2012].

The best way to understand personality disorder is in terms of an entrenched extremely maladaptive and rigid coping mechanism (can't cope/won't cope). The best outcomes for PD patients are achieved with consistent, long-term, therapeutic relationships and a readiness by the patient to address their coping mechanisms, typically with talking therapy. Medication has minimal effect and repeated emergency service responses with subsequent hospital admission are not beneficial [Gunderson, 2011].

The nature of the personality disorder is about frantically avoiding perceived isolation and abandonment, which typically manifest as becoming engaged in risky behaviour in order to prompt rescue. This can elicit 'knight in shining armour' behaviour in emergency services personnel and is in stark contrast to mental health staff who are likely to be more consistent and stick to the patient's care plan, becoming unpopular in the process. A common strategy adopted by patients with PD is to 'divide and rule' (known as splitting) to help them take control of a seemingly intolerable situation. Watch for comments relating to a comparison between how caring and understanding you are versus how bad mental health or ED staff are.

2.8 Suicide and deliberate self-harm (DSH)

In the UK, there are just under 6,000 suicides each year, 75% of whom were male [ONS, 2018a]. People who regularly self-harm will continue to be at risk of future self-harm, but not typically suicide. Although DSH is regarded as taboo and unfathomable by many people, including clinicians, it may help you to think of DSH as a method of coping with incredibly difficult feelings rather than as a serious wish to die [RCP, 2010]. People who regularly overdose and/or engage in risky behaviour that is designed to elicit a response are more at risk via misadventure or accidental death, and it is not uncommon for a coroner to give a narrative verdict in such cases. Predicting who will die by suicide is very difficult, and scales, such as the SAD PERSONS scale, do not accurately predict the risk of death by suicide [Warden, 2014; Bolton, 2012].

2.8.1 IPAP suicide risk assessment

Although suicide risk assessment tools are not recommended, it is helpful to have some guidance relating to the factors that suggest your patient is at risk. Current UK Ambulance Services Clinical Practice Guidelines recommend using 'IPAP' [JRCALC, 2019]:
- **Intent:** Any thoughts of killing self?
- **Plans:** Does the patient have a plan about how they would kill themselves?
- **Actions:** Has the patient ever attempted suicide before?
- **Protection:** Does the patient have any support, such as family and friends? Are there any factors that would stop the patient taking their own life, such as family, pets, work or religion?

2.9 Assessment of patient with mental health problems

Patients with mental health problems can still have physical illnesses, so ensure that you conduct a primary survey on all patients to identify any life-threats. Once these have been excluded, you are going to need to slow down; making and implementing a plan for a patient with a mental disorder can take time.

It is not vital that ambulance clinicians are able to fully assess and diagnose patients with mental health issues. However, it is important that clinicians are able to recognise common mental health signs, symptoms and behaviours when attempting to decide upon the need for transportation or referral of a patient. Table 21.1 shows a number of factors that should be considered in your assessment. It is not exhaustive and similarly it is not necessary for all signs and symptoms to be present. However, it is important that you gain as much information as possible and you should not be afraid to ask questions as long as you so politely and professionally. Remember, if in doubt, ask for help.

2.10 Management of patients with mental disorders

Trying to assist patients with mental disorders can feel daunting. To assist non-mental health professionals in assisting patients with mental

Table 21.1 Factors to consider during a mental health assessment.

Behaviour Observe both verbal and non-verbal signs	- Does the patient make eye contact? - Is the patient calm and relaxed or anxious, upset, aggressive, suspicious or pre-occupied? - Is the patient's body language appropriate or are they hyperactive or hypoactive?
Appearance Again, assessed through observation	- Is the patient dressed properly, are they unkempt or have poor hygiene or other evidence or poor self-care? - Are there signs of self-harm, for instance cutting marks, drug and alcohol misuse, overdose?
Speech and rapport	- Is the volume of speech normal or very loud or quiet? - Is the rate of speech normal for the situation or is it pressured or especially slow? - Is the conversation spontaneous? Does the patient talk far too much or only minimally and is it in response to questions? - Is the patient friendly and co-operative or is speech forced or monotone?
Mood/affect	- Does the patient present in a way that fits with their current mood, for instance, do they appear flat, restricted or blunted, or alternatively does their mood appear to vary quickly and seem inappropriate to the situation? - Bearing this in mind, does the patient appear elated, anxious, angry, agitated or even disinterested and lacking any motivation? - Ask the patient if they have any suicidal ideas or violent thoughts.

Cognition	- Is the patient orientated to time, person and place? - Is the patient able to retain and recall information and use it appropriately? - Is the patient able to concentrate and pay attention as would be expected for the situation? - Does the patient express a normal level of general knowledge and ability to identify familiar items, objects, people and places? - Can the patient easily follow simple instructions?

Thoughts	- Does the patient have any thoughts of self-harm, suicide or thoughts of harming others?
	- Do they appear pre-occupied or to have obsessive thoughts?
	- Do they display any unusual beliefs or delusional, unrealistic ideas about themselves, others or the world in general?
	- Are they very anxious or very low or depressed?
	- Do they describe feelings of hopelessness or appear unmotivated, even to complete small tasks like eating, drinking or appropriate levels of self-care?
	- Does the thought process of the patient flow logically and naturally within the conversation or when taking the history or is their speech 'unnatural'?
	    - Do they change subject often and quickly to unrelated topics or to whatever changes in front of them?
	    - Do their thoughts seem overly fast or unusually slow?
	    - Is their speech very fast or unusually slow?
	    - Are they very vague with answers to questions, rarely addressing or coming to a point or conclusion?
	    - Are they using nonsense words or very mixed-up sentences sometimes described as a 'word salad'?
	The following symptoms and traits are often associated with psychosis-type illness and can feel very real and very disturbing for the patient. They are less likely to be found in the very young (those under 18 years old):
	- Hallucinations
	    - Visual disturbances and visions not apparent to others; these can be described as people, animals or objects and are individual to the patient.
	    - Auditory hallucinations, often hearing voices not belonging to the patient and outside of their head. These can be derogatory, commanding or abusive.
	- Delusions:
	    - The belief of a patient that their thoughts can be read, changed or removed from their minds.
	    - The patient may feel that they themselves are not real or that the situation they are in is not real.
	    - A patient may describe feeling detached or removed from themselves akin to watching themselves or their situation from afar with little control.

Insight	- Does the patient acknowledge that they have a current mental health problem? - Do they acknowledge the need for help or further input and are they willing to comply with this? - Are they able to evaluate different treatment options and choices? - Are they able to weigh up and identify any risks to themselves or others?

disorders, a mental health first aid course was created (MHFA). The aims of MHFA are to:
- Preserve life where a person may be a danger to themselves.
- Provide help to prevent the mental health problem becoming more serious.
- Promote recovery of good mental health.
- Provide comfort to a person suffering from a mental health problem.

To achieve this, MHFA advocates a five-point action plan (ALGEE) [Pappas, 2010]:
1. Approach the person, assess and assist with any crisis.
2. Listen non-judgementally.
3. Give support and information.
4. Encourage and support the person to get appropriate professional help.
5. Encourage other supports, such as self-help, family and friends.

2.10.1 General advice

- **Don't panic:** Remain calm, professional and in control. Patients are often incredibly astute at sensing any uneasiness and will try to press your buttons or force your hand.
- **There is no rush:** Making and implementing a plan can take hours.
- **Consider their medical health:** An overdose of 1 g of amitriptyline, for example, can cause serious harm and needs addressing prior to their mental health.
- **Consider their mental health:** If patients state that their mental health is not good, consider whether an ED attendance will really benefit anyone here, apart from relieving your own anxieties (and responsibility) about this patient group. In most cases, a risk assessment can be conducted by mental health staff over the phone and a contingency plan put in place.
- **Frontline mental health staff are not there just to 'have a chat' with patients:** Several national helplines are available for that purpose such as Rethink, Saneline and the Samaritans.
- **Unless patients are detained under the MHA or they haven't got mental capacity, they cannot be made to go to the ED:** If patients refuse to travel despite your kind words and advice, make a thorough note of this, make it clear you are leaving and go. You may find that it's at this point they decide to travel.
- **Recognise when you are out of your depth:** Desperate attempts and pleas to engage can indicate you're out of your depth. If you are struggling, speak to mental health staff and see if the patient is known, if there are any current concerns and/or if there is a care plan that needs to be adhered to.
- **Establish if there is a care plan:** Many mental health patients have a care plan. Of course, you aren't going to know this because you can't see it, and patients may not be happy with it or may feel it doesn't address their needs 24/7. This is often the case with frequent callers who challenge the out-of-hours services when offered a different response from that which they receive during the daytime.
- **Don't tell people to pull themselves together:** It can reinforce any negativity or feelings of hopelessness.
- **Be objective:** It can be helpful to see how patients can contradict themselves, not so you can point it out to them and make them feel stupid, but more as a reassurance that what they're saying and what they're actually doing are two different things. For example:
  - 'I feel like killing myself tonight, but I'm seeing my GP the day after tomorrow.'
  - 'I feel like killing myself, but I'm worried about the impact it would have on my children.'
  - 'I feel like killing myself, but I'm worried I'll fail and end up disabled or in pain.'

  These are common statements people make, which paradoxically protect them from suicide, and that mental health professionals look out for during an assessment. Ensure they are documented on your patient report form.
- **Avoid disclosing too much about yourself:** It's OK to be human and personable. However, don't disclose too much about yourself or try to solve their problems. Their issues may be long-term problems and it's highly unlikely they will be solved at 03:00 by excessive personal self-disclosing.

- **Don't feel you have to fill the void:** Silences of a minute or two do not mean you're not being helpful. Be comfortable with silence; it's not up to you to have all the answers.
- **You can never be sure:** There are no absolutes in mental health and it is never possible to state with absolute certainty that a patient isn't at risk.

3 Caring for yourself and colleagues

3.1 Learning objectives

At the end of this section you will be able to:
- define mental well-being
- list factors that may have an impact on mental well-being
- define resilience in-terms of mental well-being
- describe how to improve personal mental well-being resilience
- list sources of help for mental well-being
- describe how to support a colleague's mental well-being.

3.2 Introduction

As an associate ambulance practitioner (AAP) your daily job is to help and support other people during times of crisis, but this constant exposure can have a detrimental impact on your own mental health and well-being. Research suggests that emergency service workers and volunteers are more likely to suffer mental health problems than the general workforce but are less likely to take time off work or seek help (MIND, 2015).

3.3 Mental well-being

Mental well-being describes your overall mental state and considers how the way you are feeling impacts on how you can cope with day-to-day life (MIND, 2016b). People with good mental well-being can:
- feel confident and have positive self-esteem
- build and maintain positive relationships
- live and work productively
- cope with the stresses of daily life
- adapt to changes around them.

3.3.1 Impact on mental well-being

Mental well-being can be impacted by several factors, both inside and outside of work, including (MIND, 2015):
- repeated exposure to traumatic incidents
- impact of physical injuries
- workload pressure
- suffering personal loss
- relationship problems
- financial worries
- loneliness.

3.4 Building resilience

Dealing with more difficult times in life, whether they be due to personal or work-related issues, can be challenging. The capacity to stay mentally well during these periods relies on your personal mental health 'resilience'. You can try to build resilience to deal with these difficult times by (MIND, 2015):
- talking about the way you feel
- building healthy relationships
- looking after your physical health
- doing something you enjoy
- setting yourself a challenge
- relaxing
- identifying mood triggers.

3.5 Seeking help

There will be times when you recognise either in yourself, or a colleague, that personal resilience is not enough and that further help is required. Often this decision is difficult to arrive at and can be left longer than it really should have been; emergency service staff feel they should be the ones that stay strong as it is their role to help others. Left unsupported, poor mental well-being can lead to anxiety, depression and post-traumatic stress disorder (PTSD).

Help can be sought from a range of options, outlined below.

3.5.1 Employer support

Your employer is likely to have a form of internal service for supporting staff, which may include peer counselling, a multi-faith chaplain, or schemes such as Trauma Risk Management (TRiM) or external counselling support.

3.5.2 Medical support

Your GP will be able to help. While a GP may be able to give a diagnosis and medications, this is rarely the first step. They have a range of options, including just listening to your situation, and can refer you to other treatments, such as talking therapy or counselling if appropriate.

If you are facing a more urgent situation or crisis, you can also call 111 or even visit A&E or call 999.

3.5.3 Other charities

The Samaritans provide 24-hour emotional support for anyone struggling to cope. You can call anonymously if you want, with no need to give personal details, and telephone numbers are not tracked.

3.6 Supporting a colleague

There may be occasions where you think the mental well-being of a colleague is suffering and you may want to try and help them. The charity MIND produces information on how to do this, which you should look at (MIND, 2017). In summary, you should:
- show support by asking them how they are
- ask if you can help in any way
- treat them as you normally would
- don't just talk about mental health
- show trust and respect.

It may be helpful to remind them what support and services are available to them. If there is another colleague you know they respect that has been through similar in the past, it may be useful for them to talk to each other.

Your colleague may not be ready to seek help yet, so be there for them, be patient and continue to offer support and reassurance. Remember that there will be an additional emotional stress on you, so continue to look after yourself and your own resilience.

Chapter

22 Learning Disabilities

1 Supporting the care of people with learning disabilities

1.1 Learning objectives

By the end of this section you will be able to:
- define the term 'learning disability'
- explain the needs of a person with a learning disability in emergency care situations.

1.2 Introduction

A learning disability is defined as a reduced intellectual ability and difficulty with everyday activities – for example, household tasks, socialising or managing money – that affects someone for their whole life [Mencap, 2018a]. Learning disability includes the presence of a significantly reduced ability to understand new or complex information and to learn new skills (impaired intelligence), coupled with a reduced ability to cope independently (impaired social functioning) that started before adulthood, with a lasting effect on development [DoH, 2001].

It is thought that up to 350,000 people in the UK have severe learning disabilities and this figure is increasing [NHS, 2018c].

1.3 Learning disabilities legislation and rights

We have already reviewed relevant legislation in Chapter 4, 'Legal, Ethical and Professional Issues'. However, you should be aware how this legislation applies to people with learning disabilities.

1.3.1 Legislation

Equality Act 2010
According to the Equality Act 2010, a person is disabled if a physical or mental impairment has a substantial and long-term negative effect on their ability to carry out normal daily activities [HMG, 2018d]. This definition will apply to nearly all of those suffering from a learning disability.

The Equality Act extends certain rights to those recognised as suffering from a disability [HMG, 2018e], including:
- **Employment rights:** It is against the law for employers to discriminate against a person because of a disability. All employers must make reasonable adjustments so those with disabilities are not disadvantaged.
- **Education:** It is unlawful for education providers to treat disabled students unfavourably. This may be due to direct or indirect discrimination or forms of harassment or victimisation. As with employers, education providers must make reasonable adjustments to ensure that disabled students are not discriminated against.
- **Police:** A person with a learning disability should only be interviewed when a responsible person is present. The responsible person, or 'appropriate adult', should not work for the police and should have experience of working with people with learning difficulties. The only exception to this is when a delay would result in harm to people, property or evidence.

Consent and capacity
Adults with a learning disability have the same legal rights and freedoms as anyone else [Mencap, 2018b]. Having a learning difficulty does not automatically mean a person lacks mental capacity; in fact, the majority will have full capacity. As always, you must assess your patient as the individual they are and have no pre-conceived ideas as to their potential mental ability until you have completed a formal and structured assessment.

1.3.2 Rights

As outlined above, people with learning difficulties have the same rights as all other people; these rights are detailed within the Human Rights Act 1998.

People with learning difficulties have the same right to access healthcare as all other people. However, due to a number of factors, patients with learning disabilities find it far harder to access healthcare and therefore suffer the consequences, including earlier death and poor long-term condition management, as identified by Sir Jonathan Michael [2008] in his public inquiry into accessing healthcare for those with learning difficulties.

As a health professional, you should actively promote the rights of those with learning difficulties and help them to overcome the issues they face in accessing healthcare. Depending on the situation, this may take many forms, but could include:
- supporting them in phoning the GP surgery to make an appointment
- arranging for a friend or relative to escort them to a hospital visit
- helping them to plan their journey to visit their local GP surgery.

1.4 Causes of learning disabilities

There are four main causes that are responsible for learning disabilities [Holland, 2011]:
- genetics
- events before birth
- events during birth
- events after birth.

1.4.1 Genetics

Chromosomal conditions, such as Down's syndrome or Fragile X syndrome, are not in themselves learning disabilities, but they do frequently cause learning disabilities.

1.4.2 Events before birth

Infections that a mother suffers from during pregnancy can be transmitted to the fetus, leading to developmental problems and learning disabilities. Other maternal factors, including dietary deficiencies, excessive alcohol consumption during the pregnancy and endocrine disorders such as phenylketonuria, can also cause learning disabilities.

1.4.3 Events during birth

If a baby's oxygen supply is interrupted for a significant period of time during a traumatic or difficult delivery, brain damage that will cause a learning disability may occur.

1.4.4 Events after birth

In the early years of life, a child is susceptible to many factors that may cause long-term impairment and learning disabilities as a result. Examples of this include infections, particularly meningitis or encephalitis, and traumatic injuries of the brain, sustained by falls, road traffic accidents or non-accidental injuries.

1.5 Categories of learning disabilities

Learning disabilities are categorised as mild, moderate, severe or profound [Holland, 2011]. As with all conditions, the way in which any individual is challenged by their disability will be unique to them. Many people diagnosed with learning difficulties will be able to lead largely independent lives, whereas others may need more significant help and support.

For people with mild learning difficulties, some occasional support for complex issues may be all that is required, whereas many people with profound and multiple learning disabilities will require more intense help, potentially through to round-the-clock care.

You must always assess any patient with learning difficulties as an individual. Understand how they would normally manage, and what level of support they require on a day-to-day basis. Do not assume, just because a person has a diagnosis of a learning difficulty, that they are incapable of making decisions about their own care needs.

2 Disabilities, healthcare and discrimination

2.1 Learning objectives

By the end of this section, you will be able to:
- describe how learning disabilities lead to inequality in healthcare

Disabilities, healthcare and discrimination

- describe how you may need to adapt your methods of communication when assisting a person with a learning disability
- give examples of sources of information, advice and guidance to support the well-being of people with learning disabilities
- describe how learning difficulties influence a person's vulnerability
- define hate crime and the actions to take if your patient is a victim of disability hate crime.

2.2 Inequality in healthcare

People with learning disabilities tend to have poorer health than people without a learning disability, as they are more likely to have additional health problems. This includes a higher incidence of weight-related problems, mental health issues and respiratory diseases.

As well as this, people with learning disabilities are more likely to have poor health outcomes as a result of not receiving equal healthcare. This means that people with learning difficulties die on average 16 years earlier than the general population, with approximately 1,200 people with a learning disability dying avoidably each year [Mencap, 2018c].

In 2013, the Confidential Inquiry into Premature Deaths of People with Learning Disabilities [CIPOLD, 2013] reported that, despite numerous previous reports and campaigns, reasonable adjustments are still not being made to ensure that people with learning disabilities get the best care possible.

Findings from the report included the following:
- Professionals were unaware how to adapt their practice to support patients with learning difficulties.
- Agencies caring for people with learning difficulties communicated poorly.
- Adherence to the Mental Capacity Act is generally poor, with many professionals not understanding how to apply it to people with learning difficulties.

2.3 Tackling inequality

Simple changes can make a significant difference to caring for people with learning disabilities. The principles of Mencap's 'Treat me well' campaign [Mencap, 2018d], designed to improve care for people with learning disabilities, revolves around:
- better communication
- more time
- clearer information.

Many hospitals that have signed up to the 'Treat me well' campaign will have advocates who can support patients with learning difficulties; these will often be learning disability liaison nurses.

As a healthcare professional, you should make all reasonable adjustments necessary to ensure that patients with learning disabilities receive the same standard of care as any other patients. Modifications will be unique based on the situation but, very importantly, you will need to adjust your communication techniques.

2.4 Communication

As discussed previously, every individual will be affected by their own disability in a unique way, so in order to be able to communicate effectively you need to first understand what is normal for your patient.

For a patient with mild or moderate learning difficulties, you may be able to communicate in a near-to-normal manner, just ensuring that you use language that is not overly complex or difficult to understand. For patients with more severe or profound learning difficulties, it is likely you will need to make more significant adjustments.

Patients with severe, multiple or profound learning difficulties frequently rely on non-verbal communication, including facial expressions, vocal sounds, body language and behaviour. Some may have a small range of formal communication tools including words, drawings, gestures or symbols. Others may not have reached any form of intentional communication and you may be relying on feedback from carers as to how changes in behaviour may be indicating pain or distress. In these situations, you should seek out the advice of those who know the patient best, as they may be able to better interpret signs the patient is displaying.

You should also consider the use of specialist assessment tools, such as the Abbey pain scale, which is used to assess pain in patients who cannot verbalise, and be mindful that many people with profound learning difficulties also suffer from some degree of visual and/or hearing disability [Mencap, 2008].

Some further guidelines for communicating with people who have learning difficulties include [Mencap, 2018e]:
- Find a good place to communicate in, somewhere quiet without distractions.
- If you are talking to a large group, be aware that some people may find this difficult.
- Ask open questions.
- Check with the person that you understand what they are saying: 'The TV isn't working? Have I got that right?'
- If the person wants to take you to show you something, go with them.
- Watch the person. They may tell you things by their body language and facial expressions.
- Learn from experience. You will need to be more observant and don't feel awkward about asking parents/carers for their help.
- Try drawing. Even if your drawing is not great, it might still be helpful.
- Take your time; do not rush your communication.
- Use gestures and facial expressions. If you are asking if someone is unhappy, make your facial expression unhappy to reinforce what you are saying. Do your best to do this in a natural way to avoid being patronising.
- Be aware that some people find it easier to use real objects to communicate with, but photos and pictures can really help, too.

Remember that when you meet most of your patients, it will be an emergency situation for them, even if it does not appear serious to you. They may be scared, frightened and feeling more vulnerable than usual. Try to calm your patient and reassure them. Remember that anyone, including those with learning disabilities, can react in unpredictable ways when scared and you should be prepared to respond to this and support them as required. Especially try to avoid conflict as this inevitably makes the situation worse and can lead to loss of trust.

2.5 Learning difficulties and vulnerability

People with learning difficulties are more vulnerable to harm due to their disability. As with other types of abuse, this harm could take the form of physical abuse, mental abuse, financial abuse or sexual abuse.

People with learning disabilities are also often victims of hate crimes. Disability hate crime is when a person is attacked, threatened or verbally abused as a result of their disability, or perceived disability [Disability Rights UK, 2017]. Staggeringly, as many as 88% of people with learning disabilities reported some form of bullying or harassment in the previous year [Mencap, 2013], and there have been a number of tragic cases where people with learning disabilities have been murdered as a result of their disability.

It is thought that the vast majority of hate crimes go unreported at present. As with all vulnerable people, you should do all you can to tackle a person's vulnerability and ensure their safety. Any activity that may be described as a hate crime should be reported to the police, with the consent of your patient.

Refer to Chapter 4, 'Legal, Ethical and Professional Issues', for more information on safeguarding and how to make a safeguarding referral.

2.6 Further support

In the management of an individual incident, you should look to friends, family and carers to help support your patient where possible. You may also be able to get further advice and support from:
- social workers
- support agencies.

Also consider what local expertise may be available through specialist learning disability nurses or charities such as Mencap, available at www.mencap.co.uk.

Chapter

23 Older People

1 Ageing

1.1 Learning objective

By the end of the section, you will be able to:
- describe the anatomical and physiological changes that occur as a person ages.

1.2 Introduction

Older people are generally defined as those aged over 65. However, ageing is a highly unique process and there may be patients at a lower age that suffer from the same conditions and vulnerabilities as those aged 65 and over. So, although being aged over 65 is still the most accepted definition of older people, you should likewise consider that those aged 50–64 may also suffer from the same issues, depending on the unique progression of their own disease, vulnerabilities or risk factors [NICE, 2013].

The percentage of the population classed as older is growing rapidly with 18% of the UK population currently aged over 65 and predictions indicating that by 2037 this will reach nearly 25% [ONS, 2018b]. Although there are no national statistics relating to the number of older people who call the ambulance service, around 45% of the 4,374,611 people who attended an emergency department in 2012/13, and arrived by ambulance, were over the age of 65 [HSCIC, 2014b].

1.3 Anatomy and physiology of ageing

There is no single mechanism of ageing. Instead, there are a range of mechanisms that over time result in the worsening of cell function, causing cellular damage and impairing the body's ability to repair itself. This results in a range of anatomical and physiological changes (Figure 23.1).

1.3.1 Musculoskeletal system

Bones, joints and muscles are all affected by ageing.

Bones

Bone formation is greatest in the period from birth to adolescence, but equalises with bone absorption in a person's twenties, before bone absorption becomes more dominant. This leads to a reduction in body calcium, impairing the body's ability to create bone matrix and increasing the risk of fracture. Cancellous bones, such as those found in the vertebral bodies, wrists and hips, are especially vulnerable. Calcium supplements are often prescribed as absorption of calcium from the digestive system also declines with age [Farley, 2011].

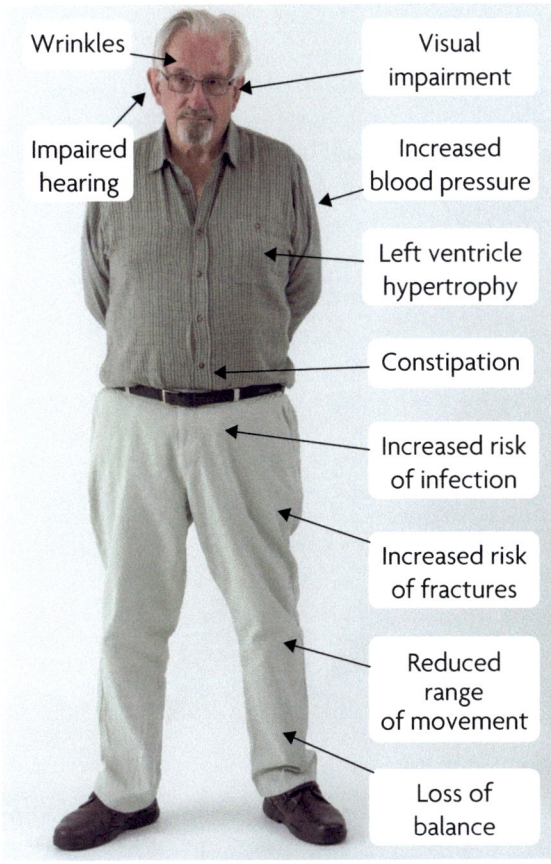

Figure 23.1 Changes related to ageing.

Joints

The loss of fluid in the fibrocartilage within the intervertebral discs results in kyphosis: the familiar stooped posture of older age, which also reduces the height of the person. With stooping comes a change in the person's centre of gravity and changes to their gait, which becomes slower, shorter and more cautious [Knight, 2008b]. Kyphosis (Figure 23.2) also means that the shape of the thoracic cavity changes, resulting in decreased space for the lungs, which can worsen respiratory conditions such as COPD.

Other joints are affected too, especially synovial joints. The reduction in synovial fluid and cartilage leads to bones coming into direct contact with each other. In addition, ligaments shorten and become less elastic and flexible, which contributes to a reduction in the joint's range of movement [Farley, 2011].

Muscles

Muscles atrophy (waste away), leading to a reduction in muscle strength and mass. The rate of decline is variable, with some muscles, such as the diaphragm, remaining unchanged, whereas the lower limbs can experience noticeable atrophy. Coupled with the decline in nervous system function, movement speed is reduced, and increased muscle rigidity results in limited movement in the neck, shoulders, hips and knees [Farley, 2011].

1.3.2 Respiratory system

The respiratory system is in steady decline from around the age of 25, following a functional peak at 20 years of age. There are a variety of external factors that adversely affect the respiratory system, including poor nutrition, lack of physical exercise and smoking [Farley, 2011]. Changes due to ageing are fairly insignificant compared to the external factors as there is usually sufficient spare capacity in lung function to offset any decline due to older age.

Airway changes

There are a number of changes in the airway itself as we age. Mucus becomes increasingly thick, leading to it lodging in the nasopharynx and causing recurrent coughs. The cilia that line the trachea and smaller airways become less effective at clearing foreign debris and pathogens which, coupled with a diminished cough reflex, increases the chance of infection [Knight, 2017].

Ventilatory changes

Respiratory function does deteriorate with age, in tandem with the decline of the musculoskeletal system. Costal cartilages become stiff, making the chest wall more rigid and difficult to ventilate. In addition, there is also gradual age-related reduction in respiratory muscle strength, primarily linked to atrophy of the muscles associated with respiration [Knight, 2017]. Shortness of breath on exertion is more common in older people due to [Farley, 2011]:

- decreasing muscle strength
- muscles being more prone to fatigue when work of breathing increases
- muscle-wasting
- decreased blood supply to the muscles of respiration.

These changes mean that the body has less capacity to respond to increased requirements for ventilation when required. These increased demands may be as a result of exercise, trauma,

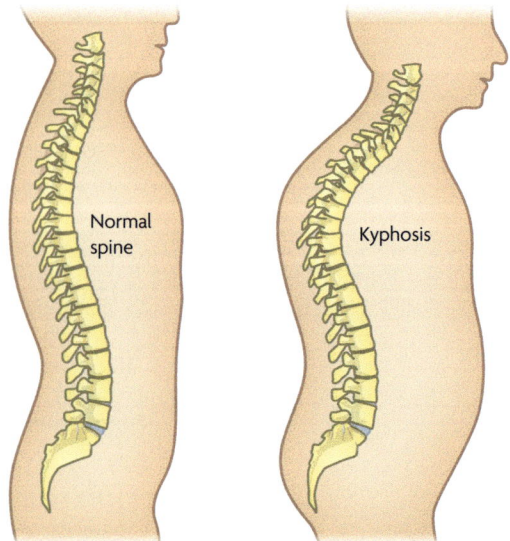

Figure 23.2 A comparison or a normal spine (left) and a spine with significant kyphosis (right).

or increased metabolic requirement due to the body fighting an infection or similar. This is especially true if the patient has a disease of the respiratory system, such as COPD, which already lowers the capacity of the ventilatory system to keep up with the body's requirements for gas exchange [Knight, 2017].

1.3.3 Cardiovascular system

Blood vessels
As the body ages, blood vessels (particularly the arteries) lose their elasticity and become less compliant. The tunica media of large arteries thickens, which makes the arteries more rigid. The inner endothelial layer, normally smooth to encourage blood flow, becomes roughened by muscle fibres that have migrated from the tunica media, which increases the resistance to blood flow [Knight, 2008a].

Systolic blood pressure increases, due to left ventricular hypertrophy (LVH) and the decrease in elasticity and diameter of the blood vessels. Smaller arteries and arterioles, along with baroreceptors, become less sensitive, leading to a sluggish response to changes in posture, such as from sitting to standing, which can cause postural hypotension [Farley, 2011].

Heart
In order to overcome the increase in systemic vascular resistance, the heart needs to pump with greater force; like all muscles that are exercised, it thickens (hypertrophies), particularly the left ventricle.

There are also changes in the electrical conduction system, with the sino-atrial node losing around 50–75% of pacemaker cells by the age of 50. Progressive fibrosis and cell death in the bundle of His leads to cardiac conduction problems such as a decrease in maximal heart rate and increase in arrhythmias [Knight, 2008a].

1.3.4 Nervous system

Brain and senses
In healthy people the ageing brain functions normally, and learning, for example, is still able to occur. However, brain weight does decline by approximately 5–10% over a lifetime with little change up to the age of 50 years. Indeed, it is not until 60 years of age and older that there is a significant reduction in weight [Farley, 2011].

An important consequence of this is the separation of the brain from the skull, which allows increased movement and stretching of the bridging veins between the brain and the outer layer of the meninges. During trauma involving the head, this can result in tearing of the veins, with subsequent subdural haemorrhage, bleeding into the subdural space [GEMS, 2015].

About 10% of neurons are lost by the age of 75, but this does not result in significant loss of mental function. However, the loss of sensory neurons leads to impaired hearing, vision, smelling, temperature regulation and appreciation of pain. In addition, as proprioception reduces, older people become increasingly reliant on visual, tactile and auditory cues to stay on their feet, which increases the risk of falling, particularly if any/all of these senses are impaired [Knight, 2008c].

Eyes
The muscles of the eyelids lose tone and elasticity and a reduction in orbital fat makes the eyes become sunken, reducing the upward gaze. The cornea flattens and thickens with age, making it duller and less transparent, increasing the risk of visual blurring. At the same time, there is a reduction in the sensitivity of the cornea, decreasing the awareness of any eye injuries. Pupil diameter declines, resulting in a reduction in light entering the eye, which adversely affects vision, particularly at night. Finally, the lens thickens and stiffens, reducing visual acuity and the ability to focus further [Farley, 2011].

Ears
Hearing loss is common, although not inevitable, with around 50% of people over 75 having hearing difficulties. High-pitched sounds and consonants are particularly affected. This may be especially noticeable for the person when there are high levels of background noise, and it makes identifying the direction of sound tricky.

Spinal cord

As the body ages, reflexes slow and there is a delayed response to stimuli because of a reduction in the numbers of conducting nerve fibres. This in turn causes a reduction in reaction time. The loss of large nerve fibres in the sympathetic nervous system contributes to the problem of postural hypotension and, overall, there is a reduction in the efficiency of the autonomic nervous system. This can result in usually well-tolerated stressors, such as heat, cold and extreme exercise, becoming harmful and even life-threatening [Farley, 2011].

1.3.5 Immune system

From a functional peak around puberty, there is a gradual reduction in immune system capacity over a person's lifetime of 5–30%, but the immune system does continue to function even in very old adults. However, older people are more likely to die of infectious diseases such as pneumonia, influenza and gastroenteritis, for example. In addition, older adults respond differently to infection than younger adults, including [Farley, 2011]:

- Fewer microorganisms are required to cause symptomatic infection.
- Confusion prior to a raised temperature is more common.
- Symptoms can be masked and/or mistaken for other diseases.
- The immune system can be compromised by medication such as steroids and anti-inflammatories.
- There is increased risk from chronic diseases such as diabetes and chronic obstructive pulmonary disease.

1.3.6 Integumentary system

The skin is probably the most visible sign of older age and all layers are affected [Farley, 2011]:
- **Epidermis:** Loss of melanocytes and other skin cells leads to decreased surface contact between the dermis and epidermis, which reduces the exchange of nutrients and other products of metabolism. In addition, the epidermis atrophies, causing roughened skin that takes longer to heal and provides less of a barrier.
- **Dermis:** This layer also atrophies, becoming thinner. In addition, there is a reduction in mast cells, which play an important role in injury and infection responses. The dramatic reduction in dermal blood vessels leads to pallor, decreased temperature and impaired thermoregulation compounded by a loss of sensory nerve endings, increasing the risk of injury.
- **Hypodermis:** A reduction in subcutaneous fat leads to increased conductive heat loss, and the redistribution of the fat leads to bony prominences, which are vulnerable to pressure ulcers and fractures following trauma. Clinically, the skin looks dry, lax and wrinkly. The wrinkles are due to a combination of gravity, decreasing subcutaneous fat and, in the face, repeated traction by facial muscles. In addition, photo-ageing caused by ultraviolet radiation from the sun increases the number of skin lesions, which are usually benign, although they can become cancerous later in life.

1.3.7 Digestive system

Food intake declines with age, with about a 10% reduction in calorific intake each decade after 50 years of age. Older people may experience altered taste, linked mainly to a decrease in the sense of smell and smell discrimination as the appeal of foods is based on its smell and taste. In addition, they are more likely to have missing teeth and poorly fitting dentures, all of which contribute to weight loss and malnutrition becoming more common. Increased intake of sugar and salt can contribute to the development of diabetes and high blood pressure [Nigam, 2008].

Muscular contractions that initiate the swallowing reflex also decline with age, leading to dysphagia and increased risk of choking. Lower down the gastrointestinal tract, there is impaired absorption of essential fats and other nutrients, while in the large intestine peristalsis slows, increasing the transit time of bowel contents, which can cause constipation. This in turn can lead to the formation of haemorrhoids due to the increased straining required to defecate [Nigam, 2008].

2 Caring for older patients

2.1 Learning objectives

By the end of this section, you will be able to:
- identify a range of common conditions associated with ageing
- describe the impact co-morbidities will have on your treatment plans
- discuss attitudes towards ageing.

2.2 Age-related conditions

The following include a range of conditions commonly associated with older patients. However, these conditions are not necessarily unique to older patients and can be seen in younger people as well in certain circumstances.

2.2.1 Parkinson's disease

Due to the death of cells in the brain, Parkinson's patients don't produce enough of the neurotransmitter dopamine. Approximately one in every 350 people in the UK suffers from the disease for which there is no cure and the underlying cause is unclear, although it is thought to be a combination of genetic and environmental factors [Parkinson's UK, 2018].

The main symptoms of Parkinson's disease are:
- tremor, rigidity and slowness of movement
- tiredness
- pain
- depression
- constipation.

Parkinson's disease is treated with a combination of medication, therapy and occasionally surgery to help alleviate symptoms and slow the progression of the disease.

Parkinson's is associated with a higher-than-average risk of developing dementia, but two-thirds remain unaffected. When it does occur, it is usually in the late stages of Parkinson's disease (Alzheimer's Society, 2018a).

2.2.2 Arthritis

Arthritis is defined as inflammation within a joint. There are many different forms of the condition, but the two most common are degenerative mechanical arthritis (osteoarthritis) and inflammatory arthritis (Figure 23.3) [Arthritis Research UK, 2018].

Degenerative forms of mechanical arthritis (osteoarthritis)

A normal joint is covered at the ends of the bone in smooth cartilage, to allow bone ends to glide across each other. In degenerative forms of arthritis, these smooth cartilage ends have been worn away. The underlying bone tries to repair this, but often

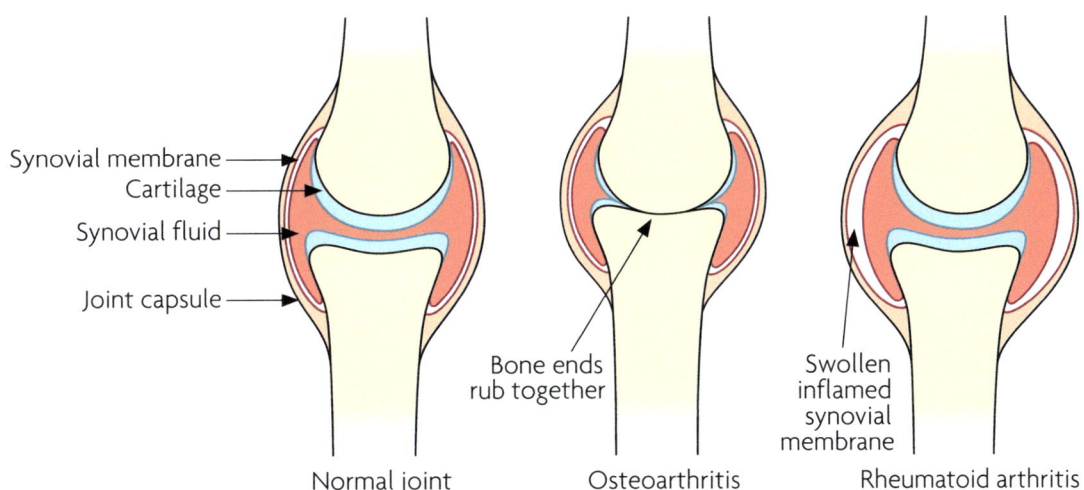

Figure 23.3 Normal and arthritic joints.

overgrows, altering the shape of the joint. This is known as osteoarthritis.

Osteoarthritis is particularly common in joints that see heavy use, including the hips and knees, base of thumb and big toe.

Inflammatory arthritis (rheumatoid arthritis)
Inflammation is a normal response as part of the body's healing process, but in patients with this form of arthritis the inflammation happens for no obvious normal reason. This is an autoimmune condition (the body's own immune system is attacking the joints). Instead of helping to repair the body, it causes damage to the joint, pain and stiffness. This type of arthritis often affects several joints at once and includes rheumatoid arthritis. As well as joint pain, other symptoms of rheumatoid arthritis include:
- tiredness
- depression
- irritability
- flu-like symptoms.

2.2.3 Osteoporosis

Bones are constantly going through a process of regenerating themselves by breaking down old matter and replacing it with new. Up to around the late twenties bone density increases slowly and from around 35 years onwards it starts (very gradually at first) to decrease as part of the natural ageing process. However, in certain people this can be accelerated and lead to weaker bones, which are more likely to fracture as a result.

Osteoporosis occurs when the mesh-like structure within bones becomes thin, causing bones to become fragile and break easily [National Osteoporosis Society, 2018]. Women are more susceptible to osteoporosis due to increased bone loss in the years following the menopause.

The main risk of osteoporosis is the increased risk of fractures from just minor forces, rather than the significant force we would normally expect to cause a fracture. Broken hips and wrists are common injuries, as is a broken neck or back in a fall from just standing height.

When assessing a patient who has a history of osteoporosis, have a very low threshold for suspecting fractures and be mindful that some clinical examination tools, such as the Canadian c-spine rule, may not be reliable in this patient group.

2.2.4 Mental illness in the elderly

Mental health is discussed in its own chapter, but it is worth considering some specific mental health challenges facing older people.

It is thought by some that mental health problems are a normal part of ageing, but this is not necessarily the case. Most older people do not develop mental health problems, and many of those that do can be helped or treated, or the onset prevented with the right action early on [MHF, 2015].

Dementia
Dementia is one of the most common causes of mental health illness in older patients and we will look at this in some detail in the next section of this chapter.

Depression
Depression is another common mental health illness in later life that makes people feel sad and lack motivation [Age UK, 2018a]. We all feel like this at times, but depression occurs when these feelings are more intense and persist for weeks, months or longer. Depression is often linked to loss, which is common as people grow older. These losses can influence people's self-esteem and feelings of value and include:
- loss of job
- loss of good health
- loss of independence
- loss of spouse or friends
- loss of social network.

As with depression at any age, a number of treatment options, including medication and talking therapies, are available. It is also possible that certain things can be done to prevent the development of depression initially.

Many elderly people are isolated and spend prolonged periods of time on their own. Arranging for appropriate social interactions can help to alleviate these feelings of isolation and prevent the development of depression in the first place.

When treating older patients, make sure you consider the risk of depression as one of your holistic assessments. Mental and physical health are closely intertwined and you should be looking to always promote an individual's mental well-being as well as their physical well-being. Groups such as Age UK offer services such as befriending; consider providing details of these services when appropriate.

2.3 Patients with co-morbidities

When treating elderly patients, it is often the case that they suffer from a number of simultaneous co-morbidities (other illnesses). For example, a patient suffering from cardiovascular disease and type 2 diabetes has two serious long-term conditions that can be life-limiting, especially if not managed correctly. They also interact with each other and can make the other disease worse. This makes caring for patients very challenging as a number of conditions may be interacting and causing varied presentation.

Many of these patients will have specialist medical or nursing support and might be under the care of a chronic condition management team, or community matron.

When dealing with patients with a range of co-morbidities, be sure to consider all of the conditions that may be influencing the current presentation; do not become fixated on just one element of the patient's illness. These cases are complex and in elderly patients, who may already have compromised immune systems or compensatory mechanisms, can represent significant dangers. Be prepared to seek early additional help and support in such situations and recognise the limitations of your own scope of practice and knowledge where necessary.

2.4 Attitudes to ageing

A positive attitude towards ageing is fundamental for ageing well and current attitudes towards ageing in society and the media may be negatively impacting on the older population [AAA, 2015].

As has already been discussed, ageing is unique to every individual and age itself is no marker for a person's independence, or ability to contribute to society. Some people will suffer from a range of age-related illnesses in their sixties whereas others will live long into their nineties with limited, if any, illness or disability.

Everyone, regardless of age, should be encouraged to live the best-quality life that they can and you must not judge anyone's ability on purely their age. Doing so would not just lead to an inaccurate assessment, but would also be considered discrimination by the Equality Act 2010.

3 Dementia

3.1 Learning objectives

By the end of this section you will be able to:
- define dementia
- explain the differences between dementia and delirium
- describe a number of strategies that can assist you when communicating with a patient with dementia
- identify a number of causes of challenging behaviour
- explain how to manage challenging behaviour.

3.2 Introduction

Dementia is not a disease in its own right. Instead, it is an umbrella term to cover a range of conditions and diseases that result in the gradual death of cells within the brain, leading to progressive cognitive decline. The most common symptoms include: memory loss, confusion, mood and personality changes, and problems with planning and performing tasks in the right order [SCIE, 2018].

Dementia is an 'organic' disorder, meaning that there is an associated physical deterioration of the brain tissue. This can be seen via a brain scan or, after death, at autopsy, though different physical changes will be seen depending on the exact type of dementia. Dementia is progressive – the damage and symptoms get worse over time. It is not a normal result of ageing [SCIE, 2018].

3.2.1 Dementia in context
It is estimated that between 600,000–800,000 people have dementia in the UK, although the majority of suffers are undiagnosed [Age UK, 2018b]. The majority of people affected by dementia are over 65, but many are younger. Two-thirds of people with dementia are women [SCIE, 2018]. It is estimated that the current cost to the UK economy stands at £26 billion a year [Alzheimer's Society, 2019].

Dementia is an increasing challenge as people are living longer. By 2025, it is estimated that the number of people in the UK living with dementia will have reached one million [NHS, 2017d].

3.3 Dementia
Dementia tends to affect sufferers in three different ways:
- **Cognitive:** As the areas of the brain responsible for cognition are damaged and the number of cells are reduced, sufferers are less able to deal with complex thought processes or store memories so easily.
- **Behavioural:** As different areas of the brain are affected, a person's behaviour may change. This is particularly seen in frontotemporal dementia where the sufferer may lose a sense of inhibition.
- **Neurological:** Physical changes to the structure of the brain mean that the brain of dementia sufferers is not able to function appropriately. A loss of brain cells and a change to the type and quantity of chemicals in the brain leads to a vast change in neurological function. In some forms, including dementia with Lewy bodies, physical signs such as shaking may develop, showing changes to the neurological system.

3.3.1 Different types of dementia
There are many different types of dementia, with Alzheimer's disease being the most common single cause in the UK, making up around two-thirds of cases, and vascular dementia coming in second. However, multiple-disease processes are even more common than single-disease processes, with Alzheimer's disease and vascular dementia, and Alzheimer's disease and Lewy bodies dementia, being common combinations [NG, 2001].

3.3.2 Causes of dementia
Different forms of dementia have different underlying causes. The most common are [Alzheimer's Society, 2018b; NHS 2017d; Age UK 2018b]:
- Alzheimer's disease
- vascular dementia
- Lewy bodies
- frontotemporal dementia.

Alzheimer's disease
In Alzheimer's disease, loss of brain cells leads to the shrinking of the brain. The cerebral cortex, the area of the brain responsible for processing thought and other complex functions including memory, calculations and some communication skills, is most affected.

Clumps of protein gather in the brain and it is thought that they are responsible for the increased rate of brain cell death. Connections between brain cells are also lost and the chemicals that normally carry signals, known as neurotransmitters, are greatly reduced, all of which leads to the cognitive impairment seen.

Vascular dementia
Vascular dementia occurs when cells are damaged as a result of a lack of blood and therefore oxygen reaching brain tissue. As people age, their vessels tend to become narrow and harden where fatty deposits develop. This process means that less blood can get through the vessels and surrounding brain tissue is starved of oxygen.

Patients who have been diagnosed with small vessel disease or have previously suffered from a stroke or a transient ischaemic attack (TIA) are at increased risk of developing vascular dementia.

Lewy bodies
Lewy bodies are small lumps of protein that develop inside brain cells. It is not known what causes them and neither is it fully understood how they damage the brain and cause dementia to

develop. Lewy bodies dementia is responsible for around 10–15% of dementia cases.

Lewy bodies dementia is closely linked to Parkinson's disease and a similar slow progression of disease will be seen. Over the years, as the brain damage becomes more significant, physical symptoms such as shaking (tremors), muscle stiffness and poor movement may develop.

Frontotemporal dementia
Frontotemporal dementia occurs when two areas of the brain, the frontal lobe and the temporal lobe, are damaged by shrinking. Although less common overall, it is one of the most common forms of dementia in those under 65 years of age, with a peak in diagnosis between 45 and 65 years of age. It is estimated that around one-fifth of cases are due to an inherited genetic mutation.

Other causes include:
- infections, including encephalitis
- some brain tumours
- lack of thyroid hormone
- head injury
- long-term alcohol abuse.

3.3.3 Disease progression

Every sufferer will have a unique disease progression. However, the main forms of dementia are all progressive, i.e. they will get worse with time. The speed at which any individual's disease progresses will vary widely and is based on many factors, including their age at time of onset, genetics and other physical and mental health factors [Alzheimer's Society, 2018b]. Patients with a history of poorly controlled heart disease or diabetes are likely to experience a faster deterioration.

The progression can be described in three broad stages:

Early (mild) stage
Dementia normally begins with mild subtle changes in a person's abilities or behaviour. The changes are often incorrectly thought to be just part of a normal ageing process and include:
- loss of memory of recent events
- mislaying items around the house
- becoming confused easily
- losing track of the day or date.

Middle (moderate) stage
As the disease progresses, changes become more obvious and a greater degree of help is required in day-to-day life. Changes may include:
- needing frequent reminders or help to eat, wash, dress and use the toilet
- becoming increasingly forgetful, especially of names
- becoming confused about where they are and trying to walk off to find somewhere else
- experiencing difficulty with perception and starting to have delusions.

Changes in behaviour are more commonly seen during this stage and sufferers can become easily upset, angry or even aggressive – perhaps because they are misinterpreting events or do not understand what is happening.

Late (severe) stage
At this stage sufferers will need increasing levels of help with daily activities and may gradually become totally dependent on others for nursing care. Loss of memory can become severe and they may not recognise people and their surroundings, though they may have occasional moments of clarity or recognition.

Behaviour changes can become very severe with restlessness, agitation and angry outbursts, particularly during periods of close personal care, usually because the sufferer does not understand what is happening.

This stage of the disease can be very distressing for both the sufferer and their family and carers and needs to be managed gently and tactfully.

3.3.4 Recognising dementia

If you attend a patient and you believe they, or someone else, may be suffering from the early stages of dementia, you should support them to seek further help.

Whilst dementia cannot be cured, there is an ever-developing range of treatments available that can help to slow the progression of the disease [NHS, 2017d].

The sooner dementia is recognised, the sooner it can be treated. This can lead to a delayed progression of the disease and the ability to provide other forms of support that may be beneficial. If you believe your patient is suffering from dementia, you should either refer them (with their consent) to an appropriate service or encourage them to visit their GP.

Receiving a diagnosis of dementia can be challenging as much stigma is still attached to the condition. Any patient who thinks they may be suffering from the disease, or who has recently been diagnosed, may need support to come to terms with this diagnosis. This is also true for the family, friends and carers of a patient with dementia. Help and advice are available from a range of services including the patient's own GP and a number of social support services and charities, including the Alzheimer's Society.

3.3.5 Living with dementia

Living with dementia is unique to every individual suffering from the disease. One of the key aims of supporting dementia patients should be to support them in retaining independence as far as possible.

As the disease progresses, more and more help may be required but this should be matched to a person's condition, and it should not immediately be assumed that they cannot make decisions for themselves, or care for themselves, just because they have a formal diagnosis of dementia.

3.3.6 Dementia and other diseases

When assessing a dementia patient, be careful not to attribute changes in their status to the ongoing deterioration of the condition without good evidence to do so. Dementia normally progresses slowly and any sudden changes should prompt you to search for a different cause. Many dementia patients will suffer from other co-morbidities (the presence of other diseases) and a detailed assessment will be required to identify any underlying illness.

You should ask those around you who are familiar with the patient for detailed information on their condition. For example, you may be asked to see a dementia patient with increased confusion. This is a common scenario and can be very difficult to manage. If the family or carers report a rapid change in cognitive state, it is unlikely that this is due to the dementia itself and is more likely a result of another disease process. What makes your assessment increasingly difficult is the confused nature of the patient, which means it can be difficult to elicit a detailed history and examination.

3.3.7 Treating patients with dementia

If working in an ambulance or urgent and unscheduled care environment, it is likely that you will frequently meet patients with dementia at various stages of the disease progression. Managing these patients may require some significant modifications to your usual approach. Although every encounter will be unique, you should consider the following guidance:

- Approach all situations in a calm manner: Your patient may be confused, scared or not understand what is happening. A calm manner on your part can help to relax your patient and make them feel safe.
- Communicate clearly and be patient: More information about communicating with dementia patients is included in the next section.
- Wherever possible and appropriate, support a patient in making their own decisions about their healthcare.
- Use relatives, friends and carers wherever possible to aid communication and to help the patient feel more relaxed by having a friendly familiar face present.
- Be compassionate: Remember that every dementia patient is different and will need different management; there is not one single way to manage 'dementia patients'.

3.3.8 Aggressive behaviour

Patients with dementia may sometimes become aggressive, either verbally or physically. This can be very distressing for the person, carers, friends and family. You should understand why this happens and how to resolve it as part of your role.

Patients with dementia have the same needs as everyone else, including comfort, social interaction, stimulation, emotional well-being and being free from pain. However, dementia patients may not understand their own needs or be able to communicate them. This can lead to frustration and in turn challenging or aggressive behaviour. For example, if a dementia patient is in pain, they may express this as anger and aggression as they cannot express the true cause of their distress.

Guidance for responding to such situations includes [Alzheimer's Society, 2018c]:
- Remain calm and avoid confrontation, as a heated response will make the situation worse.
- Reassure the person and acknowledge any feelings they are able to express.
- Listen to what they are saying.
- Try to explore what is causing the behaviour.
- Try to distract their attention if they remain angry.
- Maintain eye contact, come down to their level and try to ensure your body language and positioning is not aggressive or restrictive in any way.

3.3.9 Dementia and pain management

Pain management for dementia patients remains a difficult issue, especially for those that are not able to communicate effectively. It is well-recognised that dementia patients frequently receive inadequate pain relief [Chandler, 2014] and that is especially true of emergency care patients.

One of the key challenges is that patients are unable to express their pain, so healthcare staff tend to underestimate the amount of pain a patient is suffering and therefore do not provide adequate pain management techniques.

It is recommended that standardised assessment tools should be used to assess the level of pain that a patient is suffering if they are not able to communicate it themselves. One such tool designed for use with late-stage dementia patients is the Abbey pain scale (Figure 23.4) [Abbey, 2004].

When administering pain relief to dementia patients, you should observe for a reduction in the Abbey pain scale score. This may take time and close observation will be required.

You should be aware of the different forms of pain relief available, both pharmacological and non-pharmacological, and use them appropriately, or request help from another clinician with a broader range of analgesic options as required.

When making decisions on which pain relief to use, be sure to consider side-effects and any polypharmacy interactions. Many dementia patients will be on a large number of chronic medications, which may include pain relief medicines. Remember to act only within your scope of practice and to seek help and advice when you are unsure of the best way to proceed.

3.3.10 Dementia and discrimination

The Equality Act 2010 defines a disability as any physical or mental impairment that has a 'substantial' and 'long-term' negative effect on a person's ability to carry out normal daily activities. Clearly, dementia meets these criteria so those that suffer from it are protected by the Equality Act, which makes it illegal to discriminate against them on the basis of their disability. Nonetheless, the Alzheimer's Society (2015) identifies that dementia patients are frequently discriminated against for a broad range of reasons, including:
- **Stigma:** Dementia is still highly stigmatised, which results in a failure to understand the broad nature of the disease.
- **Impaired mental capacity:** An assumption that patients are unable to make even simple decisions so others decide for them, without having taken all reasonable steps to support the person in making the decision themselves.
- **Ageism:** Dementia is generally an illness of older persons, meaning that many symptoms are put down to 'getting old' rather than being tackled and treated appropriately.

Chapter 23 – Older People

The Abbey Pain Scale
For measurement of pain in people with dementia who cannot verbalise.

How to use scale: While observing the resident, score questions 1 to 6.

Name of resident:...

Name and designation of person completing the scale:..

Date: .... Time: ....

Latest pain relief given was.. at ....hrs.

Q1. Vocalisation
eg whimpering, groaning, crying
Absent 0   Mild 1   Moderate 2   Severe 3

Q1 [   ]

Q2. Facial expression
eg looking tense, frowning, grimacing, looking frightened
Absent 0   Mild 1   Moderate 2   Severe 3

Q2 [   ]

Q3. Change in body language
eg fidgeting, rocking, guarding part of body, withdrawn
Absent 0   Mild 1   Moderate 2   Severe 3

Q3 [   ]

Q4. Behavioural change
eg increased confusion, refusing to eat, alteration in usual patterns
Absent 0   Mild 1   Moderate 2   Severe 3

Q4 [   ]

Q5. Physiological change
eg temperature, pulse or blood pressure outside normal limits, perspiring, flushing of pallor
Absent 0   Mild 1   Moderate 2   Severe 3

Q5 [   ]

Q6. Physical changes
eg skin tears, pressure areas, arthritis, contractures, previous injuries
Absent 0   Mild 1   Moderate 2   Severe 3

Q6 [   ]

Add scores for Q1 to Q6 and record here ➔ Total pain score [   ]

Now tick the box that matches the Total Pain Score ➔

0–2 No pain	3–7 Mild	8–13 Moderate	14+ Severe

Finally, tick the box which matches the type of pain ➔

Chronic	Acute	Acute on chronic

Abbey J, De Bellis A, Piller N, Esterman A, Gilles L, Parker D, Lowcay B. The Abbey Pain Scale.
Funded by the JH & JD Gunn Medical Research Foundation 1998–2002.

Figure 23.4 The Abbey pain scale.

Source: Abbey J, Piller N, De Bellis A, Esterman A, Parker D, Gilles L and Lowcay B (2004). The Abbey pain scale: a 1-minute numerical indicator for people with end-stage dementia, *International Journal of Palliative Nursing*. 10:1, 6–13. Copyright © 2004 MA Healthcare Ltd. Reproduced by permission of MA Healthcare Ltd.

When caring for dementia patients, remember that each patient is an individual, with a unique illness and unique needs. Therefore, you must tailor your treatment so that it is uniquely appropriate for each patient you come into contact with.

3.3.11 Dementia vs delirium

If dementia can be thought of as chronic brain failure, then delirium is acute brain failure [Barrett, 2014]. Unlike dementia, it is usually temporary and there is an underlying cause which can normally be corrected, for example, an acute infection. It is a common and serious condition that is characterised by disruptions in thinking, consciousness, attention, cognition and perception. Unlike dementia, its onset is over a short period of time (typically hours to days). To complicate matters, patients with dementia can also develop delirium and this has been associated with serious complications and poor outcome, including death [Fick, 2002].

Delirium is often divided into three subtypes [Hosker, 2017]:
- **Hyperactive:** Characterised by anxiety, restlessness, irritability, anger and frustration. Patients may be easily startled and distracted, and unable to sit still. Speech can be loud, but incoherent with frequent topic-hopping.
- **Hypoactive:** Patients with hypoactive delirium are typically lethargic, apathetic, slow in movement, withdrawn, drowsy and difficult to wake.
- **Mixed:** A combination of the two other variants, with patients fluctuating between hyperactive and hypoactive delirium throughout the day.

Differentiating between delirium and dementia can be difficult, especially in the pre-hospital setting where you do not know the patient and it can be hard to clearly establish a baseline. If in doubt, it is safer to assume delirium, as this more commonly is associated with acute illness, and ensure patients receive prompt medical attention [SAS, 2014].

3.4   *Communication*

Although the principles of communication have already been covered in Chapter 3, 'Communication', there are some additional points to consider when you are caring for a patient with dementia:
- Get their attention: Approach the patient from the front so they can see you coming. Try to make eye contact and ensure they can see your face and body movements.
- Use their name: Using their name can help them understand that you are not a stranger (although this may not be true), which can be reassuring.
- Frequently remind them who you are: This can reduce anxiety and avoid the patient becoming alarmed at being treated by a stranger.
- Keep ambient noise and activity to a minimum: Reducing distractions, activity and noise will help a patient with dementia (indeed most patients) to concentrate on what you are saying.
- Don't rush: Take your time. Slowing your rate of speech can help, but increase the time spent speaking and listening. It may help if you leave brief pauses between sentences, allowing the patient time to think and respond if they wish to.
- Keep calm: Adopt a calm tone and manner to reduce distress and make the patient feel more comfortable with you. Patients with dementia maintain the ability to determine your body language even after their ability to understand speech has been lost.
- Keep things simple: Avoid jargon and speak in short and simple-to-understand sentences. When giving instructions, break down the task into simple stages. Give clear instructions; for example, rather than saying 'Sit there', you could try saying 'Sit in this blue chair, please'.
- Use the patient's preferred method of communication: Establish this early on from the patient and others who know them. This includes speaking to the patient in their first language or using communication aids such as pictures or talking mats.

3.5   *Challenging behaviour*

Many patients with dementia are placid and sweet-tempered, but over 90% will exhibit some form of challenging behaviour. This includes [Barrett, 2014]:
- sleeplessness
- wandering

- agitation
- pacing
- aggression (including spitting)
- disinhibition
- jealousy (especially sexual jealousy).

Challenging behaviour needs to be seen as a manifestation of unmet needs, which the patient may not be able to express, such as boredom, frustration and/or annoyance.

3.5.1 Managing challenging behaviour

It is important to appreciate that each patient will be slightly different, so the best way of managing challenging behaviour will need to be tailored to them. Advice from carers and/or relatives may help, but general principles include [YAS, 2013]:

- trying to find out what is the cause of the behaviour
- reducing the stress and/or demands placed on the patient
- explaining what is happening using the patient's name and saying who you are; you are likely to have to repeat this process often
- giving patients time to respond to your requests or questions
- trying not to show criticism or irritation and avoiding confrontation with patients
- watching for warning signs that they are becoming more anxious or agitated; get help if the situation does not calm down quickly
- referring to carers and/or relatives who know the patient and who will have experience in managing the patient's challenging behaviour
- avoiding making sudden movements or using a sharp tone; instead, remain calm and keep your voice low.

4 Frailty

4.1 Learning objectives

By the end of this section, you will be able to:
- define the term frailty
- describe how frailty has an impact on patients
- describe how to recognise and support patients with frailty.

4.2 Introduction

Frailty is a distinctive health state related to the ageing process in which multiple body systems gradually lose their inbuilt reserves [BGS, 2018], such that they are unable to deal with everyday or acute stresses [Xue, 2012].

Approximately 10% of patients aged over 65 are defined as suffering from frailty, rising to between a quarter and a half of those aged 85 years and older [Clegg, 2013], so this is a patient group you will frequently encounter.

4.3 Recognising frailty

Different models of recognising frailty have been proposed and as yet no single model is preferred [BGS, 2018]. One of the simpler models, known as the phenotype model [Fried, 2001], describes a distinct set of characteristics:
- unintentional weight loss
- reduced muscle strength
- reduced gait speed
- self-reported exhaustion
- low energy expenditure.

Generally, individuals with three or more of these characteristics are said to be frail, although a formal diagnosis requires a far more in-depth assessment by a GP or geriatrician.

4.4 Living with frailty

Living with frailty will be unique for each person. For some people, frailty will be the only condition they suffer from, which means they are likely to be only an occasional user of health services, until such times as they become acutely unwell. For others, frailty may be one of many long-term complex conditions they live with, meaning they are a frequent user of health services [BGS, 2018].

Frailty will mean that an individual's health reserves are diminished, so when they become unwell, they have a lesser ability to cope with acute illness/infection. As such, conditions that may normally be well-tolerated and easily treated (such as a simple respiratory tract infection) can become a life-threatening illness.

4.5 Supporting patients with frailty

You should consider whether a patient already has a diagnosis of frailty and how this might have an impact on any other health problem they are suffering from. Equally, you may also see a patient who you believe is frail, but who does not have a specific diagnosis of frailty yet.

In your management of a patient, you should consider how their frailty may have an impact on other medical conditions, and whether it leaves them at increased risk of other illness or injury. As mentioned above, what may be a simple infection to most people can quickly become life-threatening to a frail patient without the physiological reserves to combat illness.

A common situation you may encounter would be attending an older person who has fallen at home. On arrival, they may be uninjured and not requiring medical treatment, but through your initial assessment you may identify that you believe they may be suffering from frailty. In this scenario, you should seek their consent to refer them to their GP for a fuller assessment and consideration of a care and support plan to help them and, where possible, restrict the progression of their frailty.

5 Falls

5.1 Learning objectives

By the end of this section, you will be able to:
- identify the risks to older people of suffering a fall
- describe additional considerations for the assessment of an older person that has fallen
- describe the importance of a falls referral.

5.2 Introduction

Falls in older people are common, with one in three adults aged over 65 and living at home having at least one fall a year, and about half of these having more frequent falls than this [NHS, 2018e].

The causes of falls can be diverse and often complicated, they may be linked to previous conditions such as frailty, immobility and injury. Falls can also result from patients with cognitive impairment, such as dementia, forgetting their limitations or unsuitable environments or medication regimes.

Although many falls will not result in any injury, they are also the most common cause of injury-related deaths in those aged over 75 [NHS 2018b]. Falls from standing height are the most common mechanism to cause major trauma and the thorax and head are the most commonly injured areas [RCEM, 2018].

Elderly fallers represent approximately 10% of 999 calls to the ambulance services [WAS, 2018].

5.3 Assessing people who fall

People who fall should be assessed using the standard assessment process outlined in Chapter 10, 'Patient Assessment'. There are, however, a number of things that you should specifically consider as part of your assessment, including:
- Due to age-related changes and presence of other conditions such as osteoporosis, older people can suffer significant injuries from what might normally seem minor mechanisms. For example, a fall from standing height can cause severe trauma.
- A fractured neck of femur or pelvis is common; be aware how to assess for these injuries.
- Consider how medications the patient is on might complicate the situation, i.e. anticoagulants with head injuries.
- The presence of some conditions, such as diabetes, can mean that patients do not feel pain in the same way, which can result in injuries being masked.
- Consider very carefully what the cause of the fall was. Was it a simple trip over an inappropriately placed rug or furniture, or was it actually a dizzy spell caused by an underlying medical condition?
- How long has the patient been on the floor? Patients who spend a long time on the floor are at risk of conditions such as rhabdomyolysis due to breakdown of muscle tissues when they are lying on the hard ground.

If you assess someone as not needing to attend hospital, then your service may have a process in place for arranging a multifactorial falls risk assessment. This is designed to help identify and mitigate risk to the patient of suffering injuries from future falls [NICE, 2013]. Where such a pathway exists, you should seek the patient's consent to refer to one of these services. If necessary, you may also seek further guidance from other community teams, the GP, or a specialist paramedic in urgent care, depending on your local arrangements.

It is likely that a fall assessment will require the following information:

- Details of the patient and their consent for the referral.
- Why have they fallen.
- How many falls they have suffered in a recent period (often the last year).
- A basic mobility assessment.
- The number of medications a patient takes.

If appropriate, you should complete one of these referrals each time you attend a person who has fallen so that the services responsible for managing falls understand how significant the problem is.

Chapter

24 Cardiac Arrest

1 Adult basic life support

1.1 Learning objectives
By the end of this section you will be able to:
- explain the benefits of the chain of survival to basic life support
- explain common types and causes of cardiac arrest in adults
- explain the procedure for providing basic life support to adults.

1.2 Introduction
Cardiac arrest is the ultimate medical emergency, but you will have the ability to undertake the two most effective treatments for this: cardiopulmonary resuscitation (more commonly called basic life support in healthcare circles) and defibrillation. However, the role of the ambulance service is just one link in a chain that maximises the patient's chance, not only of a return of spontaneous circulation (ROSC), but also of surviving to hospital discharge neurologically intact (i.e. with normal or near-normal brain function) [Perkins, 2015]. That chain is known as the chain of survival [Nolan, 2006].

1.3 Chain of survival
The chain of survival encompasses four key principles that are required if a resuscitation is to be successful in adults (Figure 24.1) [Perkins, 2015]:
- early recognition and call for help
- early bystander cardiopulmonary resuscitation (CPR)
- early defibrillation
- post-resuscitation care.

1.3.1 Early recognition and call for help
This relies on patients and the public calling for help early and can be influenced by the ambulance service with public education and training sessions. Recognition of cardiac chest pain is particularly important as around 21–33% of patients with acute myocardial ischaemia will suffer a cardiac arrest in the first hour following onset [Müller, 2006].

1.3.2 Early CPR
Performing CPR immediately following cardiac arrest can double or triple the chance of the patient surviving [Perkins, 2015]. When a member of the public calls 999, they will be given advice on

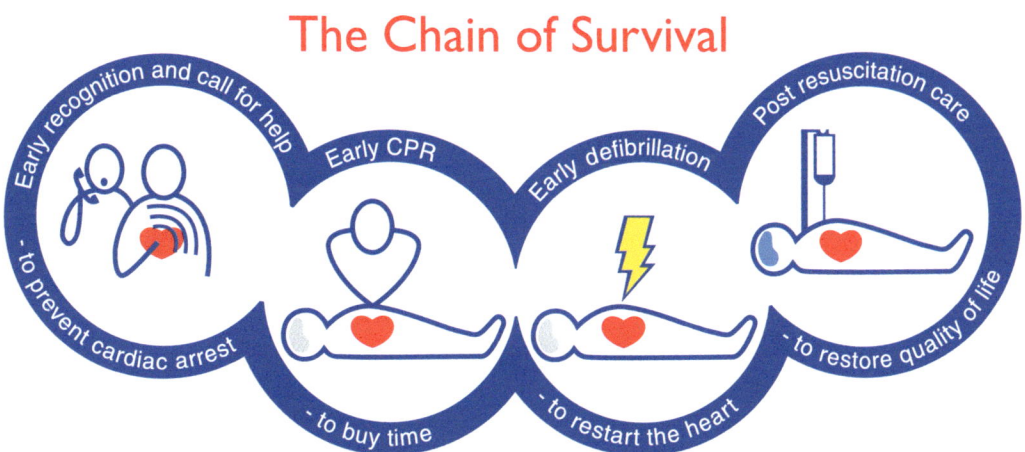

Figure 24.1 The chain of survival.
Source: Image reproduced by the kind permission of Laerdal Medical.

how to perform chest compressions only, as this has been shown to produce higher survival rates in adults than conventional CPR (chest compression and mouth-to-mouth ventilation) when performed by untrained bystanders [Hüpfl, 2010].

1.3.3 Early defibrillation

Providing good quality CPR and defibrillating in the first 3–5 minutes of a cardiac arrest can produce a survival rate of 50–75%, but, conversely, the chance of surviving to hospital discharge falls by 10–12% for every minute of delay [Perkins, 2015].

1.3.4 Post-resuscitation care

Restarting your patient's heart and palpating a pulse (ROSC) is a great feeling, but the patient is not out of the woods yet. The true measure of success is returning the patient to their pre-cardiac-arrest state, with brain function intact so that they can leave hospital. Providing post-resuscitation care on scene, en route and in hospital is crucial if this is to happen [Nolan, 2016].

1.3.5 Children

In stark contrast to adults, children usually suffer a cardiac arrest secondary to hypoxia. The outcomes from these secondary cardiac arrests are very poor and the emphasis with children is to intervene before their heart arrests [Skellett, 2016].

1.4. Causes of cardiac arrest in adults

The commonest cause of cardiac arrest in adults is an irregular heart rhythm (arrhythmia) caused by myocardial ischaemia or infarction [Nolan, 2016]. Most victims of sudden cardiac death (SCD) have a history of cardiac disease and commonly experience warning signs, such as chest pain in the hour prior to cardiac arrest [Monsieurs, 2015].

Other circulatory causes of cardiac arrest are most commonly due to hypovolaemia in patients who become suddenly ill. Of course, adults are also prone to cardiac arrests due to a primary airway or breathing problem, just like children. Ideally, you will intervene before an airway or breathing problem deteriorates into cardiac arrest [Nolan, 2016].

1.5 Adult BLS

Basic life support (BLS) refers to maintenance of airway patency, and supporting breathing and circulation, with artificial ventilation and chest compressions as required [JRCALC, 2019]. The procedure described is for a single rescuer, but tasks are usually shared when there is more than one rescuer on scene, such as when you are working as a crew.

1.5.1 Procedure

Procedure – To perform basic life support on an adult

Take the following steps to perform adult BLS [Perkins, 2015; JRCALC, 2019]:

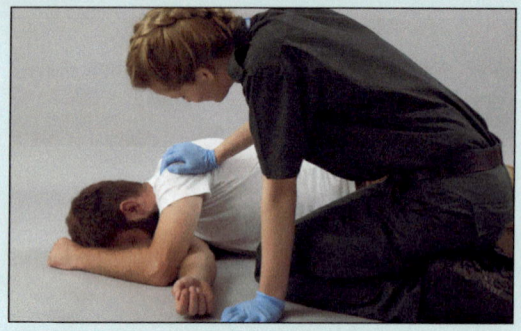

1. Ensure the scene is safe for you, your colleague, the patient and other bystanders. Check the patient to see if they are responsive by gently shaking their shoulders and asking if they are all right.

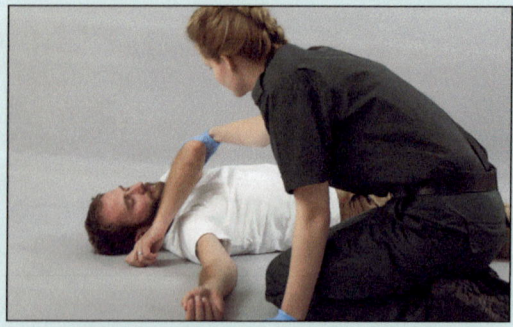

2. If the patient responds, obtain a history and undertake a further patient assessment. If the patient does not respond, inform your colleague so they can assist. Turn the patient onto their back.

Adult basic life support

Procedure – To perform basic life support on an adult – *cont*

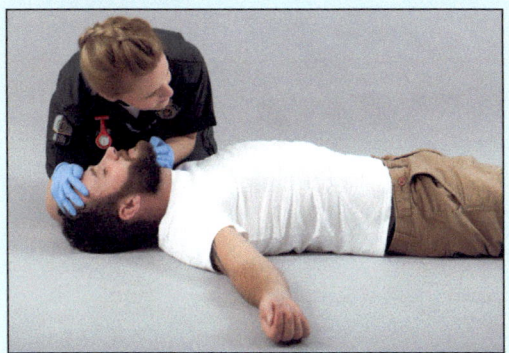

3. Open the patient's airway and look, listen and feel for breathing for no more than ten seconds. Note that agonal breathing (occasional gasps) is common immediately following cardiac arrest and should not be confused with normal breathing or taken as a sign of life. If the patient is breathing normally, place them in the recovery position.

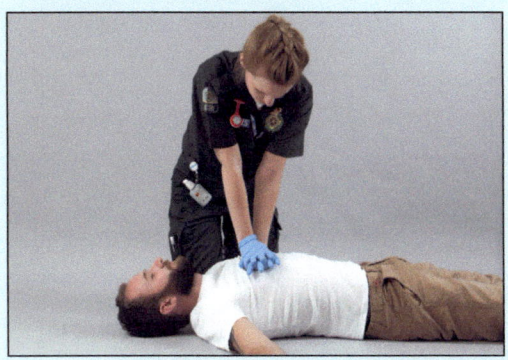

4. If the patient is not breathing normally or there are no signs of life (not moving or coughing), start chest compressions:
   - Kneel beside the patient.
   - Place the heel of one hand in the centre of the chest (lower half of the sternum).
   - Place the heel of your other hand on top of the first.
   - Interlock your fingers and ensure that pressure is not applied over the patient's ribs.

Procedure – To perform basic life support on an adult – *cont*
   - Keeping your arms straight and with you positioned directly over the patient's chest, apply downward pressure to compress the chest by 5–6 cm.
   - After each compression release the pressure on the chest, but maintain contact with the patient's skin.
   - Repeat at a rate of 100–120 compressions/minute.

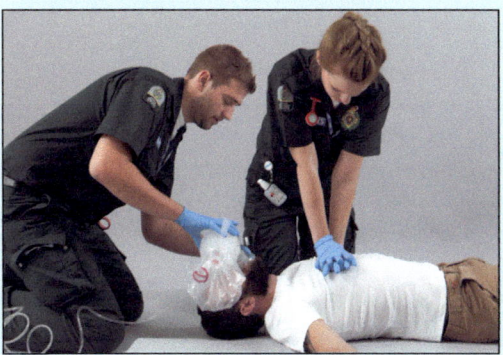

5. After 30 compressions, open the airway (you can insert an oropharyngeal airway if available) and provide two rescue breaths with a pocket mask or bag-valve-mask. If your colleague is available, they may well have already assembled the equipment and be prepared to ventilate. Each ventilation should cause the chest to rise and take about one second to deliver. Do not attempt to compress the chest while ventilation is being provided, but keep your hands in the correct position so that chest compressions can immediately resume once the ventilations have been administered.

Procedure – To perform basic life support on an adult – *cont*

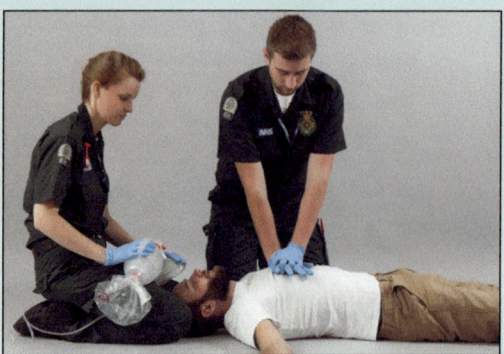

6. Continue with chest compressions and ventilations at a ratio of 30:2. You should alternate chest compressions with your colleague every two minutes, but keep the changeover time to a minimum.

2 Paediatric basic life support

2.1 Learning objectives

By the end of this section you will be able to:
- explain how the causes of cardiac arrest in children are usually different from adults
- explain the procedure for providing basic life support to paediatric patients.

2.2 Introduction

You will recall from Chapter 20, 'Children and Infants', that paediatric patients are not small adults. This is especially true of cardiac arrest where, unlike adults, who experience a primary cardiac arrest typically due to a cardiac arrhythmia, infants and children usually suffer a secondary cardiac arrest [Maconochie, 2015]. This is not the sudden event experienced by adults, but a progressive worsening of the patient's condition until they cannot continue to compensate. Outcome from secondary cardiac arrest is poor.

Paediatric basic life support (BLS) is different from that of adults, and there are also some differences between infants (paediatric patients under one year of age) and children (between one year of age and puberty), and so they are presented separately in this section.

2.3 Infant BLS

2.3.1 Procedure

Procedure – To perform basic life support on an infant

Take the following steps to perform basic life support on an infant [Maconochie, 2015; JRCALC, 2019]:

1. Ensure the scene is safe for you, your colleague, the patient and other bystanders. Check for responsiveness by placing a hand on the infant's forehead to stabilise it and tug their hair while calling their name. If they do not have hair, consider flicking the soles of their feet. Never shake an infant.

2. If the patient responds, assess the infant's ABCDE, call for assistance and reassess regularly. If they do not respond, summon additional assistance.

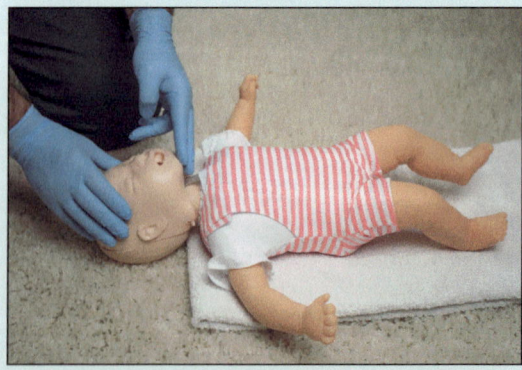

3. Open the infant's airway by placing one hand on their forehead and gently tilt it back until it is in a neutral position. Perform a chin lift by placing the fingertips of your other hand on the bony part of the lower jaw and lift upwards. Don't compress the soft tissues under the jaw as this will occlude the airway. Placing a towel under the infant's shoulders and upper body can help keep their head in a neutral position.

Paediatric basic life support

Procedure – To perform basic life support on an infant – *cont*

4. If a head tilt–chin lift is not effectively opening the airway, you can use a jaw thrust to open the airway:
   - Position yourself behind the infant.
   - Place two fingers under both angles of the jaw.
   - Rest your thumbs on the infant's cheeks.
   - Lift the jaw upwards.

5. Look, listen and feel for normal breathing by placing your face close to the infant's face:
   - Look for chest and abdominal movements.
   - Listen for airflow at the mouth and nose.
   - Feel for airflow at the mouth and nose.

6. If the infant is breathing normally, turn them on to their side and monitor their breathing.

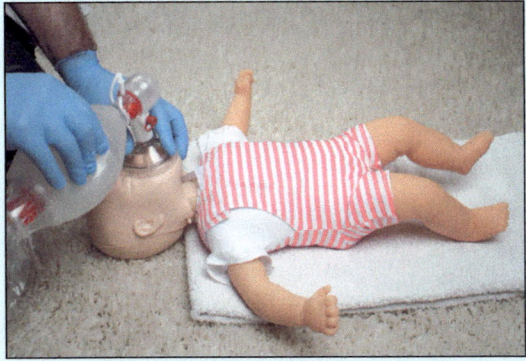

7. If the infant is not breathing normally or there are no signs of life (not moving or coughing), check for, and carefully remove, any airway obstruction and provide five rescue breaths:
   - Ensure the head is in a neutral position and apply a chin lift.
   - Either place a bag-valve-mask over the infant's mouth and nose, or take a breath and place your mouth over the mouth and nose of the infant.

Procedure – To perform basic life support on an infant – *cont*

   - Ventilate the chest steadily for one second, just enough to make the chest rise.
   - Maintain head tilt–chin lift and watch the chest fall.
   - Repeat this sequence five times.

8. If the infant's chest is not rising and falling in a similar fashion to normal breathing, open the infant's mouth and check for any visible obstruction. Do not blindly sweep in the infant's mouth. Reposition the head to ensure it is in the neutral position, using a jaw thrust if the head tilt–chin lift manoeuvre is not effective. Make no more than five attempts to achieve effective ventilation before moving on to chest compressions.

9. Check for signs of life (movement, coughing or normal breathing). If you are confident in checking for a pulse, feel for a brachial pulse in the medial aspect of the infant's arm. Unless you are sure you can feel a pulse, assume it is absent and start chest compressions. If there are signs of circulation, reassess airway and breathing and manage appropriately.

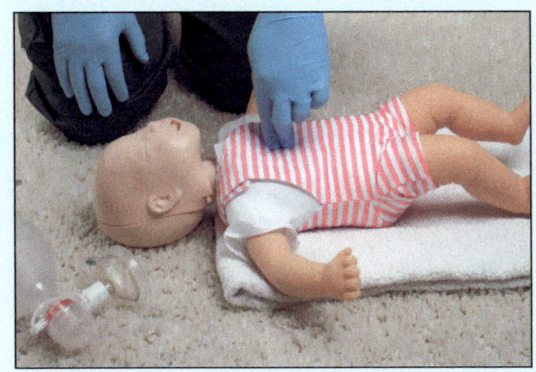

Procedure – To perform basic life support on an infant – cont

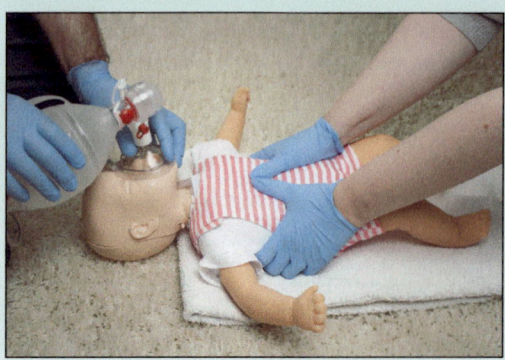

10. If there are no signs of life and/or no pulse or a pulse rate of less than 60 beats/minute, start chest compressions:
    - If you are on your own, use the tips of two fingers; otherwise, adopt the encircling technique by placing both thumbs side by side on the lower sternum and spreading the remaining fingers around to the infant's back.
    - Avoid compressing the abdomen by placing your fingers one finger's width above the xiphisternum.
    - Compress the sternum at least one-third of the depth of the chest (or by 4 cm) and then fully release the pressure while maintaining contact with the sternum.
    - Repeat the compressions at a rate of 100–120/minute for 15 compressions and then give two ventilations.
    - Continue compressions and ventilations at a ratio of 15:2 unless you are on your own, in which case a ratio of 30:2 may be easier.
    - Continue until the infant shows signs of life or you become exhausted.

2.4 Child BLS
2.4.1 Procedure

Procedure – To perform basic life support on a child

Take the following steps to perform basic life support on a child [Maconochie, 2015; JRCALC, 2019]:

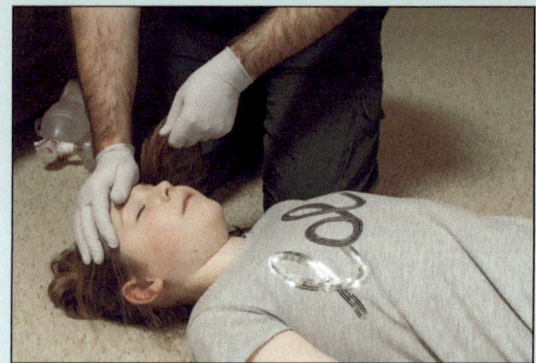

1. Ensure the scene is safe for you, your colleague, the patient and other bystanders. Check for responsiveness by placing a hand on the child's forehead to stabilise it and tug their hair while calling their name or telling them to wake up. Never shake a child.

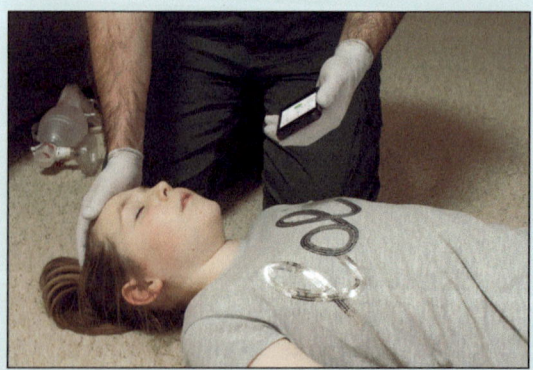

2. If the patient responds, assess the child's ABCDE, call for assistance and reassess regularly. If they do not respond, summon additional assistance.

Paediatric basic life support

Procedure – To perform basic life support on a child – *cont*

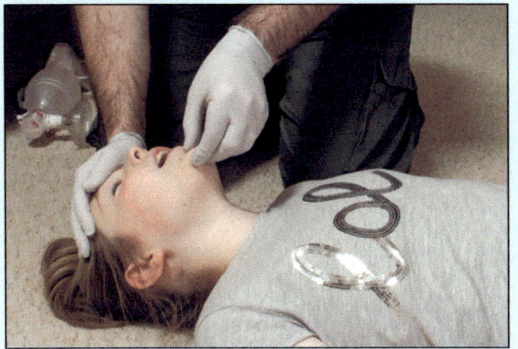

3. Open the child's airway by placing one hand on their forehead and gently tilt it back until it is in a 'sniffing' position. Perform a chin lift by placing the fingertips of your other hand on the bony part of the lower jaw and lift upwards. Don't compress the soft tissues under the jaw as this will occlude the airway. Do not use a head tilt–chin lift technique in children who you suspect have a cervical spine injury: use a jaw thrust instead.

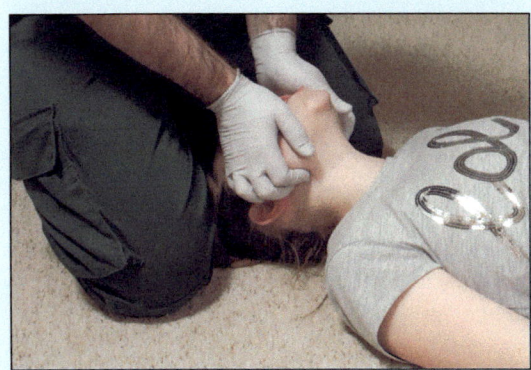

3a. If a head tilt–chin lift is not effectively opening the airway, or you suspect a cervical spine injury, use a jaw thrust to open the airway.

Procedure – To perform basic life support on a child – *cont*

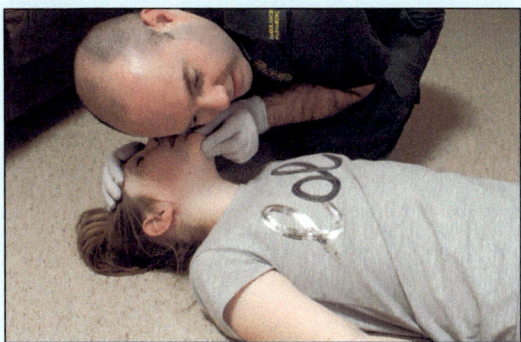

4. Look, listen and feel for normal breathing by placing your face close to the child's face:
   - Look for chest and abdominal movements.
   - Listen for airflow at the mouth and nose.
   - Feel for airflow at the mouth and nose.

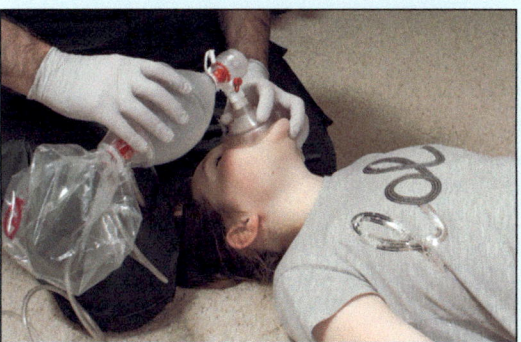

5. If the child is not breathing or there are no signs of life (not moving, no normal breathing or coughing), check for, and carefully remove, any airway obstruction that is visible and provide five rescue breaths:
   - Apply a head tilt–chin lift.
   - Either place a bag-valve-mask over the child's mouth and nose, or take a breath and place your mouth over the mouth of the child and pinch their nose to prevent air from escaping.
   - Ventilate the chest steadily for one second, just enough to make the chest rise.
   - Maintain head tilt–chin lift and watch the chest fall.
   - Repeat this sequence five times.

Chapter 24 – Cardiac Arrest

Procedure – To perform basic life support on a child – *cont*

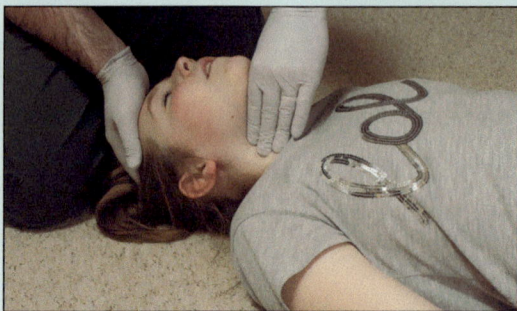

6. Check for signs of life (movement, coughing or normal breathing). If you are confident in checking for a pulse, feel for a carotid pulse at the neck. Unless you are sure you can feel a pulse, assume it is absent and start chest compressions. If there are signs of circulation, reassess airway and breathing and manage appropriately.

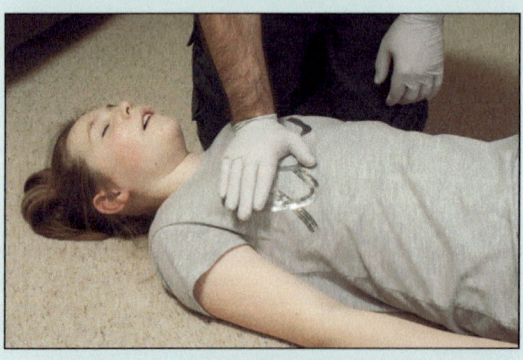

7. If there are no signs of life and/or no pulse or a pulse rate of less than 60 beats/minute, start chest compressions:
   - Position yourself at the side of the child.
   - Avoid compressing the abdomen, by locating the xiphisternum and placing the heel of one hand one finger's width above this point.
   - Lock your elbows and position your body so that your shoulders are directly over the child's chest.
   - Compress the sternum at least one-third of the depth of the chest (or by 5 cm) and then fully release the pressure while

Procedure – To perform basic life support on a child – *cont*

   maintaining contact with the sternum. If this is difficult, use the two-handed technique as you would for adults.
   - Repeat the compressions at a rate of 100–120/minute for 15 compressions and then give two ventilations.
   - Continue compressions and ventilations at a ratio of 15:2 unless you are on your own, in which case a ratio of 30:2 may be easier.
   - Continue until the child shows signs of life or you become exhausted.

3 Defibrillation

3.1 Learning objectives

By the end of this section you will be able to:
- describe the types of cardiopulmonary arrest
- recognise when it is appropriate to use a defibrillator
- explain the safety considerations when using a defibrillator.

3.2 Introduction

Heart rhythms associated with cardiac arrest are divided into shockable and non-shockable rhythms, depending on whether they should receive an electric current across the myocardium (heart muscle) to depolarise a sufficient amount of the heart muscle simultaneously and allow the normal heart pacemaker (the sinoatrial node) to resume control of the electrical conduction system. Delivering electricity to the heart in this way is known as defibrillation [Nolan, 2016].

In patients who have a shockable rhythm, the sooner they receive defibrillation, the greater the chance it will be successful and the patient will survive. However, it is equally important to ensure that defibrillation minimises the interruption of cardiopulmonary resuscitation (CPR). For each five-second delay in CPR prior to delivering a shock, the chance of the shock being successful is halved [Nolan, 2016].

3.3 Shockable rhythms

There are two shockable rhythms: ventricular fibrillation and pulseless ventricular tachycardia.

3.3.1 Ventricular fibrillation (VF)

VF is a rapid and disorganised ventricular rhythm and is never associated with a palpable pulse. On an electrocardiogram (ECG), you will not see any discernible P, QRS or T waves and complexes, and the rate of the undulations is typically between 150 and 500 [Garcia, 2004]. The height (amplitude) of the electrical activity you can see is often referred to as its coarseness (Figure 24.2). As a rule of thumb, if you find it difficult to decide whether the rhythm is VF or asystole (more on this shortly), you should not shock the patient [Soar, 2015].

3.3.2 Ventricular tachycardia

Ventricular tachycardia (VT) is known as a broad- or wide-complex tachycardia, because the QRS complexes are > 0.12 seconds in duration (typically 0.16–0.20 seconds). It usually originates from the ventricles, is monomorphic (has one shape), and has a regular rhythm at a rate of 100–300/minute (Figure 24.3) [Nolan, 2016; Garcia, 2004]. Unlike patients with VF, patients with VT may have a pulse and/or signs of life, so always check before defibrillating.

3.4 Non-shockable rhythms

As with shockable rhythms, there are two non-shockable rhythms: asystole and pulseless electrical activity. As the name implies, these are patients who will not benefit from defibrillation.

3.4.1 Asystole

Asystole is the term given to the absence of electrical activity from the heart. On an ECG, you will see a flat (isoelectric) or almost flat line (Figure 24.4) [Garcia, 2004]. A variant of asystole is an agonal rhythm, which is characterised by slow (rate of < 20/min), irregular and wide ventricular complexes, often varying in shape (morphology) [Nolan, 2016].

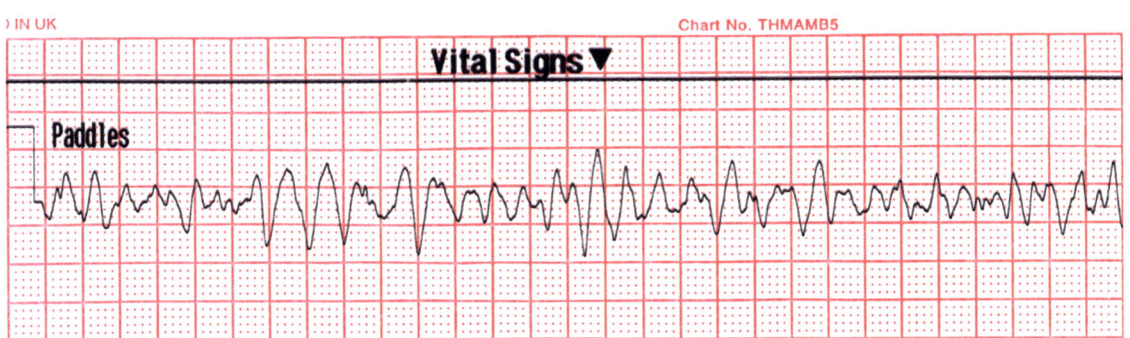

Figure 24.2 Ventricular fibrillation.

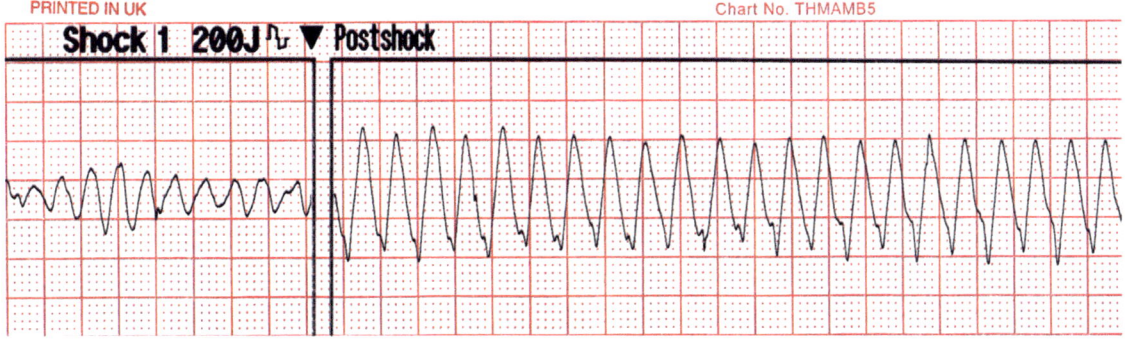

Figure 24.3 Ventricular tachycardia following a 200 J shock. The patient was in VF prior to the shock.

Chapter 24 – Cardiac Arrest

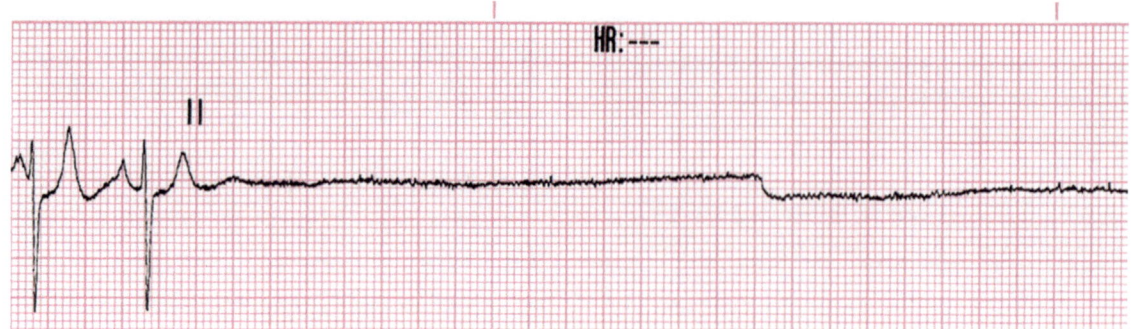

Figure 24.4 Asystole. Note the two complexes on the left-hand side of the ECG before the start of asystole. The baseline is not always completely straight in asystole.

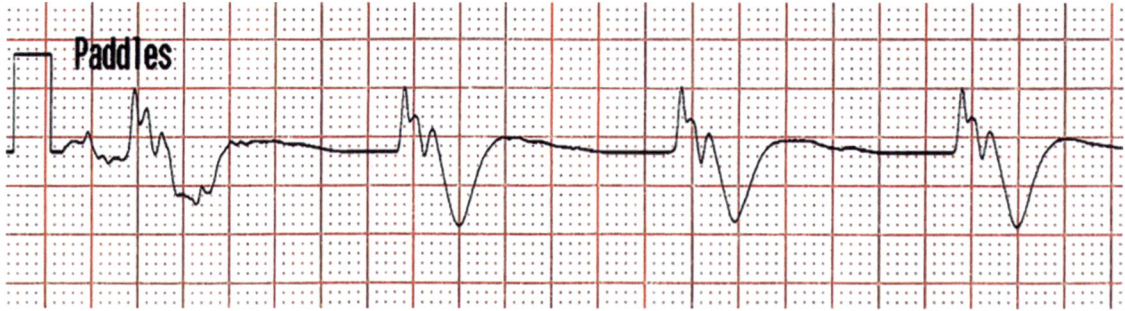

Figure 24.5 An example of an ECG showing pulseless electrical activity.

3.4.2 Pulseless electrical activity (PEA)

PEA is organised electrical activity in the absence of a palpable pulse (Figure 24.5). Typically, patients in PEA will have some mechanical myocardial activity, but it is not sufficiently strong to produce adequate cardiac output to lead to a detectable pulse or blood pressure [Nolan, 2016]. PEA is associated with a number of reversible causes that are a key component of advanced life support. As with VT, it is important to feel for a pulse and/or look for signs of life prior to determining the need for CPR.

3.5 Defibrillators

There are many brands and types of defibrillator on the market and it is important that you are familiar with the equipment you have in your workplace/ambulance. Broadly, they fall into two types: automated external defibrillators (AEDs) and manual defibrillators.

3.5.1 Automated external defibrillators (AEDs)

These 'shock boxes' are devices that provide voice and visual prompts to guide the public and healthcare professionals to defibrillate safely. AEDs are now widely available in public places such as shopping centres, sports centres, airports and railway stations [BHF, 2017]. Despite their name, some AEDs can be manually overridden by healthcare providers proficient in rhythm interpretation, but they are capable of recognising shockable and non-shockable rhythms [Nolan, 2016].

3.5.2 Manual defibrillators

The main advantage with manual defibrillation is the reduction in time for rhythm analysis. This minimises the interruption of chest compressions. In addition, manual defibrillators in the ambulance service are usually capable of other functions such as monitoring vital signs as well as being able to deliver synchronised shocks and external pacing (Figure 24.6).

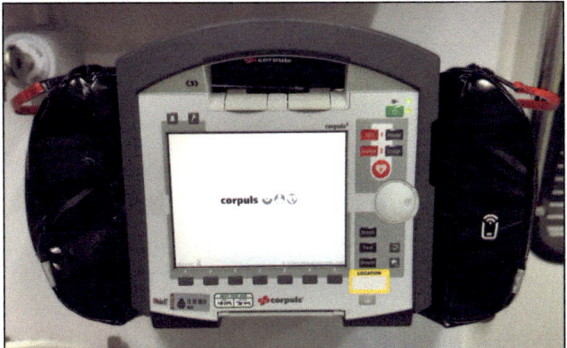

Figure 24.6 A Corpuls3 monitor/defibrillator commonly used by ambulance services.

3.5.3 Difficult environment and defibrillation

You will frequently encounter challenging environments that make resuscitation difficult. In terms of defibrillation, some of these can increase the risk of injury due to inadvertent electrocution. However, prompt defibrillation is life-saving and so it is important that you make a dynamic risk assessment and do not delay a shock unnecessarily.

Specific defibrillation scenarios include [Deakin, 2015]:
- **Wet surfaces:** This is safe as long as you are not in contact with the patient and the patient's skin (if wet) is dried to ensure good contact is made by the self-adhesive pads to the patient's chest.
- **Metal surfaces:** As before, this is safe as long as you are not in contact with the patient. Metal surfaces actually conduct any current that leaks from the pads through the metal and away from the crew and bystanders.
- **In-flight:** Defibrillation in aircraft and helicopters is safe, particularly if the patient is in contact with metal surfaces for the reason given above. Oxygen use in a confined cabin could potentially increase the risk of fire, although there are no reports of these occurring. Consider restricting oxygen use in aircraft cabins or confined spaces.

3.5.4 Safety

The only person who should receive a shock when a defibrillator is used is the patient. This can be achieved as long as members of the resuscitation team communicate well, so that everyone is well clear of the patient at the time of defibrillation.

Other ways of maximising safety include [Nolan, 2016; Deakin, 2015; Kerber, 2012]:
- Use self-adhesive pads rather than paddles.
- Do not defibrillate patients while they are in water or near an explosive or combustible environment.
- Ensure that the rescuers do not hold intravenous infusion equipment or the ambulance trolley during defibrillation.
- Wear gloves.
- Shave the patient's chest, if required, to obtain a good skin-to-electrode contact.
- Avoid placing the pads over jewellery, piercings, medication patches, wounds and tumours.
- Ensure that the pads are well away from pacemaker sites (8 cm in adults and 12 cm in children).
- Remove oxygen from the patient unless the ventilation bag is directly connected to an endotracheal tube or supraglottic airway device. It should be at least one metre away from the patient's chest.

3.5.5 Adult defibrillation

Pad placement

The standard placement for defibrillator pads is to place one just below the right clavicle, to the right of the sternum, and the other in the left mid-axillary line, about level with the V6 ECG electrode or female breast. This should ensure that it is clear of breast tissue [Soar, 2015].

Alternative positions include:
- **Anterior–posterior:** One pad is placed over the left precordium, and the other on the back, just under the left scapula (shoulder blade).
- **Posterolateral:** One pad is placed in the left mid-axillary line, level with the V6 ECG electrode or female breast, and the other over the right scapula.
- **Bi-axillary:** One pad is placed on either side of the lateral chest wall.

Chapter 24 – Cardiac Arrest

3.5.6 AED procedure (adults)

Procedure – To defibrillate using an AED
Take the following steps to defibrillate using an AED [Perkins, 2015]:

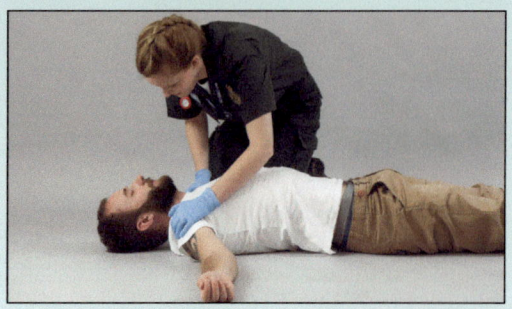

1. Check for danger and ensure that you, your colleagues, the patient and bystanders are safe. Assess the patient's responsiveness.

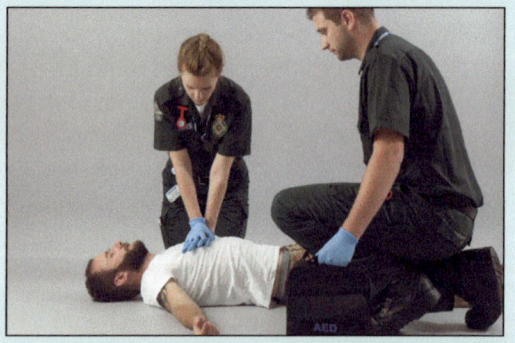

2. If the patient is unresponsive and not breathing normally, start CPR at a ratio of 30 compressions to two ventilations (30:2).

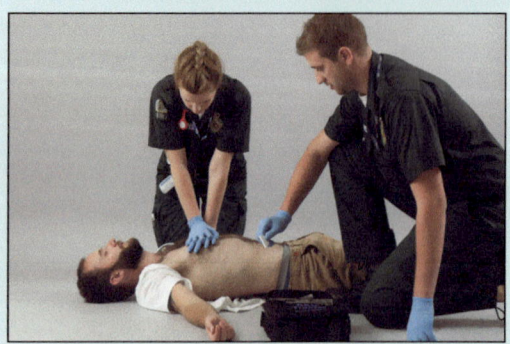

3. Bare the patient's chest and ensure that the pad sites are free from jewellery, piercings, medication patches, pacemakers, wounds and tumours. Shave the chest if required.

Procedure – To defibrillate using an AED – *cont*

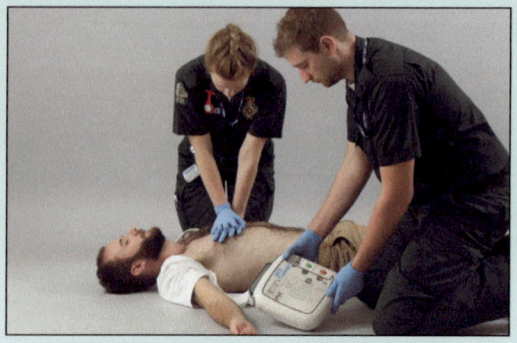

4. Switch on the AED and attach the pads to the patient, ensuring they make a good contact.

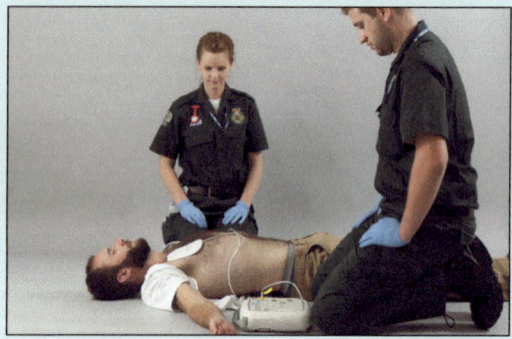

5. Follow visual/voice prompts, ensuring that no one touches the patient while the AED is analysing the rhythm.

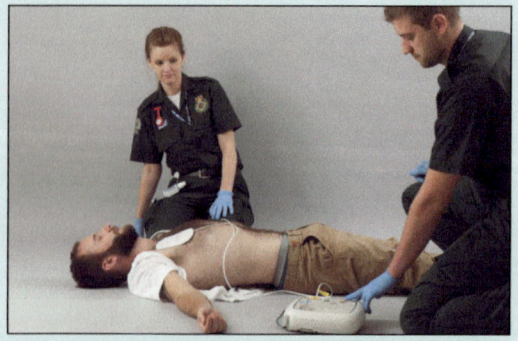

6. Shock?
   - If a shock is advised, make sure everyone is clear of the patient and push the shock button.
   - If a shock is not advised, skip to step 7.

Defibrillation

Procedure – To defibrillate using an AED – *cont*

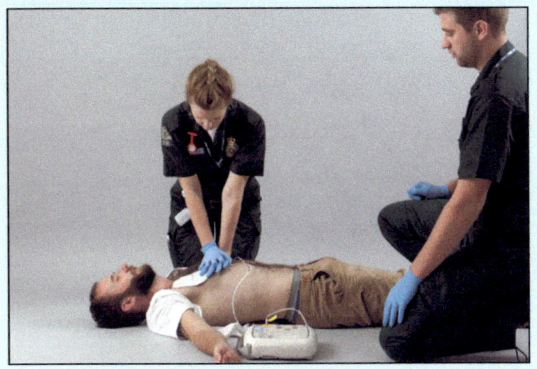

7. Immediately restart CPR at a ratio of 30:2. Follow visual/voice prompts.

3.5.7 Manual defibrillation procedure (adults)

Procedure – To manually defibrillate a patient
Take the following steps to manually defibrillate a patient [Soar, 2015]:

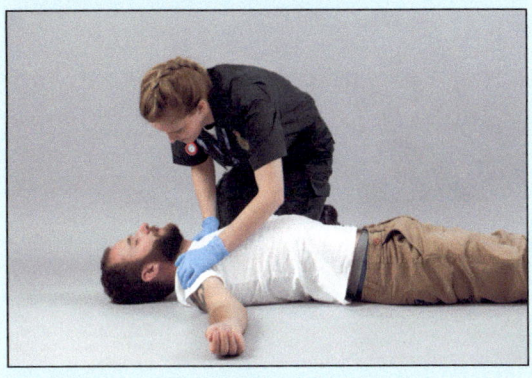

1. Ensure that the scene is safe for you, your colleagues, the patient and other bystanders. Assess the patient's responsiveness.

Procedure – To manually defibrillate a patient – *cont*

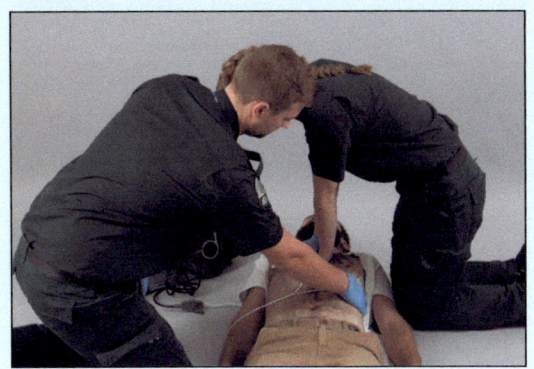

2. Confirm cardiac arrest and start chest compressions. Bare the patient's chest and ensure that the pad sites are free from jewellery, piercings, medication patches, pacemakers, wounds and tumours. Do not interrupt chest compressions while applying the self-adhesive defibrillator pads.

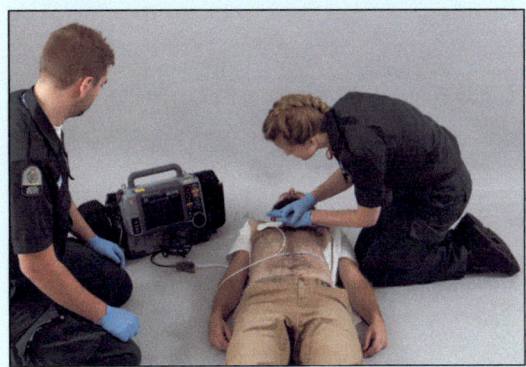

3. Plan actions before pausing chest compressions for rhythm analysis and make sure all team members know their role and the sequence of actions. Stop chest compressions for up to five seconds to analyse the rhythm. If not VF or asystole, check for a pulse and/or signs of life.

Chapter 24 – *Cardiac Arrest*

Procedure – To manually defibrillate a patient – *cont*

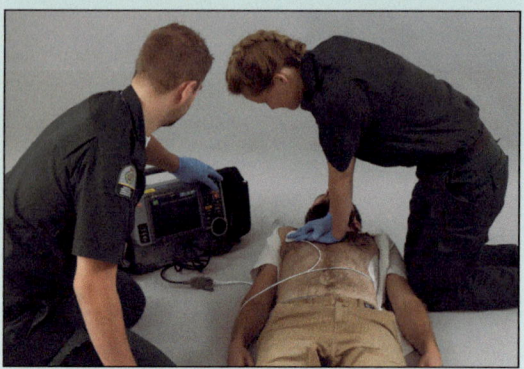

4. If VF/pulseless VT, follow instructions below. If PEA/asystole, skip to step 5.
   - Immediately resume chest compressions.
   - The designated person should charge the defibrillator according to the manufacturer's recommendation.
   - While the defibrillator is charging, everyone except for the chest compressor should stand back and move oxygen away.
   - Once the defibrillator is charged, the person defibrillating should tell the chest compressor to 'stand clear' and deliver the shock as soon as they have moved.

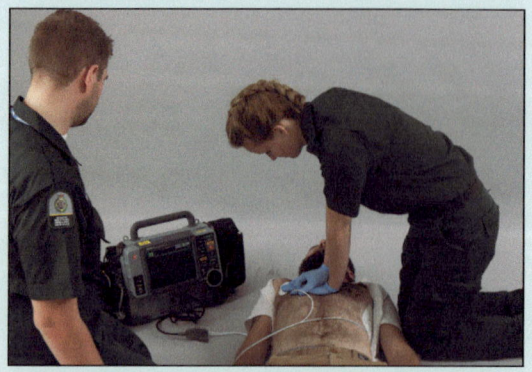

5. Restart CPR immediately at a ratio of 30:2 without checking for a pulse or assessing the rhythm.

Procedure – To manually defibrillate a patient – *cont*

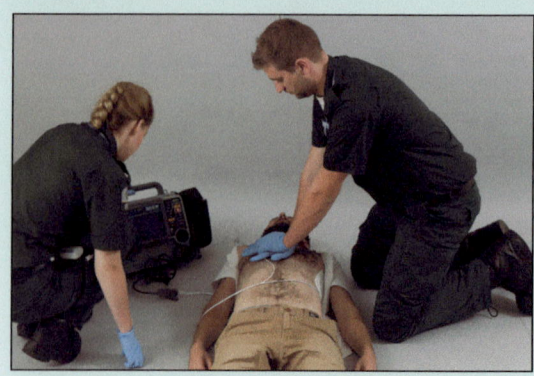

6. Continue for a further two minutes and ensure that roles are allocated as the chest compressor should be changed every two minutes. Once two minutes has elapsed, chest compressions should be briefly paused and the rhythm analysed.

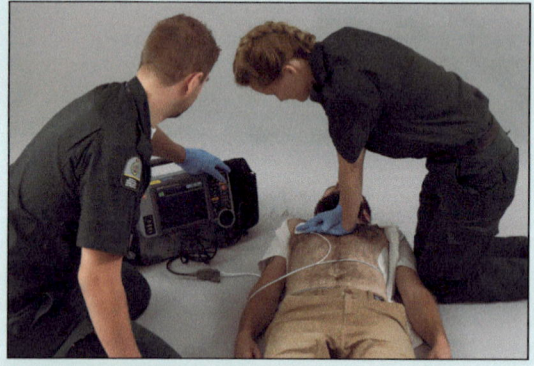

7. Repeat steps 4–6.

3.5.8 Paediatric defibrillation

Pad placement

The standard placement for defibrillator pads is to place one just below the right clavicle, to the right of the sternum, and the other in the left mid-axillary line. Adult defibrillator pads can be used on children who are over 25 kg (about eight years of age), but they must not touch each other. Use paediatric pads for children under 25 kg (under eight years of age), if available, but adult pads can be used in smaller children if there is no alternative [Maconochie, 2015].

If a sufficient gap between the defibrillator pads is not possible due to patient size, use the anterior–posterior pad placement described above.

3.5.9 AED procedure (children)

Procedure – To defibrillate a child with an AED

Take the following steps to defibrillate a child with an AED [Maconochie, 2015]:

1. Check for danger and ensure that you, your colleagues, the patient and bystanders are safe.
2. Start basic life support (BLS). If you are on your own, perform one minute of CPR before attaching the AED.
3. Bare the patient's chest and ensure that the pad sites are free from jewellery, piercings, medication patches, pacemakers, wounds and tumours.
4. Switch on the AED and attach the pads to the patient, ensuring they make a good contact. Use paediatric pads on patients under 25 kg if available.
5. Follow visual/voice prompts, ensuring that no-one touches the patient while the AED is analysing the rhythm.
6. Shock?
   - If a shock is advised, make sure everyone is clear of the patient and push the shock button.
   - If a shock is not advised, skip to step 7.
7. Immediately resume CPR at a ratio of 15:2 (30:2 if you are on your own). Follow visual/voice prompts

3.5.10 Manual defibrillation procedure (children)

Procedure – To manually defibrillate a child

Take the following steps to manually defibrillate a child [Maconochie, 2015]:

1. Ensure that the scene is safe for you, your colleague, the patient and other bystanders.
2. Start basic life support (BLS).
3. Bare the patient's chest and ensure that the pad sites are free from jewellery, piercings, medication patches, pacemakers, wounds and tumours.
4. Plan actions before pausing chest compressions for rhythm analysis and make sure all team members know their role and the sequence of actions.
5. Stop chest compressions for up to five seconds to analyse the rhythm. If not VF or asystole, check for a pulse and/or signs of life.
6. If VF/pulseless VT follow instructions below. If PEA/asystole, skip to step 7.
   - Immediately resume chest compressions.
   - The designated person should charge the defibrillator by selecting the appropriate energy (4 J/kg).
   - While the defibrillator is charging, everyone except for the chest compressor should stand back and move oxygen away.
   - Once the defibrillator is charged, the person defibrillating should tell the chest compressor to 'stand clear' and deliver the shock as soon as they have done so.
7. Restart CPR immediately at a ratio of 15:2 without checking for a pulse or assessing the rhythm.
8. Continue for a further two minutes and ensure that roles are allocated as the chest compressor should be changed every two minutes.
9. Once the two minutes are up, chest compressions should be briefly paused and the rhythm analysed.
10. Repeat steps 6–9.

4 Cardiac arrest in special circumstances

4.1 Learning objectives

By the end of this section you will be able to:
- explain the considerations for a pregnant patient in cardiac arrest
- explain the considerations for a hypothermic patient in cardiac arrest
- explain the management of a drowned patient in cardiac arrest
- explain the management of a patient who has suffered a traumatic cardiac arrest.

4.2 Introduction

In this chapter, you have been introduced to the principles and techniques of resuscitation of a patient in cardiac arrest. However, in some circumstances, the techniques need to be modified and/or alternative techniques used.

4.3 Cardiac arrest in pregnancy

The general procedure for resuscitating a pregnant patient is the same as for any other patient. However, for patients who are more than 20 weeks pregnant, there is a risk that their fetus-filled uterus can press down on the inferior vena cava and aorta, restricting venous return and leading to a reduction in cardiac output and uterine perfusion [Nolan, 2016].

To prevent this from occurring, the pregnant patient must not lie supine. In the conscious patient, the lateral position is often used, but this is not practicable in a cardiac arrest when chest compressions need to be provided. Instead, the uterus should be manually displaced to the maternal left side [Mansfield, 2018].

The CPR hand position for patients in advanced pregnancy (over 28 weeks) may need to be 2–3 cm higher on the sternum. In addition, you may not be able to place the defibrillator pads in their usual position, due to their large breasts. In these cases, use alternative pad placement, such as an anterior–posterior, or bi-axillary, placement [Deakin, 2015].

During the latter stages of pregnancy, the patient is more likely to regurgitate their stomach contents and aspirate them into the lungs, particularly with over-enthusiastic bag-valve-mask ventilation. Consider using a supraglottic airway device early on in the resuscitation and keep suction close by. Intubation is ideal, if you have a clinician capable, but anatomical changes in pregnancy can make this difficult [Mansfield, 2018].

If there is no response to CPR within five minutes, the patient should be rapidly transferred to the nearest suitable receiving hospital. An alert call should be made, making it clear that this is a maternal cardiac arrest and requesting an obstetrician in the emergency department. When initial resuscitation attempts fail, the best chance for successful resuscitation is an emergency caesarean section [JRCALC, 2019]. Note that in some areas, there may be pre-hospital critical care teams that can perform a resuscitative hysterotomy. Follow local guidance.

4.4 Cardiac arrest in hypothermic patients

In cases of moderate and severe hypothermia, signs of life can be difficult to identify. You should therefore check for breathing and a pulse for up to one minute. If the patient has a core body temperature of less than 30°C, some modification of the advanced life support algorithm is required. In these cases, a maximum of three shocks only should be administered if the patient is in VF or pulseless VT. No intravenous drugs (such as adrenaline and amiodarone) should be given until the patient has been warmed up. Once the core body temperature is over 30°C, but less than 35°C, defibrillation can continue as usual. When administering intravenous drugs, the time interval between each administration should be doubled (i.e. every 6–10 minutes). Once the patient's core body temperature is over 35°C, they can be resuscitated as normal. Post-resuscitation care is the same as for other cardiac arrest scenarios, including the use of therapeutic temperature management, if appropriate [Truhlář, 2015].

Remember that unless there is a clear indication that the cardiac arrest has been caused by a lethal injury or fatal illness, patients should be resuscitated based on the principle that 'no one is dead until warm and dead' [Truhlář, 2015].

4.5 Cardiac arrest in drowned patients

Resuscitation is difficult while in the water and should consist of ventilations only. Chest compressions are futile in deep water, so wait until the patient is on a firm surface, such as the shore or the deck of a boat [Szpilman, 2004]. The incidence of spinal injuries is very low (around 0.5%) and immobilising the spine delays effective resuscitation, so only immobilise the spine when there is a clear mechanism of injury that could cause spinal injury (such as diving into shallow water or water skiing) [Watson, 2001; Truhlář, 2015].

Get the victim out of the water as soon as possible and place them supine (on their back), with head and torso at the same level, and check for breathing. If your patient is not breathing, or is breathing abnormally, administer five rescue breaths via a bag-valve-mask connected to high-flow oxygen. Note that this is different from the usual ABC approach that the current resuscitation guidelines advocate for adults, but reflects that correction of hypoxia is the most important aspect in the management of the drowned patient. It can be difficult to differentiate post-arrest gasping from initial respiratory efforts of the drowning patient, so if you are unsure, administer ventilations and start CPR. Pulse checks are unreliable, so try to utilise other diagnostic tests if available, such as electrocardiogram (ECG) and end-tidal carbon dioxide ($EtCO_2$) monitoring. If in doubt, commence chest compressions with ventilations at a ratio of 30:2. Compression-only CPR is not advocated [Truhlář, 2015].

Regurgitation of stomach contents and inhaled water is common, so intubating early is preferable, depending on the skill level of the clinicians on scene. Supraglottic airway devices are not so useful in drowning patients, as pulmonary compliance is likely to be low, requiring the use of high inflation pressures [Truhlář, 2015]. Advanced life support follows the normal algorithm, unless the patient is hypothermic, in which case follow the guidance for hypothermic patients in cardiac arrest.

Large amounts of foam can be generated by the mixing of moving air with water and surfactant from the lungs. If this occurs, do not waste time trying to suction it, continue to provide ventilations until an appropriate clinician can intubate the patient.

Resuscitation efforts should not be stopped unless it is clear that it would be futile to continue (e.g. due to the patient sustaining massive traumatic injuries). There are no completely accurate prognostic indicators in drowning, although duration of submersion is correlated with risk of death or severe neurological impairment [Szpilman, 2012]. In water above 6°C, survival after submersion for more than 30 minutes is unlikely. At 6°C or below, survival time can be extended up to 90 minutes, although this is more likely to apply to children immersed in ice-cold water [Tipton, 2011]. As with hypothermia, the general rule is that your patient is not dead until they are warm and dead [Truhlář, 2015].

4.6 Traumatic cardiac arrest

Surviving a traumatic out-of-hospital cardiac arrest is uncommon. However, survival rates of 6–7% have been reported, so it is important to manage these patients effectively. The key to success is to identify and treat the reversible causes of traumatic cardiac arrest (TCA) [Deakin, 2015]:

- hypovolaemia
- hypoxia
- tension pneumothorax
- tamponade (cardiac).

The first three reversible causes can be addressed by most ambulance crews, and have been referred to by the acronym HOT (hypovolaemia, oxygenation and tension pneumothorax), which you might hear being used during teaching or incidents involving TCA [Lockey, 2013].

4.6.1 Management

All trauma patients in cardiac arrest should be resuscitated unless there is a clear indication that attempts would be futile (e.g. injuries incompatible with life). Patients who have suffered blunt trauma are likely to be resuscitated on scene, but those with penetrating injury must be rapidly transferred to an emergency department [JRCALC, 2019], unless there is a suitable pre-hospital critical care team available. Follow local guidance.

Follow the principles of standard trauma patient management [JRCALC, 2019]:
- **<C>:** Control catastrophic haemorrhage.
- **A:** Ensure the airway is open and clear, and insert an advanced airway as soon as possible.
- **B:** Search for and manage sucking chest wounds. A tension pneumothorax can be hard to detect, so it is likely that both sides will be decompressed by a suitably qualified clinician. Use high-flow oxygen during the resuscitation attempt.
- **C:** Hypovolaemia needs to be addressed with fluid (preferably blood). Senior clinicians on scene are likely to request repeated boluses of 0.9% saline (or blood, if available) and administer tranexamic acid.

5 Post-resuscitation care

5.1 *Learning objectives*

By the end of this section you will be able to:
- state clinical signs that indicate an ROSC
- explain the management of the post-resuscitation patient.

5.2 *Introduction*

A return of spontaneous circulation (ROSC) in a patient who you have resuscitated is a great feeling, but it is just the first step on the path to complete recovery from a cardiac arrest. A complex pathophysiological process occurs as a result of whole body ischaemia during a cardiac arrest and subsequent reperfusion when ROSC is achieved. This is known as post-cardiac arrest syndrome [Deakin, 2015].

During rhythm/pulse checks, if an organised rhythm is seen on the ECG that is compatible with a cardiac output, you should look for evidence of ROSC [Soar, 2015]:
- signs of life including purposeful movement, normal breathing or coughing
- presence of a central pulse
- a significant increase in end-tidal carbon dioxide ($EtCO_2$).

5.3 *Management*

The following steps should be taken once ROSC is achieved [Deakin, 2015; JRCALC, 2019]:
- Reassess the patient's airway and breathing:
  - Provide ventilation, if required, at a rate of 10–12 breaths/minute.
  - Oxygen therapy should be titrated to maintain an SpO_2 of 94–98%.
  - Use capnography if available and adjust ventilation to maintain normocapnia (4.6–6.0 kPa). Switch from manual to mechanical ventilation to ensure appropriate rate and tidal volume is administered.
- Reassess the patient's circulation:
  - Maintain continuous ECG monitoring and record a 12-lead ECG.
  - A senior clinician will obtain vascular access, if not already achieved.
  - Perform frequent pulse and blood pressure checks. Aim for a systolic blood pressure of 90–100mmHg. A 250 ml IV/IO bolus may be required, but follow the guidance of the senior clinician on scene.
- Check blood glucose. The target range is over 4 mmol/l but no more than 10 mmol/l.
- Aim for a core temperature no higher than 36.0°C. Do this by passively cooling the patient (i.e. don't cover the patient in blankets or heat the interior of the ambulance).
- Convulsions can occur following ROSC and will need to be managed promptly with benzodiazepine drugs such as diazepam.
- Transport:
  - Patients should be kept as flat as possible, feet first when descending stairs and placed in a 30° head-up position once in the ambulance.

- Patients with evidence of ST-segment elevation myocardial infarction (STEMI) should be transported to an appropriate facility as per local guidance.
- An alert call should be made to the receiving facility.

6 Cardiac arrest decisions

6.1 Learning objectives

By the end of this section you will be able to:
- explain when a resuscitation attempt may be stopped or not commenced
- describe the procedure for the recognition of life extinct (ROLE)
- state the management of a sudden unexpected death in an infant, child or adolescent.

6.2 When to start and stop resuscitation

Whenever there is a chance that a patient may survive from a cardiac arrest, resuscitation should be attempted unless a patient has stated, via an 'advance decision to refuse treatment' (ADRT) or Recommended Summary Plan for Emergency Care and Treatment (ReSPECT), that this should not occur, or there is a valid 'do not attempt cardiopulmonary resuscitation' (DNACPR) [JRCALC, 2019].

However, there are certain patients who have an injury or presenting condition that is unequivocally associated with death, irrespective of age [JRCALC, 2019]:
- Massive cranial and cerebral destruction.
- Hemicorporectomy (complete amputation of the body below the waist) or similar massive injury.
- Decomposition/putrefaction: Tissue damage suggests that the patient has been dead for hours, days or even longer.
- Incineration: Full thickness burns and charring covering more than 95% of the total body surface area (TBSA).
- Hypostasis: The pooling of blood in the dependent part of the body after death.
- Rigor mortis: Stiffness of the body and limbs following death.
- Fetal maceration.

6.2.1 Conditions when resuscitation can be discontinued

Even if resuscitation has been commenced, this should be stopped if any of the following are present [JRCALC, 2019]:
- A DNACPR.
- An ADRT clearly states that the patient is not to be resuscitated.
- The patient is in the final stages of a terminal illness and the senior clinician determines that CPR would not be successful even if no formal DNACPR decision has been documented.
- The patient has been submerged for more than 60 minutes (or more than 90 minutes if submerged in icy water).
- There is no realistic chance that CPR would be successful because all of the following are present:
  - At least 15 minutes have elapsed since the onset of cardiac arrest.
  - No bystander CPR was provided prior to the arrival of the ambulance service.
  - There are no exclusion factors such as drowning, hypothermia, poisoning or pregnancy.
  - The ECG shows asystole for more than 30 seconds.

6.3 End of life decisions

6.3.1 Advance care planning

In terminal conditions, death can often be anticipated, which provides patients with the opportunity to consider their wishes and preferences about future care, particularly as they are likely to be unable to do so when close to death. Unfortunately, only 5% of people put these wishes and preferences in writing by means of an advance care plan (ACP, sometimes also called a preferred priorities for care document, or treatment escalation plan) [NatCen, 2013]. The contents of an ACP are not legally binding, but any best-interests decision about patients must take into account the patient's wishes and preferences [Watson, 2009]. One example of an ACP is the Recommended Summary Plan for Emergency Care and Treatment (ReSPECT). This is a personalised plan specifying the person's recommended clinical care during an emergency when they do not have capacity to make decisions. This will include cardiac arrest and death (and takes the place of a DNACPR in this instance), but is not limited to only those events. Ask about the presence of such a plan as part of your patient assessment.

6.3.2 Advance decisions to refuse treatment (ADRTs)

ADRTs (also known as living wills) are documents that outline specific aspects of care that the patient does not wish to receive. This is then typically referred to when the patient is unable to make these wishes clear. Examples of the interventions that a patient may refuse include being ventilated, being tube-fed, receiving antibiotics and being admitted to hospital unless they are suffering from a complaint with a treatable cause.

Unlike an ACP, this is a legal document and, as long as the phrase 'even if life is at risk' is present, and the document is signed, dated and witnessed, the contents must be respected by healthcare staff. Note that treatment can only be declined and not requested, and the ADRT only comes into effect once the patient loses mental capacity [NEoLCP, 2013].

6.3.3 Do not attempt cardiopulmonary resuscitation (DNACPR) decisions

DNACPR decisions are made by a senior clinician, usually with involvement from the patient's clinical team. This will normally be a consultant, GP or suitably experienced nurse [BMA, 2007]. There are four broad situations when a DNACPR decision will be made [Dimond, 2015]:
- A mentally competent patient refuses resuscitative treatment.
- A valid advanced directive clearly states that the patient does not want CPR.
- CPR is unlikely to be successful.
- Successful CPR is possible, but the length and quality of life following resuscitation is not in the patient's best interests.

Ideally, this is written and agreed ahead of time and documentary evidence of the decision will be presented to you before you commence resuscitation. However, even if there is no formal DNACPR in place, the senior clinician can still elect not to start or continue resuscitation if the patient is in the final stages of a terminal illness and they think that CPR would not be successful. Ultimately, if you are unsure about the validity of previously made decisions, then commencing resuscitation is defendable if you believe it is in the patient's best interests. [JRCALC, 2019].

6.4 Recognition of life extinct (ROLE)

6.4.1 Action to be taken after verification of death

The actions to take following the confirmation of death will be determined by local guidelines and you should ensure that you are familiar with them. The UK Ambulance Services Clinical Practice Guidelines provide a suggested guideline (Figure 24.7) [JRCALC, 2019].

6.4.2 Preserving the scene

In the event of a death being suspicious, you must make efforts to preserve the scene, which may become part of a police investigation. A key issue of forensic scene management is Locard's Exchange Principle. This principle suggests that everyone who comes into a scene brings some trace evidence with them and takes some other evidence away; this can include DNA, skin cells, fingerprints or clothing fibres, etc. After an incident, the police may forensically search a scene for this trace evidence to help to piece together the events leading up to an accident or incident.

When working in a potential crime scene, disturb the scene as little as possible. If you need to move things, try to remember where they were before

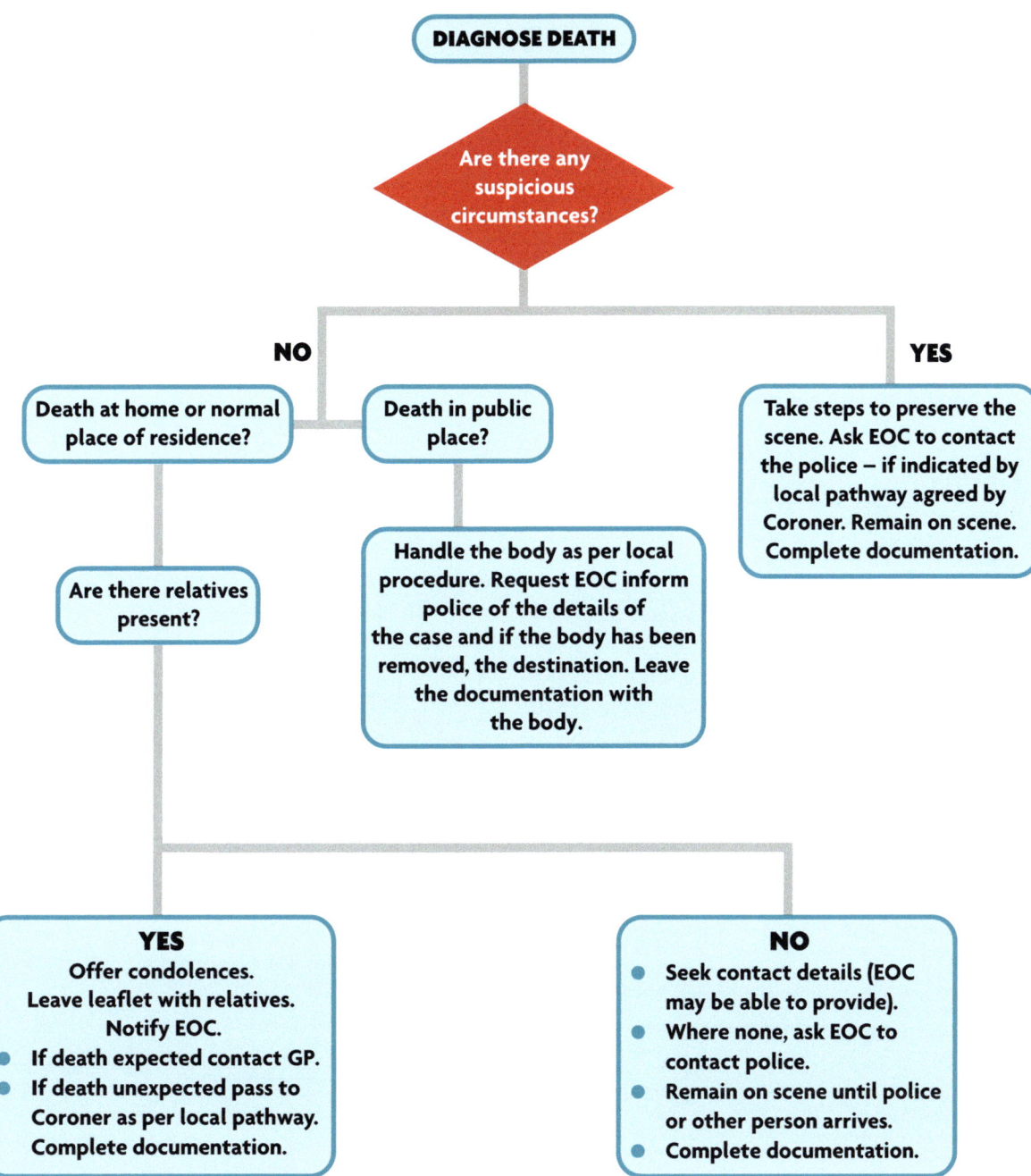

Figure 24.7 Action to be taken after verification of death.

you move them so you can relay this information to the police afterwards.

When possible, withdraw from the scene, leaving everything where it is at the point you can leave. If the patient is deceased, you should let the patient remain where they are and leave any clinical equipment you have been using where it is. You might need to cover the patient if the police are not on scene and it is raining. If this is necessary, use a foil blanket rather than a cloth blanket. Cloth blankets can contain microfibres from other environments or other patients that have not removed by the cleaning process.

6.5 Sudden unexpected death in infants, children and adolescents

Sudden unexpected death in infancy, children and adolescents (SUDICA) is a collective term covering all deaths in patients under 18 years of age. You may be familiar with the terms 'sudden unexpected death in infants' (SUDI), which incorporates 'sudden infant death syndrome' (SIDS) or cot death [Krous, 2010].

This is likely to be one of the most difficult experiences for you as an AAP, particularly as you are likely to be the first on scene. It is also going to be a devastating experience for parents. Although the vast majority of SUDICA will ultimately be attributable to natural causes, it is important that you are aware of the potential of abuse to be a cause. As such, guidelines have been developed to ensure that specialist paediatric and police involvement occurs in every case.

You should follow your local ambulance service guidelines for these cases, but there are a number of principles that are likely to apply to all services [RCP, 2016; DfE, 2015; JRCALC, 2019]:

- All infants and children should have resuscitation attempted unless there is a presenting condition unequivocally associated with death (such as hypostasis and rigor mortis).
- All infants and children should be transported to the local emergency department (ED), not a mortuary, unless the police decide that forensic evidence is required first.
- Support the family: Remember that the vast majority of these cases are due to natural causes and not abuse. Think before you speak and do not criticise the parents/carers.
- Use the infant's/child's name whenever you are referring to them.
- Avoid placing an infant/child in a body bag.
- Parents will need to accompany the infant or child to hospital. If appropriate, offer to take them in the ambulance or ensure that they have alternative means of transport and know where to go. The police may be able to assist with this.
- Don't underestimate the effect that an incident like this can have on you. Follow your ambulance service post-critical incident debriefing guidelines and seek support from your colleagues as well as formal counselling, if required.

Chapter

25 End of Life Care

1 End of life care

1.1 Learning objectives

By the end of this section you will be able to:
- define palliative care and end of life care
- describe the national guidelines for end of life care
- describe the importance of advance care planning
- describe the religious and spiritual influences on end of life care
- describe how to support relatives and carers.

1.2 Introduction

Palliative and end of life care (EoLC) are emotive topics and something you will frequently come across in your role as an associate ambulance practitioner. In recent years, the provision of palliative care has changed significantly and has a high profile in the media (not always positively) and amongst healthcare staff.

In the UK, when surveyed, the majority of people have expressed the wish that when the time comes, they would prefer to die at home [NatCen, 2013]. Despite this, over 50% of deaths occur in hospitals [DoH, 2015b].

You may previously have heard of the concept of providing a 'good death'. Exactly what a good death entails is not clear, but most would agree that, so far as possible, it includes the management of symptoms (such as pain), compassionate and competent care, the addressing of spiritual and psychological needs and, where possible, the involvement of family [Marie Curie, 2015].

EoLC is improving, but there is still more that can be done to ensure everyone who is approaching the end of their life has the death they would want.

1.3 Palliative care and end of life care

Palliative care is provided to people living with a terminal illness for which there is no cure. It can also be given to people with complex, often progressive, illnesses who need symptom control [Marie Curie, 2018a].

Palliative care is aimed at improving a person's quality of life. It does this by managing pain and other distressing symptoms, but also examines any psychological, social or spiritual needs. The family and friends of the person with the terminal illness are also supported. Palliative care does not just occur at the end of someone's life, it can begin a long time before in association with other therapies a patient may be receiving. People receiving palliative care can live for several years.

EoLC is an important part of palliative care. EoLC is for people thought to be in the last year of their life, though this can be difficult to identify; in some cases, EoLC may only be required in the last weeks or days of life. The aim of EoLC is to help people live as well as possible and to die with dignity whilst providing good symptom control [Marie Curie, 2018a].

1.4 Care of dying adults in the last days of life

The National Institute for Health and Care Excellence has published detailed guidelines on providing care for adults in the last days of life, normally thought to be the last 2–3 days [NICE, 2015c]. The guidelines are designed to improve care for end of life patients and make sure that they, and the people important to them, are included in decision-making related to their care, as well as ensuring that they are kept comfortable and maintain their dignity. There are a number of key points to these guidelines, which are briefly outlined below.

Chapter 25 – End of Life Care

1.4.1 Recognising when a person may be in the last days of life

It is not always easy to determine when a person is entering the last days of life and it can be hard for health professionals to determine this. Often the person's condition will rapidly deteriorate or even improve in their final days and hours. If it is thought that the person is in the final days/hours of life, this should be recognised so that plans can be put in place to ensure they receive the correct EoLC. As an ambulance clinician, you may be the first to recognise that a person is in the final days/hours of their life and you should communicate this with those responsible for their overall care. Other factors you should consider are:

- Does the person have unmet physiological, psychological, social and spiritual needs?
- Be aware that improvement in signs and symptoms could indicate the person is stabilising or recovering.
- Investigations and treatments should be limited to those that make a difference to care in the last few days of life.
- Seek advice from colleagues experienced in end of life care on what should happen next.

1.4.2 Communication

A person in the final stages of life should be included in the decision-making related to their care wherever possible. This should also include the relatives and others close to the patient that they wish to be involved. It is also important that all of those responsible for caring for the patient communicate together effectively to establish the person's wishes and see that they are enacted, so far as is possible.

You should not withhold information from the person if they wish to know it. Someone in their wider care team should discuss the prognosis with the person as well as the wider treatment options available. Sometimes, however, this may need to be performed by an ambulance crew, if no other professionals with a better knowledge of the patient are available.

1.4.3 Shared decision-making

Wherever possible, the person or their appointed delegate should be actively engaged in the decision-making related to their care. As part of this, you should consider the patient's capacity to make decisions and any known pre-existing wishes. Hopefully, there will be a nominated lead healthcare professional who is responsible for the overall care of the patient, and who you can contact for decision-making support. If this is not possible, then it may be necessary for the senior clinician at the scene to lead on the decision-making process, taking into account all available facts and using other sources of decision-making support where possible.

1.4.4 Maintaining hydration

If the person wishes to, and is able to do so safely, they should be offered hydration in the final days of life. In the role of the ambulance service, this may include offering small drinks or wet sponges to suck on.

Giving fluids does have risks associated with it, such as aspiration, so you should not offer fluids unless it is known to be safe for the patient to take them. If you are unsure, you should seek advice.

Fluids must not be withheld without good reason and if it is thought that a patient is unable to safely take fluid orally then other options may be available. This will be for the person's lead clinician or clinic team to decide. A lack of hydration can cause distressing symptoms and has been previously identified as an area of poor care for the EoLC patient.

1.4.5 Pharmacological interventions

Although rarely the answer in isolation, there are a number of pharmacological interventions that should be considered if required for the end of life care patient. These include medications to manage:

- pain
- breathlessness
- nausea and vomiting
- anxiety, delirium and agitation
- respiratory secretions.

Normally, these medications will be administered by the GP, end of life care team or a specialist paramedic.

End of life care

1.4.6 Anticipatory prescribing

In addition to giving medications, it is likely that the person may be prescribed some medication in anticipation of events, often in packs known as 'just in case' boxes. These include some of the medications to treat the symptoms listed above and that it is thought the patient might need at some future point.

Paramedics should be familiar with a number of these medications and can administer them as they have already been prescribed for the patient. It is likely, however, that they will seek advice from someone with more experience in end of life care before they do administer the medications. They will also ensure that the person's records have been accurately updated if any such medications do need to be administered.

1.5 Religious and spiritual influences on end of life care

Meeting the spiritual needs of people approaching the end of life is a key part of their overall holistic care [NICE, 2015c]. Patients should feel as though their spiritual needs are met at the end of life, but this has been one area identified as requiring significant development [DoH, 2008].

Every patient is likely to have different spiritual needs and the way in which these will be met will be as unique as the need itself [Cancer Research UK, 2016a].

As a healthcare professional, you should be prepared to discuss the spiritual needs of your patients as part of their overall care. Some people may want a spiritual leader to visit them, which you should arrange if possible; others may be content just to discuss their beliefs and anxieties. Give patients space to have these discussions. You may not be able to answer their concerns, but sometimes just listening can help [Marie Curie, 2017].

Consider what other sources of help might be available, including a chaplaincy service, which may be available from the local hospital, hospice or palliative care team.

1.6 Advance care planning

Advance care planning is the process of making decisions relating to an individual's care for when they become too ill to communicate their wishes or make reasoned decisions anymore [Cancer Research UK, 2016b; NHS England, 2018d; Gold Standards Framework, 2018]. It can also refer to whether a person would want to be resuscitated and how they would want their body to be handled after death.

Advance care plans (ACPs) allow for an individual to be in control of their own death and can be a great source of relief to patients who are otherwise not in control of their illness. Advance care plans allow a patient to state general principles of how they wish to be treated, what treatments they do not want to receive, and to identify who will speak for them when they are not able to do so themselves.

Advance care plans come in many forms, including:
- **Living will/advance statement of preferences:** A living will or advance statement sets out what a person wants to happen when they become too unwell to make decisions for themselves. It tends to include generic statements such as 'I would prefer to die at home in my own bed'. It can also include preferences about religious care and personal treatment. It is not legally binding, but can be a good guide to help health and social care professionals in their decision-making. If you are faced with an end of life patient who has made an advance statement, you should respect their wishes and do all you can to safely facilitate them.
- **Advance decision to refuse treatment (ADRT):** ADRTs allow a patient to state what they would not want to happen when they are no longer able to make their own decisions; they may include specific treatments, such as resuscitation. More information about ADRTs is available in Chapter 4, 'Legal, Ethical and Professional Issues'.

Other forms of advanced care planning may include a ReSPECT document, a treatment escalation plan (TEP), or a Do Not Attempt Resuscitation (DNAR) order. The patient may also have appointed a lasting power of attorney to speak for them and to make medical decisions on their behalf. See section 3.4, 'Mental capacity' of Chapter 4, 'Legal, Ethical and Professional Issues', for further details on this role.

1.7 Disclosures of patient wishes

While caring for an EoLC patient, they may express to you how they wish to be treated. These wishes should be respected, documented on your clinical records and handed over to the next level of care. If key decisions, such as whether the patient wishes to be resuscitated, are not clear, you should consider asking the patient/family/carers if this has been discussed and what the outcome was. This is particularly true if you think that death is imminent.

Any decisions communicated to you should be recorded, and where they relate to the refusal of life-saving treatment they must be documented, signed by the patient or another person in the presence of the patient, and the decision must be witnessed [DCA, 2014].

Remember that all such decisions are only binding if they are valid. For a reminder on what makes a decision valid, refer to Chapter 4, 'Legal, Ethical and Professional Issues'.

1.8 Hospices

The aim of hospice care is to improve the quality of life and well-being for palliative care patients [HospiceUK, 2018]. Hospices bring together a range of expertise in managing the common symptoms associated with incurable illnesses. These services include medical and nursing care for incurable conditions as well as pain and other symptom management. Other services may include:
- physiotherapy
- occupational therapy
- bereavement care
- respite care
- spiritual advice
- practical and financial issue support.

The benefits of hospices are that they are experienced in dealing with incurable diseases and have all the expertise, both medical and more holistic, available under one roof.

It is a misconception to believe that a person has to be dying to receive support from a hospice. Although they will support people in the final days of their illness, hospice support can start a long time before and may include a number of short admissions for symptom management, care plan creation and respite care, as appropriate.

You should be aware of the services that hospices offer and that they are generally seen as centres of excellence for palliative care. If you have a patient you believe would benefit from hospice care, you should consider discussing this with them or their GP with the patient's consent.

1.9 End of life care in the community

You will frequently be called to patients in the end of life phase in the community. Sometimes this will be to patients where there are clear plans laid out, but sometimes it may be less expected or unplanned.

In all situations, you should remember the basic principles of end of life care described above and strive towards providing a good death. Some specific considerations may include:
- Communication: At the end of life, both patients and relatives can become very anxious. Calm communication considering all the available facts will be required to ensure peace for all present.
- Consider the plans that have been made and put in place already and follow them where possible. Also consider any known overarching wishes the patient may be known to have, i.e. to avoid admission to hospital if possible.
- Symptom management is one of the most common reasons to call for an ambulance in end of life care. This may be because the patient is suffering from acute pain or shortness of breath. Managing this can rely on several different strategies, including:
  - contacting a GP or palliative care team to change a patient's medication
  - asking a senior clinician to administer 'just in case' medications, which are sometimes prescribed and left with patients in case the situation changes

- asking your paramedic colleagues if they have treatment options such as the administration of anti-sickness or pain relief medication.
- Consider asking for specialist help early. Follow your local protocols, but sources of help may include:
  - GP/out-of-hours service
  - palliative care teams
  - hospices
  - specialist paramedics.

1.10 Resuscitation in end of life care

By definition, patients who are recognised as being at the end of life are expected to die. Cardiopulmonary resuscitation is unlikely to be successful in a person suffering from a known life-limiting condition and, although CPR can be attempted on anyone, there comes a time when it is no longer in the best interests of a patient to attempt it [Dying Matters, 2018].

Dying with dignity is a big concern for many people and performing CPR with no realistic chance of survival can undermine this [GMC, 2018b], cause distress to relatives and in some circumstances provide false hope.

Hopefully, in most situations, the patient will have discussed their wishes with their GP and family in advance, and some form of advanced care planning will have been completed. If, however, no such records exist, then the senior clinician at scene may need to make a decision on the appropriateness of CPR for the patient. Your paramedic colleague may determine that it would be futile and not in the patient's best interest to resuscitate in line with their guidelines on commencing and withholding resuscitation.

1.11 Supporting carers and relatives

Caring for someone with a terminal illness can be a very challenging and demanding time. It can also be emotionally difficult and extremely stressful, especially if the carer is a friend or member of the family. Carers can feel isolated, unsupported, resentment, anger and guilt at different times when caring for someone who is dying [Marie Curie, 2018b].

Carers are experts in looking after individuals and are likely to know the patient far better than any health or social professional involved. Their well-being is of paramount importance and you should specifically consider this as part of your management. Below are some tips on how to support and involve carers in patient care [Marie Curie, 2018c; NCPC, 2012]:

- Try to involve the carer in decision-making; they know the patient and their wishes well.
- Promote respite care when appropriate: many carers will feel that they are abandoning their loved ones by letting them receive respite care, but it can be essential to allow a carer to recuperate and continue providing the best care possible for a loved one.
- Provide information about support services: make the family aware of local support, including hospices, GPs and palliative care services.

2 Bereavement

2.1 Learning objectives

By the end of this section, you will be able to:
- define bereavement, bereaved and grief
- describe the bereavement process
- identify the emotions that accompany grief
- recognise when people may need additional help coping with bereavement
- identify different sources of help for coping with bereavement
- describe when health professionals should seek help after assisting with bereavement.

2.2 Introduction

Dealing with bereavement is an inevitable factor of working in emergency healthcare. As a health professional, you should be aware of the bereavement and grieving process, and how you can support those suffering from bereavement.

We all suffer loss and the grief that goes with it at times during our life. Understanding how people

respond to this can be beneficial. Below are some definitions of words relevant to this process:
- **Bereavement:** The state of having been bereaved. Bereavement may also be defined as the time we take to adjust to having been bereaved and to cope with the grief associated with that.
- **Bereaved:** To have been deprived of a close relative or friend through their death.
- **Grief:** This is a complex set of emotions experienced after the loss of someone close [Cancer Research UK, 2016c].

2.3 Bereavement and grieving process

It is generally accepted that there are four stages to bereavement [NHS, 2017b], including:
- accepting that the loss is real
- experiencing the pain of grief
- adjusting to life without the person who has died
- putting less emotional energy into grieving and putting more into something new (moving on).

While most people will go through all these stages, how quickly and smoothly they do so will be unique to the individual; there is no right or wrong way to grieve [Marie Curie, 2014]. While there is no standard 'grief', it is likely that a bereaved person will have emotions that feel chaotic and out of control, but with time these will become less intense. A number of different grief models or theories exist, but it is likely that the person suffering from grief will experience some, if not all, of these emotions [NHS, 2017b]:
- shock and numbness
- overwhelming sadness
- tiredness or exhaustion
- anger: this can be towards the person who has died, the illness, God (or other religious figures) or others.
- guilt, for being angry, about something they said or did not say, or about not being able to stop their loved one from dying.

If relevant, you should reassure bereaved parties that these feelings are entirely normal and they will get better with time.

2.4 Referring for additional help

Everyone's experiences of grief are unique to them and will take different amounts of time to resolve. It is normal to experience a range of difficult emotions, but in some circumstances it may be beneficial to seek help. If any of the following are evident, you should recommend someone seek additional support [NHS, 2017a]:
- Unable to get out of bed.
- Self-neglect or neglect of the wider family – for example, not eating properly.
- Feeling unable to go on without the person that has been lost
- The emotion is so intense it is affecting day-to-day life – for example, being unable to face going to work or taking anger out on someone else.

It may be appropriate for you to refer someone directly for help, for instance to their GP; however, as always, respect patient autonomy and seek consent before making this referral.

2.5 Sources of help

A wide range of help and support services are available to those that have experienced bereavement. Initially a person's GP is a good place to start as they can refer them for a range of therapies or even prescribe medication if appropriate.

Most people will only need a small amount of help to assist them in progressing through the grieving process, but for some it may take a lot longer.

You should also be aware of other sources of help though, and these may include:
- the Samaritans
- charities helping people to cope with bereavement
- hospice grief support teams
- grief counsellors.

2.6 Support for health professionals

Dealing with bereavement and supporting those that have been bereaved can be emotionally draining on health professionals. Remember to look after yourself. If you find situations are playing on your mind, you cannot stop thinking about an incident you attended, are feeling anxious about going to work or generally stressed, then you should seek help for yourself.

This help is available through a number of different routes, but might include occupational health, internal counselling services, or your own GP.

References

A & Ors v East Sussex CC
A & Ors, R (on the application of) v East Sussex County Council & Anor [2003] EWHC 167 (Admin). Available at: https://www.bailii.org/ew/cases/EWHC/Admin/2003/167.html [Accessed: 12 July 2019].

AAA, 2015
Age Action Alliance, 2015. *Attitudes to Ageing*. Available at: http://ageactionalliance.org/theme/attitudes-to-ageing/ [Accessed: 12 July 2019].

AACE, 2019
Association of Ambulance Chief Executives, 2019. *Structure of UK Ambulance Services*. Available at: https://aace.org.uk/uk-ambulance-service/ [Accessed: 3 January 2019].

AAFP, 2012
American Academy of Family Physicians, 2012. *Advanced Life Support in Obstetrics: Provider Manual*. Kansas: AAFP.

AAOS, 2011
American Academy of Orthopaedic Surgeons and American College of Emergency Physicians, 2011. *Critical Care Transport*. Sudbury: Jones and Bartlett Publishers.

AAP, 2006
American Academy of Pediatrics, 2006. The Apgar Score. *Advances in Neonatal Care*, 6(4), 220–223.

AAP, 2018
American Academy of Pediatrics, 2018. *Paediatric Education for Prehospital Professionals*. Revised 3rd ed. Burlington: Jones & Bartlett Learning.

Aaronson, 2012
Aaronson PI, Ward JPT and Connolly MJ, 2012. *The Cardiovascular System at a Glance*. 4th ed. Chichester: Wiley-Blackwell.

Abbey, 2004
Abbey J, Piller N, DeBellis A et al., 2004. The Abbey pain scale: A 1-minute numerical indicator for people with end-stage dementia. *International Journal of Palliative Nursing*, 10(1), 6–13.

Abrassart, 2013
Abrassart S, Stern R and Peter R, 2013. Unstable pelvic ring injury with hemodynamic instability: What seems the best procedure choice and sequence in the initial management? *Orthopaedics and Traumatology: Surgery & Research*, 99(2), 175–182.

Adams, 2002
Adams JE, Davis GG, Heidepriem RW III et al., 2002. Analysis of the incidence of pelvic trauma in fatal automobile accidents. *American Journal of Forensic Medicine and Pathology*, 23(2), 132–136.

ADSHG, 2016
Addison's Disease Self Help Group, 2016. *Diagnosing Addison's: A guide for GPs*. Available at: https://www.addisons.org.uk/files/file/3-diagnosing-addisons-a-guide-for-gps/ [Accessed: 10 January 2019].

Adults with Incapacity (Scotland) Act 2000
The Scottish Government, 2008. *Adults with Incapacity (Scotland) Act 2000*. Available at: https://www2.gov.scot/Publications/2008/03/25120154/0 [Accessed: 12 July 2019].

Age UK, 2018a
Age UK, 2018. *Depression and Anxiety*. Available at: https://www.ageuk.org.uk/information-advice/health-wellbeing/conditions-illnesses/depression-anxiety/ [Accessed: 15 December 2018].

Age UK, 2018b
Age UK 2018. *Dementia*. Available at: https://www.ageuk.org.uk/information-advice/health-wellbeing/conditions-illnesses/dementia/ [Accessed: 15 December 2018].

Age UK, 2019
Age UK, 2019. *Safeguarding Older People from Abuse and Neglect*. Available at: https://www.ageuk.org.uk/globalassets/age-uk/documents/factsheets/fs78_safeguarding_older_people_from_abuse_fcs.pdf [Accessed: 5 January 2019].

Ahmad, 2006
Ahmad F, Cheshire N and Hamady M, 2006. Acute aortic syndrome: Pathology and therapeutic strategies. *Postgraduate Medical Journal*, 82(967), 305–312.

Airwave, 2019
Airwave, 2019. *Emergency Services Network*. Available at: https://www.airwavesolutions.co.uk/products/products-and-services/emergency-services-network/ [Accessed: 17 February 2019].

References

ALK-Abello, 2018
ALK-Abello, 2018. *Jext 150 and 300 Micrograms Solution for Injection in Pre-Filled Pen: Patient information leaflet*. Available at: https://www.medicines.org.uk/emc/files/pil.5747.pdf. [Accessed: 5 January 2019].

Allan, 2004
Allan MA and Marsh J, 2004. *History and Examination*. 2nd ed. Edinburgh: Mosby.

Allen, 2007
Allen LA and O'Connor CM, 2007. Management of acute decompensated heart failure. *Canadian Medical Association Journal*, 176(6), 797–805.

Allison, 2004
Allison K and Porter K, 2004. Consensus on the pre-hospital approach to burns patient management. *Accident and Emergency Nursing*, 12(1), 53–57.

ALSG, 2010
Advanced Life Support Group, 2010. *Pre-hospital Obstetric Emergency Training*. Chichester: Wiley-Blackwell.

ALSG, 2018
Advanced Life Support Group, 2018. *Pre-obstetric Emergency Training: A Practical Approach*. 2nd ed. Hoboken, NJ: Wiley-Blackwell.

Althaus, 1982
Althaus U, Aeberhard P, Schüpbach P et al., 1982. Management of profound accidental hypothermia with cardiorespiratory arrest. *Annals of Surgery*, 195(4), 492–495.

Alzheimer's Society, 2015
Alzheimer's Society, 2015. *Equality, Discrimination and Human Rights*. Available at: https://www.alzheimers.org.uk/about-us/policy-and-influencing/what-we-think/equality-discrimination-human-rights [Accessed: 25 July 2019].

Alzheimer's Society, 2016
Alzheimer's Society, 2016. *Deprivation of Liberty Safeguards (DoLS)*. Available at: https://www.alzheimers.org.uk/get-support/legal-financial/deprivation-liberty-safeguards-dols [Accessed: 30 December 2018].

Alzheimer's Society, 2018a
Alzheimer's Society, 2018. *Parkinson's Disease*. Available at: https://www.alzheimers.org.uk/about-dementia/types-dementia/parkinsons-disease [Accessed: 15 December 2018].

Alzheimer's Society, 2018b
Alzheimer's Society, 2018. *How Dementia Progresses*. Available at: https://www.alzheimers.org.uk/about-dementia/symptoms-and-diagnosis/how-dementia-progresses [Accessed: 15 December 2018].

Alzheimer's Society, 2018c
Alzheimer's Society, 2018. *Responding to Aggressive Behaviour*. Available at: https://www.alzheimers.org.uk/about-dementia/symptoms-and-diagnosis/symptoms/responding-aggression#content-start [Accessed: 15 December 2018].

Alzheimer's Society, 2019
Alzheimer's Society, 2019. *Dementia Tax*. Available at: https://www.alzheimers.org.uk/about-us/policy-and-influencing/what-we-think/dementia-tax [Accessed: 18 February 2019].

Ambu, 2011
Ambu, 2011. *Ambu Perfit ACE: Instructions for Use*. Denmark: Ambu D/S.

Angell-James, 1975
Angell-James JE and Daly MB, 1975. Some aspects of upper respiratory tract reflexes. *Acta Oto-laryngologica*, 79(3–4), 242–252.

Apgar, 1953
Apgar V, 1953. A proposal for a new method of evaluation of the newborn infant. *Current Researches in Anesthesia & Analgesia*, 32(4), 260–267.

Arlt, 2002
Arlt W, 2002. Quality of life in Addison's Disease – the case for DHEA replacement. *Clinical Endocrinology*, 56(5), 573–574.

Arthritis Research UK, 2018
Arthritis Research UK, 2018. *About Arthritis*. Available at: https://www.versusarthritis.org/about-arthritis/ [Accessed: 15 December 2018].

Asbury, 2014
Asbury S and Jacobs E, 2014. *Dynamic Risk Assessment: The Practical Guide to Making Risk-Based Decisions with the 3-Level Risk Management Model*. Abingdon, Oxon: Routledge.

Ashburn, 2012
Ashburn J, Harrison T, Ham J and Strote J, 2012. Emergency physician estimation of blood loss. *Western Journal of Emergency Medicine*, 13(4), 376–379.

References

Athanassiadi, 2010
Athanassiadi K et al., 2010. Prognostic factors in flail-chest patients, *European Journal of Cardio-thoracic Surgery*, 38(4): 466–471.

Austin, 2010
Austin MA, Wills KE, Blizzard L et al., 2010. Effect of high flow oxygen on mortality in chronic obstructive pulmonary disease patients in prehospital setting: Randomised controlled trial. *British Medical Journal*, 341, c5462.

Austin, 2014
Austin N, Krishnamoorthy V and Dagal A, 2014. Airway management in cervical spine injury. *International Journal of Critical Illness & Injury Science*, 4(1), 50–56.

Baile, 2000
Baile WF, 2000. SPIKES – A six-step protocol for delivering bad news: Application to the patient with cancer. *The Oncologist*, 5(4), 302–311.

Bailey, 2010
Bailey, B, 2010. Partner violence during pregnancy: Prevalence, effects, screening, and management. *International Journal of Women's Health*, 2, 183–197.

Baker, 2009
Baker SJK and Wass JAH, 2009. Addison's disease. *BMJ*, 339, (jul02 1), b2384.

Baker, 2014
Baker DDJ, 2014. The clinical presentation of toxic trauma: Assessment and diagnosis. In *Toxic Trauma*. London, Springer: 113–133.

Balvers, 2016
Balvers K, Van der Horst M, Graumans M et al., 2016. Hypothermia as a predictor for mortality in trauma patients at admittance to the Intensive Care Unit. *Journal of Emergencies, Trauma, and Shock*, 9(3), 97–102.

Band, 2011
Band RA, Gaieski DF, Hylton JH et al., 2011. Arriving by emergency medical services improves time to treatment endpoints for patients with severe sepsis or septic shock. *Academic Emergency Medicine*, 18(9), 934–940.

Barnes, 2015
Barnes J, Duffy A and Hamnett N, 2015. The Mersey Burns App: Evolving a model of validation. *Emergency Medicine Journal*, 32(8), 637–641.

Barrett, 2014
Barrett E and Burns A, 2014. *Dementia Revealed: What primary care needs to know*. Available at: https://dementiapartnerships.com/wp-content/uploads/sites/2/dementia-revealed-toolkit.pdf [Accessed: 25 July 2019].

Bartlett, 2008
Bartlett N, Yuan J, Holland AJ et al., 2008. Optimal duration of cooling for an acute scald contact burn injury in a porcine model. *Journal of Burn Care & Research: Official Publication of the American Burn Association*, 29(5), 828–834.

Battaloglu, 2015
Battaloglu E, Battaloglu E, Chu J and Porter K, 2015. Obstetrics in trauma. *Trauma*, 17(1), 17–23.

Battaloglu, 2016
Battaloglu E, McDonnell D, Chu J, Lecky F and Porter K, 2016. Epidemiology and outcomes of pregnancy and obstetric complications in trauma in the United Kingdom. *Injury*, 47(1), 184–187.

Bazarian, 2003
Bazarian JJ, Eirich MA and Salhanick SD, 2003. The relationship between pre-hospital and emergency department Glasgow Coma Scale scores. *Brain Injury*, 17(7), 553–560.

BBA, 2018
British Burns Association, 2018. *First Aid Clinical Practice Guidelines*. Available at: https://www.britishburnsassociation.org/wp-content/uploads/2017/06/BBA-First-Aid-Guideline-3.7.18.pdf [Accessed: 4 July 2019].

BCS, 2017
British Cardiovascular Society, 2017. *Recording a Standard 12-lead Electrocardiogram*. Available at: http://www.scst.org.uk/resources/SCST_ECG_Recording_Guidelines_20171.pdf [Accessed: 10 December 2018].

Beck, 1961
Beck AT, Ward CH, Mendelson M et al., 1961. An inventory for measuring depression. *Arch Gen Psychiatry*, 4(6), 561–571.

Benger, 2009
Benger J, Nolan J and Clancy M (eds), 2009. *Emergency Airway Management*. Cambridge: Cambridge University Press.

Betsy, 2012
Betsy T and Keogh JE, 2012. *Microbiology Demystified*. 2nd ed. New York: McGraw-Hill.

References

BGS, 2018
British Geriatric Society, 2018. *Frailty: What's it all about?* Available at: https://www.bgs.org.uk/resources/frailty-what's-it-all-about [Accessed: 17 February 2019].

BHF, 2017
British Heart Foundation & Resuscitation Council (UK), 2017. *A Guide to Automated External Defibrillators (AED).* Available at: https://www.resus.org.uk/publications/a-guide-to-aeds/ [Accessed: 30 December 2018].

Bickley, 2006
Bickley LS, Szilagyi PG and Bates B, 2006. *Bates' Guide to Physical Examination and History Taking.* 9th ed. Philadelphia: Lippincott Williams & Wilkins.

Blaber, 2008
Blaber A, 2008. *Foundations for Paramedic Practice: A Theoretical Perspective.* Maidenhead: Open University Press.

Bledsoe, 2014
Bledsoe BE, Porter RS and Cherry RA, 2014. *Paramedic Care: Principles and Practice.* Vol. 3. Harlow: Pearson.

Blom, 2014
Blom L and Black JJM, 2014. Major incidents. *BMJ*, 348, g1144.

BMA, 2007
British Medical Association, Resuscitation Council (UK), and Royal College of Nursing, 2007. *Decisions Relating To Cardiopulmonary Resuscitation.* Available at: https://www.resus.org.uk/dnacpr/ [Accessed: 15 July 2019].

BMA, 2014a
British Medical Association, 2014. *Safe Handover: Safe patients.* Available at: https://www.bma.org.uk/-/media/Files/PDFs/Practical%20advice%20at%20work/Contracts/safe%20handover%20safe%20patients.pdf [Accessed: 15 July 2019].

BMA, 2014b
British Medical Association, 2014. *The Law and Ethics of Abortion.* Available at: https://www.bma.org.uk/-/media/files/pdfs/employment%20advice/ethics/the-law-and-ethics-of-abortion-2018.pdf?la=en [Accessed: 15 July 2019].

BMA, 2018
British Medical Association, 2018. *Consent to Treatment Adults with Capacity.* Available at: https://www.bma.org.uk/advice/employment/ethics/medical-students-ethics-toolkit/6-consent-to-treatment-capacity [Accessed: 30 December 2018].

BOC, 2013a
BOC Healthcare, 2013. *Medical Oxygen.* Available at: http://www.bochealthcare.co.uk/internet./lh.lh.gbr/en/images/504370-healthcare%20medical%20oxygen%20integral%20valve%20cylinders%20leaflet%2006409_54069.pdf%20 [Accessed: 20 September 2018].

BOC, 2013b
BOC Healthcare, 2013. *ENTONOX® (50% nitrous oxide/50% oxygen).* Available at: http://www.bochealthcare.co.uk/en/images/504365-Healthcare%20Entonox%20Integral%20Valve%20Cylinder%20Instructions%20leaflet-04_tcm409-57216.pdf [Accessed: 20 September 2018].

Body, 2010
Body R, Carley S, Wibberley C et al., 2010. The value of symptoms and signs in the emergent diagnosis of acute coronary syndromes. *Resuscitation*, 81(3), 281–286.

Bolton, 2012
Bolton JM, Spiwak R and Sareen J, 2012. Predicting suicide attempts with the sad persons scale: A longitudinal analysis. *Journal of Clinical Psychiatry*, 73(6), e735–e741.

Booker, 2007
Booker R, 2007. Peak expiratory flow measurement. *Nursing Standard*, 21(39), 42–43.

Bose, 2006
Bose P, Regan F and Paterson-Brown S, 2006. Improving the accuracy of estimated blood loss at obstetric haemorrhage using clinical reconstructions. *BJOG: An International Journal of Obstetrics and Gynaecology*, 113(8), 919–924.

Boulton, 2018
Boulton AJ, Lewis CT, Naumann DN et al. Prehospital haemostatic dressings for trauma: A systematic review. *Emergency Medicine Journal*, 35, 449–457.

Bowers, 2007
Bowers B and Scase C, 2007. Tracheostomy: Facilitating successful discharge from hospital to home. *British Journal of Nursing*, 16(8), 476–479.

Boyett, 2009
Boyett MR, 2009. 'And the beat goes on.' The cardiac conduction system: The wiring system of the heart. *Experimental Physiology*, 94(10), 1035–1049.

Boyle, 2009
Boyle JS, Bechtel LK and Holstege CP, 2009. Management of the critically poisoned patient. *Scandinavian Journal of Trauma, Resuscitation and Emergency Medicine*, 17(1), 1–11.

References

BPAS, 2015
British Pregnancy Advisory Service, 2015. *What is Abortion?* Available at: https://www.bpas.org/abortion-care/considering-abortion/what-is-abortion/ [Accessed: 18 November 2015].

Briar, 2003
Briar C and Lasserson D, 2003. *Nervous System*. 2nd ed. London: Mosby.

Briscoe, 2006
Briscoe VJ and Davis SN, 2006. Hypoglycemia in type 1 and type 2 diabetes: physiology, pathophysiology, and management. *Clinical Diabetes*, 24(3), 115 –121.

Brophy, 2012
Brophy GM, Bell R, Claassen J et al., 2012. Guidelines for the evaluation and management of status epilepticus. *Neurocritical Care*, 17(1), 3–23.

BSI, 2011
British Standards Institution, 2011. *BS EN 1089-3:2011*. London: BSI.

BTS, 2010
Levy ML, Le Jeune I, Woodhead MA et al., 2010. Primary care summary of the British Thoracic Society guidelines for the management of community acquired pneumonia in adults: 2009 update. Endorsed by the Royal College of General Practitioners and the Primary Care Respiratory Society UK. *Primary Care Respiratory Journal*, 19(2), 21–27.

Burgess, 1990
Burgess AR, Eastridge BJ, Young JW et al., 1990. Pelvic ring disruptions: Effective classification system and treatment protocols. *Journal of Trauma*, 30(7), 848–856.

Burton, 2006
Burton JH, Harrah JD, Germann CA et al., 2006. Does end-tidal carbon dioxide monitoring detect respiratory events prior to current sedation monitoring practices? *Academic Emergency Medicine: Official Journal of the Society for Academic Emergency Medicine*, 13(5), 500–504.

Buss, 2010
Buss J and Thompson G (eds), 2010. *Auscultation Skills: Breath & Heart Sounds*. 4th ed. Philadelphia: Wolters Kluwer/Lippincott Williams & Wilkins Health.

Butz, 2015
Butz DR, Collier Z, O'Connor A, Magdziak M and Gottlieb LJ, 2015. Is palmar surface area a reliable tool to estimate burn surface areas in obese patients? *Journal of Burn Care and Research*, 36(1), 87–91.

Bydon, 2014
Bydon M and Gokaslan Z, 2014. Time to treatment of cauda equina syndrome: A time to re-evaluate our clinical decision. *World Neurosurgery*, 82(3), 344–345.

Cancer Research UK, 2016a
Cancer Research UK, 2016. *Your Spiritual Needs at the End of Life*. Available at: https://www.cancerresearchuk.org/about-cancer/coping/dying-with-cancer/making-plans/spiritual-needs [Accessed: 31 December 2018].

Cancer Research UK, 2016b
Cancer Research UK, 2016. *Care Planning*. Available at: https://www.cancerresearchuk.org/about-cancer/coping/dying-with-cancer/making-plans/care-planning [Accessed: 31 December 2018].

Cancer Research UK, 2016c
Cancer Research UK, 2016. *Coping with Grief*. Available at: https://www.cancerresearchuk.org/about-cancer/coping/dying-with-cancer/after-someone-dies/coping-with-grief [Accessed: 1 January 2019].

Canto, 2012
Canto AJ, Kiefe CI, Goldberg RJ et al., 2012. Differences in symptom presentation and hospital mortality according to type of acute myocardial infarction. *American Heart Journal*, 163(4), 572–579.

Cantwell, 2011
Cantwell R, Clutton-Brock T, Cooper G et al., 2011. Saving mothers' lives: Reviewing maternal deaths to make motherhood safer: 2006–2008. The Eighth Report of the Confidential Enquiries into Maternal Deaths in the United Kingdom. *BJOG: An International Journal of Obstetrics and Gynaecology*, 118(Supplement 1), 1–203.

Capps, 2010
Capps JA, Sharma V and Arkwright PD, 2010. Prevalence, outcome and pre-hospital management of anaphylaxis by first aiders and paramedical ambulance staff in Manchester, UK. *Resuscitation*, 81(6), 653–657.

Castledine, 2009
Castledine G and Close A, 2009. *Oxford Handbook of Adult Nursing*. Oxford, Oxford University Press.

CCI, 2017
Clement Clarke International, 2017. *Mini-wright Peak Flow Meter Instructions for Use*. Edinburgh: Clement Clarke International. Available at: https://www.haag-streit.com/fileadmin/Clement_Clarke/Peak_Expiratory_Flow/Mini-Wright_Standard/1902169-MW_Stnd_IFU.pdf [Accessed: 21 November 2018].

References

CDC, 2017
Centers for Disease Control and Prevention, 2017. *What are the Symptoms of Gynecologic Cancers?* Available at: https://www.cdc.gov/cancer/gynecologic/basic_info/symptoms.htm [Accessed: 15 July 2019].

CESA, 2018
Cauda Equina Syndrome Association, 2018. *CES Red Flag Symptoms*. Available at: https://www.ihavecaudaequina.com/about-us/red-flags/ [Accessed: 22 November 2018].

Champion, 1989
Champion HR, Sacco WJ, Copes WS et al., 1989. A revision of the trauma score. *Journal of Trauma*, 29(5), 623–629.

Chan, 2003
Chan MM, 2003. What is the effect of fingernail polish on pulse oximetry? *Chest*, 123(6), 2163–2164.

Chandler, 2014
Chandler R and Bruneau B, 2014. Barriers to the management of pain in dementia care. *Nursing Practice*, 110(28), 12–16.

Chapin, 2013
Chapin MM, Rochette LM, Annest JL et al., 2013. Nonfatal choking on food among children 14 years or younger in the United States, 2001–2009. *Pediatrics*, 132(2), 275–281.

Chapman, 2013
Chapman V and Charles C (eds), 2013. *The Midwife's Labour and Birth Handbook*, 3rd ed. Oxford: Wiley-Blackwell.

Charmandari, 2014
Charmandari E, Nicolaides NC and Chrousos GP, 2014. Adrenal insufficiency. *The Lancet*, 383(9935), 2152–2167.

Chauhan, 2018
Chauhan R, Conti BM and Keene D, 2018. Marauding terrorist attack (MTA): Prehospital considerations. *Emergency Medicine Journal: EMJ*, 35(6), 389–395.

Children Act 2004
UK Government, 2004. Children Act 2004, Section 11. Available at: http://www.legislation.gov.uk/ukpga/2004/31/section/11 [Accessed: 7 July 2019].

Chin, 2004
Chin RFM, Neville BGR and Scott RC, 2004. A systematic review of the epidemiology of status epilepticus. *European Journal of Neurology*, 11(12), 800–810.

Choi, 2014
Choi K and Hong J, 2014. Management of pelvic organ prolapse. *Korean Journal of Urology*, 55(11), 693–702.

CIPOLD, 2013
CIPOLD, 2013. *Confidential Inquiry into Premature Deaths of People with Learning Disabilities*. Reports available at: http://www.bristol.ac.uk/cipold/reports/ [Accessed: 18 December 2018].

Civil Contingencies Act 2004
UK Government, 2004. *Civil Contingencies Act 2004*. Available at: http://www.legislation.gov.uk/ukpga/2004/36/contents [Accessed: 12 November 2018].

Clarke, 2015
Clarke E, 2015. *Law and Ethics for Midwifery*. London: Routledge.

Clegg, 2013
Clegg A et al., 2013. Frailty in elderly people. *The Lancet*, 381(9868), 752–762.

Coad, 2015
Coad J and Dunstall M, 2015. *Anatomy and Physiology for Midwives*. London: Churchill Livingstone.

Connor, 2013
Connor D, Greaves I, Porter K et al., 2013. Pre-hospital spinal immobilisation: An initial consensus statement. *Emergency Medicine Journal*, 30(12), 1067–1069. Available at: https://fphc.rcsed.ac.uk/media/1764/pre-hospital-spinal-immobilisation.pdf [Accessed: 11 February 2019].

Control of Substances Hazardous to Health Regulations 2002
UK Government, 2002. *The Control of Substances Hazardous to Health Regulations 2002*. Available at: http://www.legislation.gov.uk/uksi/2002/2677/regulation/7/made [Accessed: 27 December 2018].

Cook, 2006
Cook TM and Hommers C, 2006. New airways for resuscitation? *Resuscitation*, 69(3), 371–387.

Cooper, 2012
Cooper C, 2012. *Psychiatry at a Glance*. 5th ed. Chichester: Wiley-Blackwell.

CoP, 2015
College of Paramedics, 2015. *Paramedic Career Framework*. 3rd ed. Available at: https://www.collegeofparamedics.co.uk/downloads/Post-Reg_Career_Framework_3rd_Edition.pdf [Accessed: 3 January 2019].

Corcoran, 2013
Corcoran N, 2013. *Communicating Health: Strategies for Health Promotion*. 2nd ed. Los Angeles: Sage Publications.

References

Corwell, 2014
Corwell B, Knight B, Olivieri L et al., 2014. Current diagnosis and treatment of hyperglycemic emergencies. *Emergency Medicine Clinics of North America*, 32(2), 437–452.

CQC, 2015
Care Quality Commission, 2015. *Regulation 20: Duty of Candour*. Available at: http://www.cqc.org.uk/sites/default/files/20150327_duty_of_candour_guidance_final.pdf [Accessed: 23 November 2018].

Crawford, 2018
Crawford S, 2018. Changing the system — Major trauma patients and their outcomes in the NHS (England) 2008–17. *EClinicalMedicine*, 4(5), 3.

Crook, 2013
Crook J and Taylor RM, 2013. The agreement of fingertip and sternum capillary refill time in children. *Archives of Disease in Childhood*, 98(4), 265–268.

Cryer, 2008
Cryer PE, 2008. The barrier of hypoglycemia in diabetes. *Diabetes*, 57(12), 3169–3176.

CSCB, 2014
Coventry Safeguarding Children Board, 2014. *Serious Case Review: Daniel Pelka*. Available at: https://www.lgiu.org.uk/wp-content/uploads/2013/10/Daniel-Pelka-Serious-Case-Review-Coventry-LSCB.pdf [Accessed: 21 January 2019].

Cure the NHS, 2014
Cure the NHS, 2014. *Cure the NHS Campaign*. Available at: http://www.curethenhs.co.uk/cure-the-nhs-campaign/%20 [Accessed: 15 July 2019].

Cuttle, 2008
Cuttle L, Kempf M, Kravchuk O et al., 2008. The optimal temperature of first aid treatment for partial thickness burn injuries. *Wound Repair and Regeneration: Official Publication of the Wound Healing Society [and] the European Tissue Repair Society*, 16(5), 626–634.

Cuttle, 2009
Cuttle L, Pearn J, McMillan JR et al., 2009. A review of first aid treatments for burn injuries. *Burns*, 35(6), 768–775.

Czura, 2011
Czura CJ, 2011. Merinoff Symposium 2010: Sepsis – speaking with one voice. *Molecular Medicine*, 17(1–2), 2–3.

Daniels, 2011
Daniels R, Nutbeam T, McNamara G et al., 2011. The sepsis six and the severe sepsis resuscitation bundle: A prospective observational cohort study. *Emergency Medicine Journal*, 28(6), 507–512.

Data Protection Act, 1998
UK Government, 1998. *Data Protection Act 1998*. London: The Stationery Office.

Datta, 2006
Datta A and Tipton M, 2006. Respiratory responses to cold water immersion: Neural pathways, interactions, and clinical consequences awake and asleep. *Journal of Applied Physiology*, 100(6), 2057–2064.

Daughters of Eve, 2018
Daughters of Eve, 2018. *Reversing FGM*. Available at: http://www.dofeve.org/reversing-fgm.html [Accessed: 29 December 2018].

DCA, 2014
Department for Constitutional Affairs, 2014. *Mental Capacity Act Code of Practice*. Available at: https://www.gov.uk/government/publications/mental-capacity-act-code-of-practice [Accessed: 5 January 2019].

Deakin, 2015
Deakin C, Jewkes F, Lockey D et al., 2015. *Prehospital Resuscitation*. Available at: https://www.resus.org.uk/resuscitation-guidelines/prehospital-resuscitation/ [Accessed: 9 November 2015].

Deary, 1993
Deary IJ, Hepburn DA, MacLeod KM et al., 1993. Partitioning the symptoms of hypoglycaemia using multi-sample confirmatory factor analysis. *Diabetologia*, 36(8), 771–777.

Dekker, 2018
Dekker R, 2018. *Evidence on: Birthing Positions*. Available at: https://evidencebasedbirth.com/evidence-birthing-positions/ [Accessed: 29 December 2018].

DfE, 2015
Department for Education, 2015. *Working Together to Safeguard Children*. Available at: https://www.gov.uk/government/publications/working-together-to-safeguard-children--2 [Accessed: 21 January 2019].

DfE, 2017
Department for Education, 2017. *Safeguarding and Radicalization*. Available at: https://assets.publishing.service.gov.uk/government/uploads/system/uploads/attachment_data/file/635262/Safeguarding_and_Radicalisation.pdf [Accessed: 17 February 2019].

References

Dickson, 2017
Dickson JM, Peacock, M, Grünewald, RA, Howlett S, Bissell P, Reuber M, 2017. Non-epileptic attack disorder: the importance of diagnosis and treatment. *BMJ Case Reports, 2017*. Available at: https://doi.org/10.1136/bcr-2016-218278 [Accessed: 4 December 2018].

Dieckmann, 2010
Dieckmann RA, Brownstein D and Gausche-Hill M, 2010. The pediatric assessment triangle: a novel approach for the rapid evaluation of children. *Pediatric Emergency Care*, 26(4), 312–315.

Dimond, 2015
Dimond MB, 2015. *Legal Aspects of Nursing*. 7th ed. Harlow, United Kingdom: Pearson.

Disability Rights UK, 2017
Disability Rights UK, 2017. *Stop Disability Hate Crime*. Available at: https://www.disabilityrightsuk.org/how-we-can-help/independent-living/stop-disability-hate-crime [Accessed: 18 December 2018].

Dixon, 2009
Dixon M, Carmody N and O'Donnell C, 2009. The effectiveness of supraglottic airway devices in pre-hospital basic life support airway management. *Emergency Medicine Journal*, 26(10), 4.

Dobson, 2009
Dobson T, Jensen J, Karim S et al., 2009. Correlation of paramedic administration of furosemide with emergency physician diagnosis of congestive heart failure. *Journal of Emergency Primary Health Care*, 7(3), 3.

DoH, 2000
Department of Health, 2000. *No Secrets: Guidance on protecting vulnerable adults in care*. Available at: https://www.gov.uk/government/publications/no-secrets-guidance-on-protecting-vulnerable-adults-in-care [Accessed: 21 January 2019].

DoH, 2001
Department of Health, 2001. *Valuing People*. Available at: https://www.gov.uk/government/uploads/system/uploads/attachment_data/file/250877/5086.pdf [Accessed: 14 June 2019].

DoH, 2003
Department of Health, 2003. *Confidentiality: NHS Code of Practice*. Available at: https://www.gov.uk/government/publications/confidentiality-nhs-code-of-practice [Accessed: 8 December 2018].

DoH, 2005
Department of Health Emergency Preparedness Division, 2005. *NHS Emergency Planning Guidance 2005*. Available at: https://webarchive.nationalarchives.gov.uk/20080817111334/http://www.dh.gov.uk/en/Publicationsandstatistics/Publications/PublicationsPolicyAndGuidance/DH_4121072 [Accessed: 15 October 2018].

DoH, 2006
Department of Health, 2006. *Medical Gases: Health technical memorandum 02-01: Medical gas pipeline systems*. Available at: https://assets.publishing.service.gov.uk/government/uploads/system/uploads/attachment_data/file/153575/HTM_02-01_Part_A.pdf [Accessed: 20 September 2018].

DoH, 2007
Department of Health, 2007. *Mass Casualties Incidents: A framework for planning*. Available at: https://webarchive.nationalarchives.gov.uk/20130124035118/http://www.dh.gov.uk/prod_consum_dh/groups/dh_digitalassets/@dh/@en/documents/digitalasset/dh_073397.pdf [Accessed: 4 July 2019].

DoH, 2008
Department of Health, 2008. *End of Life Care Strategy*. Available at: https://www.gov.uk/government/uploads/system/uploads/attachment_data/file/136431/End_of_life_strategy.pdf [Accessed: 18 July 2019].

DoH, 2009a
Department of Health and Health Protection Agency, 2009. *Pandemic (H1N1) 2009 Influenza*. Available at: https://www.gov.uk/government/publications/pandemic-flu-infection-control-ambulance-services [Accessed: 22 December 2018].

DoH, 2009b
Department of Health, 2009. *Reference Guide to Consent for Examination Or Treatment*. Available at: https://www.gov.uk/government/publications/reference-guide-to-consent-for-examination-or-treatment-second-edition [Accessed: 5 January 2019].

DoH, 2010a
Department of Health, 2010. *Essence of Care 2010: Benchmarks for the Fundamental Aspects of Care: Benchmarks for Personal Hygiene*. London: The Stationery Office.

DoH, 2010b
Australian Government, Department of Health, 2010. *Personal Hygiene*. Available at: http://www.health.gov.au/internet/publications/publishing.nsf/content/ohp-enhealth-manual-atsi-cnt-l-ohp-enhealth-manual-atsi-cnt-l-ch3-ohp-enhealth-manual-atsi-cnt-l-ch3.7 [Accessed: 21 December 2018].

References

DoH, 2010c
Department of Health, 2010. *Ambulance Guidelines: Reducing infection through effective practice in the pre-hospital environment*. Available at: http://aace.org.uk/wp-content/uploads/2011/11/New-DH-Guidelines-Reducing-HCAIs.pdf [Accessed: 22 December 2018].

DoH, 2013a
Department of Health, 2013. *Managing Healthcare Fire Safety*. Available at: https://www.gov.uk/government/publications/managing-healthcare-fire-safety [Accessed: 28 July 2019].

DoH, 2013b
Department of Health, 2013. *Health Technical Memorandum 07-01: Safe management of healthcare waste*. Available at: https://www.gov.uk/government/uploads/system/uploads/attachment_data/file/167976/HTM_07-01_Final.pdf [Accessed: 28 November 2018].

DoH, 2013c
Department of Health, 2013. *Winterbourne View Hospital: Department of Health Review and Response*. Available at: https://www.gov.uk/government/publications/winterbourne-view-hospital-department-of-health-review-and-response [Accessed: 21 January 2019].

DoH, 2014
Department of Health and Concordat Signatories, 2014. *Mental Health Crisis Care Concordat*. Available at: https://s16878.pcdn.co/wp-content/uploads/2014/04/36353_Mental_Health_Crisis_accessible.pdf. [Accessed: 20 January 2018].

DoH, 2015a
Department of Health, 2015. *NHS Constitution for England*. Available at: https://www.gov.uk/government/publications/the-nhs-constitution-for-england/the-nhs-constitution-for-england [Accessed: 18 January 2019].

DoH, 2015b
Department of Health, 2015. *2010 to 2015 Government Policy: End of Life Care*. Available at: https://www.gov.uk/government/publications/2010-to-2015-government-policy-end-of-life-care [Accessed: 18 January 2019].

DoH, 2015c
Department of Health, 2015. *Mental Health Act 1983: Code of Practice*. Available at: https://www.gov.uk/government/uploads/system/uploads/attachment_data/file/435512/M HA_Code_of_Practice.PDF [Accessed: 23 June 2019].

Dougherty, 2008
Dougherty L, 2008. *Intravenous Therapy Nursing Practice Second Edition*. 2nd ed. Oxford: Wiley-Blackwell.

Dougherty, 2015
Dougherty L, Lister S and West-Oram A, 2015. *Royal Marsden Manual of Clinical Nursing Procedures*. 9th ed. Hoboken: John Wiley & Sons Inc.

Douglas, 2005
Douglas G, Nicol EF, Robertson C et al., 2005. *Macleod's Clinical Examination*. 11th ed. Edinburgh: Elsevier Churchill Livingstone.

Drake, 2015
Drake RL, Vogl W, Mitchell AWM and Gray H, 2015. *Gray's Anatomy for Students*. 3rd ed. Philadelphia, PA: Churchill Livingstone/Elsevier.

Dunn, 2005
Dunn L, 2005. Pneumonia: Classification, diagnosis and nursing management. *Nursing Standard*, 19(42), 50–54.

Durrer, 2003
Durrer B, Brugger H, Syme D et al., 2003. The medical on-site treatment of hypothermia: ICAR-MEDCOM recommendation. *High Altitude Medicine & Biology*, 4(1), 99–103.

DWI, 2012
Drinking Water Inspectorate, 2012. *Legislation*. Available at: http://dwi.defra.gov.uk/stakeholders/guidance-and-codes-of-practice/WS(WQ)-regs-england2010.pdf [Accessed: 27 December 2018].

Dying Matters, 2018
Dying Matters, 2018. *The Resuscitation Conversation*. Available at: https://www.dyingmatters.org/gp_page/resuscitation-conversation [Accessed: 31 December 2018].

Dykes, 2002
Dykes M, 2002. *Crash Course: Anatomy*. 2nd ed. London: Mosby.

Eastridge, 2007
Eastridge BJ, Salinas J, McManus JG et al., 2007. Hypotension begins at 110 mmHg: Redefining 'hypotension' with data. *Journal of Trauma: Injury, Infection, and Critical Care*, 63(2), 291–299.

EC, 2013
European Commission, 2013. *Chemicals at Work – A new labelling system*. Available at: https://osha.europa.eu/en/file/49187/ [Accessed: 21 December 2018].

References

ECA, 2017
European Chemicals Agency, 2017. *Guidance on Labelling and Packaging in Accordance with Regulation (EC) No 1272/2008*. Available at: https://echa.europa.eu/regulations/clp/labelling [Accessed: 21 December 2018].

EEAST, 2014
East of England Ambulance Service, 2014. *Clinical Manual 2014*. Bridgwater: Class Professional Publishing.

Elliott, 2011
Elliott J and Heller S, 2011. Hypoglycaemia unawareness. *Practical Diabetes International*, 28(5), 227–232.

Enoch, 2009
Enoch S, Roshan A and Shah M, 2009. Emergency and early management of burns and scalds. *BMJ*, 338, b1037–b1037.

EPT, 2015
Ectopic Pregnancy Trust, 2015. *Reasons for an Ectopic Pregnancy*. Available at: http://www.ectopic.org.uk/patients/reasons-for-an-ectopic-pregnancy/ [Accessed: 11 November 2018].

Equality Act 2010
UK Government, 2010. *Equality Act 2010*. Available at: http://www.legislation.gov.uk/ukpga/2010/15/contents [Accessed: 11 July 2019].

Evans, 2012
Evans JDW and Sutton P, 2012. *Cardiovascular System*. Edinburgh: Mosby/Elsevier.

Eve Appeal, 2019
The Eve Appeal, 2019. *Gynaecological Cancers*. Available at: https://www.eveappeal.org.uk/gynaecological-cancers/ [Accessed: 18 July 2019].

Fairbank, 2014
Fairbank J and Mallen C, 2014. Cauda equina syndrome: Implications for primary care. *British Journal of General Practice*, 64(619), 67–68.

Falk, 2003
Falk E and Thuesen L, 2003. Pathology of coronary microembolisation and no reflow. *Heart*, 89(9), 983–985.

Farley, 2011
Farley A and Hendry C, 2011. *The Physiological Effects of Ageing*. Chichester: Wiley-Blackwell.

Feber, 2006
Feber T, 2006. Tracheostomy care for community nurses: basic principles. *British Journal of Community Nursing*, 11(5), 186–193.

Ferno, 2006
Ferno-Washington, 2006. *Scoop EXL Stretcher Series User Manual*, Wilmington: Ferno-Washington.

Ferreira, 2005
Ferreira J and Stanley L, 2005. *Evaluation of Manual Handling Tasks Involving the Use of Carry Chairs by UK Ambulance Personnel*. Sudbury: HSE Books.

Fick, 2002
Fick DM, Agostini JV and Inouye SK, 2002. Delirium superimposed on dementia: A systematic review. *Journal of the American Geriatrics Society*, 50(10), 1723–1732.

Findlay, 2007
Findlay G et al., *Trauma: Who Cares?* Available at: http://www.ncepod.org.uk/2007report2/Downloads/SIP_report.pdf [Accessed: 23 July 2019].

Food Safety Act 1990
UK Government, 1990. *Food Safety Act 1990*. Available at: http://www.legislation.gov.uk/ukpga/1990/16/contents [Accessed: 27 July 2019].

Fouche, 2014
Fouche PF, Simpson PM, Bendall J et al., 2014. Airways in out-of-hospital cardiac arrest: Systematic review and meta-analysis. *Prehospital Emergency Care*, 18(2), 244–256.

FPHC, 2017
Faculty of Pre-Hospital Care, 2017. *Position Statement on the Application of Tourniquets*. Available at: https://fphc.rcsed.ac.uk/media/2398/position-statement-on-the-application-of-tourniquets-july-2017.pdf [Accessed: 28 February 2019].

FPHC, 2018
Faculty of Pre-Hospital Care, 2018. *Corrosive Substance Attack*. Available at: https://fphc.rcsed.ac.uk/media/2490/corrosive-substance-attack_28032018.pdf [Accessed: 16 February 2019].

Francis, 2013
Francis R, 2013. *Final Report – Mid Staffordshire NHS Foundation Trust Public Inquiry*. Available at: http://webarchive.nationalarchives.gov.uk/20150407084003/http://www.midstaffspublicinquiry.com/report [Accessed: 31 December 2014].

Francis, 2015
Francis R, 2015. *Freedom to Speak Up Review*. Available at: https://freedomtospeakup.org.uk/wp-content/uploads/2014/07/f2su_web.pdf [Accessed: 15 February 2019].

References

Frank, 2010
Frank M, Schmucker U, Stengel D et al., 2010. Proper estimation of blood loss on scene of trauma: Tool or tale? *Journal of Trauma: Injury, Infection, and Critical Care*, 69(5), 1191–1195.

Fraser, 2012
Fraser D and Cooper M, 2012. *Myles Textbook for Midwives*. 15th ed. London: Churchill Livingstone Elsevier.

Freyenhagen, 2009
Freyenhagen F, 2009. Personal autonomy and mental capacity. *Psychiatry*, 8(12), 465–467.

Fried, 2001
Fried LP et al., 2001. Frailty in older adults: Evidence for a phenotype. *Journals of Gerontology Series A: Biological Sciences and Medical Sciences*, 56(3), 146–156.

Frykberg, 1988
Frykberg ER and Tepas JJ, 1988. Terrorist bombings: Lessons learned from Belfast to Beirut. *Annals of Surgery*, 208(5), 569–576.

Fuchs, 2012
Fuchs S, Yamamoto L, American Academy of Pediatrics et al., 2012. *APLS: The Pediatric Emergency Medicine Resource*. Burlington, MA: Jones & Bartlett Learning.

Gabbe, 2011
Gabbe BJ, de Steiger R, Esser M et al., 2011. Predictors of mortality following severe pelvic ring fracture: Results of a population-based study. *Injury*, 42(10), 985–991.

Garcia, 2004
Garcia TB and Miller GT, 2004. *Arrhythmia Recognition: The Art of Interpretation*. Sudbury: Jones and Bartlett Publishers.

Garcia, 2015
Garcia TB, 2015. *12-Lead ECG: The Art of Interpretation*. 2nd ed. Burlington, MA: Jones & Bartlett Learning.

Gardner, 2010
Gardner A, Gardner E and Morley T, 2010. Cauda equina syndrome: A review of the current clinical and medico-legal position. *European Spine Journal*, 20(5), 690–697.

Garlapati, 2012
Garlapati AK and Ashwood N, 2012. An overview of pelvic ring disruption. *Trauma*, 14(2), 169–178.

Geerts, 2012
Geerts BF, van den Bergh L, Stijnen T et al., 2012. Comprehensive review: Is it better to use the Trendelenburg position or passive leg raising for the initial treatment of hypovolemia? *Journal of Clinical Anesthesia*, 24(8), 688–674.

GEMS, 2015
Snyder DR, American Geriatrics Society and National Association of Emergency Medical Technicians (US), 2015. *Geriatric Education for Emergency Medical Services: (GEMS)*. 2nd ed. Burlington, MA: Jones & Bartlett Learning.

Gibbs, 1988
Gibbs G, 1988. *Learning by Doing: A Guide to Teaching and Learning Methods*. London: FEU.

Ginsberg, 2004
Ginsberg L, 2004. *Lecture Notes: Neurology*. 8th ed. Oxford: Wiley-Blackwell.

Gitelman, 2008
Gitelman A, Hishmeh S, Morelli BN et al., 2008. Cauda equina syndrome: A comprehensive review. *American Journal of Orthopedics*, 37(11), 556–562.

GMC, 2018a
General Medical Council, 2018. *Decision Making and Consent*. Available at: https://www.gmc-uk.org/-/media/ethical-guidance/related-pdf-items/consent-draft-guidance/consent-draft-guidance.pdf?la=en&hash=920B435518160455840473FA316D7BEEBDFBB332 [Accessed: 30 December 2018].

GMC, 2018b
General Medical Council, 2018. *Cardiopulmonary Resuscitation (CPR)*. Available at: https://www.gmc-uk.org/ethical-guidance/ethical-guidance-for-doctors/treatment-and-care-towards-the-end-of-life/cardiopulmonary-resuscitation-cpr [Accessed: 31 December 2018].

GMC, 2019
General Medical Council, 2019. *Disclosing Patients' Personal Information: A framework*. Available at: https://www.gmc-uk.org/ethical-guidance/ethical-guidance-for-doctors/confidentiality/disclosing-patients-personal-information-a-framework#paragraph-17 [Accessed: 4 January 2019].

Goldberg, 2007
Goldberg A, Southern DA, Galbraith PD et al., 2007. Coronary dominance and prognosis of patients with acute coronary syndrome. *American Heart Journal*, 154(6), 1116–1122.

Golden, 1997
Golden FSC, David GC and Tipton MJ et al., 1997. *Review of Rescue and Immediate Post-immersion Problems: A Medical/Ergonomic Viewpoint*. Sudbury: HSE Books.

References

Gold Standards Framework, 2018
The Gold Standards Framework, 2018. *Advanced Care Planning*. Available at: http://www.goldstandardsframework.org.uk/advance-care-planning [Accessed: 31 December 2018].

Gowens, 2018
Gowens P et al., 2018. Consensus statement: A framework for safe and effective intubation by paramedics. *British Paramedic Journal*, 3(1), 23–27.

Graveling, 2009
Graveling AJ and Frier BM, 2009. Hypoglycaemia: An overview. *Primary Care Diabetes*, 3(3), 131–139.

Gray, 2013
Gray A, Ward K, Lees F et al., 2013. The epidemiology of adults with severe sepsis and septic shock in Scottish emergency departments. *Emergency Medicine Journal*, 30(5), 397–401.

Greaves, 2008
Greaves I, Porter K, Ryan J et al., 2008. *Trauma Care Manual*. 2nd ed. London: Hodder Arnold.

Greaves, 2010
Greaves I, Porter K and Smith J, 2010. *Practical Prehospital Care: The Principles and Practice of Immediate Care*. London: Churchill Livingstone.

Greaves, 2019
Greaves I, Porter K and Wright C, 2019. *Trauma Care Pre-Hospital Manual*. Boca Raton: CRC Press.

Green and Tones, 2015
Green J, Tones K, Cross R and Woodall J, 2015. *Health Promotion*. London: Sage Publications.

Gregory, 2010a
Gregory P, Ward A and Sanders MJ, 2010. *Sanders' Paramedic Textbook*. Edinburgh: Mosby.

Gregory, 2010b
Gregory P, 2010. *Manual of Clinical Paramedic Procedures*. Chichester: Wiley-Blackwell.

Gruenberg, 2008
Gruenberg B, 2008. *Birth Emergency Skills Training: Manual for Out-Of-Hospital Midwives*. Duncannon: Birth Muse Press.

Guly, 2010
Guly HR, Bouamra O, Little R et al., 2010. Testing the validity of the ATLS classification of hypovolaemic shock. *Resuscitation*, 81(9), 1142–1147.

Gunderson, 2011
Gunderson JG, 2011. Borderline personality disorder. *New England Journal of Medicine*, 364(21), 2037–2042.

Gupta, 2009
Gupta A, Taly AB, Srivastava A et al., 2009. Non-traumatic spinal cord lesions: Epidemiology, complications, neurological and functional outcome of rehabilitation. *Spinal Cord*, 47(4), 307–311.

Haider, 2009
Haider AH et al., 2009. Mechanism of injury predicts patient mortality and impairment after blunt trauma, *Journal of Surgical Research*, 153(1), 138–142.

Halliwell, 2011
Halliwell D, Jones P, Ryan L and Clark R, 2011. The revision of the primary survey: A 2011 review. *Journal of Paramedic Practice*, 3(7), 366–374.

Hammell, 2009
Hammell CL and Henning JD, 2009. Prehospital management of severe traumatic brain injury. *BMJ*, 338, b1683.

Harbison, 2003
Harbison J, Hossain O, Jenkinson D et al., 2003. Diagnostic accuracy of stroke referrals from primary care, emergency room physicians, and ambulance staff using the face arm speech test. *Stroke*, 34(1), 71–76.

Harrison, 2007
Harrison P, 2007. *Managing Spinal Cord Injury: The First 48 Hours*. Milton Keynes: Spinal Injuries Association.

Hart, 2006
Hart CA and Thomson APJ, 2006. Meningococcal disease and its management in children. *BMJ*, 333(7570), 685–690.

Hartwell, 2016
Hartwell Medical, 2016. *Evac-U-Splint Application Guidelines*. Available at: https://www.hartwellmedical.com/pdfs/EVAC-U-SPLINT_AppGuide_AGEV_10-16.pdf [Accessed: 14 February 2019].

Hasler, 2011a
Hasler RM, Nuesch E, Jüni P et al., 2011. Systolic blood pressure below 110 mmHg is associated with increased mortality in blunt major trauma patients: Multicentre cohort study. *Resuscitation*, 82(9), 1202–1207.

Hasler, 2011b
Hasler RM, Exadaktylos AK, Bouamra O et al., 2011. Epidemiology and predictors of spinal injury in adult major

References

trauma patients: European cohort study. *European Spine Journal*, 20(12), 2174–2180.

Hasler, 2012
Hasler RM, Nuesch E, Jüni P et al., 2012. Systolic blood pressure below 110 mmHg is associated with increased mortality in penetrating major trauma patients: multicentre cohort study. *Resuscitation*, 83(4), 476–481.

Hazardous Waste Regulations 2005
UK Government, 2005. *The Hazardous Waste (England and Wales) Regulations 2005*. Available at: http://www.legislation.gov.uk/uksi/2005/894/contents/made [Accessed: July 2019].

HC, 2009
The Healthcare Commission, 2009. *Investigation into Mid Staffordshire NHS Foundation Trust*. Available at: http://webarchive.nationalarchives.gov.uk/20110504135228/http://www.cqc.org.uk/_db/_documents/investigation_into_mid_staffordshire_nhs_foundation_trust.pdf [Accessed: 31 July 2019].

HCPC, 2014
Health and Care Professions Council, 2014. *Standards of Proficiency – Paramedics*. Available at: http://www.hcpc-uk.org.uk/publications/standards/index.asp?id=48%20 [Accessed: 27 December 2018].

HCPC, 2016
Health and Care Professions Council, 2016. *Standards of Conduct, Performance and Ethics*. Available at: https://www.hcpc-uk.org/standards/standards-of-conduct-performance-and-ethics/ [Accessed: 28 December 2018].

HCPC, 2018
Health and Care Professions Council, 2018. *New Threshold for Paramedic Registration*. Available at: https://www.hcpc-uk.org/news-and-events/blog/2018/new-threshold-for-paramedic-registration/ [Accessed: 3 January 2019].

Health and Safety at Work etc. Act 1974
UK Government, 1974. *Health and Safety at Work etc. Act 1974*. Available at: http://www.legislation.gov.uk/ukpga/1974/37 [Accessed: 27 December 2014].

Health and Social Care Act 2008
UK Government, 2008. *Health and Social Care Act 2008*. Available at: http://www.legislation.gov.uk/ukpga/2008/14/contents [Accessed: 27 July 2019].

Hellesen, 2018
Hellesen A, Bratland E and Husebye, ES, 2018. Autoimmune Addison's disease – An update on pathogenesis. *Annales d'Endocrinologie*, 79(3), 157–163.

Helm, 2003
Helm M, Schuster R, Hauke J et al., 2003. Tight control of prehospital ventilation by capnography in major trauma victims. *British Journal of Anaesthesia*, 90(3), 327–332.

Hettiaratchy, 2004
Hettiaratchy S and Papini R, 2004. Initial management of a major burn: II – assessment and resuscitation. *BMJ*, 329(7457), 101–103.

Hickin, 2015
Hickin S, Renshaw J, Williams R and Patel H, 2015. *Respiratory System*. London: Mosby.

Hinkelbein, 2007
Hinkelbein J, Genzwuerker HV, Sogl R et al., 2007. Effect of nail polish on oxygen saturation determined by pulse oximetry in critically ill patients. *Resuscitation*, 72(1), 82–91.

HMFSIPS, 1998
HM Fire Service Inspectorate Publications Section, 1998. *Fire Service Manual*. Vol. 1, No. 1. London: The Stationery Office.

HMG, 2006
HM Government, 2006. *Making Your Premises Safe*. Available at: https://www.gov.uk/government/publications/making-your-premises-safe-from-fire [Accessed: 28 July 2019].

HMG, 2018a
HM Government, 2018. *CONTEST: The United Kingdom's Strategy for Countering Terrorism*. Available at: https://assets.publishing.service.gov.uk/government/uploads/system/uploads/attachment_data/file/716907/140618_CCS207_CCS0218929798-1_CONTEST_3.0_WEB.pdf [Accessed: 4 January 2019].

HMG, 2018b
HM Government, 2018. *Health and Safety Executive*. Available at: https://www.gov.uk/government/organisations/health-and-safety-executive [Accessed: 23 December 2018].

HMG, 2018c
HM Government, 2018. *Public Health England: About us*. Available at: https://www.gov.uk/government/organisations/public-health-england/about [Accessed: 23 December 2018].

References

HMG, 2018d
HM Government, 2018. *Definition of Disability under the Equality Act 2010*. Available at: https://www.gov.uk/definition-of-disability-under-equality-act-2010 [Accessed: 16 December 2018].

HMG, 2018e
HM Government, 2018. *Disability Rights*. Available at: https://www.gov.uk/rights-disabled-person [Accessed: 16 December 2018].

Hodgetts, 2006
Hodgetts TJ, Mahoney PF, Russell MQ et al., 2006. ABC to <C>ABC: Redefining the military trauma paradigm. *Emergency Medicine Journal*, 23(10), 745–746.

Holland, 2011
Holland K, 2011. *Factsheet: Learning disabilities*. Available at: http://www.bild.org.uk/EasySiteWeb/GatewayLink.aspx?alId=2522 [Accessed: 14 July 2019].

Holt, 2010
Holt TA, 2010. *ABC of Diabetes*. 6th ed. Chichester: Wiley-Blackwell/BMJ.

Home Office, 2015
Home Office, 2015. *Initial Operational Repsonse to a CBRN Incident*. Available at: https://www.jesip.org.uk/uploads/media/pdf/CBRN%20JOPs/IOR_Guidance_V2_July_2015.pdf [Accessed 5 January 2019].

Home Office, 2017
Home Office, 2017. *Fire Statistics: England April 2015 to March 2016*. Available at: https://assets.publishing.service.gov.uk/government/uploads/system/uploads/attachment_data/file/611182/fire-statistics-england-1516-hosb0517.pdf [Accessed: 16 February 2019].

Hosker, 2017
Hosker C, 2017. *Hypoactive Delirium*. Available at: https://www.bmj.com/content/357/bmj.j2047.full [Accessed: 2 January 2019].

HospiceUK, 2018
HospiceUK, 2018. *What is Hospice Care?* Available at: https://www.hospiceuk.org/about-hospice-care/what-is-hospice-care [Accessed: 31 December 2018].

Howlett, 2011
Howlett JG, 2011. Acute heart failure: Sections learned so far. *Canadian Journal of Cardiology*, 27(3), 284–295.

HPA, 2009a
Health Protection Agency, 2009. *Generic Incident Management*. Available at: http://webarchive.nationalarchives.gov.uk/20140714084352/http://www.hpa.org.uk/webc/hpawebfile/hpaweb_c/1194947395416 [Accessed: 5 July 2019].

HPA, 2009b
Health Protection Agency, 2009. *ORCHIDS Project: Optimisation through research of chemical incident decontamination systems*. Available at: http://www.orchidsproject.eu/index.html [Accessed: 6 July 2019].

HSCIC, 2014a
Health and Social Care Information Centre, 2014. *Caldicott Guardians*. Available at: http://systems.hscic.gov.uk/infogov/caldicott [Accessed: 8 July 2019].

HSCIC, 2014b
Health and Social Care Information Centre, 2014. *Accident and Emergency Attendances in England – 2012–13*. Available at: http://hscic.gov.uk/catalogue/pub13464/acci-emer-atte-eng-2012-13-data.xls [Accessed: 23 July 2019].

HSE, 2003
Health and Safety Executive, 2003. *The Principles of Good Manual Handling: Achieving a consensus*. Available at: http://www.hse.gov.uk/research/rrpdf/rr097.pdf [Accessed: 21 July 2019].

HSE, 2009a
Health and Safety Executive, 2009. *Health and Safety Law*. Available at: http://www.hse.gov.uk/pubns/law.pdf [Accessed: 29 July 2019].

HSE, 2009b
Health and Safety Executive, 2009. *Evidence-based review of the Current Guidance on First Aid Measures for Suspension Trauma*. Available at: http://www.hse.gov.uk/research/rrpdf/rr708.pdf [Accessed: 20 July 2019].

HSE, 2011
Health and Safety Executive, 2011. *Risk Factors Associated with Pushing and Pulling Loads*. Available at: http://www.hse.gov.uk/msd/pushpull/risks.htm [Accessed: 21 July 2019].

HSE, 2012
Health and Safety Executive, 2012. *Manual Handling at Work*. Available at: http://www.hse.gov.uk/pubns/indg143.pdf [Accessed: 21 July 2019].

References

HSE, 2013a
Health and Safety Executive, 2013. *Oxygen Use in the Workplace*. Available at: http://www.hse.gov.uk/pubns/indg459.pdf [Accessed: 20 September 2018].

HSE, 2013b
Health and Safety Executive, 2013. *Managing for Health and Safety*. Available at: http://www.hse.gov.uk/pubns/priced/hsg65.pdf [Accessed: 29 July 2019].

HSE, 2013c
Health and Safety Executive, 2013. *Control of Substances Hazardous to Health: Approved Code of Practice*. Available at: http://www.hse.gov.uk/pubns/priced/l5.pdf [Accessed: 29 July 2019].

HSE, 2013d
Health and Safety Executive, 2013. *Personal Protective Equipment (PPE) at Work*. Available at: http://www.hse.gov.uk/pubns/indg174.pdf [Accessed: 29 July 2019].

HSE, 2014a
Health and Safety Executive, 2014. *Safe Use of Work Equipment*. Available at: http://www.hse.gov.uk/pubns/priced/l22.pdf [Accessed: 29 July 2019].

HSE, 2014b
Health and Safety Executive, 2014. *The Health and Safety Toolbox*. Available at: http://www.hse.gov.uk/pubns/books/hsg268.htm [Accessed: 7 December 2018].

HSE, 2015a
Health and Safety Executive, 2015. *Managing the Risks From Skin Exposure.* Available at: http://www.hse.gov.uk/skin/professional/managerisk.htm [Accessed: 23 July 2019].

HSE, 2015b
Health and Safety Executive, 2015. *Methods of Decontamination*. Available at: http://www.hse.gov.uk/biosafety/blood-borne-viruses/methods-of-decontamination.htm [Accessed: 28 July 2019].

HSE, 2015c
Health and Safety Executive, 2015. *Sharps Injuries*. Available at: http://www.hse.gov.uk/healthservices/needlesticks/ [Accessed: 28 July 2019].

HSE, 2015d
Health and Safety Executive, 2015. *Laundry Treatment at High and Low Temperatures*. Available at: http://www.hse.gov.uk/biosafety/blood-borne-viruses/laundry-treatments.htm [Accessed: 28 July 2019].

HSE, 2016
Health and Safety Executive, 2016. *Manual Handling Operations Regulations 1992: Guidance on Regulations*. Available at: http://www.hse.gov.uk/pubns/priced/l23.pdf [Accessed: 10 December 2018].

HSE, 2017a
Health and Safety Executive, 2017. *Tackling Work-related Stress Using the Management Standards Approach*. Available at: http://www.hse.gov.uk/pubns/wbk01.pdf [Accessed: 27 December 2018].

HSE, 2017b
Health and Safety Executive, 2017. *Carriage of Dangerous Goods Manual*. Available at: http://www.hse.gov.uk/cdg/manual/index.htm [Accessed: 28 December 2018].

HSE, 2018a
Health and Safety Executive, 2018. *Risk – Controlling the risks in the workplace*. Available at: http://www.hse.gov.uk/risk/controlling-risks.htm [Accessed: 23 December 2018].

HSE, 2018b
Health and Safety Executive, 2018. *Decide Who Might Be Harmed and How*. Available at: http://www.hse.gov.uk/risk/decide-who-might-be-harmed.htm [Accessed: 23 December 2018].

HSE, 2018c
Health and Safety Executive, 2018. *Evaluate the Risks*. Available at: http://www.hse.gov.uk/risk/evaluate-the-risks.htm [Accessed: 23 December 2018].

HSE, 2018d
Health and Safety Executive, 2018. *Management of Risk When Planning Work: The right priorities*. Available at: http://www.hse.gov.uk/construction/lwit/assets/downloads/hierarchy-risk-controls.pdf [Accessed: 23 December 2018].

HSE, 2018e
Health and Safety Executive, 2018. *Record Your Significant Findings*. Available at: http://www.hse.gov.uk/risk/record-your-findings-and-implement-them.htm [Accessed: 23 December 2018].

HSE, 2018f
Health and Safety Executive, 2018. *Review Your Risk Assessment and Update if Necessary*. Available at: http://www.hse.gov.uk/risk/review-your-assessment.htm [Accessed: 23 December 2018].

References

HSE, 2018g
Health and Safety Executive, 2018. *Managing Legionella in Hot and Cold Water Systems*. Available at: http://www.hse.gov.uk/healthservices/legionella.htm [Accessed: 27 December 2018].

HSE, 2018h
Health and Safety Executive, 2018. *Signs of Stress*. Available at: http://www.hse.gov.uk/stress/signs.htm [Accessed: 2 December 2018].

HSE, 2019a
HSE, 2019. *The Ambulance Service*. London: HSE. Available at: https://www.hse.gov.uk/healthservices/casestudies/ambulance.htm [Accessed: 29 July 2019].

HSE, 2019b
HSE, 2019. *Work-related Contact Dermatitis in the Health Services*. London: HSE. Available at: https://www.hse.gov.uk/skin/employ/highrisk/healthcare.htm [Accessed: 29 July 2019].

Human Rights Act 1988
UK Government 1988, *Human Rights Act 1998*. Available at: http://www.legislation.gov.uk/ukpga/1998/42/contents [Accessed: 31 July 2019].

Hüpfl, 2010
Hüpfl M, Selig HF and Nagele P, 2010. Chest-compression-only versus standard cardiopulmonary resuscitation: A meta-analysis. *The Lancet*, 376(9752), 1552–1557.

Husebye, 2009
Husebye E and Løvås K, 2009. Pathogenesis of primary adrenal insufficiency. *Best Practice & Research Clinical Endocrinology & Metabolism*, 23(2), 147–157.

Iacono, 2005
Iacono L and Lyons K, 2005. Making GCS as easy as 1, 2, 3, 4, 5, 6. *Journal of Trauma Nursing*, 12(3), 77–81.

Ibanez, 2018
Ibanez B, James S, Agewall, S et al., 2018. 2017 ESC Guidelines for the management of acute myocardial infarction in patients presenting with ST-segment elevation. The Task Force for the management of acute myocardial infarction in patients presenting with ST-segment elevation of the European Society of Cardiology (ESC). *European Heart Journal*, 39(2), 119–177.

Idris, 2003
Idris AH, Berg RA, Bierens J et al., 2003. Recommended guidelines for uniform reporting of data from drowning. *Circulation*, 108(20), 2565–2574.

Intersurgical, 2017
Intersurgical, 2017. *I-gel® Aupraglottic Airway from Intersurgical: An introduction*. Available at: https://www.youtube.com/watch?time_continue=216&v=Z0962B8axAY [Accessed: 3 December 2018].

ILAE, 1993
International League Against Epilepsy, 1993. Guidelines for epidemiologic studies on epilepsy. *Epilepsia*, 34(4), 592–596.

Innes, 2018
Innes JA, Dover AR, Fairhurst K, Britton R and Danielson E, 2018. *Macleod's Clinical Examination*. 14th ed. Edinburgh: Elsevier.

Ireland, 2011
Ireland S, Endacott R, Cameron P et al., 2011. The incidence and significance of accidental hypothermia in major trauma – A prospective observational study. *Resuscitation*, 82(3), 300–306.

ISWP, 2016
Intercollegiate Stroke Working Party, 2016. *National Clinical Guideline for Stroke*. Available at: https://www.strokeaudit.org/SupportFiles/Documents/Guidelines/2016-National-Clinical-Guideline-for-Stroke-5t-(1).aspx [Accessed: 4 December 2018].

Jalo, 2009
Jalo M, Magennis P, Ridout F et al., 2009. The second UK National Facial Injury Survey: The demography, aetiology, nature of injury and treatment. *British Journal of Oral and Maxillofacial Surgery*, 47(7), e58.

James, 2011
James B, 2011. *Lecture Notes: Ophthalmology*. 11th ed. Chichester: Wiley-Blackwell.

Jasper, 2003
Jasper M, 2003. *Beginning Reflective Practice*. Cheltenham: Nelson Thornes.

JCO, 2010
Judicial Communications Office, 2010. *Coroner's Inquests into the London Bombings of 7 July 2005: Hearing transcripts*. Available at: http://webarchive.nationalarchives.gov.uk/20120216072438/http:/7julyinquests.independent.gov.uk/hearing_transcripts/09122010am.htm [Accessed: 28 July 2019].

Jenkins, 2008
Jenkins JL, McCarthy M, Sauer L et al., 2008. Mass-casualty triage: Time for an evidence-based approach. *Prehospital Disaster Medicine*, 23(1), 3–8.

References

JESIP, 2016
Joint Emergency Services Interoperability Programme, 2016. Joint Doctrine: The interoperability framework. Available at: https://www.jesip.org.uk/joint-doctrine [Accessed: 21 December 2018].

JESIP, 2019
JESIP, 2019. *JESIP: The programme*. Available at: https://www.jesip.org.uk/jesip-the-programme [Accessed: 3 January 2018].

Johns, 1994
Johns C, 1994. Nuances of reflection. *Journal of Clinical Nursing*, 3(2), 71–75.

Johnson, 2004
Johnson S and Henderson SO, 2004. Myth: The Trendelenburg position improves circulation in cases of shock. *CJEM*, 6(1), 48–49.

Johnson, 2012
Johnson G and Hill-Smith I, 2012. *The Minor Illness Manual*. London: Radcliffe Publishing.

Jolles, 2002
Jolles S, 2002. Paul Langerhans. *Journal of Clinical Pathology*, 55(4), 243.

Jorolemon, 2018
Jorolemon MR and Krywko DM, 2018. Blast injuries. *StatPearls*, 2018 Jan–. Available at: https://www.ncbi.nlm.nih.gov/books/NBK430914/ [Accessed: 17 February 2019].

JRCALC, 2019
Joint Royal Colleges Ambulance Liaison Committee and Association of Ambulance Chief Executives, 2019. *JRCALC Clinical Guidelines 2019*. Bridgwater: Class Professional Publishing.

Judd, 1993
Judd C and Park B, 1993. Definition and assessment of accuracy in social stereotypes. *Psychological Review*, 100(1), 109–128.

Kaeser, 2010
Kaeser P-F and Kawasaki A, 2010. Disorders of pupillary structure and function. *Neurologic Clinics*, 28(3), 657–677.

Kalson, 2012
Kalson NS, Jenks T, Woodford M et al., 2012. Burns represent a significant proportion of the total serious trauma workload in England and Wales. *Burns: Journal of the International Society for Burn Injuries*, 38(3), 330–339.

Kanter, 2013
Kanter J and Kruse-Jarres R, 2013. Management of sickle cell disease from childhood through adulthood. *Blood Reviews*, 27(6), 279–287.

Kapit, 2001
Kapit W and Elson LM, 2001. *The Anatomy Coloring Book*. 3rd ed. London: Benjamin Cummings.

Kauffman, 2014
Kauffman M, 2014. *History and Physical Examination: A Common Sense Approach*. Burlington, MA: Jones & Bartlett Learning.

Kehoe, 2015
Kehoe A, Smith JE, Edwards A et al., 2015. The changing face of major trauma in the UK. *Emergency Medicine Journal*, 32(12), 911–915.

Kelder, 2011
Kelder JC, Cramer MJ, van Wijngaarden J et al., 2011. The diagnostic value of physical examination and additional testing in primary care patients with suspected heart failure. *Circulation*, 124(25), 2865–2873.

Kelly, 2004
Kelly AC, Upex A and Bateman DN, 2004. Comparison of consciousness level assessment in the poisoned patient using the alert/verbal/painful/unresponsive scale and the Glasgow Coma Scale. *Annals of Emergency Medicine*, 44(2), 108–113.

Kerber, 2012
Kerber RE, 2012. Hands-on defibrillation – the end of 'I'm clear, you're clear, we're all clear'? *Journal of the American Heart Association*, 1(5), 1–3.

Kilner, 2002
Kilner T, 2002. Triage decisions of prehospital emergency health care providers, using a multiple casualty scenario paper exercise. *Emergency Medicine Journal*, 19(4), 348–353.

King, 2014
King D, Morton R and Bevan C, 2014. How to use capillary refill time. *Archives of Disease in Childhood – Education & Practice Edition*, 99(3), 111–116.

Kligfield, 2007
Kligfield P, Gettes LS, Bailey JJ et al., 2007. Recommendations for the standardization and interpretation of the electrocardiogram. Part I: the electrocardiogram and its technology. A scientific statement from the American Heart Association Electrocardiography and Arrhythmias Committee, Council on Clinical Cardiology; the American

References

College of Cardiology Foundation; and the Heart Rhythm Society, endorsed by the International Society for Computerized Electrocardiology. *Journal of the American College of Cardiology*, 49(10), 1109–1127.

Knight, 2008a
Knight J and Nigam Y, 2008. Exploring the anatomy and physiology of ageing. Part 1 – the cardiovascular system. *Nursing Times*, 104(31), 26–27.

Knight, 2008b
Knight J and Nigam Y, 2008. Exploring the anatomy and physiology of ageing. Part 10 – muscles and bone. *Nursing Times*, 104(48), 22–23.

Knight, 2008c
Knight J and Nigam Y, 2008. Exploring the anatomy and physiology of ageing. Part 5 – the nervous system. *Nursing Times*, 104(35), 18–19.

Knight, 2017
Knight J and Nigam Y, 2017. Anatomy and physiology of ageing 2: the respiratory system. *Nursing Times* [online], 113(3), 53–55. Available at: https://www.nursingtimes.net/roles/older-people-nurses/anatomy-and-physiology-of-ageing-2-the-respiratory-system/7016004.article [Accessed: 15 December 2018].

Knops, 2011
Knops SP, Schep NW, Spoor CW et al., 2011. Comparison of three different pelvic circumferential compression devices: A biomechanical cadaver study. *Journal of Bone and Joint Surgery*, 93(3), 230–240.

Kodali, 2013
Kodali BS, 2013. Capnography outside the operating rooms. *Anesthesiology*, 118(1), 192–201.

Konstantinides, 2014
Konstantinides SV, Torbicki A, Agnelli G, et al., 2014. 2014 ESC Guidelines on the diagnosis and management of acute pulmonary embolism: The Task Force for the Diagnosis and Management of Acute Pulmonary Embolism of the European Society of Cardiology (ESC). Endorsed by the European Respiratory Society (ERS). *European Heart Journal*, 35(43), 3033–3069k.

Kovacs, 2011
Kovacs G and Law JA, 2011. *Airway Management in Emergencies*. 2nd ed. Shelton: McGraw-Hill Medical.

Krassioukov, 2012
Krassioukov A, 2012. Autonomic dysreflexia. *Clinical Journal of Sport Medicine*, 22(1), 39–45.

Krell, 2006
Krell J, McCoy M, Sparto P et al., 2006. Comparison of the Ferno Scoop Stretcher with the long backboard for spinal immobilization. *Prehospital Emergency Care*, 10(1), 46–51.

Krous, 2010
Krous H, 2010. Sudden unexpected death in infancy and the dilemma of defining the sudden infant death syndrome. *Current Pediatric Reviews*, 6(1), 5–12.

Kuhajda, 2014
Kuhajda I, Zarogoulidis K, Kougioumtzi I et al., 2014. Penetrating trauma. *Journal of Thoracic Disease*, 6(Suppl 4), 461–465.

Kumar, 2012
Kumar P and Clark M, 2012. *Kumar And Clark's Clinical Medicine*, 8th ed. Edinburgh: Saunders.

Kusakabe, 2013
Kusakabe T, 2013. Cauda equina syndrome. *Orthopaedics and Trauma*, 27(4), 215–219.

Lange, 2010
Lange RT, Iverson GL, Brubacher JR et al., 2010. Effect of blood alcohol level on Glasgow Coma Scale scores following traumatic brain injury. *Brain Injury*, 24(7/8), 919–927.

Layon, 2009
Layon AJ and Modell JH, 2009. Drowning: Update 2009. *Anesthesiology*, 110(6), 1390–1401.

Leath, 2015
Leath C and Lowery WJ, 2017. Assessment of acute abdomen. *BMJ Best Practice*. Available at: https://bestpractice.bmj.com/topics/en-gb/503 [Accessed: 12 April 2019].

Le Fort, 1901
Le Fort, 1901. Etude experimentale sur les fractures de la machoire superieure.

Lee, 2007a
Lee C, Revell M, Porter K et al., 2007. The prehospital management of chest injuries: A consensus statement. Faculty of Pre-hospital Care, Royal College of Surgeons of Edinburgh. *Emergency Medicine Journal*, 24(3), 220–224.

Lee, 2007b
Lee C, Porter KM and Hodgetts TJ, 2007. Tourniquet use in the civilian prehospital setting. *Emergency Medicine Journal*, 24(8), 584–587.

Lee, 2007c
Lee C and Porter K, 2007. The prehospital management of pelvic fractures. *Emergency Medicine Journal*, 24(2), 130–133.

Lee, 2011
Lee JK and Vadas P, 2011. Anaphylaxis: mechanisms and management. *Clinical & Experimental Allergy*, 41(7), 923–938.

Leech, 2016
Leech C et al., 2016. The pre-hospital management of life-threatening chest injuries: A consensus statement. *Trauma*, 19(1), 54–62.

Leenen, 2010
Leenen L, 2010. Pelvic fractures: Soft tissue trauma. *European Journal of Trauma and Emergency Surgery*, 36(2), 117–123.

Leigh-Smith, 2005
Leigh-Smith S and Harris T, 2005. Tension pneumothorax – Time for a re-think? *Emergency Medicine Journal*, 22(1), 8–16.

Lencean, 2003
Lencean, SM, 2003. Classification of spinal injuries based on the essential traumatic spinal mechanisms, *Spinal Cord*, 41, 385–396.

Lerner, 2011
Lerner EB et al., 2011. Does mechanism of injury predict trauma center need? *Prehospital Emergency Care*, 15(4), 518–525.

Levitan, 2000
Levitan RM, Sather SD and Ochroch EA, 2000. Demystifying direct laryngoscopy and intubation. *Hospital Physician*, 36(5), 47–56.

Levitan, 2006
Levitan RM, Kinkle WC, Levin WJ et al., 2006. Laryngeal view during laryngoscopy: a randomized trial comparing cricoid pressure, backward-upward-rightward pressure, and bimanual laryngoscopy. *Annals of Emergency Medicine*, 47(6), 548–555.

Lewin, 2008
Lewin J and Maconochie I, 2008. Capillary refill time in adults. *Emergency Medicine Journal*, 25(6), 325–326.

Lipman, 2014
Lipman GS, Eifling K, Ellis MA, Gaudio, FG, Otten, EM and Grissom CK, 2014. Wilderness Medical Society practice guidelines for the prevention and treatment of heat-related illness: 2014 update. *Wilderness & Environmental Medicine*, 25(4), 55–65.

Lisk, 2014
Lisk R and Yeong K, 2014. Reducing mortality from hip fractures: a systematic quality improvement programme. *BMJ Quality Improvement Reports*, 3(1), 1–6.

Lissauer, 2007
Lissauer T and Clayden G, 2007. *Illustrated Textbook of Paediatrics*. 3rd ed. Edinburgh: Mosby.

Lockey, 2013
Lockey DJ, Lyon RM and Davies GE, 2013. Development of a simple algorithm to guide the effective management of traumatic cardiac arrest. *Resuscitation*, 84(6), 738–742.

LOLER, 1998
UK Government, 1998. *The Lifting Operations and Lifting Equipment Regulations*. Available at: http://www.legislation.gov.uk/uksi/1998/2307/contents/made [Accessed: 21 August 2014].

Longmore, 2014
Longmore M, Wilkinson I, Baldwin A et al., 2014. *Oxford Handbook of Clinical Medicine*. 9th ed. Oxford: Oxford University Press.

Lonnecker, 2001
Lonnecker S and Schoder V, 2001. Hypothermia after burn injury – influence of pre-hospital management. *Der Chirurg*, 72(2), 164–167.

Lord, 2005
Lord SR and Davis PR, 2005. Drowning, near drowning and immersion syndrome. *Journal of the Royal Army Medical Corps*, 151(4), 250–255.

Louwen, 2016
Louwen F, Daviss B, Johnson K and Reitter A, 2016. Does breech delivery in an upright position instead of on the back improve outcomes and avoid cesareans? *International Journal of Obstetrics and Gynaecology*, 136(2), 151–161.

Lunt, 2010
Lunt H, Florkowski C, Bignall M et al., 2010. Capillary glucose meter accuracy and sources of error in the ambulatory setting. *New Zealand Medical Journal*, 123(1310), 74–85.

Lupsa, 2014
Lupsa BC and Inzucchi SE, 2014. Diabetic ketoacidosis and hyperosmolar hyperglycemic syndrome. In: Loriaux L (ed.), *Endocrine Emergencies*. Totowa, NJ: Humana Press, 15–31.

MacDuff, 2010
MacDuff A, Arnold A and Harvey J, 2010. Management of spontaneous pneumothorax: British Thoracic Society

References

pleural disease guideline 2010. *Thorax*, 65(Supplement 2), ii18–ii31.

Macfarlane, 2014
Macfarlane A and Dorkenoo E, 2014. *Female Genital Mutilation in England and Wales: updated statistical estimates of the numbers of affected women living in England and Wales and girls at risk. Interim report on provisional estimates*. Available at: http://openaccess.city.ac.uk/3865/1/Female%20Genital%20Mutilation%20in%20England%20and%20Wales.pdf [Accessed: 16 July 2019].

Mackway-Jones, 2012
Mackway-Jones K, Carley S and Advanced Life Support Group, 2012. *Major Incident Medical Management and Support: The Practical Approach at the Scene*. Chichester: Wiley-Blackwell.

Macleod, 2005
Douglas G, Nicol EF, Robertson C et al., 2005. *Macleod's Clinical Examination*. 11th ed. Edinburgh: Elsevier Churchill Livingstone.

Maconochie, 2015
Maconochie IK, Bingham R, Eich C et al., 2015. European resuscitation council guidelines for resuscitation 2015. Section 6. Paediatric life support. *Resuscitation*, 95, 223–248.

Magill-Cuerden, 2011
Magill-Cuerden J and MacDonald S, 2011. *Mayes' Midwifery: A Textbook for Midwives*. Edinburgh: Bailliere-Tindall.

Magowan, 2014
Magowan B, Owen P and Thomson A, 2014. *Clinical Obstetrics and Gynaecology*. Oxford: Elsevier Health Services.

Magner, 2004
Magner JJ, 2004. Heart failure. *British Journal of Anaesthesia*, 93(1), 74–85.

Mahon, 2013
Mahon A, Jenkins K, and Burnapp L, 2013. *Oxford Handbook of Renal Nursing*. Oxford: Oxford University Press.

Maissan, 2018
Maissan IM, Ketelaars R, Vlottes B, Hoeks SE, Hartog D and Stolker R, 2018. Increase in intracranial pressure by application of a rigid cervical collar: A pilot study in healthy volunteers. *European Journal of Emergency Medicine*, 25(6), 24–28.

Management of Health and Safety at Work Regulations 1999
UK Government, 1999. *The Management of Health and Safety at Work Regulations 1999*. Available at: http://www.legislation.gov.uk/uksi/1999/3242/contents/made [Accessed: 29 July 2019].

Mancia, 2013
Mancia G, Fagard R, Narkiewicz K et al., 2013. 2013 ESH/ESC Guidelines for the management of arterial hypertension. The Task Force for the Management of Arterial Hypertension of the European Society of Hypertension (ESH) and of the European Society of Cardiology (ESC). *European Heart Journal*, 34(28), 2159–2219.

Mangar Health, 2016
Mangar Health, 2016. *Camel User Instructions*. Available at: https://mangarhealth.com/uk/wp-content/uploads/sites/2/2016/09/M10337-Issue-5-Camel-User-Instructions.pdf [Accessed 5 January 2019].

Mangar International, 2016
Mangar International, 2016. *ELK User Instructions and Warranty*. Available at: https://mangarhealth.com/uk/wp-content/uploads/sites/2/2016/09/ME0117-Issue-7-ELK-User-Instructions.pdf [Accessed: 20 December 2014].

Mansfield, 2018
Mansfield A, Association of Ambulance Chief Executives, and Joint Royal Colleges Ambulance Liaison Committee, 2018. *Emergency Birth in the Community*. Bridgwater: Class Professional Publishing.

Manual Handling Operations Regulations 1992
UK Government, 1992. *The Manual Handling Operations Regulations 1992*. Available at: http://www.hse.gov.uk/pubns/priced/l23.pdf [Accessed: 29 December 2014].

Marie Curie, 2014
Marie Curie, 2014. *Stages of Grief and Grieving in Your Own Way*. Available at: https://www.mariecurie.org.uk/help/support/bereaved-family-friends/dealing-grief/grieving-your-way [Accessed: 1 January 2019].

Marie Curie, 2015
Marie Curie, 2015. *An Answer to the Question of What is a Good Death?* Available at: https://www.mariecurie.org.uk/blog/what-is-a-good-death/48655 [Accessed: 31 December 2018].

Marie Curie, 2017
Marie Curie, 2017. *Spirituality at the End of Life*. Available at: https://www.mariecurie.org.uk/professionals/palliative-care-knowledge-zone/individual-needs/spirituality-end-life [Accessed: 31 December 2018].

Marie Curie, 2018a
Marie Curie, 2018. *What are Palliative Care and End of Life Care?* Available at: https://www.mariecurie.org.uk/help/

support/diagnosed/recent-diagnosis/palliative-care-end-of-life-care# [Accessed: 31 December 2018].

Marie Curie, 2018b
Marie Curie, 2018. *Life After Caring*. Available at: https://www.mariecurie.org.uk/help/support/being-there/end-of-life-preparation/life-after-caring [Accessed: 1 January 2019].

Marie Curie, 2018c
Marie Curie, 2018. *Becoming a Carer*. Available at: https://www.mariecurie.org.uk/help/support/being-there/helping-someone-cope/carer-role [Accessed: 1 January 2019].

Marie Stopes, 2019
Marie Stopes UK, 2019. *Surgical Abortion*. Available at: http://www.mariestopes.org.uk/abortion-services/surgical-abortion/ [Accessed: 17 February 2019].

Marieb, 2013
Marieb E and Hoehn K, 2013. *Human Anatomy and Physiology*. New York: Pearson.

Martineau, 2006
Martineau L and Shek PN, 2006. Evaluation of a bi-layer wound dressing for burn care: I. Cooling and wound healing properties. *Burns*, 32(1), 70–76.

Matis, 2008
Matis G and Birbilis T, 2008. The Glasgow Coma Scale – a brief review. Past, present, future. *Acta Neurologica Belgica*, 108(3), 75–89.

May, 2007
May P and Trethewy C, 2007. Practice makes perfect? Evaluation of cricoid pressure task training for use within the algorithm for rapid sequence induction in critical care. *Emergency Medicine Australasia*, 19(3), 207–212.

McCormack, 2010
McCormack R, Strauss EJ, Alwattar BJ et al., 2010. Diagnosis and management of pelvic fractures. *Bulletin of the NYU Hospital for Joint Diseases*, 68(4), 281–291.

McCullough, 2014
McCullough A, Haycock J, Forward D and Moran C, 2014. Major trauma networks in England. *British Journal of Anaesthesia*, 113(2), 202–206.

McGrath, 2012
McGrath BA, Bates L, Atkinson D et al., 2012. Multidisciplinary guidelines for the management of tracheostomy and laryngectomy airway emergencies: Tracheostomy management guidelines. *Anaesthesia*, 67(9), 1025–1041.

McMurray, 2012
McMurray JJV, Adamopoulos S, Anker SD et al., 2012. ESC guidelines for the diagnosis and treatment of acute and chronic heart failure 2012: The Task Force for the Diagnosis and Treatment of Acute and Chronic Heart Failure 2012 of the European Society of Cardiology. Developed in collaboration with the Heart Failure Association (HFA) of the ESC. *European Heart Journal*, 33(14), 1787–1847.

Medicines Act 1968
UK Government, 1968. *Medicines Act 1968*. Available at: http://www.legislation.gov.uk/ukpga/1968/67 [Accessed: 13 July 2019].

Mehta, 2014
Mehta A and Hoffbrand V, 2014. *Haematology at a Glance*. 4th ed. Chichester: Wiley-Blackwell.

Meldrum, 1973
Meldrum BS and Horton RW, 1973. Physiology of status epilepticus in primates. *Archives of Neurology*, 28(1), 1–9.

Mencap, 2008
Mencap, 2008. *About Profound and Multiple Learning Disabilities*. Available at: https://www.mencap.org.uk/sites/default/files/2016-11/PMLD%20factsheet%20about%20profound%20and%20multiple%20learning%20disabilities.pdf [Accessed: 4 July 2019].

Mencap, 2013
Mencap, 2013. *Four Things You Probably Didn't Know About Disability Hate Crime*. Available at: https://www.mencap.org.uk/blog/four-things-you-probably-didnt-know-about-disability-hate-crime [Accessed: 6 July 2019].

Mencap, 2018a
Mencap, 2018. *What is a Learning Disability?* Available online: https://www.mencap.org.uk/learning-disability-explained/what-learning-disability [Accessed: 16 December 2018].

Mencap, 2018b
Mencap, 2018. *The Mental Capacity Act*. Available at: https://www.mencap.org.uk/advice-and-support/mental-capacity-act [Accessed: 18 December 2018].

Mencap, 2018c
Mencap, 2018. *Health – what we think*. Available at: https://www.mencap.org.uk/about-us/what-we-think/health-what-we-think [Accessed: 18 December 2018].

Mencap, 2018d
Mencap, 2018. *Treat Me Well*. Available at: https://www.mencap.org.uk/get-involved/campaign-mencap/current-campaigns/treat-me-well [Accessed: 18 December 2018].

References

Mencap, 2018e
Mencap, 2018. *Communicating with People with a Learning Disability*. Available at: https://www.mencap.org.uk/learning-disability-explained/communicating-people-learning-disability [Accessed: 18 December 2018].

Mental Capacity Act 2005
UK Government, 2005. *Mental Capacity Act 2005*. Available at: http://www.legislation.gov.uk/ukpga/2005/9/contents [Accessed: 5 July 2019].

Mental Health Network, 2014
Mental Health Network, 2014. *Positive and Proactive Care*. Available at: https://www.nhsconfed.org/-/media/Confederation/Files/Publications/Documents/Positive-and-proactive-care.pdf?dl=1 [Accessed: 16 July 2019].

Mercer, 2007
Mercer JS, Erickson-Owens DA, Graves B et al., 2007. Evidence-based practices for the fetal to newborn transition. *Journal of Midwifery & Women's Health*, 52(3), 262–272.

Met Police, 2018
Metropolitan Police, 2018. *What is Domestic Abuse?* Available at: https://www.met.police.uk/advice/advice-and-information/daa/domestic-abuse/what-is-domestic-abuse/ [Accessed: 4 January 2019].

MHF, 2015
Mental Health Foundation, 2015. *How to Look After Your Mental Health in Later Life*. Available at: https://www.mentalhealth.org.uk/publications/how-to-in-later-life [Accessed: 6 July 2019].

MHRA, 2014
Medicines and Healthcare Regulatory Agency, 2014. *Rules for the Sale, Supply and Administration of Medicines for Specific Healthcare Professionals*. Available at: https://www.gov.uk/government/publications/rules-for-the-sale-supply-and-administration-of-medicines/rules-for-the-sale-supply-and-administration-of-medicines-for-specific-healthcare-professionals [Accessed: 12 January 2019].

Michael, 2008
Michael J, 2008. *Healthcare for All: Report of the independent inquiry into access to healthcare for people with learning disabilities*. Available at: https://webarchive.nationalarchives.gov.uk/20130105064250/http://www.dh.gov.uk/en/Publicationsandstatistics/Publications/PublicationsPolicyAndGuidance/DH_099255. [Accessed: 12 July 2019].

Middleton, 2012
Middleton PM, 2012. Practical use of the Glasgow Coma Scale: A comprehensive narrative review of GCS methodology. *Australasian Emergency Nursing Journal*, 15(3), 170–183.

MIND, 2013
MIND, 2013. *Mental Health Crisis Care: Physical Restraint in Crisis. A report on physical restraint in hospital settings in England*. https://www.mind.org.uk/media/197120/physical_restraint_final_web_version.pdf [Accessed: 5 January 2019].

MIND, 2015
MIND, 2015. *Ambulance: How to Manage Your Mental Wellbeing*. Available at: https://www.mind.org.uk/media/23702012/managing-mental-wellbeing-ambulance_3_new_update.pdf [Accessed: 8 April 2019].

MIND, 2016a
MIND, 2016. *How to Increase Your Self-esteem*. Available at: https://www.mind.org.uk/information-support/types-of-mental-health-problems/self-esteem/#.XC9IM6d0d-U [Accessed: 4 January 2019].

MIND, 2016b
MIND, 2016. *How to Improve Your Mental Wellbeing*. Available at: https://www.mind.org.uk/38566.aspx#.WbUVwLGZOu4 [Accessed: 30 January 2018].

MIND, 2017
MIND, 2017. *Ambulance: Supporting a Colleague With a Mental Health Problem*. Available at: https://www.mind.org.uk/media/16772202/supporting-a-colleague-ambulance_new-images-2017.pdf [Accessed: 8 April 2019].

MIND, 2019a
MIND, 2019. *Terms You Need to Know*. Available at: https://www.mind.org.uk/information-support/legal-rights/sectioning/terms-you-need-to-know/#.XENUCc_7RTY [Accessed: 19 January 2019].

MIND, 2019b
MIND, 2019. *Sections 135 & 136*. Available at: https://www.mind.org.uk/information-support/legal-rights/police-and-mental-health/sections-135-136/#.XENVlc_7RTY [Accessed: 19 January 2019].

Misuse of Drugs Act 1971
UK Government, 1971. *Misuse of Drugs Act 1971*. Available at: http://www.legislation.gov.uk/ukpga/1971/38/contents [Accessed: 13 July 2019].

References

Misuse of Drugs Regulations 2001
UK Government, 2001. *The Misuse of Drugs Regulations 2001*. Available at: http://www.legislation.gov.uk/uksi/2001/3998/contents/made [Accessed: 13 July 2019].

Mittal, 2009
Mittal R, Vermani E, Tweedie I et al., 2009. Critical care in the emergency department: Traumatic brain injury. *Emergency Medicine Journal*, 26(7), 513–517.

Modell, 1999
Modell JH, Bellefleur M and David JH, 1999. Drowning without aspiration: Is this an appropriate diagnosis? *Journal of Forensic Sciences*, 44, 1119–1123.

Monga, 2011
Monga A and Dobbs S, 2011. *Gynaecology by Ten Teachers*. Oxford: CRC Press.

Monsieurs, 2015
Monsieurs KG, Nolan JP, Bossaert LL et al., 2015. European resuscitation council guidelines for resuscitation 2015. section 1. executive summary. *Resuscitation*, 95, 1–80.

Montalescot, 2013
Montalescot G, Sechtem U, Achenbach S et al., 2013. 2013 ESC guidelines on the management of stable coronary artery disease. The Task Force on the Management of Stable Coronary Artery Disease of the European Society of Cardiology. *European Heart Journal*, 34(38), 2949–3003.

Moore, 2005
Moore C and Woollard M, 2005. Dextrose 10% or 50% in the treatment of hypoglycaemia out of hospital? A randomised controlled trial. *Emergency Medicine Journal*, 22(7), 512–515.

Moorhouse, 2007
Moorhouse I, Thurgood A, Walker N et al., 2007. A realistic model for catastrophic external haemorrhage training. *Journal of the Royal Army Medical Corps*, 153(2), 99–101.

Moppett, 2007
Moppett IK, 2007. Traumatic brain injury: Assessment, resuscitation and early management. *British Journal of Anaesthesia*, 99(1), 18–31.

Moritz, 1947
Moritz AR and Henriques FC, 1947. Studies of thermal injury. *American Journal of Pathology*, 23(5), 695–720.

Moye, 2007
Moye J and Marson DC, 2007. Assessment of decision-making capacity in older adults: An emerging area of practice and research. *Journals of Gerontology. Series B, Psychological Sciences and Social Sciences*, 62(1), 3–11.

Muehlberger, 2010
Muehlberger T, Ottomann C, Toman N et al., 2010. Emergency pre-hospital care of burn patients. *The Surgeon*, 8(2), 101–104.

Mukherjee, 2008
Mukherjee S and Bhide A, 2008. Antepartum haemorrhage. *Obstetrics, Gynaecology & Reproductive Medicine*, 18(12), 335–339.

Müller, 2006
Müller D, Agrawal R and Arntz H-R, 2006. How sudden is sudden cardiac death? *Circulation*, 114(11), 1146–1150.

Murakami, 2003
Murakami K and Traber DL, 2003. Pathophysiological basis of smoke inhalation injury. *Physiology*, 18(3), 125–129.

Muraro, 2014
Muraro A, Roberts G, Worm M et al., 2014. Anaphylaxis: guidelines from the European Academy of Allergy and Clinical Immunology. *Allergy*, 69(8), 1026–1045.

Murray, 2015
Murray L, Little M, Pascu O and Hoggett KA, 2015. *Toxicology Handbook*. 3rd ed. London: Churchill Livingstone.

Mutschler, 2013
Mutschler M, Nienaber U, Brockamp T et al., 2013. A critical reappraisal of the ATLS classification of hypovolaemic shock: does it really reflect clinical reality? *Resuscitation*, 84(3), 309–313.

Mutschler, 2014
Mutschler M, Nienaber U, Müntzberg M et al., 2014. Assessment of hypovolaemic shock at scene: Is the PHTLS classification of hypovolaemic shock really valid? *Emergency Medicine Journal*, 31(1), 35–40.

NAEMT, 2019
National Association of Emergency Medical Technicians and College of Paramedics, 2019. *Advanced Medical Life Support*: UK edition. 2nd ed. Boston: Jones & Bartlett Learning.

NAEMT, 2020
National Association of Emergency Medical Technicians and American College of Surgeons, 2020. *PHTLS: Prehospital Trauma Life Support*. 9th ed. Burlington, MA: Jones & Bartlett Learning.

References

NAGSPE, 2013
National Advisory Group on the Safety of Patients in England, 2013. *A Promise To Learn – A commitment to act.* Available at: https://assets.publishing.service.gov.uk/government/uploads/system/uploads/attachment_data/file/226703/Berwick_Report.pdf [Accessed: 19 February 2019].

NAO, 2010
National Audit Office, 2010. *Progress in Improving Stroke Care: Department of Health.* London: The Stationery Office.

NAR, 2019
North American Rescue, 2019. *CAT Gen 7 Instructions for Use.* Available at: https://www.narescue.com/fileuploader/download/download/?d=1&file=custom%2Fupload%2FCAT_Gen7_Instructions.pdf_1456237633.pdf [Accessed: 28 February 2019].

NARU, 2013
National Ambulance Service Medical Directors Group, 2013. *Triage Sieve.* Available at: http://naru.org.uk/wp-content/uploads/2014/02/NARU-TRIAGE-SIEVE-JU5A304D.pdf [Accessed: 21 December 2018].

NARU, 2015a
National Ambulance Resilience Unit, 2015. *National Ambulance Service Command and Control Guidance.* Available at: http://naru.org.uk/documents/national-ambulance-service-command-control-guidance/ [Accessed: 1 July 2019].

NARU, 2015b
National Ambulance Resilience Unit, 2015. *Major Incident Initial Action Cards – Oct 2015.* Available at: https://naru.org.uk/documents/major-incident-initial-action-cards/ [Accessed: 21 December 2018].

NARU, 2017a
National Ambulance Resilience Unit, 2017. *Initial Operational Response – Aide Memoire.* Available at: https://naru.org.uk/wp-content/uploads/2018/03/IOR-REMOVE-AIDE-MEMOIRE.pdf [Accessed: 21 December 2018].

NARU, 2017b
National Ambulance Resilience Unit, 2017. *Corrosive Substance Attacks: NHS offers public advice on how to respond.* Available at: https://naru.org.uk/acid-attacks-nhs-offers-public-advice-respond/ [Accessed: 28 February 2019].

NARU, 2019
National Ambulance Resilience Unit, 2019. National Inter-Agency Liaison Officer. Available at: https://narueducationcentre.org.uk/courses/national-inter-agency-liaison-officer-nilo-2/ [Accessed: 3 January 2019].

Naseem, 2018
Naseem H et al., 2018. An assessment of pelvic binder placement at a UK major trauma centre. *Annals of the Royal College of Surgeons of England,* 100(2), 101–105.

NatCen, 2013
NatCen Social Research, 2013. *British Social Attitudes Research for Dying Matters.* Available at: https://www.dyingmatters.org/sites/default/files/BSA30_Full_Report.pdf [Accessed: 4 July 2019].

Nater, 2014
Nater A and Fehlings MG, 2014. The timing of decompressive spinal surgery in cauda equina syndrome: A perspective statement. *World Neurosurgery,* 83(1), 19–22.

National Institute for Clinical Development, 2017
National Institute for Clinical Development, 2017. *Healthcare-associated Infections: Prevention and control in primary and community care.* Available at: https://www.nice.org.uk/guidance/cg139/chapter/1-Guidance#standard-principles [Accessed: 23 December 2018].

National Osteoporosis Society, 2018
National Osteoporosis Society, 2018. *What is Osteoporosis and What Does it Do?* Available at: https://nos.org.uk/about-osteoporosis/what-is-osteoporosis/ [Accessed: 15 December 2018].

NBCG, 2008
National Burn Care Group, 2008. *UK Burn Injury Data 1986–2007.* UK: UK National Burn Care Group.

NCEC, 2017
National Chemical Emergency Centre, 2017. *Dangerous Goods Emergency Action Code List 2017.* Norwich: The Stationery Office.

NCPC, 2012
National Council for Palliative Care, 2012. *Who Cares? Support for carers of people approaching the end of life.* Available at: http://www.ncpc.org.uk/sites/default/files/Who_Cares_Conference_Report.pdf [Accessed: 6 December 2018].

NEAS, 2014
North East Ambulance Service NHS Trust, 2014. *Clinical Handbook 2014.* Bridgwater: Class Professional Publishing.

Neligan, 2010
Neligan A and Shorvon SD, 2010. Frequency and prognosis of convulsive status epilepticus of different causes: A systematic review. *Archives of Neurology,* 67(8), 931–940.

References

Nellist, 2013
Nellist E and Lethbridge K, 2013. The need for paramedics to be able to identify cauda equina syndrome. *Journal of Paramedic Practice*, 5(7), 376–379.

NEoLCP, 2013
National End of Life Care Programme, 2013. *Improvement Hub – Advance Decisions to Refuse Treatment: A Guide for Health and Social Care Professionals.* Available at: https://www.england.nhs.uk/improvement-hub/publication/advance-decisions-to-refuse-treatment-a-guide-for-health-and-social-care-professionals/ [Accessed: 6 December 2018].

NG, 2001
Neuropathology Group of the Medical Research Council Cognitive Function and Ageing Study, 2001. Pathological correlates of late-onset dementia in a multicentre, community-based population in England and Wales. Neuropathology Group of the Medical Research Council Cognitive Function and Ageing Study (MRC CFAS). *The Lancet*, 357(9251), 169–175.

NHSCAG, 2010
NHS Clinical Advisory Groups Report, 2010. *Regional Networks for Major Trauma*. Available at: http://www.uhs.nhs.uk/Media/SUHTInternet/Services/Emergencymedicine/Regionalnetworksformajortrauma.pdf [Accessed: 23 July 2019].

NHS, 2016
NHS, 2016. *Overview: Hip Fracture*. Available at: https://www.nhs.uk/conditions/hip-fracture/ [Accessed: 17 February 2019].

NHS, 2017a
NHS, 2017. *Domestic Abuse and Violence*. Available at: https://www.nhs.uk/live-well/healthy-body/getting-help-for-domestic-violence/ [Accessed: 4 January 2019].

NHS, 2017b
NHS, 2017. *Coping With Bereavement*. Available at: https://www.nhs.uk/conditions/stress-anxiety-depression/coping-with-bereavement/ [Accessed: 1 January 2019].

NHS, 2017c
NHS, 2017. *Nosebleed*. Available at: https://www.nhs.uk/conditions/nosebleed/ [Accessed: 11 February 2019].

NHS, 2017d
NHS, 2017. *Dementia Guide*. Available at: https://www.nhs.uk/conditions/dementia/about/ [Accessed: 18 February 2019].

NHS, 2018a
NHS, 2018. *Norovirus (vomiting bug)*. Available at: https://www.nhs.uk/conditions/norovirus/ [Accessed: 23 December 2018].

NHS, 2018b
NHS, 2018. *Moodzone*. Available at: https://www.nhs.uk/conditions/stress-anxiety-depression/understanding-stress/ [Accessed: 27 December 2018].

NHS, 2018c
National Health Service, 2018. *Heavy Periods*. Available at: https://www.nhs.uk/conditions/heavy-periods/ [Accessed: 29 December 2018].

NHS, 2018d
NHS, 2018. *Overview: Learning Disabilities*. Available at: https://www.nhs.uk/conditions/learning-disabilities/ [Accessed: 16 December 2018].

NHS, 2018e
NHS, 2018. *Overview: Falls*. Available at: https://www.nhs.uk/conditions/falls/ [Accessed: 16 December 2018].

NHS Choices, 2015
NHS Choices, 2015. *Abuse and Neglect of Vulnerable Adults*. Available at: http://www.nhs.uk/conditions/social-care-and-support-guide/pages/vulnerable-people-abuse-safeguarding.aspx [Accessed: 21 July 2019].

NHS Digital, 2016
NHS Digital, 2016. *Adult Psychiatric Morbidity Survey: Survey of Mental Health and Wellbeing, England, 2014*. Available at: https://digital.nhs.uk/data-and-information/publications/statistical/adult-psychiatric-morbidity-survey/adult-psychiatric-morbidity-survey-survey-of-mental-health-and-wellbeing-england-2014 [Accessed: 16 July 2019].

NHS Digital, 2017
NHS Digital, 2017. *Data on Written Complaints in the NHS*. Available at: https://files.digital.nhs.uk/pdf/l/a/data_on_written_complaints_in_the_nhs_2016-17_report.pdf [Accessed: 27 December 2018].

NHS Digital, 2018a
NHS Digital, 2018. *Hospital Admitted Patient Care Activity, 2017–18*. Available at: https://digital.nhs.uk/data-and-information/publications/statistical/hospital-admitted-patient-care-activity/2017-18 [Accessed: 22 November 2018].

NHS Digital, 2018b
NHS Digital, 2018. *Codes of Practice for Handling Information in Health and Care*. Available at:

References

https://digital.nhs.uk/data-and-information/looking-after-information/data-security-and-information-governance/codes-of-practice-for-handling-information-in-health-and-care [Accessed: 4 July 2019].

NHS Digital, 2018c
NHS Digital, 2018. *A Guide to Confidentiality in Health and Social Care*. Available at: https://digital.nhs.uk/data-and-information/looking-after-information/data-security-and-information-governance/codes-of-practice-for-handling-information-in-health-and-care/a-guide-to-confidentiality-in-health-and-social-care [Accessed: 30 December 2018].

NHS Employers, 2017
NHS Employers, 2017. *Occupational Health*. Available at: https://www.nhsemployers.org/your-workforce/retain-and-improve/staff-experience/health-work-and-wellbeing/protecting-staff-and-preventing-ill-health/partnership-working-across-your-organisation/occupational-health [Accessed: 27 December 2018].

NHS England, 2013a
NHS England, 2013. *A Guide to the FFP3 Respirator*. Available at: https://www.fullsupporthealthcare.com/wp-content/uploads/2016/07/HSE-Respirator-Mask-Guidance.pdf [Accessed: 4 July 2019].

NHS England, 2013b
NHS England, 2013. *NHS Standard Contract for Specialised Burns Care*. Available at: https://www.england.nhs.uk/wp-content/uploads/2014/04/d06-spec-burn-care-0414.pdf [Accessed: 16 February 2019].

NHS England, 2013c
NHS England, 2013. *NHS Standard Contract for Spinal Cord Injuries*. Available at: https://www.england.nhs.uk/commissioning/wp-content/uploads/sites/12/2014/04/d13-spinal-cord-0414.pdf [Accessed: 11 February 2019].

NHS England, 2017
NHS England, 2017. *Emergency Preparedness, Resilience and Response (EPRR)*. Available at: https://www.england.nhs.uk/ourwork/eprr/ [Accessed: 21 December 2018].

NHS England, 2018a
NHS England, 2018. *Ambulance Response Programme Review*. Available at: https://www.england.nhs.uk/wp-content/uploads/2018/10/ambulance-response-programme-review.pdf [Accessed: 3 January 2019].

NHS England, 2018b
NHS England, 2018. *Statistical Note: Ambulance Quality Indicators (AQI)*. Available at: https://www.england.nhs.uk/statistics/wp-content/uploads/sites/2/2018/12/20181213-Ambulance-Quality-Indicators-Statistical-Note.pdf [Accessed: 3 January 2019].

NHS England, 2018c
NHS England, 2018. *Confidentiality Policy*. Available at: https://www.england.nhs.uk/wp-content/uploads/2016/12/confidentiality-policy-v4.pdf [Accessed: 4 January 2019].

NHS England, 2018d
NHS England, 2018. *My Future Wishes: Advanced Care Planning (ACP) for people with dementia in all care settings*. Available at: https://www.england.nhs.uk/wp-content/uploads/2018/04/my-future-wishes-advance-care-planning-for-people-with-dementia.pdf [Accessed: 31 December 2018].

NHS England, 2019a
NHS England, 2019. *The 6Cs*. Available at: https://www.england.nhs.uk/leadingchange/about/the-6cs/ [Accessed: 5 January 2019].

NHS England, 2019b
NHS England, 2019. *Equality Delivery System*. Available at: https://www.england.nhs.uk/about/equality/equality-hub/eds/ [Accessed: 4 January 2019].

NHS England, 2019c
NHS England, 2019. *Equality, Diversity and Health Inequalities*. Available at: https://www.england.nhs.uk/about/equality/ [Accessed: 4 January 2019].

NHS Equality and Diversity Council, 2017
NHS Equality and Diversity Council, 2017. *Annual Report 2016/17*. Available at: https://www.england.nhs.uk/wp-content/uploads/2017/09/nhs-edc-annual-report-16-17.pdf [Accessed: 5 January 2019].

NHS Improvement, 2018
NHS Improvement, 2018. *Guidance for Boards on Freedom to Speak Up in NHS Trusts and NHS Foundation Trusts*. Available at: https://improvement.nhs.uk/documents/2468/Freedom_to_speak_up_guidance_May2018.pdf [Accessed: 30 December 2018].

NHS Institute for Innovation and Improvement, 2010
NHS Institute for Innovation and Improvement, 2010. *Safer Care SBAR*. Available at: https://www.england.nhs.uk/improvement-hub/wp-content/uploads/sites/44/2017/11/SBAR-Implementation-and-Training-Guide.pdf [Accessed: 19 February 2019].

References

NICE, 2004
National Institute for Health and Care Excellence, 2004. *Self-harm in Over 8s: Short-term management and prevention of recurrence*. Available at: https://www.nice.org.uk/guidance/cg16 [Accessed: 15 January 2019].

NICE, 2009
National Institute for Health and Clinical Excellence, 2009. *NICE Interventional Procedure Guidance [IPG280]: Infracoccygeal sacropexy using mesh for uterine prolapse repair*. London: NICE.

NICE, 2012
National Institute for Health and Care Excellence, 2012. *Health Inequalities and Population Health*. Available at: https://www.nice.org.uk/advice/lgb4/chapter/Introduction [Accessed: 10 July 2019].

NICE, 2013
National Institute for Health and Care Excellence, 2013. *Falls: Assessment and prevention of falls in older people*. Available at: http://www.nice.org.uk/guidance/cg161/evidence/falls-full-guidance-190033741 [Accessed: 29 July 2019].

NICE, 2014
National Institute for Health and Care Excellence, 2014. *Head Injury: Assessment and early management*. Available at: http://www.nice.org.uk/guidance/cg176/ [Accessed: 5 July 2019].

NICE, 2015a
National Institute for Health and Care Excellence, 2015. *Menorrhagia*. Available at: https://cks.nice.org.uk/menorrhagia#!topicSummary [Accessed 6 July 2019].

NICE, 2015b
National Institute for Health and Care Excellence, 2015. *Meningitis (bacterial) and meningococcal septicaemia in under 16s: recognition, diagnosis and management*. Available at: https://www.nice.org.uk/guidance/cg102 [Accessed: 22 November 2018].

NICE, 2015c
National Institute for Health and Care Excellence, 2018. *NG31: Care of dying adults in the last days of life*. Available at: https://www.nice.org.uk/guidance/ng31/chapter/Recommendations#pharmacological-interventions [Accessed 31 December 2018].

NICE, 2015d
National Institute for Health and Care Excellence, 2015. *Chronic kidney disease in adults: assessment and management*. Available at: https://www.nice.org.uk/guidance/cg182 [17 January 2019].

NICE, 2016a
National Institute for Health and Care Excellence, 2016. *Pneumonia in Adults*. Available at: https://www.nice.org.uk/guidance/qs110 [Accessed: 19 December 2018].

NICE, 2016b
National Institute for Health and Care Excellence, 2016. *Stable Angina: Management*. Available at: https://www.nice.org.uk/guidance/cg126 [Accessed: 11 December 2018]

NICE, 2016c
National Institute for Health and Care Excellence, 2016. *Diabetes (type 1 and type 2) in children and young people: Diagnosis and management*. Available at: https://www.nice.org.uk/guidance/ng18/chapter/1-Recommendations#type-1-diabetes [Accessed: 14 December 2018].

NICE, 2016d
National Institute for Health and Care Excellence, 2016. *Type 1 Diabetes in Adults: Diagnosis and management*. Available at: https://www.nice.org.uk/guidance/ng17/chapter/1-Recommendations#blood-glucose-management-2 [Accessed: 14 December 2018].

NICE, 2016e
National Institute for Health and Care Excellence, 2016. *Major Trauma: Service delivery*. Available at: https://www.nice.org.uk/guidance/ng40/chapter/recommendations#prehospital-triage [Accessed: 5 January 2019].

NICE, 2016f
National Institute for Health and Care Excellence, 2016. *Major trauma: assessment and initial management*. Available at: https://www.nice.org.uk/guidance/ng39/chapter/recommendations#management-of-haemorrhage-in-prehospital-and-hospital-settings [Accessed: 9 July 2019].

NICE, 2016g
National Institute for Health and Care Excellence, 2016. *Mersey Burns for Calculating Fluid Resuscitation Volume When Managing Burns*. Available at: https://www.nice.org.uk/advice/mib58/resources/mersey-burns-for-calculating-fluid-resuscitation-volume-when-managing-burns-pdf-63499233245893 [Accessed: 16 February 2019].

NICE, 2016h
National Institute for Health and Care Excellence, 2016. *Sprains and Strains – NICE CKS*. Available at: https://cks.

References

nice.org.uk/sprains-and-strains#!scenario [Accessed: 29 July 2019].

NICE, 2017a
National Institute of Clinical Excellence, 2017. *Child Maltreatment: When to suspect maltreatment in under 18s*. Available at: https://www.nice.org.uk/guidance/cg89/chapter/Introduction [Accessed: 5 January 2019].

NICE, 2017b
National Institute for Health and Care Excellence, 2017. *Clinical Guideline CG139: Healthcare-associated infections: Prevention and control in primary and community care*. Available at: https://www.nice.org.uk/guidance/cg139/chapter/1-Guidance#standard-principles [Accessed: 27 December 2018].

NICE, 2017c
National Institute for Health and Care Excellence, 2017. *Hip Fracture: Management*. Available at: https://www.nice.org.uk/guidance/cg124/informationforpublic [Accessed: 17 February 2019].

NICE, 2017d
National Institute for Health and Care Excellence, 2017. *Fracture (complex): Assessment and management.* Available at: https://www.nice.org.uk/guidance/ng37/ifp/chapter/pelvic-fractures#pelvic-binders [Accessed: 16 February 2019].

NICE, 2018
National Institute for Health and Care Excellence, 2018. *Chronic Obstructive Pulmonary Disease in over 16s: Diagnosis and management*. Available at: https://www.nice.org.uk/guidance/ng115 [Accessed: 18 December 2018].

NICE, 2019
National Institute for Health and Care Excellence, 2019. *Hypertension in Pregnancy: The management of hypertensive disorders during pregnancy*. https://www.nice.org.uk/guidance/ng133 [Accessed: 26 July 2019].

Nickerson, 2007
Nickerson E, 2007. *Crash Course: Infectious Diseases*. Edinburgh: Mosby/Elsevier.

Nienaber, 2012
Nienaber CA and Powell JT, 2012. Management of acute aortic syndromes. *European Heart Journal*, 33(1), 26–35.

Nigam, 2008
Nigam Y and Knight J, 2008. Exploring the anatomy and physiology of ageing. Part 3 – the digestive system. *Nursing Times*, 104(33), 22–23.

NIHR, 2012
National Institute for Health Research, 2012. *Diversity and Inclusion: What's it about and why is it important for public involvement in research?* Available at: https://www.invo.org.uk/wp-content/uploads/2012/10/INVOLVEDiversityandInclusionOct2012.pdf [Accessed: 4 July 2019].

Ninis, 2010
Ninis N, Nadel S and Glennie L, 2010. *Sections from Research for Doctors in Training*. 3rd ed. Bristol: Meningitis Research Foundation.

NNBC, 2012
National Network for Burn Care, 2012. National Burn Care Referral Guidelines, NNBC. Available at: https://www.britishburnassociation.org/wp-content/uploads/2018/02/National-Burn-Care-Referral-Guidance-2012.pdf [Accessed: 10 July 2019].

Nolan, 2006
Nolan J, Soar J and Eikeland H, 2006. The chain of survival. *Resuscitation*, 71(3), 270–271.

Nolan, 2010
Nolan JP, Soar J, Zideman DA et al., 2010. European Resuscitation Council guidelines for resuscitation 2010 section 1. Executive summary. *Resuscitation*, 81(10), 1219–1276.

Nolan, 2016
Nolan, J and Resuscitation Council (UK), 2016. *Advanced Life Support*, 7th ed. London: Resuscitation Council (UK).

Noppen, 2010
Noppen M, 2010. Spontaneous pneumothorax: epidemiology, pathophysiology and cause. *European Respiratory Review*, 19(117), 217–219.

NPIS, 2019
National Poisons Information Service, 2019. *Poisoning with an Unknown Substance*. Available at: https://www.toxbase.org/upload/Toxidromes%2031%20May%202019.pdf [Accessed: 29 July 2019].

NPSA, 2007a
National Patient Safety Agency, 2007. *Healthcare Risk Assessment Made Easy*. Available at: http://www.nrls.npsa.nhs.uk/resources/?entryid45=59825 [Accessed: 9 July 2019].

NPSA, 2007b
National Patient Safety Agency, 2007. *Safer Practice Notice: Colour coding of hospital cleaning materials and equipment*.

Available at: http://www.nrls.npsa.nhs.uk/EasySiteWeb/getresource.axd?AssetID=60088&type=full&servicetype=Attachment [Accessed: 28 July 2019].

NPSA, 2008
National Patient Safety Agency, 2008. *Risk Matrix for Risk Managers*. Available at: http://www.npsa.nhs.uk/nrls/improvingpatientsafety/patient-safety-tools-and-guidance/risk-assessment-guides/risk-matrix-for-risk-managers/ [Accessed: 9 July 2019].

NSPCC, 2014
National Society for the Prevention of Cruelty to Children, 2014. *Culture and Faith: Learning from case reviews*. Available at: https://learning.nspcc.org.uk/media/1332/learning-from-case-reviews_culture-and-faith.pdf [Accessed: 5 January 2019].

NSPCC, 2018
National Society for the Prevention of Cruelty to Children, 2018. *How Safe Are Our Children?* Available at: https://learning.nspcc.org.uk/media/1067/how-safe-are-our-children-2018.pdf [Accessed: 6 January 2019].

NSPCC, 2019
National Society for the Prevention of Cruelty to Children, 2019. *Female Genital Mutilation (FGM)*. Available at: https://www.nspcc.org.uk/preventing-abuse/child-abuse-and-neglect/female-genital-mutilation-fgm/ [Accessed: 5 January 2019].

NTSP, 2014
National Tracheostomy Safety Project (Great Britain), 2014. *Comprehensive Tracheostomy Care: The National Tracheostomy Safety Project Manual*, McGrath BA (ed.). Chichester: John Wiley & Sons.

Nutbeam, 2013
Nutbeam T and Boylan M, 2013. *ABC of Prehospital Emergency Medicine*. Chichester: John Wiley & Sons.

NZGG, 2007
New Zealand Guidelines Group, 2007. *Management of Burns and Scalds in Primary Care*. Wellington: Accident Compensation Corporation.

O'Brien, 2003
O'Brien E, Asmar R, Beilin L et al., 2003. European society of hypertension recommendations for conventional, ambulatory and home blood pressure measurement. *Journal of Hypertension*, 21(5), 821–848.

O'Donnell, 2010
O'Donnell MJ, Xavier D, Liu L et al., 2010. Risk factors for ischaemic and intracerebral haemorrhagic stroke in 22 countries (the INTERSTROKE study): A case-control study. *The Lancet*, 376(9735), 112–123.

O'Driscoll, 2017
O'Driscoll BR, Howard LS, Earis J, Mak V, British Thoracic Society Emergency Oxygen Guideline Group, and BTS Emergency Oxygen Guideline Development Group, 2017. BTS guideline for oxygen use in adults in healthcare and emergency settings. *Thorax*, 72(Suppl 1), ii1–ii90.

ONS, 2013
Office for National Statistics, 2013. *Births in England and Wales by Characteristics of Birth 2, 2012*. Available at: https://www.ons.gov.uk/peoplepopulationandcommunity/birthsdeathsandmarriages/livebirths/bulletins/characteristicsofbirth2/2013-11-21 [Accessed: 3 July 2019].

ONS, 2017
Office for National Statistics, 2017. *Deaths Registered in England and Wales*. Available at: https://www.ons.gov.uk/peoplepopulationandcommunity/birthsdeathsandmarriages/deaths/datasets/deathsregisteredinenglandandwalesseriesdrreferencetables [Accessed: 3 October 2018].

ONS, 2018a
Office for National Statistics, 2018. *Suicides in the UK*. Available at: https://www.ons.gov.uk/peoplepopulationandcommunity/birthsdeathsandmarriages/deaths/bulletins/suicidesintheunitedkingdom/2017registrations [Accessed: 19 January 2019].

ONS, 2018b
Office for National Statistics, 2018. *Overview of the UK Population: November 2018*.
https://www.ons.gov.uk/peoplepopulationandcommunity/populationandmigration/populationestimates/articles/overviewoftheukpopulation/november2018 [Accessed: 12 December 2018].

Orlowski, 1989
Orlowski JP, Abulleil MM and Phillips JM, 1989. The hemodynamic and cardiovascular effects of near-drowning in hypotonic, isotonic, or hypertonic solutions. *Annals of Emergency Medicine*, 18(10), 1044–1049.

Osler, 2012
Osler W, 2012. Pneumonia part 1: Pathology, presentation and prevention. *British Journal of Nursing*, 21(2), 103–106.

References

Oyetunji, 2011
Oyetunji TA, Chang DC, Crompton JG et al., 2011. Redefining hypotension in the elderly: Normotension is not reassuring. *Archives of Surgery*, 146(7), 865–869.

Paiva, 2010
Paiva M, Piedade S and Gaspar Â, 2010. Toothpaste-induced anaphylaxis caused by mint (mentha) allergy. *Allergy*, 65(9), 1201–1202.

Paliwal, 2014
Paliwal P, Ali S, Bradshaw S et al., 2014. Management of type III female genital mutilation in Birmingham, UK: A retrospective audit. *Midwifery*, 30(3), 282–288.

Panesar, 2013
Panesar SS, Javad S, de Silva D et al., 2013. The epidemiology of anaphylaxis in Europe: A systematic review. *Allergy*, 68(11), 1353–1361.

Pante, 2010
Pante MD and American Academy of Orthopaedic Surgeons, 2010. *Advanced Assessment and Treatment of Trauma*. Sudbury: Jones and Bartlett Publishers.

Papadopoulos, 2006
Papadopoulos IN, Kanakaris N, Bonovas S et al., 2006. Auditing 655 fatalities with pelvic fractures by autopsy as a basis to evaluate trauma care. *Journal of the American College of Surgeons*, 203(1), 30–43.

Pappas, 2010
Pappas R and Frize M, 2010. *Intellectual Disability: Mental Health First Aid Manual*. Available at: https://mhfa.com.au/sites/default/files/2nd-Edn-ID-MHFA-Manual-Sept-2012-small.pdf [Accessed: 23 July 2019].

Parkinson's UK, 2018
Parkinson's UK, 2018. *What Causes Parkinson's?* Available at: https://www.parkinsons.org.uk/information-and-support/what-causes-parkinsons [Accessed: 15 December 2018].

Pasquel, 2014
Pasquel FJ, and Umpierrez GE, 2014. Hyperosmolar hyperglycemic state: A historic review of the clinical presentation, diagnosis, and treatment. *Diabetes Care*, 37(11), 3124–3131.

Patel, 2016
Patel S et al., 2016. Patterns of maxillofacial trauma in a major UK trauma centre – A 4 year retrospective review, *British Journal of Oral and Maxillofacial Surgery*, 54(10), e151.

Paterson-Brown & Howell, 2016
Paterson-Brown S and Howell, C (eds.), 2016. *Managing Obstetric Emergencies and Trauma: The MOET Course Manual*. 3rd ed. Cambridge: Cambridge University Press.

Paul, 1998
Paul A, 1998. *Where Bias Begins: The Truth About Stereotypes*. Available at: https://www.psychologytoday.com/articles/199805/where-bias-begins-the-truth-about-stereotypes [Accessed: 31 July 2019].

Peña, 2012
Peña SB and Larrard AR, 2012. Does the Trendelenburg position affect hemodynamics? A systematic review. *Emergencias*, 24, 143–150.

Perkins, 2015
Perkins GD, Handley AJ, Koster RW et al., 2015. European Resuscitation Council guidelines for resuscitation 2015. Section 2. Adult basic life support and automated external defibrillation. *Resuscitation*, 95, 81–99.

Perry, 2008
Perry M and Morris C, 2008. Advanced trauma life support (ATLS) and facial trauma: Can one size fit all? Part 2: ATLS, maxillofacial injuries and airway management dilemmas. *International Journal of Oral and Maxillofacial Surgery*, 37(4), 309–320.

Personal Protective Equipment at Work Regulations 1992
UK Government, 1992. *The Personal Protective Equipment at Work Regulations 1992*. Available at: http://www.legislation.gov.uk/uksi/1992/2966/regulation/4/made [Accessed: 29 July 2019].

Physio-Control, 2009
Physio-Control, 2009. *LifePak 15 Monitor/defibrillator Operating Instructions*. Available at: http://moodle.999cpd.com/%20http://www.physio-control.com/uploadedfiles/physio85/contents/emergency_medical_care/products/operating_instructions/lifepak15_operatinginstructions_3306222-002.pdf [Accessed: 11 July 2019].

Pickard, 2011
Pickard A, Karlen W, Ansermino JM. Capillary refill time: Is it still a useful clinical sign? *Anesthesia & Analgesia*, 113(1), 120–123.

References

PIE, 2014
Picker Institute Europe, 2014. *NHS Staff Surveys – 2013 results*. Available at: http://www.nhsstaffsurveys.com/page/1006/latest-results/2013-results/ [Accessed: 8 July 2019].

Piette, 2006
Piette MHA and De Letter EA, 2006. Drowning: Still a difficult autopsy diagnosis. *Forensic Science International*, 163(1/2), 1–9.

Piirilä, 1995
Piirilä P and Sovijärvi ARA, 1995. Crackles: Recording, analysis and clinical significance. *European Respiratory Journal*, 8(12), 2139–2148.

Pilbery, 2016
Pilbery R, Caroline NL, American Academy of Orthopaedic Surgeons et al., 2016. *Nancy Caroline's Emergency Care in the Streets*. 7th ed. Burlington: Jones & Bartlett Learning.

Pokorná, 2010
Pokorná M, Necas E, Kratochvíl J et al., 2010. A sudden increase in partial pressure end-tidal carbon dioxide ($PETCO_2$) at the moment of return of spontaneous circulation. *Journal of Emergency Medicine*, 38(5), 614–621.

Porth, 2014
Porth C, 2014. *Essentials of Pathophysiology: Concepts of Altered States*. 4th ed. Philadelphia: Lippincott Williams and Wilkins.

Prasarn, 2014
Prasarn ML, Horodyski M, Scott NE et al., 2014. Motion generated in the unstable upper cervical spine during head tilt–chin lift and jaw thrust manoeuvres. *The Spine Journal*, 14(4), 609–614.

Preston, 2004
Preston ST and Hegadoren K, 2004. Glass contamination in parenterally administered medication. *Journal of Advanced Nursing*, 48(3), 266–270.

Prien, 1988
Prien T and Traber DL, 1988. Toxic smoke compounds and inhalation injury – a review. *Burns, Including Thermal Injury*, 14(6), 451–460.

Prometheus Medical, 2018
Prometheus Medica, 2018. *Prometheus Traction Splint Instructions for Use*. Available at: https://www.prometheusmedical.co.uk/sites/default/files/equipment-pdfs/Traction%20Device%20IFU%20Single%20Use%20v2.pdf [Accessed: 16 February 2019].

PROMPT, 2017
Winter C, Draycott T, Muchatuta N and Crofts J (eds.), 2017. *PROMPT Course Manual*. 3rd ed. Cambridge: Cambridge University Press.

Provision and Use of Work Equipment Regulations 1998
UK Government, 1998. *The Provision and Use of Work Equipment Regulations 1998*. Available at: http://www.legislation.gov.uk/uksi/1998/2306/contents/made [Accessed: 29 July 2019].

Prussin, 2006
Prussin C and Metcalfe DD, 2006. 5. IgE, mast cells, basophils, and eosinophils. *Journal of Allergy and Clinical Immunology*, 117(2, Supplement 2), S450–S456.

Public Health England, 2016
Public Health England, 2016. *Meningococcal: The green book*. Available at: https://www.gov.uk/government/publications/meningococcal-the-green-book-chapter-22 [Accessed: 23 July 2019].

Public Health England, 2017
Public Health England, 2017. *Understanding Health Inequalities in England*. Available at: https://publichealthmatters.blog.gov.uk/2017/07/13/understanding-health-inequalities-in-england/ [Accessed: 4 January 2019].

Public Health England, 2018a
Public Health England, 2018. *First Stroke Estimates in England: 2007 to 2016*. Available at: https://www.gov.uk/government/publications/first-stroke-estimates-in-england-2007-to-2016 [Accessed: 22 July 2019].

Public Health England, 2018b
Public Health England, 2018. *Clinical Governance*. Available at: https://www.gov.uk/government/publications/newborn-hearing-screening-programme-nhsp-operational-guidance/4-clinical-governance [Accessed: 4 January 2019].

Public Health England, 2018c
Public Health England, 2018. *Invasive Meningococcal Disease in England: Annual laboratory confirmed reports for epidemiological year 2017 to 2018*. Available at: https://assets.publishing.service.gov.uk/government/uploads/system/uploads/attachment_data/file/751821/hpr3818_IMD.pdf [Accessed: 29 July 2019].

Public Health England, 2019
Public Health England, 2019. *Meningococcal Disease: Guidance, data and analysis*. Available at:

References

https://www. gov.uk/government/collections/meningococcal-disease-guidance-data-and-analysis [Accessed: 29 July 2019].

Pumphrey, 2000
Pumphrey R, 2000. Sections for management of anaphylaxis from a study of fatal reactions. *Clinical & Experimental Allergy*, 30(8), 1144–1150.

Purcell, 2016
Purcell D, 2016. *Minor Injuries: A Clinical Guide*. 3rd ed. London: Elsevier.

PYNG Medical, 2014
PYNG Medical, 2014. *T-POD Responder Training Session*. Available at: http://www.pyng.com/wp-content/uploads/2014/09/T-PODResponder-Training-PowerPoint-Presentation.pdf [Accessed: 16 February 2019].

QAS, 2018a
Queensland Ambulance Service, 2018. *Clinical Practice Manual*. Available at: https://ambulance.qld.gov.au/clinical.html [Accessed: 3 December 2018].

QAS, 2018b
Queensland Ambulance Service, 2018. *Clinical Practice Procedures: Trauma/helmet removal*. Available at: https://www.ambulance.qld.gov.au/docs/clinical/cpp/CPP_Helmet%20removal.pdf [Accessed: 12 February 2019].

Ramanath, 2009
Ramanath VS, Oh JK, Sundt TM et al., 2009. Acute aortic syndromes and thoracic aortic aneurysm. *Mayo Clinic Proceedings*, 84(5), 465–481.

Rana, 2018
Rana N, Kc A, Malqvist M, Subedi K and Anderson, 2018. Effect of delayed cord clamping of term on neurodevelopment at 12 months: A randomised controlled trial. *Neonatology*, 115(1), 36–42.

Ranasinghe, 2011
Ranasinghe AM, Strong D, Boland B et al., 2011. Acute aortic dissection. *BMJ*, 343, d4487–d4487.

Randle, 2009
Randle J, Coffey F and Bradbury M, 2009. *Oxford Handbook of Clinical Skills in Adult Nursing*. Oxford: Oxford University Press.

RCEM, 2018
Royal College of Emergency Medicine, 2018. *Silver Trauma*. Available at: https://www.rcemlearning.co.uk/foamed/silver-trauma/ [Accessed: 7 January 2019].

RCGP, 2018a
Royal College of General Practitioners, 2018. *Person-Centered Care Toolkit*. Available at: https://www.rcgp.org.uk/clinical-and-research/resources/toolkits/person-centred-care-toolkit.aspx [Accessed: 30 December 2018].

RCGP, 2018b
Royal College of General Practitioners 2018. *Flowchart for Infants/Children under 16 years with Suspected UTI*. Available at: https://assets.publishing.service.gov.uk/government/uploads/system/uploads/attachment_data/file/755891/PHE_UTI_flowchart_-_children.pdf [Accessed: 17 January 2019].

RCN, 2017
Royal College of Nursing, 2017. *Clinical Governance: Five key themes*. Available at: https://www.rcn.org.uk/clinical-topics/clinical-governance/five-key-themes [Accessed: 4 January 2019].

RCN, 2018
Royal College of Nursing, 2018. *Barriers to Communication*. Available at: https://rcni.com/hosted-content/rcn/first-steps/barriers-to-communication [Accessed: 27 November 2018].

RCOG, 2012
Royal College of Obstetricians and Gynaecologists, 2012. *Shoulder Dystocia (Green-top 42)*. Available at: https://www.rcog.org.uk/en/guidelines-research-services/guidelines/gtg42/ [Accessed 4 August 2018].

RCOG, 2013
Royal College of Obstetricians and Gynaecologists, 2013. *Information For You: Pelvic organ prolapse*. London: RCOG. Available at: https://www.rcog.org.uk/globalassets/documents/patients/patient-information-leaflets/gynaecology/pi-pelvic-organ-prolapse.pdf [Accessed: 16 July 2019].

RCP, 2010
Royal College of Psychiatrists, 2010. *Self-harm, Suicide and Risk: Helping people who self-harm*. Available at: https://www.rcpsych.ac.uk/docs/default-source/improving-care/better-mh-policy/college-reports/college-report-cr158.pdf?sfvrsn=fcf95b93_2 [Accessed: 19 January 2019].

RCP, 2017
Royal College of Physicians, 2017. *National Early Warning Score (NEWS) 2*. London: RCP. Available at: https://www.rcplondon.ac.uk/projects/outputs/national-early-warning-score-news-2 [Accessed: 12 July 2019].

References

RCP, 2016
The Royal College of Pathologists and Royal College of Paediatrics and Child Health, 2016. *Sudden Unexpected Death in Infancy and Childhood.* Available at: https://www.rcpath.org/asset/874AE50E-C754-4933-995A804E0EF728A4/ [Accessed: 6 December 2018].

RCPCH, 2015
Royal College of Paediatrics and Child Health, 2015. *The Physical Signs of Child Abuse.* London: RCPCH.

Rees, 2003
Rees DC, Olujohungbe AD, Parker NE et al., 2003. Guidelines for the management of the acute painful crisis in sickle cell disease. *British Journal of Haematology*, 120(5), 744–752.

RNLI, 2017
Royal National Lifeboat Institution, 2017. *RNLI 2017 Operational Statistics.* Available at: https://rnli.org/-/media/rnli/downloads/170073_annual_ops_stats_report_lr.pdf [Accessed: 5 December 2018].

Roberts, 2003a
Roberts K and Smith A, 2003. Outcome of diabetic patients treated in the prehospital arena after a hypoglycaemic episode, and an exploration of treat and release protocols: A review of the literature. *Emergency Medicine Journal*, 20(3), 274–276.

Roberts, 2003b
Roberts K and Porter K, 2003. How do you size a nasopharyngeal airway. *Resuscitation*, 56(1), 19–23.

Roberts, 2014
Roberts JR, Custalow, Thomsen et al., 2014. *Roberts and Hedges' Clinical Procedures in Emergency Medicine.* 6th ed. New York: Elsevier.

Rodgers, 2004
Rodgers H, Greenaway J, Davies T et al., 2004. Risk factors for first-ever stroke in older people in the north east of England: A population-based study. *Stroke*, 35(1), 7–11.

Roguin, 2006
Roguin A, 2006. Rene Theophile Hyacinthe Laënnec (1781–1826): The man behind the stethoscope. *Clinical Medicine & Research*, 4(3), 230–235.

Rolfe, 2001
Rolfe G, Freshwater D and Jasper M, 2001. *Critical Reflective Practice in Nursing and the Helping Professions.* Basingstoke: Palgrave Macmillan.

Root, 2009
Root T, 2009. OpthoBook. Available at: http://www.ophthobook.com/pdfvault/OpthoBook_1.0.pdf [Accessed: 4 December 2018].

Ross, 2014
Ross S, 2014. *Rapid Infection Control Nursing.* Chichester: Wiley-Blackwell.

Sakai, 2014
Sakai T, Kitamura T, Iwami T et al., 2014. Effectiveness of prehospital Magill forceps use for out-of-hospital cardiac arrest due to foreign body airway obstruction in Osaka City. *Scandinavian Journal of Trauma, Resuscitation and Emergency Medicine*, 22. Available at: http://www.ncbi.nlm.nih.gov/pmc/articles/PMC4156961/ [Accessed: 14 July 2019].

SAM, 2019
SAM Medical, 2019. *SAM Pelvic Sling II: Training.* Available at: https://www.sammedical.com/assets/uploads/SLI-PED-G-01_FEB-2018-STATIC-sm.pdf [Accessed: 16 February 2019].

SAS, 2014
Scottish Ambulance Service, 2014. *Dementia Learning Resource.* Available at: https://www.nes.scot.nhs.uk/media/3064028/scottish_ambulance_service.pdf [Accessed: 15 July 2019].

Savage, 2011
Savage MW, Dhatariya KK, Kilvert A et al., 2011. Joint British Diabetes Societies guideline for the management of diabetic ketoacidosis: Diabetic ketoacidosis guidelines. *Diabetic Medicine*, 28(5), 508–515.

Saver, 2006
Saver JL, 2006. Time is brain – quantified. *Stroke*, 37(1), 263–266.

SBNS, 2009
The Society of British Neurological Surgeons, 2009. *Standards of Care for Established and Suspected Cauda Equina Syndrome.* Available at: www.sbns.org.uk/index.php/download_file/view/131/87 [Accessed: July 2019].

SCAS, 2018
South Coast Ambulance Service, 2018. *Infection Prevention, Control and Decontamination Policy and Procedures.* Available at: https://www.scas.nhs.uk/wp-content/uploads/Infection-prevention-control-and-decontamination-policy.pdf [Accessed: 27 December 2018].

References

SCAS, 2019
South Central Ambulance Service, 2019. *Community and Co-responders*. Available at: https://www.scas.nhs.uk/our-services/community-and-co-responders/ [Accessed: 3 January 2019].

Schmitt, 2002
Schmitt HJ and Mang H, 2002. Head and neck elevation beyond the sniffing position improves laryngeal view in cases of difficult direct laryngoscopy. *Journal of Clinical Anesthesia*, 14(5), 335–338.

SCIE, 2018
Social Care Institute for Excellence (SCIE), 2018. *About Dementia: What is dementia?* Available at: https://www.scie.org.uk/dementia/about/ [Accessed: 15 December 2018].

Scott, 2013
Scott I, Porter K, Laird C, Greaves I and Bloch M, 2013. *The Prehospital Management of Pelvic Fractures: Initial consensus statement*. Available at: https://fphc.rcsed.ac.uk/media/1765/the-pre-hospital-management-of-pelvic-fractures.pdf [Accessed: 17 July 2019].

Scott, 2015
Scott AR, the Joint British Diabetes Societies (JBDS) for Inpatient Care and the JBDS hyperosmolar hyperglycaemic guidelines group, 2015. Management of hyperosmolar hyperglycaemic state in adults with diabetes. *Diabetic Medicine*, 32(6), 714–724.

Scott, 2017
Scott TE et al., 2017. Primary blast lung injury: A review. *British Journal of Anaesthesia*, 118(3), 311–316.

Sharma, 2008
Sharma A and Jindal P, 2008. Principles of diagnosis and management of traumatic pneumothorax. *Journal of Emergencies, Trauma and Shock*, 1(1), 34–41.

Shattock, 2012
Shattock MJ and Tipton MJ, 2012. 'Autonomic conflict': A different way to die during cold water immersion? *Journal of Physiology*, 590(14), 3219–3230.

Sheridan, 2012
Sheridan R, 2012. *Burns: A Practical Approach to Immediate Treatment and Long-term Care*. London: Manson Publishing.

Shivaji, 2014
Shivaji T et al., 2014. The epidemiology of hospital treated traumatic brain injury in Scotland, *BMC Neurology*, 14(2), 1–7.

Siada, 2017
Siada SS et al., 2017. Current outcomes of blunt open pelvic fractures: How modern advances in trauma care may decrease mortality, *Acute Care Open*, 2(1), e000136.

SIGN/BTS, 2016
Scottish Intercollegiate Guidelines Network and British Thoracic Society, 2016. *British Guideline on the Management of Asthma: A national clinical guideline*. Available at: https://www.brit-thoracic.org.uk/document-library/clinical-information/asthma/btssign-asthma-guideline-2016/ [Accessed: 18 December 2018].

Silver, 2003
Silver A, 2003. *Module 4: 12-Lead ECG Theory. Fast Track to Thrombolysis*. Roche.

Simon, 2010
Simon C, 2010. *Oxford Handbook of General Practice*. 3rd ed. Oxford Handbooks. Oxford: Oxford University Press.

Simons, 2001
Simons FER, Gu X and Simons KJ, 2001. Epinephrine absorption in adults: Intramuscular versus subcutaneous injection. *Journal of Allergy and Clinical Immunology*, 108(5), 871–873.

Simons, 2007
Simons FER, Frew AJ. Ansotegui IJ et al., 2007. Risk assessment in anaphylaxis: Current and future approaches. *Journal of Allergy and Clinical Immunology*, 120(1, Supplement), S2–S24.

Singer, 2006
Singer AJ, Freidman B, Modi P et al., 2006. The effect of a commercially available burn-cooling blanket on core body temperatures in volunteers. *Academic Emergency Medicine*, 13(6), 686–690.

Singer, 2010
Singer AJ, Taira BR, Thode Jr HC et al., 2010. The association between hypothermia, prehospital cooling, and mortality in burn victims. *Academic Emergency Medicine*, 17(4), 456–459.

Singer, 2016
Singer M, Deutschman CS, Seymour CW et al., 2016. The third international consensus definitions for sepsis and septic shock (sepsis-3). *JAMA*, 315(8), 801–810.

SJA, SAA, BRC, 2016
St. John Ambulance, St. Andrew's First Aid, British Red Cross, 2016. *First Aid Manual*. Revised 10th ed. London: Dorling Kindersley.

References

Skellett, 2016
Skellett S, Hampshire S, Bingham R et al., 2016. *European Paediatric Advanced Life Support*. 4th ed. London: RC(UK).

Smith, 2011
Smith J (ed.), 2011. *The Guide to the Handling of People: A Systems Approach*. Teddington: BackCare.

Smith, 2013
Smith LA, Price N, Simonite V et al., 2013. Incidence of and risk factors for perineal trauma: A prospective observational study. *BMC Pregnancy and Childbirth*, 13(1), 59.

Smith, 2018
Smith RP, 2018. The clinical classification and causes of menorrhagia. In RP Smith (ed.), *Dysmenorrhea and Menorrhagia: A Clinician's Guide*. Cham: Springer International Publishing.

Smiths Medical, 2014
Smiths Medical, 2014. *paraPac plus Model 310 Ventilator*. Luton: Smiths Medical International Ltd.

Smithson, 2012
Smithson H and Walker MC, 2012. *ABC of Epilepsy*. Chichester: John Wiley & Sons.

Smithuis, 2008
Smithuis R and Willems T, 2008. *Coronary Anatomy and Anomalies. The radiology assistant*. Available at: http://www.radiologyassistant.nl/en/p48275120e2ed5 [Accessed: 4 July 2019].

Soar, 2008
Soar J, Pumphrey R, Cant A et al., 2008. Emergency treatment of anaphylactic reactions – guidelines for healthcare providers. *Resuscitation*, 77(2), 157–169.

Soar, 2010
Soar J, Perkins GD, Abbas G et al., 2010. European Resuscitation Council guidelines for resuscitation 2010. Section 8. Cardiac arrest in special circumstances: electrolyte abnormalities, poisoning, drowning, accidental hypothermia, hyperthermia, asthma, anaphylaxis, cardiac surgery, trauma, pregnancy, electrocution. *Resuscitation*, 81(10), 1400–1433.

Soar, 2015
Soar J, Nolan JP, Böttiger BW et al., 2015. European Resuscitation Council guidelines for resuscitation 2015. Section 3. Adult advanced life support. *Resuscitation*, 95, 100–147.

Soroudi, 2007
Soroudi A, Shipp HE, Stepanski BM et al., 2007. Adult foreign body airway obstruction in the prehospital setting. *Prehospital Emergency Care*, 11(1), 25–29.

Spiteri, 1988
Spiteri MA, Cook DG and Clarke SW, 1988. Reliability of eliciting physical signs in examination of the chest. *The Lancet*, 1(8590), 873–875.

Stefanopoulos, 2014
Stefanopoulos P, Hadjigeorgiou G, Filippakis K and Gyftokostas D, 2014. Gunshot wounds: A review of ballistics related to penetrating trauma. *Journal of Acute Disease*, 3(3), 178–185.

Stewart, 2013
Stewart M, 2013. Bet 3: Pelvic circumferential compression devices for haemorrhage control: Panacea or myth? *Emergency Medicine Journal*, 30(5), 425–426.

Studnek, 2012
Studnek JR, Artho MR, Garner Jr CL et al., 2012. The impact of emergency medical services on the ED care of severe sepsis. *American Journal of Emergency Medicine*, 30(1), 51–56.

Stuke, 2007
Stuke L, Diaz-Arrastia R, Gentilello LM et al., 2007. Effect of alcohol on Glasgow Coma Scale in head-injured patients. *Annals of Surgery*, 245(4), 651–655.

Survivors Trust, 2012
The Survivors Trust, 2012. *Sexual Assault Referral Centres (SARCS)*. Available at: http://www.thesurvivorstrust.org/sarc/ [Accessed: 17 July 2019].

SWAST, 2016
South Western Ambulance Services NHS Foundation Trust, 2016. *Infection Prevention and Control*. Available at: https://www.swast.nhs.uk/assets/1/ipcpolicy.pdf [Accessed: 27 December 2018].

Szpilman, 2004
Szpilman D and Soares M, 2004. In-water resuscitation – is it worthwhile? *Resuscitation*, 63(1), 25–31.

Szpilman, 2012
Szpilman D, Bierens JJLM, Handley AJ et al., 2012. Drowning. *New England Journal of Medicine*, 366(22), 2102–2110.

Talley, 2006
Talley NJ and O'Connor S, 2006. *Clinical Examination: A Systematic Guide to Physical Diagnosis*. 5th ed. London: Elsevier.

References

Tannahill, 2008
Tannahill A, 2008. Health promotion: The Tannahill model revisited. *Public Health*, 122(12), 1387–1391.

Tapson, 2008
Tapson VF, 2008. Acute pulmonary embolism. *New England Journal of Medicine*, 358(10), 1037–1052.

TARN, 2017
The Trauma Audit & Research Network, 2017. *Major Trauma in Older People*. Available at: https://www.tarn.ac.uk/Content.aspx?c=3793 [Accessed: 28 February 2019].

Teasdale, 1974
Teasdale G and Jennett B, 1974. Assessment of coma and impaired consciousness. *The Lancet*, 304(7872), 81–84.

Teasdale, 2014
Teasdale G, Allen D, Brennan P, McElhinney E and Mackinnon L, 2014. *The Glasgow Coma Scale: An update after 40 years*. Nursing Times, 110, 12–16.

Teasdale, 2015
Teasdale G, 2015. *Glasgow Coma Scale: Do it this way*. Available at: https://www.glasgowcomascale.org/downloads/GCS-Assessment-Aid-English.pdf?v=3 [Accessed: 4 December 2018].

Teleflex, 2013
Teleflex, 2013. *Using the LMA MAD Nasal Intranasal Mucosal Atomization Device*. Available at: https://www.teleflex.com/usa/product-areas/ems/intranasal-drug-delivery/mad-nasal-atomization-device/AN_ATM_MAD-Nasal-Usage_Guide_AI_2012-1528.pdf [Accessed: 24 October 2018].

Teleflex, 2017
Teleflex, 2017. *Arrow EZ-IO Education*. Available at: https://www.teleflex.com/usa/clinical-resources/ez-io/ [Accessed: 24 October 2018].

Thadepalli, 2002
Thadepalli H, 2002. Women gave birth to the stethoscope: Laennec's introduction of the art of auscultation of the lung. *Clinical Infectious Diseases*, 35(5), 587–588.

Thomassen, 2009
Thomassen O, Skaiaa SC, Brattebo G et al., 2009. Does the horizontal position increase risk of rescue death following suspension trauma? *Emergency Medicine Journal*, 26(12), 896–898.

Thompson, 2006
Thompson MJ, Ninis N, Perera R et al., 2006. Clinical recognition of meningococcal disease in children and adolescents. *The Lancet*, 367(9508), 397–403.

Thompson, 2008
Thompson G and Sciarra J (eds), 2008. *Wound Care Made Incredibly Visual*. Ambler: Lippincott Williams and Wilkins.

Thrumurthy, 2012
Thrumurthy SG, Karthikesalingam A, Patterson BO et al., 2012. The diagnosis and management of aortic dissection. *BMJ*, 344, d8290–d8290.

Tipton, 2011
Tipton MJ and Golden FSC, 2011. A proposed decision-making guide for the search, rescue and resuscitation of submersion (head under) victims based on expert opinion. *Resuscitation*, 82(7), 819–824.

Toon, 2010
Toon MH, Maybauer MO, Greenwood JE et al., 2010. Management of acute smoke inhalation injury. *Critical Care and Resuscitation: Journal of the Australasian Academy of Critical Care Medicine*, 12(1), 53–61.

Tortora, 2017
Tortora GJ and Derrickson BH, 2017. *Principles of Anatomy and Physiology*. 15th ed. Hoboken: John Wiley Inc.

Tovey, 2008
Tovey, G, 2008. *Nutcases: Medical Law*. London: Sweet & Maxwell.

Truhlář, 2015
Truhlář A, Deakin CD, Soar J et al., 2015. European resuscitation council guidelines for resuscitation 2015. Section 4. Cardiac arrest in special circumstances. *Resuscitation*, 95, 148–201.

UCL Institute of Health Equity, 2010
UCL Institute of Health Equity, 2010. *Fair Society, Healthy Lives: The Marmot Review*. Available at: http://www.instituteofhealthequity.org/resources-reports/fair-society-healthy-lives-the-marmot-review [Accessed: 24 July 2019].

UK Fire Service Resources, 2019
UK Fire Service Resources, 2019. *Vehicle Fires*. Available at: https://www.fireservice.co.uk/safety/vehicle-fires/ [Accessed: 29 July 2019].

UK Government, 1983
UK Government, 1983. *Mental Health Act 1983*. Available at: https://www.legislation.gov.uk/ukpga/1983/20/contents. [Accessed: 19 January 2019].

UK Government, 2007
UK Government, 2007. *Mental Health Act 2007*. Available at: https://www.legislation.gov.uk/ukpga/2007/12/contents. [Accessed: 20 January 2019].

References

UK Government, 2015
UK Government, 2015. *Inequalities in Health and Life Expectancies Persist.* Available at: https://www.gov.uk/government/news/inequalities-in-health-and-life-expectancies-persist [Accessed: 3 March 2019].

UK Government, 2017a
UK Government, 2017. *Chapter 5: Inequality in health.* Available at: https://www.gov.uk/government/publications/health-profile-for-england/chapter-5-inequality-in-health [Accessed: 3 March 2019].

UK Government, 2017b
UK Government, 2017. *Home Secretary Announces Action Plan to Tackle Acid Attacks.* Available at: https://www.gov.uk/government/news/home-secretary-announces-action-plan-to-tackle-acid-attacks [Accessed: 16 February 2019].

UK Government, 2018
UK Government, 2018. *NHS Foundation Trust Directory.* Available at: https://www.gov.uk/government/publications/nhs-foundation-trust-directory/nhs-foundation-trust-directory#what-are-foundation-trusts [Accessed: 3 January 2019].

UKST, 2017
United Kingdom Sepsis Trust, 2017. *The Sepsis Manual.* Available at: https://sepsistrust.org/wp-content/uploads/2018/06/Sepsis_Manual_2017_web_download.pdf [Accessed 30 June 2019].

UNICEF, 2013
UNICEF, 2013. *Female Genital Mutilation/Cutting.* Available at: https://www.unicef.org/cbsc/files/UNICEF_FGM_report_July_2013_Hi_res.pdf [Accessed: 24 July 2019].

UNICEF, 2018
UNICEF, 2018. *What You Need to Know About Female Genital Mutilation.* Available at: https://www.unicef.org/protection/57929_endFGM.html [Accessed: 5 January 2019].

Vaidya, 2016
Vaidya, R et al., 2016. Patients with pelvic fractures from blunt trauma. What is the cause of mortality and when? *American Journal of Surgery*, 211(3), 495–500.

Valensi, 2011
Valensi P, Lorgis L and Cottin Y, 2011. Prevalence, incidence, predictive factors and prognosis of silent myocardial infarction: A review of the literature. *Archives of Cardiovascular Diseases*, 104(3), 178–188.

Van Ness-Otunnu, 2013
Van Ness-Otunnu R and Hack JB, 2013. Hyperglycemic crisis. *Journal of Emergency Medicine*, 45(5), 797–805.

Vause, 2005
Vause S and Saroya DK, 2005. Functions of the placenta. *Anaesthesia & Intensive Care Medicine*, 6(3), 77–80.

Venema, 2010
Venema AM, Groothoff JW and Bierens JJLM, 2010. The role of bystanders during rescue and resuscitation of drowning victims. *Resuscitation*, 81(4), 434–439.

Walfish, 2009
Walfish M, Neuman A and Wlody D, 2009. Maternal haemorrhage. *British Journal of Anaesthesia*, 103 (Supplement 1), i47–i56.

Walker, 2006
Walker A, James C, Bannister M et al., 2006. Evaluation of a diabetes referral pathway for the management of hypoglycaemia following emergency contact with the ambulance service to a diabetes specialist nurse team. *Emergency Medicine Journal*, 23(6), 449–451.

Wallis, 2006
Wallis LA and Carley S, 2006. Comparison of paediatric major incident primary triage tools. *Emergency Medicine Journal*, 23(6), 475–478.

Walls, 2012
Walls RM and Murphy MF (eds), 2012. *Manual of Emergency Airway Management*. 4th ed. Philadelphia: Wolters Kluwer/Lippincott Williams & Wilkins Health.

Walters, 2005
Walters TJ and Mabry RL, 2005. Issues related to the use of tourniquets on the battlefield. *Military Medicine*, 170(9), 770–775.

Warden, 2014
Warden S, Spiwak R, Sareen J et al., 2014. The sad persons scale for suicide risk assessment: A systematic review. *Archives of Suicide Research*, 18(4), 313–26.

Wardrope, 2008
Wardrope J, Driscoll P, Laird JC et al., 2008. *Community Emergency Medicine*. London: Churchill Livingstone.

WAS, 2018
Welsh Ambulance Service, 2018. *Falls Pathway*. Available at: https://www.ambulance.wales.nhs.uk/Default.aspx?pageId=205&lan=en [Accessed: 16 December 2018].

Waterhouse, 2009
Waterhouse C, 2009. The use of painful stimulus in relation to Glasgow Coma Scale observations. *British Journal of Neuroscience Nursing*, 5(5), 209–215.

References

Watson, 2001
Watson RS, Cummings P, Quan L et al., 2001. Cervical spine injuries among submersion victims. *Journal of Trauma*, 51(4), 658–662.

Watson, 2009
Watson MS (ed.), 2009. *Oxford Handbook of Palliative Care*. 2nd ed. Oxford: Oxford University Press.

Waugh, 2011
Waugh A and Grant A. 2011. *Ross and Wilson: Anatomy and Physiology in Health and Illness*. London: Churchill Livingstone Elsevier.

Wells, 2001
Wells LC, Smith JC, Weston VC et al., 2001. The child with a non-blanching rash: How likely is meningococcal disease? *Archives of Disease in Childhood*, 85(3), 218–222.

Weston, 2014
Weston D, 2014. *Fundamentals of Infection Prevention and Control: Theory and Practice*. 2nd ed. Chichester: John Wiley & Sons.

Whitaker, 2011
Whitaker DK, 2011. Time for capnography – everywhere. *Anaesthesia*, 66(7), 544–549.

White, 2010
White K and Arlt W, 2010. Adrenal crisis in treated addison's disease: A predictable but under-managed event. *European Journal of Endocrinology*, 162(1), 115–120.

WHO, 1996
World Health Organization, 1996. *Care in Normal Birth: A practical approach*. London: WHO.

WHO, 1999
World Health Organization, 1999. *Definition, Diagnosis and Classification of Diabetes Mellitus and its Complications*. Available at: https://apps.who.int/iris/bitstream/handle/10665/66040/WHO_NCD_NCS_99.2.pdf?sequence=1 [Accessed: 4 July 2019].

WHO, 2008
World Health Organization, 2008. *Classification of Female Genital Mutilation*. Available at: https://www.who.int/reproductivehealth/topics/fgm/overview/en/. [Accessed: 15 February 2019].

WHO, 2009a
World Health Organization, 2009. *WHO Guidelines on Hand Hygiene in Health Care: First Global Patient Safety Challenge: Clean Care is Safer Care. Patient Safety*. Geneva: World Health Organization.

WHO, 2009b
World Health Organization, 2009. *WHO Guidelines for Safe Surgery 2009: Safe Surgery Saves Lives*. Available at: http://apps.who.int/iris/bitstream/10665/44185/1/9789241598552_eng.pdf [Accessed: 21 January 2018].

WHO, 2011
World Health Organization, 2011. *Pulse Oximetry Training Manual*. Available at: https://www.who.int/patientsafety/safesurgery/pulse_oximetry/who_ps_pulse_oxymetry_training_manual_en.pdf?ua=1 [Accessed: 18 December 2018].

WHO, 2012
World Health Organization, 2012. *WHO Recommendations for the Prevention and Treatment of Postpartum Haemorrhage*. Geneva: World Health Organization, Available at: http://apps.who.int/iris/bitstream/10665/75411/1/9789241548502_eng.pdf?ua=1 [Accessed: 3 July 2019].

WHO, 2013
World Health Organization, 2013. *What Health Challenges Do Preterm Babies Face?* Available at: http://www.who.int/features/qa/preterm_health_challenges/en/ [Accessed: 16 July 2019].

WHO, 2014a
World Health Organization, 2014. *Preterm Birth*. Available at: http://www.who.int/mediacentre/factsheets/fs363/en/ [Accessed: 16 July 2019].

WHO, 2014b
World Health Organization 2014. *Mental Health: A state of well-being*. Available at: http://www.who.int/features/factfiles/mental_health/en/ [Accessed: 11 July 2019].

WHO, 2018
World Health Organization, 2018. *Infection Prevention and Control*. Available at: https://www.who.int/infection-prevention/about/en/ [Accessed: 23 December 2018].

Wijdicks, 2010
Wijdicks EFM, 2010. The bare essentials: Coma. *Practical Neurology*, 10(1), 51–60.

Williams, 2013
Williams TA, Finn J, Celenza A et al., 2013. Paramedic identification of acute pulmonary edema in a metropolitan ambulance service. *Prehospital Emergency Care*, 17(3), 339–347.

Women's Aid, 2019
Women's Aid, 2019. *What is Coercive Control?* Available at: https://www.womensaid.org.uk/information-support/what-is-domestic-abuse/coercive-control/ [Accessed: 17 February 2019].

Wyllie, 2015
Wyllie J, Bruinenberg J, Roehr CC et al., 2015. European resuscitation council guidelines for resuscitation 2015. Section 7: Resuscitation and support of transition of babies at birth. *Resuscitation*, 95, 249–263.

Xue, 2012
Xue QL, 2011. The frailty syndrome: Definition and natural history. *Clinics in Geriatric Medicine*, 27(1), 1–15.

Yan, 2014
Yan EB, Satgunaseelan L, Paul E et al., 2014. Post-traumatic hypoxia is associated with prolonged cerebral cytokine production, higher serum biomarker levels, and poor outcome in patients with severe traumatic brain injury. *Journal of Neurotrauma*, 31(7), 618–629.

Yarmus, 2019
Yarmus L and Akulian J, 2019. *Pneumothorax – Symptoms, diagnosis and treatment, BMJ Best Practice*. Available at: https://bestpractice.bmj.com/topics/en-gb/504/ [Accessed: 29 July 2019].

YAS, 2013
Yorkshire Ambulance Service NHS Trust, 2013. *Dementia Learning Resource for Ambulance Staff*. Available at: https://dementiapartnerships.com/resource/dementia-learning-resource-for-ambulance-staff/ [Accessed: 15 July 2019].

Yoon, 2013
Yoon, JS et al., 2013. Tension pneumothorax, is it a really life-threatening condition?, *Journal of Cardiothoracic Surgery*, 15(8), 197.

Young, 2019
Young GB, 2019. *Assessment of Coma*. Available at: https://bestpractice.bmj.com/topics/en-gb/417 [Accessed: 18 July 2019].

Zabir, 2008
Zabir AF, Choy CY and Rushdan R, 2008. Glass particle contamination of parenteral preparations of intravenous drugs in anaesthetic practice: Original research. *Southern African Journal of Anaesthesia and Analgesia*, 14(3), 17–19.

Zideman, 2015
Zideman DA, De Buck EDJ, Singletary EM et al., 2015. European resuscitation council guidelines for resuscitation 2015. Section 9. First aid. *Resuscitation*, 95, 278–287.

Zuercher, 2009
Zuercher M, Ummenhofer W, Baltussen A et al., 2009. The use of Glasgow Coma Scale in injury assessment: A critical review. *Brain Injury*, 23(5), 371–384.

Glossary

Medical terminology can be rather overwhelming at first. This glossary will provide an explanation of various terms.

Anterior
The front surface of the body, or situated nearer to the front of the body (particularly if comparing the position of one structure to another).

Arrhythmia
A problem with the rate or rhythm of the heartbeat.

Aspiration
Fluid or solid entering the lower respiratory tract (larynx and below).

Aspirin
Aspirin has an anti-platelet action which reduces clot formation and has analgesic (pain-relieving), antipyretic (temperature reducing) and anti-inflammatory actions.

Atelectasis
A collapse of lung tissue affecting all or part of a lung, and preventing the absorption of oxygen into the blood supply.

Auscultation
The technique of listening to sounds within the body using a stethoscope.

Autoimmune disease
Autoimmune diseases arise from an abnormal immune response of the body against itself, i.e. against substances and tissues that are normally present in the body.

Avulsion
An injury that occurs when a body structure is forcibly detached from its normal point of insertion by a traumatic force.

Battles sign
Bruising behind the ears, which can indicate a skull fracture.

Body mass index
Body mass index (BMI) is defined as a person's weight divided by the square of their height in metres (kg/m^2). This can be adjusted for age and gender, and supplemented with waist circumference measurements, if appropriate. A patient with a BMI of 2529.9 kg/m^2 is considered to be overweight, and if over 30 kg/m^2, obese.

Bradycardia
Slow heart rate.

Brittle asthma
Brittle asthma is a rare form of severe asthma which can result in very serious and often life-threatening attacks.

BVM
Bag-valve-mask.

Cachexia
A state of very severe weakness and ill-health involving multi-system problems such as muscle wasting, anaemia and difficulties with circulation.

Care Quality Commission
An independent health and adult social care regulator for England. Its job is to make sure health and social care services provide people with safe, effective, compassionate, high-quality care. It does this by monitoring, inspecting and regulating services to make sure they meet fundamental standards of quality and safety.

Cartilage
Cartilage is a flexible connective tissue found in areas of the body, including the joints between bones, the ribcage, the ear, the nose, the bronchial tubes and the intervertebral discs. It is not as hard and rigid as bone but is stiffer and less flexible than muscle. It does not contain blood vessels, so grows and repairs slowly.

Catastrophic haemorrhage
Bleeding severe enough to cause exsanguination, i.e. blood loss causing death, typically within minutes, or less.

Cauda equine syndrome
A condition caused by a prolapse of the lumbar disc causing the roots of the lumbosacral nerve to be compressed. This causes pain, loss of feeling in the lumbar region and problems with bladder and bowel function.

Choking
A mechanical obstruction of the airway occurring anywhere between the mouth and carina.

Circadian rhythms
Circadian rhythms are physical, mental and behavioural changes that follow an approximate 24-hour cycle, responding primarily to light and darkness in a person's environment.

Glossary

Cognitive function
A person's ability to process thoughts. It encompasses memories, perception, thinking and reasoning.

Compartment syndrome
Increased pressure with a confined anatomical space due to an injury, causing reduction of blood flow. This leads to pain and tissue damage sometimes leading to loss of the affected limb or organ.

Connective tissue
Basic tissue type that binds, supports and separates other tissue and organs.

Crepitus
The grating, crackling or popping sounds and sensations experienced under the skin and joints, or a crackling sensation due to the presence of air under the skin. A type of crepitus, bone crepitus, can be heard and felt when two fragments of a fracture are moved against each other.

Distal
Further from the point of attachment of a limb.

Dysphagia
Difficulty swallowing.

Dysphasia
Language disorder marked by a deficiency in the generation of speech, and sometimes also in its comprehension, due to brain disease or damage.

Dyspnoea
Difficulty breathing.

Endometriosis
The presence of cells of the endometrium outside the womb, causing pain and bleeding. Endometriosis can have a negative effect on a woman's ability to conceive.

$EtCO_2$
End-tidal carbon dioxide. The measurement of carbon dioxide at the end of expiration.

Fetal maceration
Degeneration and eventual disintegration of the body of a deceased unborn baby.

Focal
Affecting a specific region of the body. For example, a focal neurological deficit may result in a weakness or paralysis of a limb following an impairment of nerve, spinal cord, or brain function.

Furosemide
A commonly used diuretic (water tablet) from the group known as loop diuretics.

GFR
Abbreviation for glomerular filtration rate, also the name of a test which indicates how effectively the kidneys get rid of waste by measuring the number of millilitres of blood the kidneys are able to filter in one minute.

Glasgow Coma Scale score
The Glasgow Coma Scale (GCS) was developed in 1974 as a way of objectively testing the level of consciousness in brain-injured patients and to improve communication between healthcare professionals. It was originally a 14-point score, but the division of limb flexion into withdrawal and abnormal flexion led to the 15-point score familiar today. Although designed for in-hospital use, it is now routinely used by the ambulance service and is an important marker for the early management of traumatic brain injury (TBI).

Glucosuria
Presence of glucose in the urine.

Haematoma
A blood clot that has formed outside a blood vessel (artery or vein).

Haemolysis
Alteration or destruction of the red blood cells leading to release of the oxygen-carrying pigment haemoglobin.

Haemoptysis
Coughing up or spitting of blood from the lungs.

Humerus
The long bone of the upper arm, reaching from shoulder to elbow.

Hyperkalaemia
Too high a level of potassium in the blood.

Hypernatraemia
Too high a level of sodium in the blood.

Hypokalaemia
An insufficient level of potassium in the blood.

Hyponatraemia
An insufficient level of sodium in the blood.

Glossary

Ileus
A partial or complete blockage of the intestine, usually the small intestine.

Intercostal
Between the ribs.

Intramural haematoma
A haematoma that forms within the wall of an organ such as the bladder.

Ketonaemia
The presence of ketone bodies in the blood.

Korotkoff sounds
Turbulent blood flow that can be heard when using the manual auscultatory technique to record blood pressure. Named after a Russian surgeon, Nikolai Korotkoff, who first described them in 1905.

Kussmaul breathing
Breathing that is abnormally deep and rapid, sighing. It can be a sign of diabetic ketoacidosis, or sometimes of kidney failure. Named after the nineteenth century Strasbourg physician Adolph Kussmaul.

Lateral
Of, at, towards, or from the side or sides.

Ligand
An organic molecule which binds to a protein or nucleic acid, or to a tracer element such as an isotope.

Loop diuretics
Diuretics (water tablets) that work by inhibiting the absorption of sodium and chloride not only in the proximal and distal tubules of the kidney but also in the loop of Henle. Furosemide is an example of this class of diuretic.

Meconium
A dark green substance in the intestine of a full-term fetus, also the primary constituent of the first faeces passed by a newborn.

Medial
Towards or at the midline of the body.

METHANE
The mnemonic METHANE is designed to provide the initial communication surrounding details of a major incident. It consists of:
- **M**ajor incident declared or standby. The person making the report should be explicit whether this is a major incident declaration or a standby in anticipation of the occurrence of a major incident
- **E**xact location of the incident. Where possible the grid reference or GPS co-ordinates should be included, along with any landmarks or iconic sites
- **T**ype of incident. What is the exact nature of the incident? For example rail, chemical, road or terrorist
- **H**azards. What hazards are known to be present or could potentially manifest themselves?
- **A**ccess and egress. What are the agreed or best routes to and from the scene?
- **N**umber of casualties. How many casualties are there and, if possible to determine, what are the level and severity of injuries?
- **E**mergency services. Which emergency services are present and which are required? Include specialist resource request if known.

Microorganism
A very small organism that lives outside and inside larger organisms such as the human body.

Multiparity
Having given birth to more than two babies.

Necrosis
Death of body tissue.

Oedema
An abnormal build-up of fluid, mainly water, in the body. People with kidney failure are prone to fluid overload, leading to oedema.

Oliguria
Abnormally reduced production of urine.

OPA
Oropharyngeal airway. A curved plastic tube, with a reinforced flange at one end and designed so that it fits between the tongue and hard palate to help keep the airway open.

OPQRST
- **O** Onset. When did it (the presenting complaint) start?
- **P** Provocation/palliation. What makes it worse/better? Include self-treatment such as taking analgesia
- **Q** Quality. How does the patient describe their symptom, particularly pain? Is it sharp or dull, for example?
- **R** Region/radiation/referral. Where is the symptom located? In the case of pain, does it stay in one place

(can the patient point to it with one finger) or does it go elsewhere?
- **S** Severity. On a scale of 0 to 10, where 0 is no pain and 10 is the worst pain imaginable, what score does the patient give it now?
- **T** Time. How long has the patient had it and if it has been relieved, when did this occur? In the case of pain, also consider whether the pain is intermittent (comes and goes).

Osmotic diuresis
Osmosis is the process by which water moves from a weaker to a stronger solution through tiny holes in a semi-permeable membrane. Osmotic diuresis occurs when increased passing of urine is caused by the presence of non-absorbable, osmotically active substances in the renal tubules.

Osteomyelitis
A destructive infection of the bone, usually bacterial in origin.

Oxytocic
A drug or other substance that promotes labour by stimulating the uterus to contract.

Palpable
Able to be touched or felt.

Panda eyes
Bruising around both eyes that can be a sign of skull fracture.

Partial pressure
In a mixture of gases, each gas has a partial pressure which is the hypothetical pressure of that gas if it alone occupied the volume of the mixture at the same temperature. The total pressure of the gas mixture is the sum of the partial pressures of each individual gas in the mixture.

Percussion
A method of tapping on a surface to determine the underlying structure. It is used in clinical examinations to assess the condition of the thorax or abdomen.

Pitting oedema
Swelling or oedema which, if pressed with a finger, shows a visible indent.

Pleuritic chest pain
Chest pain that is usually sharp and stabbing, localised to a specific area of the chest (the patient can often point to the pain with a finger) and made worse by coughing and deep inspiration.

Polypharmacy
The administration of large numbers of prescription drugs at the same time.

Polyuria
The passing of large quantities of urine due to excess glucose in the bloodstream. It is a symptom of untreated diabetes.

Posterior
Further back in position; of or nearer the rear or hind end.

Primary assessment
A swift patient assessment and management process, which can be completed within 60–90 seconds. It is designed to be a stepwise approach, meaning that any abnormalities identified in one step should be addressed before moving on to the next.

Precordium
The area over the heart and lower thorax.

Primiparity
Having only given birth once before.

Proprioception
The sense of the relative position of neighbouring parts of the body and strength of effort being employed in movement.

Proximal
Located nearer to the centre of the body or the point of attachment.

Pruritis
Itching or irritation. For example, pruritus vulvae is irritation of the vulva (the genital area in women) which is caused by an infection that occurs because of an excess of sugar in the urine and is often an early sign of diabetes.

Psychomotor
Physical behaviour that is the result of conscious mental processes.

Pulse oximetry
The technique of measuring the oxygen saturation of the haemoglobin in the blood.

Recession
In an anatomical context, the drawing away of a tissue (or part of a tissue) from its normal position.

Rigors
Shaking or exaggerated shivering which usually occurs in response to a high temperature.

Glossary

SADs
Supraglottic Airway Devices. Airway devices that sit just above the glottis. The most common SAD is the laryngeal mask airway.

SAMPLE
An acronym for:
- **S** Signs and symptoms of the presenting complaint
- **A** Allergies (particularly to medication but food allergies might be relevant)
- **M** Medications
- **P** Past medical history
- **L** Last oral intake
- **E** Events that led to the current illness or injury

Scope of practice
The area or areas of a person's profession where they have the knowledge, skill and experience to practise safely and effectively.

SOCRATES
- **S** Site
- **O** Onset
- **C** Character. Same as Quality above
- **R** Radiation
- **A** Association. Are there any other signs and symptoms associated with the presenting complaint?
- **T** Timing
- **E** Exacerbating/relieving factors
- **S** Severity

Splanchnic
Referring to organs in the abdominal cavity.

Stridor
High-pitched (usually) inspiratory breath sound, indicating upper airway narrowing.

Superior
Located above or directed upward. In human anatomy, situated nearer to the top of the head (vertex). Opposite of inferior.

Supine
Lying face up, usually referring to a patient who is lying on their back.

Surfactant
A substance made up of lipids and proteins and produced in the lungs. It forms a coating over the surface of the alveoli to stabilise them and enable them to function effectively.

Sympathomimetic
An agent that produces an effect similar to that of the sympathetic nervous system.

Tachycardia
Rapid heart rate.

Tachypnoea
Rapid breathing rate.

Thoracentesis
A procedure to remove fluid (usually via a hollow needle) from the chest for analysis.

Thoracotomy
An incision of the chest wall.

TILE
- **T**ask. Consider if the lift:
  - Involves holding the load away from the body Involves long distances
  - Requires strenuous effort or twisting
- **I**ndividual. Consider whether the lift:
  - Requires specialist training
  - Presents a hazard
  - If you and your colleagues are capable of performing the lift
- **L**oad. Is the load:
  - Heavy
  - Difficult to get hold of
  - Unstable
  - Unpredictable
  - Harmful
  - Likely to grab out when alarmed at being carried down the stairs
- **E**nvironment. Determine the presence of:
  - Constraints on posture, e.g. low ceiling, confined spaces
  - Poor, uneven flooring
  - Hot/cold/wet weather
  - Poor lighting
  - Noise.

Trendelenburg position
Trolley positioned with the feet-end of the trolley raised, and the head-end lowered.

Trismus
A spasm of the jaw muscles that makes it difficult to open the mouth. Also called lockjaw.

Turgor
Condition of normal tension in a cell or group of cells, such as the skin.

Urticaria
(Also called nettle rash or hives.) Swelling of the superficial layers of the skin, usually as a result of an allergic reaction. The characteristic itchy lumps (called weals or hives) last for only a few hours.

Viscus
Any large organ in the interior of the abdomen.

Index

AACE, see Association of Ambulance Chief Executives (AACE)
AAPs, see associate ambulance practitioners (AAPs)
Abbey pain scale 375, 449–450, 461
ABCDE assessment 141
abdomen
    assessment 328, 330
    injuries 340–341
    pan in pregnancy 402
abdominal cavity 340
abnormal capnograms 205
abrasion, see grazes (abrasion)
abrasion (grazes), 325–326
abrasions 369
abuse
    child 50
    domestic violence and 53
    escalating concerns 55
    female genital mutilation 52
    financial 52
    forms of 51–52
    neglect 52
    physical 51
    psychological/emotional 51
    sexual 51–52
    of vulnerable adults 50
Accu-Chek Aviva blood glucose meter 292–294
ACE, see Ambu Perfit adjustable collar for extrication (ACE)
acid burns 370
acidosis 290
ACP, see advance care planning (ACP)
acrocyanosis 431
ACS, see acute coronary syndromes (ACS)
ACTH, see adrenocorticotrophic hormone (ACTH)
acute abdomen
    abdominal cavity 300–302
    abdominal pain 302–303
        management of 303–304
    digestive system 302
    locating abdominal organs 302
acute chest syndrome 249
acute coronary syndromes (ACS)
    aspirin 241
    assessment of 240–241
    glyceryl trinitrate 241–242
    management of 242
    pathophysiology 240
acute heart failure (AHF) 243
acute myocardial ischaemia 467
acute smoke inhalation injury 369
Addison's disease 294
    adrenal crisis 294
    management of 295
    signs and symptoms 294–295

adenoids 150
adjuncts, airway 160–162
adrenal cortex 286–287
adrenal glands 286–288
adrenaline 281
    administration of 118
adrenocorticotrophic hormone (ACTH) 287–288
ADRT, see advance decision to refuse treatment (ADRT)
adult basic life support 467–470
adult defibrillation 477
advance care planning (ACP) 485–486
advance care planning 491–492
advance decision to refuse treatment (ADRT) 38, 486, 491
advance statement of preferences, see living will
Advanced Medical Priority Dispatch System 8
advanced paramedics 11
AEDs, see automated external defibrillators (AEDs)
affective, see mood (affective) disorders
afferent pupillary defect 262
age-related changes 465
ageing, see older people
aggressive behaviour 460–461
agonal rhythm 475
AHF, see acute heart failure (AHF)
AIC, see ambulance incident commander (AIC)
Airflo compressor 97
Airflo Plus compressor 98
Airwave network 21–22
airway
    adjuncts 160–167
    anatomy 149–152
    assessment 142
    assisting the paramedic 373
    bronchi 152
    children and infants 425, 431
    choking in adults 171–173
    choking in paediatrics 173–175
    head tilt–chin lift 154
    jaw thrust 154–156
    laryngectomy 170–171
    laryngopharynx 150–151
    larynx 151–152
    lower 151
    lungs 152
    management 152–167
    management, maxillofacial injuries 333–334
    manual airway manoeuvres 154–158
    mouth 149–150
    nasopharynx 150
    newborn 420
    nose 149
    older people 452
    oral cavity 150

Index

oropharyngeal airway (OPA) 160–161
oropharynx 150
paediatric 173–174
pharynx 150
recovery position 156–158
respiratory system, structures of 149
smoke inhalation 369
suction 158
suction catheters 158–160
trachea 152
tracheal intubation 373–378
tracheostomies 167–171
tracheostomy 170
trauma 327–328
traumatic brain injury 331
triple airway manoeuvre 156
upper 149
alcohol consumption 27
alcohol handrub, hand hygiene with 68–70
alcohol-resistant organisms 68
alkali burns 370
allergies 144
ALSG score 405
alternative care providers 9–10
alveoli 178
   gas exchange 179–180
Alzheimer's disease 458
Ambu Perfit adjustable collar for extrication (ACE)
   sitting position 351–353
   supine position 353
ambulance incident commander (AIC) 130
ambulance service, see also major incidents
   call for help 8
   clinical leadership roles 11–12
   clinical roles 10–11
   command and control roles 12–13
   handling aids 89
   legislation and guidelines 113
   major accidents command and control 129–131
   onward care 9–10
   organisational structure 7
   patient-centred care in 34
   response 8–9
   response programme call categories 9
   response to 999 call 7–8
   role in major accidents 128–129
   triage 8
   types of waste from activity 77
   working relationships 13
ambulance trolley 110–112
AMHP, see approved mental health professional (AMHP)
ammonia 369
ampoules, drawing medication from 114–116
anaphylaxis
   ABCDE assessment 281
   auto-injectors 281
   emergency management of 280

Jext auto-injector 281–282
   management 281–282
   signs and symptoms 280–281
anatomy and physiology 393
   of adrenal glands 286–288
   of pancreas 285–286
aneroid sphygmomanometer 229
angina 240
anisocoria 262
ANS, see autonomic nervous system (ANS)
antepartum haemorrhage (APH) 402–404
anti-proteases 213
anti-radicalisation 55–56
anticipatory prescribing, end of life care 491
antihistamines 281
anxiety 439
aorta 221, 244
aortic dissection 244–246
APH, see antepartum haemorrhage (APH)
approved mental health professional (AMHP) 437
aprons 73
   removing 74–75
   wearing 41
arachnoid 254
arm weakness 262
arteries, see also aorta; coronary artery disease
   blood pressure in 220
   coronary 219–220
   structure 220
   supplying brain 266
arterioles 220
arthritis, in older people 455
aspiration
   cardiac arrest in pregnancy 482
   diabetes mellitus 289
   drowning 275
   heat stroke 275
   last oral intake 145
   suction 159
   tracheostomy 168
aspirin 241, 335
   administration of 117
assisted ventilation, see also bag-valve-mask ventilation; basic life support (BLS); breathing
   bag-valve-mask 189–190
   cardiac arrest in adults 468–470
   cardiac arrest in child 472–474
   cardiac arrest in drowned patients 483
   cardiac arrest in infants 470–472
   cardiac arrest in pregnancy 482
   choking in adults 173
   choking in paediatrics 174
   chronic obstructive pulmonary disease 214
   drowning 275
   facial shields 188
   gastric distension 187
   mouth-to-mask 188–189

Index

mouth-to-mouth 187–188
Pneupac ParaPAC ventilator 190
pressure-compensated flowmeter 191–192
respiratory rate 200
Schrader outlet 191–192
tracheostomy 168–175
assisting the paramedic
   intraosseous cannulation 384–392
   intravenous cannulation 378–382
   intravenous drug administration 378–392
   intravenous infusion, preparing 382–384
   tracheal intubation 373–378
associate ambulance practitioners (AAPs) 10–11
associated neurons 257–258
Association of Ambulance Chief Executives (AACE) 7
asthma
   assessment of severity 209
   defined 208
   life-threatening 211
   management of 211
   medication 208–209
   pathophysiology 208
   preventer inhalers 208
   reliever inhalers 209
   signs and symptoms 209
asystole 152, 475–476
atherosclerosis 239
ATMIST model 19
atria 218
atrial kick 219
attitudes
   to ageing 457
   factors influencing 26–27
auscultation
   absent sounds 207
   added (adventitious) sounds 206–207
   breath sounds 206–207
   chest 207–208
   children and infants 430, 432
   normal breath sounds 206
   stethoscope 204–206
   in trauma 330
auscultatory blood pressure measurement 229
auto-injectors 281
automated blood pressure measurement 229
automated external defibrillators (AEDs) 476, 478–479, 481
autonomic conflict 275
autonomic nervous system
   older people 454
autonomic nervous system (ANS) 256–257
autoregulation 254
AVPU mnemonic 434
AVPU score 143, 145
axon 251, 252

Bachmann bundle 219
bacteria 66
bag-valve-mask (BVM) ventilation 189–190
   newborn 420
   one-person ventilation 189
   two-person ventilation 190
bag-valve-mask ventilation, children and infants 433
banana board, see transfer board (banana board)
banana board (transfer board) 101
'bare below elbows' policy 73
bariatric patients, manual handling 91–92
barotrauma 337
basic life support (BLS)
   adult 468–470
   child 472–474
   infant 470–472
   newborn 419–421
   paediatric 470–474
   procedure 468–474
Battle's sign (panda eyes) 331
bereavement
   defined 493–494
   and grieving process 494
   referring for additional help 494
   sources of help 494
   support for health professionals 495
best-interest decisions 35, 38
bimanual laryngoscopy 377
biological spillage 79
biomechanics 88
bipolar affective disorder 440
blanketing on carry chair 108–110
blast injury 318
blastocyst 399
bleeding 320–321
   assessment 321
   blood loss, estimating 321
   catastrophic haemorrhage management 322
   haemostatic agents 325
   management 321–322
   non-catastrophic haemorrhage 322
   procedure 323–325
   sources of 321
   tourniquets 323
   in trauma 328
blistering 371
blood clots, see thrombi (blood clots)
blood loss
   estimating 321
   signs of 328–329
blood pressure (BP)
   children and infants 426
   diastolic 228
   Korotkoff sounds 229
   measurement of 229–231
   non-invasive blood pressure 229
   normal range 229
   in older people 453
   pregnancy 399

Index

systolic 228
and triage 133
values 229
blood sugar 143, 288
measurement 292–294
blood sugar measurement 292–295
blood vessels
arteries 220
older people 453
structure 220–221
veins 220
BLS, *see* basic life support (BLS)
blue-light transfer 370
blunt trauma 313
abdominal injuries 341
abdominal injury 317
contusion 325
to eye 334
flail chest 340
head injuries 315
pneumothorax 337
spinal injuries 337
bones
assessment 328
older people 451
box splints 357–358
Boyle's Law 179
BP, *see* blood pressure (BP)
brachial pulse 226–227
bradycardia
causes of 227
children and infants 152, 433
drowning 275
spinal injuries 336
brain
arachnoid 254
arteries supplying 266
autoregulation 254
brain stem 253
cerebellum 253
cerebrospinal fluid 254
cerebrum 253
cranial nerves 254–255
diencephalon 253
dura 254
eye 257–259
functions of 253
hypothalamus 254
medulla oblongata 253
meninges 254
midbrain 253
older people 453
pia 254
pons 253
thalamus 254
trauma 315
brain damage, learning disabilities and 448

brain stem 253
breasts, electrocardiogram of 235
breath sound, *see* crackles (breath sound); wheezes (breath sounds)
breathing
air pressure 178–179
assessment of 143, 200–208
assisted ventilation 187–190
asthma 208–212
auscultation 204–208
automatic control 180
capnography 203–204
carbon dioxide 180
children and infants 425–426, 431–432
chronic obstructive pulmonary disease 212–214
common respiratory conditions 208–216
control of 180
diffusion 179–180
Entonox 196–200
expiration 179
external respiration 177
forceful breathing 179
gas exchange 179–180
inspiration 179
internal respiration 177
laryngectomy 171
lungs 177–178
management, maxillofacial injuries 334
mechanical ventilation 190–192
mechanics of 178–180
newborn 420
oxygen administration 192–195
oxygen physiology 180–181
oxygen saturations 200–202
peak flow 202–203
pneumonia 214–215
pulmonary embolism 215–216
pulmonary ventilation 177
pulse oximetry 200–201
respiratory rate 200
stethoscope 204–206
tracheostomy 170
trauma 328
using medical gases 181–200
voluntary (conscious) control 180
work of 430
breech presentation 415–417
bronchi 152, 177, 178
bronchial breath sounds 206
bronchodilators 214
bronchovesicular breath sounds 206
'bronze' commanders, *see* operational commanders
bruises, *see* contusion (bruises)
bruises (contusion) 326
buccal tablets 117
bundle of His 219, 453
burns

545

Index

ABC approach for 369
assessment of 366–367
cardiac arrest 485
chemical 370
classification 367
defined 366
electrical injuries 371
history of 366
impact of 371
radiation 370–371
requiring transport to hospital 367–368
'rule of nines' 366
sources of 366
thermal 368–370
types of 366
BURP manoeuvre 377
'but for' principle 28
BVM, see bag-valve-mask (BVM) ventilation

CAD, see coronary artery disease (CAD)
calcium 451
Canadian c-spine rule 456
cancellous bones 451
cannulas 379
CAP, see community-acquired pneumonia (CAP)
capacity, consent and 447
capillaries 220
capillary refill time (CRT) 433
    assessment in children 228
    defined 227–228
    factors affecting 228
    neonates 228
    recording 228
capnogram 203
capnography 169, 170, 171, 203–204
capnometry 203
carbon dioxide
    capnography 203
    gas exchange 179
carbon monoxide (CO), smoke inhalation 369
cardiac arrest
    adult basic life support 467–470
    cardiopulmonary resuscitation 467
    chain of survival 467–468
    chest compression 469–470, 471, 474, 479–480
    child basic life support 472–474
    children 468
    decisions 485–488
    defibrillation 474–481
    in drowned patients 483
    end of life decisions 485–486
    hypothermia and 482–483
    infant basic life support 470–474
    paediatric basic life support 470–474
    post-resuscitation care 468, 484–485
    in pregnancy 482
    recognition and call for help 467

recognition of life extinct 486–488
start and stop resuscitation 485
sudden unexpected death in infancy, children and adolescents 488
traumatic 483–484
cardiac arrhythmia, drowning 277
cardiac cycle
    atrial systole 221–222
    relaxation period 222
    ventricular systole 222
cardiac failure 430
cardiac output, pregnancy 399
cardiogeni shock c 247
cardiopulmonary resuscitation (CPR) 493
    cardiac arrest 467, 468
    drowning 276
cardiovascular system
    arteries 221
    atrial systole 221–222
    blood vessels 220–221
    cardiac cycle 221–222
    coronary arteries 215–220
    electrical conduction pathway 218–219
    electrocardiograms 222–223
    functions of 217
    heart 217–220
    older people 453
    relaxation period 222
    veins 221
    ventricular systole 222
cardiovascular system disorders 239–249
Care Quality Commission (CQC) 7, 30, 65, 66
carotid pulse 225, 226, 474
carry chair
    blanketing on 108–110
    transporting patient on 106–108
carry chair, see carry chair
carry sheet 101
casualty clearing officer (CCO) 131
casualty clearing station (CCS) 131
CAT tourniquet 323–324
catastrophic haemorrhage 142
    management 321–322
    primary survey 327
    treating and triaging 134
catastrophic incidents 128
catheter
    mounts 189
    suction 158–160
catheter-filter-capnography 373
cauda equina syndrome (CES) 268–269
causation 28
cavitation 314
CCO, see casualty clearing officer (CCO)
CCS, see casualty clearing station (CCS)
CDM, see clinical development manager (CDM)
cell body 252

Index

central nervous system (CNS)
   anatomy and physiology 251–253
   autonomic nervous system 256–257
   brain 253–255
   functions of 251
   information transfer and processing 251
   motor function 251
   neurons and neuroglia 252–253
   older people 453–454
   sensory function (perception) 251
   somatic nervous system 256
   spinal cord 255
central pain stimulus 260–261
cerebellum 253
cerebral cortex 336
cerebral hypoxia 275
cerebral perfusion pressure (CPP) 254
cerebrospinal fluid (CSF), 254
cerebrum 253
cervical collars 351
CES, see cauda equina syndrome (CES)
chain of infection 67
chain of survival 467–468
challenging behaviour 463–464
chemical, biological, radiological, nuclear, explosive CBRN(e) event 125, 126, 136
chemical burns 370
   eye injuries 334
chemical control 180
chemical energy 314
chemoreceptors 180
Chemsafe 135
chest assessment 328, 330
chest compression 469–470, 471, 474, 479–480
chest compressions 420–421
chest pain 467
child abuse 50, 428
child basic life support 472–474
child sexual exploitation 52
childbirth, normal, see also obstetrics
   complications 413–419
   equipment for 408–409
Children Act 2004, 135
children and infants
   abnormal airway sounds 430, 431
   abnormal positioning 430, 431
   accessory muscle use 432
   acrocyanosis 431
   airway 425, 431
   appearance 430
   assessment of
      infants 428
      pre-school 429
      school-age 429
      teenagers 429
      toddlers 428–429
   breathing 425–426, 431–432
   capillary refill time 228, 433
   cardiac arrest 470–474
   cardiac failure 430
   chain of survival 467
   choking 173–175
   circulation 426, 433–444
   circulation to skin 430
   cognitive development of infants 427
   cognitive development of pre-school 427
   cognitive development of school-age 427
   cognitive development of teenagers 427
   cognitive development of toddlers 427
   cyanosis 431
   developmental approach 428–429
   disability 434–435
   end-organ perfusion 434
   exposure/environment 435
   face and mouth 425
   flaring 430, 432
   fluid replacement 434
   general impression 430–431
   head bobbing 432
   heart rate 433
   hypoxia 470
   initial assessment and management 428–435
   major incidents 134–135
   meningococcal disease 264
   mottling 431
   nose and pharynx 425
   pallor 431
   positive-pressure ventilation 425
   primary survey 430–435
   pulse oximetry 433
   pulse volume 433
   recession 430, 432
   respiratory failure 430
   sick infant and child, recognising 429
   skin perfusion 433–434
   status epilepticus 264
   suction 431
   use of inhaler with spacer 118
   work of breathing 430
ChloraPrep 380
choking
   in adults 171–173
   algorithm 173
   causes 172
   conscious and 172, 174–175
   defined 171
   management 172–174
   paediatric airway 173–174
   recognition 172, 174
   signs of 174
   unconscious and 172–173, 175
chordae tendineae 218
chorionic villi 399
chronic bronchitis 213

Index

chronic obstructive pulmonary disease (COPD)
   crackles 206
   defined 212–213
   management of 214
   older people 453
   oxygen and 213
   pathophysiology 213
   sepsis and 284
   severe episode of 213
   signs and symptoms 213–214
   Venturi mask 186
cigarette smoking
   chronic obstructive pulmonary disease/chronic bronchitis/emphysema 212–214
   community-acquired pneumonia 214
   and fire risk 82
   and pre-term labour 418–419
circulation
   arteries 225
   assessment 143
   assessment of 225–239
   blood vessels 220–221
   cardiac cycle 221–222
   cardiovascular system disorders 239–249
   cardiovascular system, *see* cardiovascular system
   children and infants 426, 433–434
   coronary arteries 219–220
   heart 217–220
   lymphatic system and immunity 223–225
   management, maxillofacial injuries 334
   pulse 225–227
   trauma 328
   veins 221
circum-rescue collapse 276
Civil Contingencies Act 2004, 125, 134
Classification, Labelling and Packaging of Substances and Mixtures (CLP) Regulation 135
cleaning 78
   defined 76
   schedules 78
cleaning equipment, storage of 79
Clinell wipes 78–79
clinical development manager (CDM), 12
clinical governance 47–48
clinical leadership roles 11–12
clinical risk, defined 61
clinical roles 10–11
Clostridium difficile 68
CLP, *see* Classification, Labelling and Packaging of Substances and Mixtures (CLP) Regulation
CN, *see* cranial nerves (CN)
CNS, *see* central nervous system (CNS)
CO, *see* carbon monoxide (CO)
co-morbidities 460
coercive control 53
cognitive impairment 465
cold shock 275

College of Paramedics 7
colonisation 64
colour, assessment of newborn 419
coma 269–270
combustible materials, and fire risk 82
command and control roles 12–13
common toxidromes 296–297
communicating consent 35
communication
   age and 18
   barriers to 18
   basic model of 16
   with different people 15
   electronic devices 21–23
   electronic patient records 23
   emotions and 18
   end of life care 490, 492
   evacuate, disrobe and decontaminate, hazardous materials 139
   handover 19–20
   health and safety 61
   language 16, 18
   learning disabilities 449–450
   mobile data terminals 23
   modified model of 16
   non-verbal 17
   older people 463
   paralinguistic features of 16–17
   practical 19–21
   pre-alert 20
   principles of 2–3, 15–19
   radios 21–23
   record keeping 19
   sensory impairments and 18
   social context 17
   verbal 16–17
   vocabulary 16
   written 17
community-acquired pneumonia (CAP) 214
community responders 10
community treatment order (CTO) 439
complaints 29
conduction 271
confidentiality
   accessing information 43
   consent and 42
   disclosure, making 43–44
   electronic record-keeping 42
   maintaining 42–44
   patient-identifiable information 41
   physical records 42
   security of information 42–43
   sharing information 42
confirming tube placement 377–378
consent
   best-interest decisions 34
   communicating 34

Index

before sharing information 42
unable to gain 44
valid 34–35
consent and capacity 447
consolidation 214–215
constipation 454
consultant paramedic 11–12
contact dermatitis 72
CONTEST strategies 55–56
contiguous leads 236
contraction, uterine 403
Control of Substances Hazardous to Health Regulations 2002, 60, 65
contusion (bruises) 325
conus medullaris 255
convection 271
convulsions
   absence 263
   complex partial 263
   febrile 263
   generalised 263
   management of 264
   non-epileptic attack disorder 264
   partial (focal) 263
   patient's own buccal midazolam 264–265
   post-ictal phase 264
   pre-eclampsia 405
   after return of spontaneous circulation 484
   simple partial 263
   status epilepticus 264
   tonic-clonic 263
cooling 369–370
COPD, see chronic obstructive pulmonary disease (COPD)
corneal abrasion 334
coronary artery disease (CAD) 239
coroner, sharing information 44
Corpuls3 monitor/defibrillator 477
corticotropin-releasing hormone (CRH) 287–288
costal cartilages 452
counter-terrorism 55–56
County Hospital 25–26
CPP, see cerebral perfusion pressure (CPP)
CPR, see cardiopulmonary resuscitation (CPR)
CQC, see Care Quality Commission (CQC)
crackles (breath sound) 206
cranial nerves (CN) 254–255
crash helmet removal 356–357
CRH, see corticotropin-releasing hormone (CRH)
cricoid pressure, see Sellick's manoeuvre (cricoid pressure)
cricoid pressure (Sellick's manoeuvre) 377
critical care paramedics (CCPs), see specialist paramedic – critical care
CRT, see capillary refill time (CRT)
CSCATTT mnemonic 129
CSF, see cerebrospinal fluid (CSF)
CTO, see community treatment order (CTO)
culture, on abuse 50–51

Cushing's triad 331
cut, see incision (cut)
cut (incision) 326
cyanosis 431

danger labels 136, 138
Dangerous Preparations Directive (DPD) 135
Dangerous Substances Directive (DSD) 135
DCA, see double-crewed ambulance (DCA)
DCT, see Henle/distal convoluted tubule (DCT)
decompensation, signs of 433, 434
decontamination 76–77
   biological spillage 79
   defined 76
   national cleaning colour code 77–78
   personal protective equipment for 79
   procedure 78–79
   storage of cleaning equipment 79
deep vein thrombosis (DVT) 215
defibrillation
   adult 477
   in aircraft and helicopters 477
   asystole 475–476
   automated external defibrillators 476, 478–479, 481
   Corpuls3 monitor/defibrillator 477
   defined 474
   difficult environment and 477
   early 467–468
   manual defibrillators 476–477, 479–480, 481
   in metal surfaces 477
   non-shockable rhythms 475–476
   paediatric 480–481
   pulseless electrical activity 476
   safety 477
   shockable rhythms 475
   ventricular fibrillation 475
   ventricular tachycardia 475
   in wet surfaces 477
defibrillators
   automated external defibrillators 476, 478–479, 481
   Corpuls3 monitor/defibrillator 477
   manual defibrillators 476–477, 478, 481
delirium 440
   dementia vs 463
delusional disorders 440
dementia
   aggressive behaviour 460–461
   behavioural 458
   causes of 458–459
      Alzheimer's disease 458
      frontotemporal dementia 459
      Lewy bodies 458–459
      vascular dementia 458
   cognitive 458
   in context 458
   defined 457–458
   different types of 458

Index

and discrimination 461–463
living with 450
neurological 458
other diseases 460
and pain management 461
progression 459
recognising 459–460
treatment of 463
vs delirium 463
dendrites 252
depression 439, 440–441
Deprivation of Liberty Safeguards (DoLS) 38
dermal papillae 320
dermis 320, 368
    effect of ageing 454
Dextrogel 289
diabetes 288–290, 465
diabetes mellitus
    blood sugar measurement 292–294
    causes/risk of 288
    diabetic emergencies 282
    hypoglycaemia 288–290
    severe hyperglycaemia 290–292
    type 1, 288
    type 2, 288
diabetic ketoacidosis (DKA) 290
diaphragm 452
diazepam 114
diencephalon 253
diffusion 179–180
digestive system 301
direct contact burns 368
disability
    arm weakness 262
    assessment of 143, 259–263
    children and infants 434–435
    coma 269–270
    convulsions 263–265
    defined 461
    disorders of nervous system 263–270
    face, arm, speech test 262–263
    facial palsy 262
    Glasgow Coma Scale 259
    management, maxillofacial injuries 334
    meningococcal disease 266–268
    nervous system 251–259
    paralysis 269
    pupillary response 262
    speech impairment 262
    stroke 265–266
    trauma 329
disclosure
    abuse 53
    consent 43–44
discrimination 45
dislocations, fractures and 344–346
dissociative shock 247

distributive shock 247
diversity 44–45
DKA, *see* diabetic ketoacidosis (DKA)
DNACPR, *see* do not attempt cardiopulmonary resuscitation (DNACPR) decisions
DNAR, *see* Do Not Attempt Resuscitation (DNAR) order
do not attempt cardiopulmonary resuscitation (DNACPR) decisions 486
Do Not Attempt Resuscitation (DNAR) order 491
DoLS, *see* Deprivation of Liberty Safeguards (DoLS)
domestic violence and abuse 53
DOPES 378
double-crewed ambulance (DCA) 131
DPD, *see* Dangerous Preparations Directive (DPD)
DRA, *see* dynamic risk assessment (DRA)
drowning
    aspiration 273
    autonomic conflict 275
    cardiac arrest in 483
    cardiac arrhythmia 277
    circum-rescue collapse 276
    defined 275
    hypothermia 483
    hypoxia 483
    management 276–277
    pathophysiology 275–276
drug administration 114–121
    drawing medication form ampoule 114–116
    intramuscular drugs 118–120
    intranasal drugs 120–121
    legislation and guidelines 113–114
    nebulised drugs 117–118
    oral medication 117
    routes of 114
dry-drowning 275
DSD, *see* Dangerous Substances Directive (DSD)
DSH, *see* suicide and deliberate self-harm (DSH)
dura 254
duty of
    candour 30
    care vs patient rights 27
DVT, *see* deep vein thrombosis (DVT)
DWI 65
dying with dignity 493
dynamic risk assessment (DRA) 62, 63–64, 123, 124
dysphagia 454
dyspnoea 216

E, *see* chemical, biological, radiological, nuclear, explosive CBRN(e) event
ears, older people 453
ECG, *see* electrocardiogram (ECG)
eclampsia 405
ectopic pregnancy 402
ED, *see* emergency department (ED)
education 447
electrical conduction pathway 218–219

Index

electrical energy 314
electrical injuries 371
electrical wiring or equipment, and fire risk 82
electrocardiogram (ECG) 3, 222–223
    12-lead ECG interpretation 235
    artefact 231–232
    breasts 235
    calibration 231
    complex 223
    components of 223
    contiguous leads 236
    left bundle branch block (LBBB) 237–239
    'normal' 12-lead 236
    paper 231
    recording 231–239
    signs of heart attack 4
    STEMI (ST-segment elevation myocardial infarction) recognition 237
electrocardiogram, electrical injuries 371
electronic communication devices 21–23
electronic patient clinical records (EPCRs) 23
electronic record-keeping 42
electronic thermometer 273, 274
emergency 125, 127
    defined 125
emergency caesarean section 482
emergency call
    12-lead ECG 3–4
    ambulance service, response to 7–8
    arriving on scene 2
    clean up 6
    communication, principles of 2–3
    emergency operations centre 1–2
    hospital arrival 5
    manual handling 4
    paramedic, assisting 4–5
    patient assessment 3
    patient history 3
    prepare for next call 6
emergency care assistants (ECAs), *see* support workers
emergency department (ED) 298
emergency medical technicians (EMTs), *see* associate ambulance practitioners
emergency operations centre (EOC) 1–2, 125, 136, 298
emergency preparedness, resilience and response (EPRR) 127
emergency situations
    mental capacity in 36–37
emphysema 213
employment rights 447
end of life care (EoLC) 489–493
    of adults 489–490
    advance care planning 491–492
    anticipatory prescribing 491
    bereavement and grieving process 494
    communication 490
    in community 492–493
    disclosure of patient wishes 492
    health professionals, support for 495
    help and support sources 494
    hospices 492
    hydration, maintaining 490
    palliative care and 489
    pharmacological interventions 490
    recognising person in last days of life 490
    referring for additional help 494
    religious and spiritual influences 491
    resuscitation in 493
    shared decision-making 490
    supporting carers and relatives 493
end-of-life-decisions 485–486
end-organ perfusion 434
end-tidal CO_2 ($EtCO_2$) 203
endocardium 217
endocrine system 284–285
endocrine system disorders 284–295
endometrium 399
endothelium 220
endotracheal intubation 153
    and tracheostomy 171
endotracheal tubes 189
energy 314–315
energy transfer during trauma 314–315
enteric nervous system 256
enteric plexus 252
Entonox 182, 196, 410
    action 198
    after administering oxygen 195–196
    administration 198–199
    caution 198
    contra-indications 198
    cylinder 196
    dosage and administration 198
    indications 198
    preparing for administration 196–197
    preparing new cylinder for use 184–185
    side-effects 198
    after use 199–200
entry route, pathogen 67
EOC, *see* emergency operations centre (EOC)
EoLC, *see* end of life care (EoLC)
EPCRs, *see* electronic patient clinical records (EPCRs)
epicardium 217
epidermis 319–320
    damage to 368
    effect of ageing 454
epiglottis 149, 150, 151, 168, 174
epinephrine, *see* adrenaline
EpiPen 281
epistaxis, *see* nosebleed
EPRR, *see* emergency preparedness, resilience and response (EPRR)
Equality Act 2010, 46, 447, 461
equality and diversity 44–45
    discrimination 45

Index

self-esteem 45
self-image 45
equipment officer 131
erythema (reddening) 367
erythrocytes, see red blood cells (erythrocytes)
Escherichia coli (E. coli) 66
ethnicity, diabetes and 288
evaporation 271
exit route, pathogen 67
exposure/environment
    assessment 143
    autonomic conflict 275
    children and infants 435
    drowning 275–277
    extremes of temperature 271–274
    heat-loss mechanisms 271
    heat-promoting mechanisms 271
    heat-related illness 272–273
    hypothermia 271–272
    scene assessment 124
    trauma 329
external genitalia 393–394
extra resources, scene assessment 125
extremities, assessment 330
extrication board 356
eye 257–259
eye protection 73
    removing 74–75
    wearing 74
eyes
    Glasgow Coma Scale 261
    injuries, management 334–335
    older people 453

face
    children and infants 425
face, arm, speech test (FAST) 262–263, 334
face masks 73
    removing 74–75
    wearing 74
facial injuries, see maxillofacial injuries
facial palsy 262
facial shields ventilation 188
facial structures and injuries 332–333
Faculty of Pre-Hospital Care 7
fallopian tube 399
falls
    older people 465–466
fascicles 219
FAST, see face, arm, speech test (FAST)
febrile convulsions 263
female circumcision/cutting, see female genital mutilation
female genital mutilation (FGM) 52, 396, 397
Ferno Compact 2 carry chair 106
fertilisation and implantation 399
fever 267
FGM, see female genital mutilation (FGM)

fibrous cap 239
filtering face piece (FFP3) mask 73
financial abuse 52
fir tree connector 185
fire, defined 82
fire prevention 82
fire safety 81, 187
    actions in case of fire 82–83
    fire alarm 82
    fire prevention 82
    fire triangle 82
    vehicle fires 83
first-aid techniques, skeletal immobilisation 347–350
fissures 177
flail chest 340
flame burns 368
flammable gases and liquids, and fire risk 82
fluid administration set 382
food poisoning/food allergies 145
Food Safety Act 1990, 65
forceful breathing 179
foreign body, removal 172
fowler position, trolley 111
fracture, see also pelvis
    and dislocations 344–346
    older people 451
    pelvic 360–361
    skull 315
    types of 345
fractured neck 465
frailty
    defined 464
    living with 464
    recognising 464
    supporting patients with 465
Francis report 26, 29
Freedom to Speak Up (FTSU) policy 30
friction burns 369
frontotemporal dementia 459
FTSU, see Freedom to Speak Up (FTSU) policy
fundal height 401
fundal massage 417
fungi 66

ganglia 251
gas exchange 179–180
gastric distension 187
gastroenteritis 454
GCS, see Glasgow Coma Scale (GCS)
general impression 142
general impression, primary survey 327
general sales list medicines (GSL) 113
generalised convulsion 405
genetics, diabetes and 288
genetics, learning disabilities and 448
Gibbs' reflective cycle 30
    action plan 32

analysis 32
conclusion 32
description 31
evaluation 32
feelings 31–32
Glasgow Coma Scale (GCS) 133
    disability 259
    eye opening 261
    motor response 261–262
    pain stimulus 260–262
    recording 259–262
    secondary survey 145
    stroke patients 224
    trapezius pinch 260
    in trauma 312
    trauma 329
    verbal response 261
gloves 72–73
    removing 74–75
    wearing 74
glucagon, administration of 118
glucocorticoids 287–288
Glucogel 289
glucose 290–291
glyceryl trinitrate (GTN) 240
glyceryl trinitrate 241–242
goggles 73, 74, 75
'gold' commanders, *see* strategic commanders
grazes (abrasion), 325
grey matter 254
grieving process 494
grunting 432
GSL, *see* general sales list medicines (GSL)
GTN, *see* glyceryl trinitrate (GTN)
gunshot 314, 326
gynaecological cancers 424
gynaecological emergencies 421–422

haemodialysis 308–310
haemoglobin (Hb) 248
haemophilia 335
haemorrhage
    catastrophic 142
haemorrhage, *see also* bleeding
    catastrophic 322, 327
    non-catastrophic 322
    post-partum 417–418
haemorrhoids 454
haemostatic agents 325
haemothorax 340
hand hygiene 68
    with alcohol handrub 68–70
    handwashing 70–72
    skincare 72
hand-operated suction device 158
handling aids 89
handover process
    medical 19–20
    trauma 20
handrub, hand hygiene with 68–70
hands, colour of 143
handwashing 70–72
HART, *see* hazardous area response team (HART)
hate crime, defined 450
hazard assessment 139
Hazard Identification Number (HIN) 125
hazard warning panel 136
hazardous area response team (HART) 11
    chemical burns 370
    hazardous materials 135, 136
    radiation burns 370–371
    suspension trauma 342
    trauma 327
hazardous area response team leader 131
hazardous area response teams (HART), scene assessment 124
hazardous materials 60
    ambulance crew actions at scene 136–139
    assessment 139
    CLP pictograms 136
    danger labels 136, 138
    evacuate, disrobe and decontaminate 139
    international journeys 136
    labelling 135–136
    transporting 136
Hazardous Waste Regulations 2005, 65
hazards
    defined 61
    identification of 62
Hb, *see* haemoglobin (Hb)
HC, *see* Healthcare Commission (HC)
HCAI, *see* healthcare-associated infection (HCAI)
HCPC, *see* Health and Care Professions Council (HCPC)
head
    assessment 329
    bobbing 414, 430
    injures
        in older people 453
    management 331
    pathophysiology 331
    recognition 330–331
head tilt–chin lift manoeuvre 154
'head-to-toe' assessment 146–147
Health and Care Professions Council (HCPC) 7, 28
health and safety
    communicating 61
    Control of Substances Hazardous to Health Regulations 2002, 60
    emergency services 58–59
    fire safety 81–83
    Health and Safety at Work, etc. Act 1974, 57–58
    infection prevention and control 64–81
    Lifting Operations and Lifting Equipment Regulations 1998, 59
    Management of Health and Safety at Work Regulations 1999, 58

Index

Manual Handling Operations Regulations 1992, 58–59
Personal Protective Equipment at Work Regulations 1992, 59–60
policies and legislation 57–61
Provision and Use of Work Equipment Regulations 1998, 59
reason for matters 60–61
regulatory bodies 60
risk assessment 61–64
stress 83–84
Health and Safety at Work, etc. Act 1974 (HSWA) 57–58, 65
Health and Safety Executive (2016) 60, 85
Health and Social Care Act 2008 65
health inequalities 33
health professionals, support for 495
health promotion 34
health protection agencies 66
healthcare-associated infection (HCAI) 64
Healthcare Commission (HC) 25
healthcare professional
    6Cs 26
    additional sources of support 30
    complaints about 29
    County Hospital, Stafford 25–26
    duty of candour 30
    duty of care vs patient rights 27
    failure to achieve standards 29
    freedom to speak up 30
    Gibbs' reflective cycle 30–32
    negligence 27–28
    provision of 32–33
        person-centred care 33
    reflection 30–32
    scope of practice and standards 28
    values and attitudes 26–27
    values-based healthcare 25–27
    whistleblowing 29–30
healthcare waste
    from ambulance service activity 77
    domestic waste 75, 76
    infectious/potentially infectious waste 75, 76
    management 75–76
    offensive/hygiene waste 75, 76
    sharps 75, 76
    storing and handling 76
    types of 75–76
hearing, in older people 453
heart
    atrioventricular node 219
    bundle of His 219
    cardiac cycle 221–222
    chambers of 219
    coronary arteries 219–220
    electrical conduction pathway 218–219
    fascicles 219
    isovolumetric contraction 222
    left atrium 218
    left bundle branch 219
    left coronary artery 220
    left ventricle 218
    older people 453
    pericardium 217
    relaxation period 222
    right atrium 218
    right bundle branch 219
    right coronary artery 219–220
    right ventricle 218
    semilunar valves 222
    sinoatrial node 218–219
    ventricular systole 222
    wall 217
heart failure
    assessment of 243
    history, signs and symptoms 244
    management of 243–244
heart rate
    assessment of newborn 419
    children and infants 426, 433
    maternal 399
heat exhaustion 273
heat-loss mechanisms 271
heat-promoting mechanisms 271
heat-related illness 272–273
    heat exhaustion 272
    heat stress 272
    heat stroke 272–273
    management 273
heat stress 273
heat stroke 272–273
heavy menstrual bleeding 422
helmet removal 356–357
hemiplegia 269
Henle/distal convoluted tubule (DCT) 305, 307
herniated disc 85, 86f
HHS, see hyperosmolar hyperglycaemic state or syndrome (HHS)
HIN, see Hazard Identification Number (HIN)
history-taking 143–145
HONK, see hyperosmolar non-ketotic coma (HONK)
hospice care 492
hospital-acquired infection 64
HSWA, see Health and Safety at Work, etc. Act 1974 (HSWA)
Human Rights Act 1998 32, 46
hydration, maintaining 490
hydrocortisone 281
hydrogen chloride 369
hydrogen cyanide 369
hyperflexion injuries 315
hyperglycaemic crisis, see severe hyperglycaemia
hyperketonaemia 290
hyperosmolar hyperglycaemic state or syndrome (HHS) 290
hyperosmolar non-ketotic coma (HONK) 290
hypertension
    defined 229
    in pregnancy 405
hypervolaemia 276–277
Hypo-Fit 289

Index

hypodermis 320
    effect of ageing 454
hypoglycaemia 143
    management 289–290
    signs and symptoms 288–291, 289
hypotension
    defined 229
    postural 453
    spinal injuries 336
hypothalamus 254, 336
hypothermia 143, 271–272
    cardiac arrest and 482
    defined 271
    in drowning 277, 483
    management 272
    stages of 272
    thermal burns 370
    trauma 327, 329
hypovolaemia 228, 277, 399
    diabetes mellitus 290
    maxillofacial injuries 333
    in pregnancy 399
hypovolaemic shock 246–247
hypoxia
    causes of 337
    children and infants 431, 470
    drowning 483
    suction 159
    traumatic brain injury 331

ICP, *see* intracranial pressure (ICP)
IDDM, *see* insulin-dependent diabetes (IDDM)
IHD, *see* ischaemic heart disease (IHD)
IMCA, *see* independent mental capacity advocate (IMCA)
immune system
    older people 453
incident reporting system 81
incision, *see* cut (incision)
incision (cut) 326
independent mental capacity advocate (IMCA) 38
inequality in healthcare 449
infant basic life support 470–474
infection prevention and control 64
    bacteria 66
    chain of infection 67
    decontamination process 76–79
    fungi 66
    hand hygiene 68–72
    handling linen and laundry 80
    health protection agencies 66
    legionella bacteria 81
    managing healthcare waste 75–76
    microorganisms 66–67
    occupational health 81
    organisations, impact on 65
    own and patient's health 64–65
    parasites 67
    personal hygiene 68
    personal protective equipment 72–75
    regulations and legislation 65
    regulators and other bodies 66
    reporting incidents 81
    sharps injury 80–81
    splash contamination 81
    standard principles 67
    viruses 66
    World Health Organization 66
inflammatory arthritis 455, 456
inflation breaths 420
influenza 454
information governance, defined 41
information transfer and processing, central nervous system 251
infra-red tympanic thermometer 274
inhaler and spacer 118
insulin-dependent diabetes (IDDM) 288
integumentary system (skin)
    anatomy and physiology 319–320
    cross-section of 319
    dermis 320
    epidermis 319–320
    hypodermis 320
    older people 453
    physiology 320
interatrial septum 218
intercostal recession, newborn with 432
internal genitalia 394–396
international journeys, hazardous materials 136
interoperability 127
interventricular septum 218
intervertebral discs 452
intracranial pressure (ICP) 254
intramuscular drugs, administration of 118–120
intranasal drugs, administration of 120–121
intraosseous (IO) 384
intraosseous cannulation
    equipment 384–385
    procedure for 386–392
intravenous (IV) 384
intravenous cannulation
    alternative to 384
    cannulas 379
    equipment 379
    procedure for 379–382
intravenous drug administration
    intraosseous cannulation 384–392
    intravenous cannulation 378–382
    intravenous infusion, preparing 382–384
intravenous infusion, preparing 382–384
IO, *see* intraosseous (IO)
IPAP suicide risk assessment 442
ipratropium 117, 214, 281
ischaemic heart disease (IHD) 239
isovolumetric contraction 222
IV, *see* intravenous (IV)

Index

jaw thrust manoeuvre 154–156
JESIP, *see* Joint Emergency Services Interoperability Principles (JESIP) principles
Jext auto-injector 281–282
joint decision model 127
Joint Emergency Services Interoperability Principles (JESIP) principles 127
Joints, older people 452

Kendrick Traction Device (KTD) 364–365
kinetic energy 314
Korotkoff sounds 229
KTD, *see* Kendrick Traction Device (KTD)
kyphosis 452

labelling hazardous materials 135–136
labour, stages of 407–408
laceration, *see* tear (laceration)
laceration (tear) 326
lacunae 399
Langerhans cells 320
language 16, 18
Language Line 18
laryngectomy
  help and equipment 171
  management of 170–171
  stoma patency 171
laryngectomy, vs. tracheostomy 167
laryngopharynx 150–151
laryngoscope blades and handle 374–375
laryngospasm 275
larynx 151–152
last oral intake 145
lasting power of attorney (LPA) 38
LBBB, *see* left bundle branch block (LBBB)
learning disabilities
  categories of 448
  causes of 448
  communication 449–450
  defined 447
  further support 450
  healthcare and discrimination 448–449
  inequality in healthcare 449
  legislation 447
  rights 447–448
  tackling inequality 449
  and vulnerability 450
left bundle branch block (LBBB) 235, 237–239
left ventricular hypertrophy (LVH) 453
legal responsibility, manual handling 87
legionella bacteria 81
level of consciousness (LOC) 295, 434
level of consciousness 143, 145
Lewy bodies 458–459
lifting cushion 97–99
Lifting Operations and Lifting Equipment Regulations 1998 (LOLER) 59, 89

lifting/handling, procedure 90–91
linen and laundry, handling 80
Little's area 335
living wills, *see* advance decisions to refuse treatment
load
  defined 85
  reducing 87–88
loading officer 131
lobes 177
lobules 177
LOC, *see* level of consciousness (LOC)
local authorities, sharing information 44
LOLER, *see* Lifting Operations and Lifting Equipment Regulations 1998 (LOLER)
loss of consciousness (LOC), *see* coma
low-kneeling position 100
lower limbs
  injuries 343
  older people 452
  raising position, trolley 112
  splints 357
LPA, *see* lasting power of attorney (LPA)
lumbar vertebra 255
Lund and Browder charts 367
lungs 152, 177–178
  in older people 452
LVH, *see* left ventricular hypertrophy (LVH)
lymphatic system 224
lymphatic system and immunity
  anatomy and physiology 223–224
  autoimmune disease 225
  immunity 224–225
    non-specific immunity 224
    specific immunity 225

Macintosh blade 374
maculopapular rash 267
MAD, *see* mucosal atomiser device (MAD)
Magill forceps 375
major incidents 125, 128
  ambulance service, role of 128–129
  attendant's role 132
  casualty clearing station 131
  causes of 128
  CBRN(e) 125, 126, 136
  classification of 128
  command structure 132
  driver's role 132–133
  emergency 125, 127
  first crew on scene 131–133
  incident command and control 129–131
  interoperability 127
  JESIP principles 127
  joint decision model 127
  major, mass and catastrophic incidents 128
  METHANE communication model 128
  situational awareness, shared 127

Index

subsequent crews on scene 133
tourniquets 323
triage 133–135
major trauma centre (MTC) 311
major trauma triage tool 312, 313
male reproductive system 398–399
Management of Health and Safety at Work Regulations 1999 (MHSWR) 58, 87
mandible 332–333
Mangar Camel 98–99
Mangar ELK lifting cushion 92, 95–98
manic depression, see bipolar affective disorder
manual defibrillators 476–477, 479–480, 481
manual handling 4, see also moving and handling equipment and techniques
    bariatric patients 91–92
    biomechanics 88
    defined 85
    general principles 88–89
    guideline weights for lifting and lowering 89
    handling aids 89
    help and support 92
    herniated disc 85, 86
    lifting equipment regulations 59
    lifting/handling, procedure 90–91
    patients refusing aids 88
    poor, consequences of 85–86
    regulations 58–59
    risk assessment 87–88
    team handling 91
Manual Handling Operations Regulations 1992 (MHOR) 58–59, 87, 89
manual in-line stabilisation (MILS) 350
MAP, see mean arterial pressure (MAP)
marauding terrorist attack (MTA) 128
marauding terrorist firearms attack (MTFA) 128
mass casualties 128
mass incidents 128
maternity packs 408
Mauriceau-Smellie-Veit manoeuvre 415
maxilla 332
maxillofacial injuries 331
    airway management 333–334
    breathing management 334
    circulation management 334
    disability management 334
    eye injuries 334–335
    facial structures and injuries 332–333
    Le Fort I 332
    Le Fort II 332
    Le Fort III 332
    management 333
    mandible 332–333
    maxilla 332
    nosebleed 335
    orbit 332
    soft tissue 333
    teeth 333
MCA, see Mental Capacity Act 2005 (MCA)
McRobert's position 414, 417
MDTs, see mobile data terminals (MDTs)
mean arterial pressure (MAP) 254
mechanical arthritis 455–456
mechanical suction device 159
mechanical ventilation
    Pneupac ParaPAC ventilator 190
    pressure-compensated flowmeter 191–192
    procedure 191
    Schrader outlet 191–192
mechanism of injury (MOI) 123, 327
    abdomen 317
    blast injury 318
    defined 313
    energy 314–319
    head 315
    kinetics 313–314
    pelvis 317–318
    spine 315–316
    suspension trauma 318
    thorax 317
mediastinum 152, 217
medical director 12
medical gases, safe use of 181–182
    assisted ventilation 187–190
    cylinder components 183–184
    cylinder storage 182–183
    Entonox 196–200
    Firesafe 187
    integrated valve cylinders 183
    mechanical ventilation 190–192
    medium concentration mask 186
    nasal cannulae 187
    nebuliser 187
    non-rebreathe mask 189
    oxygen 192–195
    oxygen, administration of 185–187
    oxygen delivery devices 186–187
    preparation of new cylinder 184–185
    safety checks 184
    Venturi mask 186
medical handover 19–20
medical history, past 144–145
medical/surgical emergencies
    acute abdomen 300–304
    Addison's disease 294–295
    anaphylaxis 279–282
    diabetes 288–290
    endocrine system disorders 284–295
    poisoning 295–299
    sepsis 282–283
    urinary system disorders 304–310
medication 144
medication and talking therapies 456

Index

Medicines Act 1968, 113
medium concentration mask 186
medulla oblongata 253
melanocytes, loss of 454
meninges 254
meningism 268
meningococcal disease
   fever 267
   maculopapular rash 267
   management 268
   meningism 268
   pathophysiology 266–267
   petechial non-blanching rash 267
   rash 267–268
   sepsis and shock 267
   signs and symptoms 267
menstrual cycle 396
mental capacity 35–36
   advance decision to refuse treatment 38
   assessing 36–37
   'best interests' decisions making 38
   caring for restrained patient 40
   code of practice 36
   deprivation of liberty safeguards 38
   in emergency situations 37
   further support and raising concerns 40
   independent mental capacity advocate 38
   lack of capacity 35, 37
   lasting power of attorney 38
   Mental Capacity Act 2005 code of practice 36
   refusal of treatment 37–38
   supporting patients with capacity assessments 37
   use of restraint 39–40
mental disorders 439–440
   assessment of patient with mental health problems 442, 443
   bipolar affective disorder 440
   defined 437
   delirium 440
   depression 440–441
   general advice 444–445
   IPAP suicide risk assessment 442
   management of 442, 444
   mood (affective) disorders 440–441
   neurotic, stress-related and somatoform disorders 441
   organic disorders 440
   panic disorder 441
   personality disorders 441
   schizophrenia and delusional disorders 440
   suicide and deliberate self-harm 441–442
mental health
   approved mental health professional 437
   assessment of patient with mental health problems 442
   community treatment orders 439
   defined 437
   guiding principles 438
   legislation and codes of practice 437–439
   mental disorders, see mental disorders

Mental Health Act 1983 (as amended 2007) (MHA) 437–439
   mental well-being 445–446
   nearest relative 438
   section 12 doctor 437
   transporting patients 439
mental health first aid (MHFA) 444
mental illness 455–456
mental well-being
   defined 445
   employer support 445
   impact on 445
   medical support 446
   resilience 445
   seeking help 445
   supporting colleague 446
Merkel cells 320
Mersey Burns app 367
metabolic rate 426
METHANE communication model 128
methicillin-resistant *Staphylococcus aureus* (MRSA) 66
MHA, see Mental Health Act 1983 (as amended 2007) (MHA)
MHFA, see mental health first aid (MHFA)
MHOR, see Manual Handling Operations Regulations 1992 (MHOR)
MHSWR, see Management of Health and Safety at Work Regulations 1999 (MHSWR)
microorganisms 66–67
midbrain 253
MILS, see manual in-line stabilisation (MILS)
miscarriage 405
misoprostol 417
Misuse of Drugs Act 1971, 113–114
Misuse of Drugs Regulations 2001, 114
mitral valve 218
mobile data terminals (MDTs) 23
MOI, see mechanism of injury (MOI)
monoplegia 269
mood (affective) disorders 440–441
morphine 114
motor function, central nervous system 251
mouth
   airway 149–150
   children and infants 425
mouth-to-mask ventilation 188–189
mouth-to-mouth ventilation 187–188
moving and handling equipment and techniques
   ambulance trolley 110–112
   carry chair, see carry chair
   Mangar Camel 98–99
   Mangar ELK lifting cushion 95–98
   one-chair method 92–94
   patient transfer board 104–106
   patients fall in confined space 99–101
   patients in bed 104–106
   patients on floor 92–101
   seated patients 101–104
   sitting to sitting transfer 101–103

Index

sitting to standing transfer 103–104
two-chair method 94–95
MRSA, see methicillin-resistant Staphylococcus aureus (MRSA)
MTA, see marauding terrorist attack (MTA)
MTC, see major trauma centre (MTC)
MTFA, see marauding terrorist firearms attack (MTFA)
mucosal atomiser device (MAD) 120–121
mucosal burns 369
multiple births 418
muscle cramps 272
muscle tone, assessment of newborn 419–420
muscles, older people 452
musculoskeletal injuries
    examination 344
    fractures and dislocations 344–346
    history 343–344
    sprains and strains 347
musculoskeletal system, older people 451–452
myocardium 217

naloxone, administration of 120
NARU, see National Ambulance Resilience Unit (NARU)
nasal cannulae 187
nasal flaring 430
naso-oropharyngeal burns 369
nasopharyngeal airway 150
nasopharyngeal airways (NPAs), facial injuries 334
nasopharynx 150
National Advisory Group on the Safety of Patients in England 29
National Ambulance Resilience Unit (NARU) 123
national cleaning colour code 77–78
National Early Warning Score (NEWS2) 145–146, 284
National Institute for Health and Care Excellence (NICE) 7, 298
National Institute for Health and Care Excellence 489
national inter-agency liaison officer (NILO) 13, 131
National Network for Burn Care (NNBC) 367
nature of illness (NOI) 123
NEAD, see non-epileptic attack disorder (NEAD)
nearest relative 438
nebulised drugs, administration of 117–118
nebuliser 187
neck assessment 329
negligence 27–28, 52
neuroglia 252–253
neurons 251, 252–253
    loss with age 453
neurotic, stress-related and somatoform disorders 441
newborn life support 419–421
Newton's laws of motion 314
NHS Digital 7
NHS Improvement 7
NHS Pathways 8
NIBP, see non-invasive blood pressure (NIBP)
NICE, see National Institute for Health and Care Excellence (NICE)
NIDDM, see non-insulin dependent diabetes (NIDDM)

NILO, see national inter-agency liaison officer (NILO)
999 call, see emergency call
NNBC, see National Network for Burn Care (NNBC)
NOI, see nature of illness (NOI)
non-accidental injury (NAI), see physical abuse
non-catastrophic haemorrhage 322
non-epileptic attack disorder (NEAD) 264
non-insulin dependent diabetes (NIDDM) 288
non-invasive blood pressure (NIBP) 229
non-neural tissue 285
non-parenteral routes, drug administration 114
non-rebreathe mask 186, 192
non-ST-segment elevation myocardial infarction (NSTEMI) 240
non-verbal communication 17
'normal' 12-lead 236
'normal' female anatomy 393
Normocapnia, post-resuscitation care 398
nose
    airway 149
    children and infants 425
nosebleed management 335–336
notifiable diseases, sharing information 44
NPAs, see nasopharyngeal airways (NPAs)
NSTEMI, see non-ST-segment elevation myocardial infarction (NSTEMI)
nuclear energy 314
number of patients, scene assessment 124–125

obesity, diabetes and 288
obstetrics and gynaecology
    anatomy and physiology 393
    antepartum haemorrhage 402
    APGAR 412
    breech presentation 415–417
    cardiac arrest in pregnancy 482
    childbirth complications 413–419
    cord prolapse 413–414
    ectopic pregnancy 402
    equipment for childbirth 408–409
    external genitalia 393–394
    female genital mutilation 396
    gynaecological cancers 424
    gynaecological emergencies 421–422
    heavy menstrual bleeding 422
    internal genitalia 394–396
    male reproductive system 398–399
    management of
        first stage of labour 409
        second stage of labour 409–412
    maternal physiology 399
    maternity packs 408
    menstrual cycle 396
    miscarriage 405
    multiple births 418
    normal childbirth 407–413
    normal fertilisation and implantation 399
    normal pregnancy 399

Index

placenta praevia 403–404
placental abruption 402–403
post-partum haemorrhage 417–418
pre-eclampsia 405
pre-term labour 418–419
pregnancy, termination of 422–423
pregnancy, trauma in 406–407
pregnant woman, assessing 400–402
reproduction 393
resuscitation equipment 408–409
shoulder dystocia 414–415
stages of labour 407–408
terminology and abbreviations 399–400
uterine prolapse 423–424
uterine rupture 404
vaginal tissue damage 422
obstructive shock 247
occupational health 81
oedema
    pre-eclampsia 405
    smoke inhalation 369
older people
    age-related conditions 455–457
    ageing 451
    airway 452
    arthritis 455–456
    attitudes 457
    blood vessels 453
    bones 451
    brain and senses 453
    cardiovascular system 453
    challenging behaviour 463–465
    communication 463
    dementia 457–464
    digestive system 454
    ears 453
    eyes 453
    falls 465
    frailty 464–465
    heart 453
    immune system 454
    integumentary system 454
    joints 452
    mental illness 455–456
    muscles 452
    musculoskeletal system 451–452
    nervous system 453–454
    osteoporosis 456
    parkinson's disease 455
    patients with co-morbidities 457
    respiratory system 451–452
    spinal cord 454
    ventilatory changes 452–453
oliguria 267
one-chair method 92–94
onward care 9–10
OPA, see oropharyngeal airway (OPA)

open pneumothorax 337–338
operational commander 12, 130
oral cavity 150
oral intake, last 145
oral medication, administration of 117
orbit 332
oropharyngeal airway (OPA) 160–162, 431
    facial injuries 334
oropharynx 150
orthopaedic (scoop) stretcher 354–355
osteoarthritis 455–456
osteoporosis 456, 465
out-of-hospita 300
ovarian egg 399
over-triaging 134
oxygen 177, 192–195
    administration 192–195
    antepartum haemorrhage 402–404
    assisted ventilation 187, 194
    bag-valve-mask ventilation 189–190
    cautions 192
    children and infants 426
    and chronic obstructive pulmonary disease 213
    contra-indication 192
    controlled/low-dose 192
    cylinder 183
    delivery devices 185–187
    dosage and administration 192, 195
    drowning 276
    ectopic pregnancy 402
    fires and explosions 182
    Firesafe 187
    high levels 192, 193
    in hypoxaemic condition 195
    indications 192
    miscarriage 405
    moderate levels 193
    preparing new cylinder for use 184–185
    saturations 200–202
    side-effects 192
    traumatic brain injury 331
    after use 195–196
oxygen delivery devices 185–187
oxygen physiology 180–181
oxygen saturations 200–202
    pulse oximetry 200–201
    recording 201–202
oxygen transport 181
oxyhaemoglobin 200

P, see pharmacy medicines (P)
paediatric assessment triangle (PAT) 430
paediatric basic life support 470–474
paediatric defibrillation 480–481
paediatric face mask 171
pain management, dementia and 461

Index

pain stimulus 260–261
palliative care 489
palm-to-palm hold 104
pancreas 285–286
panda eyes (Battle's sign) 331
panic disorder 441
paralysis 269
paramedic, assisting 4–5
paramedics 11
paraplegia 269
parasites 67
parasympathetic nervous system 256–257
parenteral routes, drug administration 114
parietal pleura 152, 337
parking officer 131
Parkinson's disease 455
partial pressure of arterial oxygen (PaO_2) 180, 181
PAT, see Paediatric assessment triangle (PAT)
pathogen 67
patient assessment 3, 141
    ABCDE approach 141
    airway 142
    allergies 144
    blood sugar 143
    breathing 143
    catastrophic haemorrhage 142
    circulation 143
    disability 143
    exposure 143
    general impression 142
    'head-to-toe' assessment 146–147
    history-taking 143–145
    last oral intake 145
    level of consciousness 143
    past medical history 144–145
    medication 144
    National Early Warning Score 145–146
    presenting complaint 143–144
    primary survey 141–143
    pupils 143
    reassessment 147
    responsiveness 142
    SAMPLE history 144
    secondary survey 145–147
    vital signs 145
patient-identifiable information 41
patient privacy 143
patient rights, duty of care vs 27
patient transfer board 104–106
patient wishes, disclosure of 492
patients fall in confined space 99–101
patients in bed, moving and handling 104–106
patients on floor, moving and handling 92–101
PCT, see proximal convoluted (tightly coiled) tubule (PCT)
PE, see pulmonary embolism (PE)
PEA, see pulseless electrical activity (PEA)
peak expiratory flow rate (PEFR/PEF) 202–203

pelvic binders 342, see pelvic splints
pelvic splints 360–363
    SAM Pelvic Sling II 361–362
    T-POD device 262–263
pelvis
    anterior–posterior compression fractures 318
    assessment 328, 330
    combined mechanical fractures 318
    injuries 317–318, 342
    lateral compression fractures 318
    pelvic binders 342
    pelvic ring fracture 317–318
    types of fracture 318
    vertical shear fractures 318
penetrating trauma 313
    abdominal injuries 341
    energy transfer 314–315
    haemothorax 340
    pneumothorax 337
    spinal injuries 336
perception, see sensory function (perception), central nervous system
pericardium 217
peripheral chemoreceptors 180
peripheral nervous system (PNS) 251–252
peripheral pain stimulus 261
peripheral vasoconstriction 430
peristalsis 454
peritoneal dialysis 308, 310
peritoneum 340
person-centred care 33
personal hygiene 68
personal protective equipment (PPE)
    aprons 73
    for decontamination 79
    eye protection 73
    face masks 73
    gloves 72–73
    infection prevention and control 72–75
    regulations 59–60
    removing 74–75
    sleeve protectors 73–74
    storing and handling healthcare waste 76
    trauma 327
    wearing 74–75
Personal Protective Equipment at Work Regulations 1992, 59–60
personality disorders 441
petechial non-blanching rash 267
pharmaceutical adviser 12
pharmacological interventions, end of life care 490
pharmacy medicines (P) 113
pharyngeal tonsil 150
pharynx 150
    children and infants 425
phenylketonuria 448
photo-ageing 454
photoreceptor cells 257–258

Index

physical abuse 51
physical records 42
pia 254
placenta 399, 403, 408
placenta praevia 403–404
    placental abruption and 404
placental abruption 402–403
    placenta praevia and 404
plasma 220
platelets (thrombocytes) 220
pleura 152
pleuritic chest pain 216
pneumonia 454
    advice 215
    breath sounds in 215
    community-acquired pneumonia 214
    CRB-65 severity score 215
    defined 214
    management 215
    pathophysiology 214–215
    signs and symptoms 215
    transport 215
pneumothorax, *see also* open pneumothorax; tension pneumothorax
    assessment 338–339
    causes of hypoxia 337
    management 339
PNS, *see* peripheral nervous system (PNS)
poisoning
    assessment and management
        antidotes 299
        decontamination 298–299
        disposition 299–300
        enhanced elimination 299
        investigations 298
        resuscitation 297–298
        risk assessment 298
        supportive care and monitoring 298
    toxidromes 295
police 447
police, sharing information 43–44
POM, *see* prescription-only medicines (POM)
pons 253
position of patient 142
positioning, trolley 111–112
positive-pressure ventilation
    infant 425
post-cardiac arrest syndrome 484
post-ictal phase 264
post-partum haemorrhage (PPH) 417–418
post-resuscitation care 468
    management of 484–485
postural hypotension 453
posture, lifting/handling 90
pPCI, *see* primary percutaneous coronary intervention (pPCI)
PPE, *see* personal protective equipment (PPE)
PPH, *see* post-partum haemorrhage (PPH)

pre-alert 20
pre-eclampsia 405
pre-planned major events 128
pre-term infant 421
pre-term labour 418–419
pregnancy, *see* obstetrics and gynaecology
    cardiac arrest in 482
    termination of 422–423
    trauma in 406–407
prescription-only medicines (POM) 113
presenting complaint 143–144
PREVENT strategy 56
primary percutaneous coronary intervention (pPCI) 242
primary survey 141–143
primary triage officer 131
primigravida 404
proprioception 453
proteases 213
proteinuria 405
Provision and Use of Work Equipment Regulations 1998 (PUWER) 59, 89
proximal convoluted (tightly coiled) tubule (PCT) 305, 307
proximal humerus, EZ-IO in 386–389
proximal tibia, EZ-IO in 390–392
pseudo-seizures, *see* non-epileptic attack disorder
psychological/emotional abuse 51
public interest, sharing information 44
pulmonary embolism (PE)
    defined 215
    management 216
    pathophysiology 216
    risk factors 215–216
    signs and symptoms 216
pulmonary ventilation 177
pulse
    assessment 143, 225–239
    brachial pulse 226–227
    carotid pulse 225, 226
    locations 225–227
    radial pulse 226
    rate 227
    recording 227
    rhythm 227
    volume and character 227
    weak ('thready') 227
pulse oximetry 200–201
    children and infants 433
pulse volume 433
pulseless electrical activity (PEA) 476
puncture, *see* stab (puncture)
puncture (stab) 326
pupillary reactions 262
pupillary response 262
pupils 143
    children and infants 434

Purkinje fibres 219
PUWER, see Provision and Use of Work Equipment Regulations 1998 (PUWER)

quadriplegia 269

radial pulse 226
radiation 271
radiation burns 370–371
radicalisation 56
radio communication 21–23
rash 267–268
RBC, see red blood cell (RBC)
REAP, see Resourcing Escalatory Action Plan (REAP)
reassessment 147
recognition of life extinct (ROLE) 486–488
record keeping, communication and 19
recovery position 156–158
recumbent position, trolley 111
red blood cell (RBC) 247, 248
red blood cells (erythrocytes) 220
reddening, see erythema (reddening)
referrals, safeguarding 54–55
reflection 30–32
reflex bradycardia 425
reflexes, in older people 454
refusal of treatment 37
regulatory bodies 60
rehydration 273
religious and spiritual influences, on end of life care 91
repolarisation 222
reporting incidents 81
reservoir 67
resilience 445
Resourcing Escalatory Action Plan (REAP) 61
ReSPECT document 491
respiration
    assessment 330
    assessment of newborn 419
respiratory failure 430
respiratory rate 200
respiratory system
    air pressure 178–179
    alveoli 178
    bronchi 152, 177, 178
    conducting portion 177
    control of breathing 180
    diffusion 179–180
    expiration 179
    external respiration 177
    forceful breathing 179
    gas exchange 179–180
    inspiration 179
    internal respiration 177
    laryngopharynx 150–151
    lobes 177
    lobules 177
    lungs 152, 177–178
    mouth 149–150
    nasopharynx 150
    nose 149
    older people 451–452
    oropharynx 150
    pulmonary ventilation 177
    respiration 177
    respiratory portion 177
    structures of 149
    trachea 152
response to 999 call 7–8
response, types of
    hear and treat 8
    physical response 8–9
resuscitation equipment 408–409
resuscitation in end of life care 493
resuscitation, of newborn 420
resuscitation, start and stop 485
return of spontaneous circulation (ROSC) 484
rheumatoid arthritis 456
rhinovirus 66
ribs of infants 426
risk assessment 61–62
    how and to whom 52
    evaluation of risk 62–63
    identification of hazards 62
    manual handling 87–88
    precautions 63
    recording findings and proposed actions 63–64
    reducing risk 87–88
    review and update 64
    risk matrix 62
risk, defined 61
road traffic collisions
    abdominal injuries 342
    head injuries 330
    maxillofacial injuries 331
    pelvic injuries 342
    spinal injuries 336
    thoracic injuries 337
road traffic collisions (RTC) 313
ROLE, see recognition of life extinct (ROLE)
ROSC, see return of spontaneous circulation (ROSC)
RTC, see road traffic collisions (RTC)

SAD, see supraglottic airway device (SAD)
safeguarding
    abusers of vulnerable adults 50
    child abuse 50
    cultural influences 50–51
    defined 49
    domestic violence and abuse 53
    female genital mutilation 52
    financial abuse 52
    forms of abuse 51–52
    learning from previous cases 49–50

Index

management of 53–54
neglect 52
physical abuse 51
psychological/emotional abuse 51
referrals 54–55
sexual abuse 51–52
urgent concern, reporting 54
vulnerability 50–51
safety officer 131
safety, scene assessment 123
salbutamol 118, 214, 281
SAM Pelvic Sling II 361–362
SAMPLE history 144
SARS, *see* severe acute respiratory syndrome (SARS)
saturation of haemoglobin (SaO2) 181
scalds 368
SCD, *see* sickle cell disease (SCD)
scene assessment
    cause 123–124
    dynamic risk assessment model 124
    environment 124
    extra resources 125
    number of patients 124–125
    safety 123
SCENE mnemonic 123, 327
schizophrenia 440
Schrader outlet 184, 191
Schrader valve 169
SCI, *see* spinal cord injuries (SCI)
scoop, *see* orthopaedic (scoop) stretcher
seated patients, moving and handling 101–104
secondary survey 145–147
section 12 doctor 437
Sellick's manoeuvre (cricoid pressure) 377
semi-recumbent position, trolley 111
semilunar valves 222
senses, older people 453
sensory function (perception), central nervous system 251
sepsis 267, 282–284
    management 284
    pre-hospital screening tool 283
    recognition 284
    risk factors for 282–284
septic shock 282
septicaemia 267
severe acute respiratory syndrome (SARS) 73
severe hyperglycaemia 290–392
    diabetic ketoacidosis 290–291
    hyperosmolar hyperglycaemic state 291
    pathophysiology 290
    signs and symptoms 291–292
sexual abuse 51–52
shared decision-making 490
sharps bins 78
sharps injury 80
shock 267, 478, 481
    blood sugar measurement 292

cardiogenic 247
defined 246
dissociative 247
distributive 247
hypovolaemic 246–247
management of 247
obstructive 247
shortness of breath on exertion (SOBOE) 452
shoulder dystocia 414–415
sick infant and child, recognising 429
sickle cell disease (SCD) 247–249
'silver' commanders, *see* tactical commanders
sitting to sitting transfer 101–103
sitting to standing transfer 103–104
situational awareness, shared 127
skeletal immobilisation
    cervical collars 351–354
    crash helmet removal 356–357
    extrication board 356
    first-aid techniques 347–350
    manual in-line stabilisation 350
    orthopaedic (scoop) stretcher 354–356
    spinal immobilisation 350–357
    splints 357–365
    triangular bandages 347–350
skin, *see* integumentary system (skin)
skin cancer 371
skin perfusion 433–434
skincare 72
skull 315
slapper bands 134
sleeve protectors 73–74
slide sheet 101
slipped disc 85
smoke inhalation 368
Snellen chart 335
'sniffing the morning air' position 375
SOBOE, *see* shortness of breath on exertion (SOBOE)
social services, role of 55
SOCRATES 144
sodium chloride 409
soft tissue 333
SOFTT-W tourniquet 324–325
somatic nervous system 256
spacer device for inhalers 208–209
SPCC, *see* Specialist paramedic – critical care (SPCC)
Specialist paramedic – critical care (SPCC) 11
Specialist paramedic – urgent care (SPUC) 11
speech impairment 262
spinal cord 255
    older people 453
spinal cord injuries (SCI)
    management 337
    pathophysiology 336
    recognition 336
    risk factors 336
spinal immobilisation

Index

cervical collars 351
crash helmet removal 356–357
extrication board 356
manual in-line stabilisation 350
orthopaedic (scoop) stretcher 354–355
spinal injuries
  combination 317
  compression 317
  extension 316
  flexion 315
  flexion with rotation 316
spiritual needs, on end of life care 91
splash contamination 81
splints 357
  box 357–358
  pelvic 360–363
  traction 364–365
  vacuum 359–360
spontaneous abortion, see miscarriage
sprains 347
springing 147
SPUC, see Specialist paramedic – urgent care (SPUC)
ST-segment elevation myocardial infarction (STEMI) 237, 240, 485
stab, see puncture (stab)
stab (puncture) 326
stab wound 314
stable angina 240
standards of conduct, performance and ethics 28
standards of education and training 28
standards of proficiency 28
staphylococcus 66
status epilepticus 264
STEMI, see ST-segment elevation myocardial infarction (STEMI)
STEP 1-2-3 Plus method 125
sterilisation 76
stethoscope 204–206
strains 347
strategic commander 13, 129
stress
  management 84
  primary sources at work 83
  signs of 83–84
stretchers, manual handling 87, 88
stridor 431
stroke
  acute stroke 266
  anatomy and physiology 265
  assessment and management of 266
  ischaemic 265–266
  risk factors 265
  types of 265–266
sublingual tablets 117
suction catheters 158–160
sudden unexpected death in infancy, children and adolescents (SUDICA) 488
SUDICA, see sudden unexpected death in infancy, children and adolescents (SUDICA)

suicide and deliberate self-harm (DSH) 441–442
sunburn 370, 371
superficial fascia, see hypodermis
support workers (SWs) 10
supraglottic airway device (SAD) 153, 170, 189, 482
surgical face mask 73
susceptible host 67
suspension trauma 318, 342
SWs, see support workers (SWs)
sympathetic nervous system 256–257, 275
  older people 454
symphysis pubis 414
symptom management, in end of life care 492
synovial joints 452
syntometrine 417
systolic blood pressure, older people 453

T-POD device 362–363
tachycardia
  causes of 227
  children and infants 433
  in pregnancy 399
tachypnoea 216, 432
tackling inequality 449
tactical commander 12–13, 129–130
TBI, see traumatic brain injury (TBI)
TBSA, see total body surface area (TBSA), of burn
TCA, see traumatic cardiac arrest (TCA)
team handling 91
tear, see laceration (tear)
tear (laceration) 326
teeth 333
temperature, extremes of
  assessment of 273–274
  heat exhaustion 272
  heat stress 272
  heat stroke 272–273
  hypothermia 271–272
  thermoregulation 271, 454
temperature, thermoregulation 454
tension pneumothorax 338, 434
TEP, see treatment escalation plan (TEP)
terrorist attack 125
  marauding 128
thalamus 254
thermal burns
  management of 369–370
  pathophysiology of 367–369
  zones of 368
thermal energy 314
thermoregulation 271, 454
thoracic injuries
  flail chest 340, 341
  haemothorax 340
  pneumothorax 337–339
thrombi (blood clots) 216
thrombin 418

Index

thrombocytes, *see* platelets (thrombocytes)
TICLS mnemonic 430
tightly coiled, *see* proximal convoluted (tightly coiled) tubule (PCT)
TILEE acronym 87
time-critical problems 402–403
tissue, after birth 417
tone, uterine 417
tongue 149–150
total body surface area (TBSA), of burn 366–367
tourniquets 323
    CAT tourniquet 323–324
    SOFTT-W tourniquet 324–325
TOXBASE 135, 298
toxidrome signs 299
trachea 152
tracheal intubation 373–378
    assisting the paramedic 373–378
    BURP manoeuvre 377
    confirming tube placement 377–378
    DOPES 378
    equipment 373–375
    procedure for 375–376
    Sellick's manoeuvre 377
    tracheal intubation 373–378
tracheal tube 373–374
tracheostomy 67
    airway and breathing 169
    with cuffed/uncuffed tubes 168
    with fenestrated tubes 169
    help and equipment 169
    with inner cannulas 168–169
    patency 169–170
    speaking valves 170
    tubes 168–170
    vs. laryngectomy 167
traction splints 364–365
transfer board (banana board) 101
transient ischaemic attack 265
translator 18
transmission route 67
trapezius pinch 260
trauma
    abdominal injuries 317, 340–341
    assessment and management 326–347
    blast injury 318
    bleeding 320–322
    burns 366–371
    cervical collars 351
    close-range gunshot wound 315
    compression 317
    crash helmet removal 356–357
    defined 311
    energy 314
    energy transfer 314–315
    extension 316
    extrication board 356
    first-aid techniques 347
    flexion 315–316
    flexion with rotation 315
    to genital tract during childbirth 418
    head injuries 330–331
    kinetics 313–314
    major trauma triage tool 312, 313
    manual in-line stabilisation 350
    maxillofacial injuries 331–336
    mechanism of injury 312, 313–319
    mechanisms causing injury 315–319
    musculoskeletal injuries 342–347
    networks 311
    orthopaedic (scoop) stretcher 354–355
    pelvic binders 342, 343
    pelvic fracture 318, 342
    pelvis 317–318
    primary survey 327–329
    scene assessment 327
    secondary survey 329–330
    skeletal immobilisation 347–365
    spinal immobilisation 350–357
    spinal injuries 336–337
    splints 357–365
    suspension 318, 342
    thoracic injuries 317, 337–340
    triangular bandages 348
    types of 313
    wounds 320–326, 325–326
trauma handover 20
Trauma Risk Management (TRiM) 445
traumatic brain injury (TBI)
    common causes of 330
    Glasgow Coma Scale 259
    management 331
    signs and symptoms of 330–331
traumatic cardiac arrest (TCA) 483–484
'Treat me well' campaign 449
treatment escalation plan (TEP) 491
trendelenburg position, trolley 112
triage 8
    over- and under-triaging 134
    recording findings 134
    treating and triaging 134
    triage sieve and sort 133–134
    vulnerable populations 134–135
triage label 134
Triage Revised Trauma System 133
triage sieve 133–134
triage sort 133–134
triangular bandages 347
    arm sling 347–349
    elevated sling 349–350
TRiM, *see* Trauma Risk Management (TRiM)
triple airway manoeuvre 156
tunica externa 221
tunica intima 220

Index

tunica media 220
turtle neck sign 414
12-lead ECG interpretation 235
two-chair method 94–95
tympanic thermometer 272

UA, see unstable angina (UA)
under-triaging 134
unstable angina (UA) 240
upper airway 149
upright position, trolley 111
urgent concern, reporting 54
urinary system disorders 304–310
    anatomy and physiology 305–307
    renal dialysis 308–310
    urinary tract infections 307–308
urinary tract infection (UTI) 307, 308
uterine atony 417
uterine contraction 403
uterine prolapse 423–424
uterine rupture 404
uterus 482
UTI, see urinary tract infection (UTI)

vacuum splints 359–360
vaginal bleeding 402
vaginal tissue damage 422
valid consent 34–35
valleculae 150
values-based healthcare 25–27
varicella-zoster virus (VZV) 66
vascular dementia 458
vaso-occlusive crisis 248–249
vehicle fires 83
veins 220
vena cava 218
venous thromboembolism (VTE) 215
ventilatory changes, older people 452–453
ventricles 218
ventricular fibrillation (VF) 475
ventricular tachycardia (VT) 475
Venturi mask 186
verbal communication 16–17
vertebrae encapsulate 255
vesicular breath sounds 206–207
VF, see ventricular fibrillation (VF)
viruses 66
visceral pleura 152, 337
vision, in older people 453
vital signs 145
vocabulary 16
voluntary nervous system, see somatic nervous system
VT, see ventricular tachycardia (VT)
VTE, see venous thromboembolism (VTE)
vulnerability 50–51
    learning difficulties and 450
vulnerable populations, major incidents 134–135
VZV, see varicella-zoster virus (VZV)

warfarin 335
waveform capnography 378
wellbeing, risk of, sharing information 44
wheezes (breath sounds) 206–207, 432
whistleblowing 29
white matter 254
WHO, see World Health Organization (WHO)
work equipment, defined 59
work of breathing 430
    pregnancy 399
working relationships, building 13
World Health Organization (WHO) 15, 396
    definition of metal disorder 439
    healthcare 32
    infection prevention and control 66
    procedure for hand hygiene 68–70
    procedure for handwashing 70–72
wounds 325–326
    categories 325
    management 326
written communication 17

Other Titles of Interest

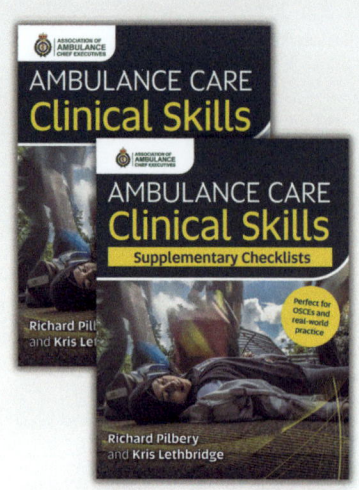

Ambulance Care Clinical Skills & Supplementary Checklists

Richard Pilbery and Kris Lethbridge

ISBN: 9781801611848

Ambulance Care Clinical Skills is a practical guide to over 80 prehospital procedures, with step-by-step instructions, full-colour illustrations and evidence-based explanations. It supports confidence and competence in areas such as patient assessment, airway management, trauma and cardiac arrest, with supplementary checklists for skills sessions and OSCE preparation.

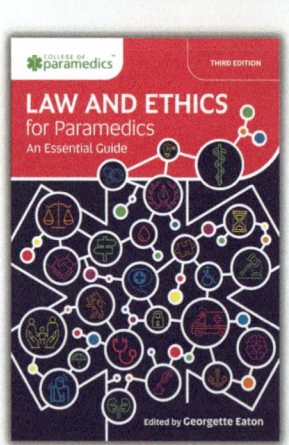

Law and Ethics for Paramedics

Georgette Eaton

ISBN: 9781801610131

This comprehensive third edition equips paramedics with essential ethical and legal knowledge, updated case law, applied ethics, and real-world examples - empowering confident, professional decision-making and excellence in patient care aligned with HCPC standards.

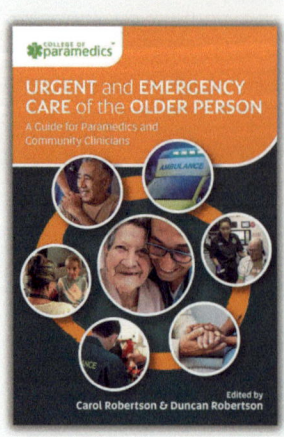

Urgent and Emergency Care of the Older Person

Carol Robertson and Duncan Robertson

ISBN: 9781859599860

Older adults form a growing share of emergency service users, demanding greater understanding and person-centred care. This resource equips clinicians to deliver evidence-based, age-appropriate practice aligned with UK priorities and guidelines.